FIRST AID FOR THE®
USMLE Step 2 CK

Eighth Edition

TAO LE, MD, MHS
Associate Clinical Professor of Medicine and Pediatrics
Chief, Section of Allergy and Immunology
Department of Medicine
University of Louisville

VIKAS BHUSHAN, MD
Diagnostic Radiologist

NATHAN WILLIAM SKELLEY, MD
Resident, Department of Orthopaedic Surgery
Washington University in St. Louis School of Medicine
Barnes-Jewish Hospital
St. Louis, Missouri

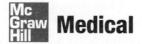 **Medicine**

New York   Chicago   San Francisco   Lisbon   London   Madrid   Mexico City
Milan   New Delhi   San Juan   Seoul   Singapore   Sydney   Toronto

First Aid for the® USMLE Step 2 CK, Eighth Edition

Copyright © 2012, 2010, 2007 by Tao Le. All rights reserved. Printed in the United States of America. Except as permitted under the United States Copyright Act of 1976, no part of this publication may be reproduced or distributed in any form or by any means, or stored in a data base or retrieval system, without the prior written permission of the publisher.

Previous editions copyright © 2006, 2003, 2001 by the McGraw-Hill Companies, Inc; copyright © 1999, 1996 by Appleton & Lange.

First Aid for the® is a registered trademark of the McGraw-Hill Companies, Inc.

5 6 7 8 9 0   DOW/DOW   16 15 14

ISBN 978-0-07-176137-6
MHID 0-07-176137-3
ISSN 1532-320X

NOTICE

Medicine is an ever-changing science. As new research and clinical experience broaden our knowledge, changes in treatment and drug therapy are required. The authors and the publisher of this work have checked with sources believed to be reliable in their efforts to provide information that is complete and generally in accord with the standards accepted at the time of publication. However, in view of the possibility of human error or changes in medical sciences, neither the authors nor the publisher nor any other party who has been involved in the preparation or publication of this work warrants that the information contained herein is in every respect accurate or complete, and they disclaim all responsibility for any errors or omissions or for the results obtained from use of the information contained in this work. Readers are encouraged to confirm the information contained herein with other sources. For example and in particular, readers are advised to check the product information sheet included in the package of each drug they plan to administer to be certain that the information contained in this work is accurate and that changes have not been made in the recommended dose or in the contraindications for administration. This recommendation is of particular importance in connection with new or infrequently used drugs.

This book was set in Electra LH by Rainbow Graphics.
The editors were Catherine A. Johnson and Peter J. Boyle.
The production supervisor was Jeffrey Herzich.
Project management was provided by Rainbow Graphics.
The art manager was Armen Ovsepyan.
RR Donnelley was printer and binder.

This book is printed on acid-free paper.

McGraw-Hill books are available at special quantity discounts to use as premiums and sales promotions, or for use in corporate training programs. To contact a representative please e-mail us at bulksales@mcgraw-hill.com.

To our families, friends, and loved ones, who supported
and assisted in the task of assembling this guide.

and

To the contributors to this and future editions, who took time to share
their knowledge, insight, and humor for the benefit of students.

Contents

CONTRIBUTING AUTHORS

Peter DeBartolo, MD
Resident, Department of Emergency Medicine
Maricopa Medical Center

Whitney Green, MD
Resident, Department of Pathology
The Johns Hopkins Hospital

Mark Jensen
University of Rochester School of Medicine
Class of 2012

Anisha Khaitan, MD
Resident, Department of Pediatrics
The Children's Hospital of Philadelphia

Richard Pollock, MD
Resident, Department of Anesthesiology
The Johns Hopkins Hospital

Jessica Schiffman, MD/MPH candidate
Harvard School of Public Health
Class of 2011
Johns Hopkins University
Class of 2012

Jason Solus, MD
Resident, Department of Pathology
Massachusetts General Hospital

Sophia Strike, MD
Resident, Department of Orthopaedic Surgery
The Johns Hopkins Hospital

Allison Leigh Tsao, MD
Resident, Department of Medicine
The Johns Hopkins Hospital

IMAGE EDITOR

S. Jarrett Wrenn, MD, PhD
Resident, Department of Radiology and Biomedical Imaging
University of California, San Francisco

WEB CONTRIBUTOR

Lauren Rothkopf, MD
Resident, Department of Internal Medicine
Beth Israel Deaconess Medical Center

FACULTY REVIEWERS

Kia Afshar, MD
Fellow, Division of Cardiology
Cleveland Clinic Foundation

Eric Darius Balighian, MD
Instructor, Department of Pediatrics
Saint Agnes and Johns Hopkins Hospital

David Cosgrove, MD
Assistant Professor, Department of Medical Oncology
Johns Hopkins University School of Medicine

Sameer Dhalla, MD
Postdoctoral Fellow, Division of Gastroenterology and Hepatology
Johns Hopkins University School of Medicine

Mark Hughes, MD, MA
Assistant Professor, Division of General Internal Medicine
Johns Hopkins University School of Medicine
Core Faculty, Berman Institute of Bioethics

Nancy Hueppchen, MD
Assistant Professor, Department of Gynecology/Obstetrics
Johns Hopkins University School of Medicine

Adrianna Jackson, MD
Resident, Department of Dermatology
Johns Hopkins University School of Medicine

Tina Latimer, MD, MPH
Assistant Program Director, Emergency Medicine Residency
Johns Hopkins University School of Medicine

Susan W. Lehmann, MD
Faculty, Department of Psychiatry and Behavioral Sciences
Johns Hopkins University School of Medicine

Michael Levy, MD, PhD
Assistant Professor, Department of Neurology
Johns Hopkins University School of Medicine

Murray A. Mittleman, MD, DrPH
Director, Cardiovascular Epidemiology Research Unit
Beth Israel Deaconess Medical Center

Kendall Moseley, MD
Instructor, Division of Endocrinology and Metabolism
The Johns Hopkins Hospital

Adam Spivak, MD
Instructor, Department of Medicine
Johns Hopkins University School of Medicine

R. Scott Stephens, MD
Faculty, Division of Pulmonary and Critical Care Medicine
Johns Hopkins University School of Medicine

Miho J. Tanaka, MD
Orthopaedic Fellow, Sports Medicine and Shoulder Service
Hospital for Special Surgery

Sumeska Thavarajah, MD
Assistant Professor, Division of Nephrology
Johns Hopkins Bayview Medical Center

Preface

With the eighth edition of *First Aid for the USMLE Step 2 CK*, we continue our commitment to providing students with the most useful and up-to-date preparation guide for the USMLE Step 2 CK. The eighth edition represents a thorough revision in many ways and includes:

- An all-new color design for better learning.
- New, innovative flash cards embedded in the margins to reinforce key concepts.
- Hundreds of new color images and illustrations throughout the text.
- A revised and updated exam preparation guide for the USMLE Step 2 CK that includes updated study and test-taking strategies for the FRED v2 computer-based testing (CBT) format.
- Revisions and new material based on student experience with recent administrations of the USMLE Step 2 CK.
- Concise summaries of more than 1000 heavily tested clinical topics written for fast, high-yield studying.
- An updated "rapid review" that tests your knowledge of each topic for last-minute cramming.
- A completely revised, in-depth guide to clinical science review and sample examination books.

The eighth edition would not have been possible without the help of the many students and faculty members who contributed their feedback and suggestions. We invite students and faculty to continue sharing their thoughts and ideas to help us improve *First Aid for the USMLE Step 2 CK*. (See How to Contribute, p. xiii.)

Tao Le
Louisville

Vikas Bhushan
Los Angeles

Nathan Skelley
St. Louis

Acknowledgments

This has been a collaborative project from the start. We gratefully acknowledge the thoughtful comments, corrections, and advice of the many medical students, international medical graduates, and faculty who have supported the authors in the continuing development of *First Aid for the USMLE Step 2 CK*.

For support and encouragement throughout the process, we are grateful to Thao Pham, Selina Franklin, and Louise Petersen. Thanks also to those who supported the authors through the revision process.

Thanks to our publisher, McGraw-Hill, for the valuable assistance of their staff. For enthusiasm, support, and commitment to this challenging project, thanks to our editor, Catherine Johnson. For outstanding editorial work, we thank Andrea Fellows. A special thanks to Rainbow Graphics, especially David Hommel, Tina Castle, and Susan Cooper, for remarkable editorial and production work, and to Ravish Amin for creating the web survey. Thanks to Elizabeth Sanders and Ashley Pound for the interior design.

For contributions and corrections, we thank Brad Barlow, Pravir Baxi, Carolyn Botros, Sarah Chamberlain, Marla Davis, Jennifer Dias, Christina Dornshuld, Scott Drutman, David Durand, Parastu Emrani, Michael Galabi, Christian Ghattas, Juan Gonzalez, Will Grover, Felipe T. Guillen, Arum Kim, Daniel Kim, Gabriel Kleinman, Nicholas Kotch, Tim LaBonte, David Levy, Christina Li, Michael Lin, Jon Lindquist, Brian J. Manfredi, Edgar Manzanera, David Margolius, Geronimo Mendoza, Karl Migally, Esmy Mohm, Dania Molla-Hosseini, Tareq Nassar, Meg Park, Jennifer Parker, Erin Perko, Kendall Riley, Nelson Royall, Eshan Sapra, Layli Sanaee, Heather Scoffone, Stephen Seedial, Malik Shahid, Joshua Sloan, Versha Srivastasa, Matthew Stewart, Sharon Tsay, Shannon Toohey, Kenneth Visalli, Amanda Weinmann, Melisa Wong, Suzanna Yadgarov, and Dustin Yoon.

Thanks to Steve Albrechta, Maureen Ayers Looby, Erika Bernardo, Rachel Burkard, Lindsey Chmielewski, Hector Colon, Erin Conboy, Abigail Dennis, Christine DeSanno, Conor Dolehide, Christina Dornshuld, Travis Dunn, Dan Falvey, William A. Fields, Kristin Gehrking, Marlow Griggs, Michelle Harper, Kristin Huntoon, Benjamin Johnson, Emily Johnson, Gina Johnson, Nicholas Jubert, Dejah Judelson, Landon Karren, Harris Khan, Alexander Kim, Sarah Liebe, Christina Lohbeck, Patrick Looser, Brandon Mauldin, Mitch McKenzie, Michelle Miller, Charles Newlin, Jordan Lee Nordquist, Sara Olmanson, Jonathan James Olson, Andrea Paulson, Monica Pena, Susan Pleasants, Vanessa Raabe, Petra Rahaman, Justin Schulte, Erin Seidel, Michael Silverstein, Rebecca Stepan, Gary Tsai, Lydia I. Turnbull, and Liz Wasson for submitting book reviews.

Tao Le
Louisville

Vikas Bhushan
Los Angeles

Nathan Skelley
St. Louis

How to Contribute

In our effort to continue to produce a high-yield review source for the Step 2 CK exam, we invite you to submit any suggestions or corrections. We also offer paid internships in medical education and publishing ranging from three months to one year (see below for details). Please send us your suggestions for

- Study and test-taking strategies for the Step 2 CK exam
- New facts, mnemonics, diagrams, and illustrations
- Low-yield topics to remove

For each entry incorporated into the next edition, you will receive a $10 gift certificate as well as personal acknowledgment in the next edition. Diagrams, tables, partial entries, updates, corrections, and study hints are also appreciated, and significant contributions will be compensated at the discretion of the authors. Also let us know about material in this edition that you feel is low yield and should be deleted.

The preferred way to submit entries, suggestions, or corrections is via our blog:

www.firstaidteam.com

We are also reachable by e-mail at firstaidteam@yahoo.com.

NOTE TO CONTRIBUTORS

All entries become property of the authors and are subject to editing and reviewing. Please verify all data and spellings carefully. In the event that similar or duplicate entries are received, only the first entry received will be used. Include a reference to a standard textbook to facilitate verification of the fact. Please follow the style, punctuation, and format of this edition if possible.

INTERNSHIP OPPORTUNITIES

The author team is pleased to offer part-time and full-time paid internships in medical education and publishing to motivated physicians. Internships may range from three months (eg, a summer) up to a full year. Participants will have an opportunity to author, edit, and earn academic credit on a wide variety of projects, including the popular First Aid series. Writing/editing experience, familiarity with Microsoft Word, and Internet access are desired. For more information, e-mail a résumé or a short description of your experience along with a cover letter to firstaidteam@yahoo.com.

How to Use This Book

We have made many improvements and added several new features to this edition of *First Aid for the USMLE Step 2 CK*. In particular, we have added more tables, charts, and images throughout the text to facilitate studying. We encourage you to read all aspects of the text to learn the material in context; however, when you get closer to test day, focus on the high-yield bolded text and comments in the margins of each page. These features have many of the "buzzwords" you should be looking for on exam day. Finally, we have included new vignette questions to periodically test your knowledge of key concepts. These questions are located in the lower or upper right corner of certain pages. To prevent peeking at the answers, you'll find the answer on the back of the same page in the lower or upper left corner. These questions are not always representative of test questions.

To **simulate** the actual test day and to properly judge your true understanding of the material, you can use the USMLERx Step 2 CK Qmax question test bank (www.usmlerx.com), which was developed by the First Aid author team. The test bank and this text are more than enough to allow many students to ace the exam. However, if you are constantly on the move while preparing for this exam or need some extra practice, use the USMLERx Step 2 CK mobile application for mobile devices.

To **broaden** your learning strategy, you can **integrate** your First Aid study with *First Aid Cases for the USMLE Step 2 CK* and *First Aid Q&A for the USMLE Step 2 CK*. Please note that *First Aid Q&A* draws a portion of its questions from USMLERx. *First Aid Cases* and *First Aid Q&A* are organized to match *First Aid for the USMLE Step 2 CK* **chapter for chapter.** After reviewing a chapter within *First Aid*, you can **review cases** on the same topics and then **test your knowledge** in the corresponding chapters of *First Aid Cases* and *First Aid Q&A*. *First Aid Q&A* is also available as an iPhone app. Additional materials may also be found in the Review Resources section of this book. Good luck!

GUIDE TO EFFICIENT EXAM PREPARATION

Introduction

The United States Medical Licensing Examination (USMLE) Step 2 allows you to pull together your clinical experience on the wards with the numerous "factoids" and classical disease presentations that you have memorized over the years. Whereas Step 1 stresses basic disease mechanisms and principles, Step 2 places more emphasis on clinical diagnosis and management, disease pathogenesis, and preventive medicine. The Step 2 examination is now composed of two parts:

- The Step 2 Clinical Knowledge examination (Step 2 CK)
- The Step 2 Clinical Skills examination (Step 2 CS)

The USMLE Step 2 CK is the second of three examinations that you must pass in order to become a licensed physician in the United States. The computerized Step 2 CK is a 1-day (9-hour) multiple-choice examination.

Students are also required to take the Step 2 CS, which is a 1-day live examination in which students examine 12 standardized patients. For more information on this examination, please refer to *First Aid for the USMLE Step 2 CS.* Information about the Step 2 CS format and about eligibility, registration, and scoring can be found at www.nbme.org.

The information found in this section as well as in the remainder of the book will address only the Step 2 CK.

KEY FACT

The goal of the Step 2 CK is to apply your knowledge of medical facts to clinical scenarios you may encounter as a resident.

USMLE Step 2 CK—Computer-Based Testing Basics

HOW WILL THE CBT BE STRUCTURED?

The Step 2 CK is a computer-based test (CBT) administered by Prometric, Inc. It is a 1-day examination with approximately 352 questions divided into eight 60-minute blocks of 44 questions each, administered in a single 9-hour testing session. The Step 2 CK uses the same **FRED v2** software program as that used on the USMLE Step 1 examination.

There are three question styles that predominate throughout the examination. The most common format is **Single One Best Answer** questions. This is the traditional multiple-choice format in which you are tasked with selecting the "most correct" answer. Another common style is **Matching Sets.** These questions consist of a series of questions related to a similar topic or prompt. Finally, **"Sequential Item Sets"** have been introduced to the examination. These are sets of multiple-choice questions that are related and must all be answered in order without skipping a question in the set along the way. As you answer questions in a given set, the previous answers become locked and cannot be changed. These are the only questions on the USMLE examination that are locked in such a way. There will be no more than five Sequential Item Sets within each USMLE Step 2 CK examination.

During the time allotted for each block on the USMLE Step 2 CK, the examinee can answer test questions in any order as well as review responses and change answers (with the exception of responses within the Sequential Item Sets described above). However, under no circumstances can examinees go back and change answers from previous blocks. Once an examinee finishes a block, he or she must click on a screen icon in order to continue to the next block. Time not used during a testing block will be added to the examinee's overall break time, but it cannot be used to complete other testing blocks.

TESTING CONDITIONS: WHAT WILL THE CBT BE LIKE?

Even if you're familiar with computer-based testing and the Prometric test centers, FRED v2 is a new testing format that you should access from the USMLE CD-ROM or Web site (www.usmle.org) and try out prior to the examination. If you familiarize yourself with the FRED v2 testing interface ahead of time, you can skip the 15-minute tutorial offered on examination day and add those minutes to your allotted break time of 45 minutes.

For security reasons, examinees are not allowed to bring personal electronic equipment into the testing area—which means that watches (even analog), cellular telephones, and electronic paging devices are all prohibited. Food and beverages are prohibited as well. The proctor will assign you a small locker in which you can store your belongings and any food you bring for the day. Examinees will also be given two ($8'' \times 11''$) laminated writing surfaces, pens, and erasers for note taking and for recording their test Candidate Identification Number (CIN). These materials must be returned after the examination. Testing centers are monitored by audio and video surveillance equipment.

You should become familiar with a typical question screen. A window to the left displays all the questions in the block and shows you the unanswered questions (marked with an "i"). Some questions will contain figures, color illustrations, audio, or video adjacent to the question. Although the contrast and brightness of the screen can be adjusted, there are no other ways to manipulate the picture (eg, zooming or panning). Larger images are accessed with an "**exhibit**" button. The examinee can also call up a window displaying normal **lab values.** You may **mark** questions to review at a later time by clicking the check mark at the top of the screen. The **annotation** feature functions like the provided dry erase sheets and allows you to jot down notes during the examination. Play with the **highlighting/strike-out** and annotation features with the vignettes and multiple answers.

You should also do a few practice blocks to determine which tools actually help you process questions more efficiently and accurately. If you find that you are not using the marking, annotation, or highlighting tools, then **keyboard shortcuts** can save you time over using a mouse. Headphones are provided for listening to audio and blocking outside noise. Alternatively, examinees can bring soft earplugs to block excess noise. These earplugs must be examined by Prometric staff before you are allowed to take them into the testing area.

WHAT DOES THE CBT FORMAT MEAN FOR ME?

The CBT format is the same format as that used on the USMLE Step 1. If you are uncomfortable with this testing format, spend some time playing with a Windows-based system and pointing and clicking icons or buttons with a mouse.

The USMLE also offers students an opportunity to take a simulated test, or practice session, at a Prometric center. The session is divided into three 1-hour blocks of 50 test items each. The 143 Step 2 CK sample test items that

KEY FACT

Expect to spend up to 9 hours at the test center.

KEY FACT

Keyboard shortcuts:
- A–E—Letter choices.
- Enter or Spacebar—Move to the next question.
- Esc—Exit pop-up Lab and Exhibit windows.
- Alt-T—Countdown and time-elapsed clocks for current session and overall test.

are available on the CD-ROM or on the USMLE Web site (www.usmle.org) are the same as those used at CBT practice sessions. **No new items are presented.** The cost is about $52 for U.S. and Canadian students but is higher for international students. Students receive a printed percent-correct score after completing the session. No explanations of questions are provided. You may register for a practice session online at www.usmle.org.

The National Board of Medical Examiners (NBME) provides another option for students to assess their Step 2 CK knowledge with the Comprehensive Clinical Science Self-Assessment (CCSSA) test. This test is available on the NBME Web site in several versions for $50 (or $60 for expanded feedback). The content of the CCSSA items resembles that of the USMLE Step 2 CK. Upon completion of the CCSSA, users will be provided with a performance profile indicating their strengths and weaknesses. This feedback is intended for use as a study tool only and is not necessarily an indicator of Step 2 CK performance. For more information on the CCSSA examination, visit the NBME's Web site at www.nbme.org and click on the link for "NBME Web-based Self-Assessment Service."

HOW DO I REGISTER TO TAKE THE EXAMINATION?

Information on Step 2 CK format, content, and registration requirements can be found on the USMLE Web site. To register for the examination in the United States and Canada, apply online at the NBME Web site (www.nbme.org). A printable version of the application is also available on this site. The preliminary registration process for the USMLE Step 2 CK is as follows:

- Complete a registration form and send your examination fees to the NBME (online).
- Select a 3-month block in which you wish to be tested (eg, June/July/August).
- Attach a passport-type photo to your completed application form.
- Complete a Certification of Identification and Authorization Form. This form must be signed by an official at your medical school (eg, the registrar's office) to verify your identity. It is valid for 5 years, allowing you to use only your USMLE identification number for future transactions.
- Send your certified application form to the NMBE for processing. (Applications may be submitted more than 6 months before the test date, but examinees will not receive their scheduling permits until 6 months prior to the eligibility period.)
- The NBME will process your application within 4–6 weeks and will send you a slip of paper that will serve as your scheduling permit.
- Once you have received your scheduling permit, decide when and where you would like to take the examination. For a list of Prometric locations nearest you, visit www.prometric.com.
- Call Prometric's toll-free number or visit www.prometric.com to arrange a time to take the examination.
- The Step 2 CK is offered on a year-round basis except for the first 2 weeks in January. For the most up-to-date information on available testing days at your preferred testing location, refer to www.usmle.org.

The scheduling permit you receive from the NBME will contain the following important information:

- Your USMLE identification number.
- The eligibility period in which you may take the examination.

- Your "scheduling number," which you will need to make your examination appointment with Prometric.
- Your CIN, which you must enter at your Prometric workstation in order to access the examination.

Prometric has no access to the codes and will not be able to supply these numbers, so **do not lose your permit!** You will not be allowed to take the Step 2 CK unless you present your permit along with an unexpired, government-issued photo identification that contains your signature (eg, driver's license, passport). Make sure the name on your photo ID exactly matches the name that appears on your scheduling permit.

KEY FACT

Because the Step 2 CK examination is scheduled on a "first-come, first-served" basis, you should be sure to call Prometric as soon as you receive your scheduling permit.

WHAT IF I NEED TO RESCHEDULE THE EXAMINATION?

You can change your date and/or center within your 3-month period without charge by contacting Prometric. If space is available, you may reschedule up to 5 days before your test date. If you need to reschedule outside your initial 3-month period, you can apply for a single 3-month extension (eg, April/May/June can be extended through July/August/September) after your eligibility period has begun (visit www.nbme.org for more information). This extension currently costs $65. For other rescheduling needs, you must submit a new application along with another application fee.

WHAT ABOUT TIME?

Time is of special interest on the CBT examination. Here is a breakdown of the examination schedule:

Tutorial	15 minutes
60-minute question blocks (44 questions per block)	8 hours
Break time (includes time for lunch)	45 minutes
Total test time	9 hours

The computer will keep track of how much time has elapsed during the examination. However, the computer will show you only how much time you have remaining in a given block. Therefore, it is up to you to determine if you are pacing yourself properly.

The computer will not warn you if you are spending more than the 45 minutes allotted for break time. The break time includes not only the usual concept of a break—when you leave the testing area—but also the time it takes for you to make the transition to the next block, such as entering your CIN or even taking a quick stretch. **If you do exceed the 45-minute break time, the time to complete the last block of the test will be reduced.** However, you can elect not to use all of your break time, or you can gain extra break time either by skipping the tutorial or by finishing a block ahead of the allotted time.

NEW SECURITY MEASURES

Smile! In early 2009, the NBME initiated a new check-in/check-out process that includes electronic capture of your fingerprints and photograph. These measures are intended to increase security by preventing fraud, thereby safeguarding the integrity of the examination. The new procedures also decrease the amount of time needed to check in and out of the examination throughout the day, thereby maximizing your break time. However, you still need to sign out and sign in with the Test Center Log when exiting and entering the testing area.

IF I LEAVE DURING THE EXAMINATION, WHAT HAPPENS TO MY SCORE?

You are considered to have started the examination once you have entered your CIN onto the computer screen. In order to receive an official score, however, you must finish the entire examination. This means that you must start and either finish or run out of time for each block of the examination. If you do not complete all the question blocks, your examination will be documented on your USMLE score transcript as an incomplete attempt, but no actual score will be reported.

The examination ends when all blocks have been completed or time has expired. As you leave the testing center, you will receive a written test-completion notice to document your completion of the examination.

WHAT TYPES OF QUESTIONS ARE ASKED?

The Step 2 CK is an integrated examination that tests understanding of normal conditions, disease categories, and physician tasks. Almost all questions on the examination are case based. A substantial amount of extraneous information may be given, or a clinical scenario may be followed by a question that could be answered without actually requiring that you read the case. It is your job to determine which information is superfluous and which is pertinent to the case at hand. Content areas include internal medicine, OB/GYN, pediatrics, preventive services, psychiatry, surgery, and other areas relevant to the provision of care under supervision. Physician tasks are distributed as follows:

- Establishing a diagnosis (25–40%)
- Understanding the mechanisms of disease (20–35%)
- Applying principles of management (15–25%)
- Promoting preventive medicine and health maintenance (15–25%)

Most questions on the examination have a **Single Best Answer** format, but some **Matching Sets** and Sequential Item Sets will be found throughout the examination. Regardless of the question format, the part of the vignette that actually asks the question—the **stem**—is usually found at the end of the scenario and generally relates to the physician task. From student experience, there are a few stems that are consistently addressed throughout the examination:

- What is the most likely diagnosis? (40%)
- Which of the following is the most appropriate initial step in management? (20%)
- Which of the following is the most appropriate next step in management? (20%)
- Which of the following is the most likely cause of . . . ? (5%)
- Which of the following is the most likely pathogen . . . ? (3%)
- Which of the following would most likely prevent . . . ? (2%)
- Other (10%)

Additional examination tips are as follows:

- Note the age and race of the patient in each clinical scenario. When ethnicity is given, it is often relevant. Know these well (see high-yield facts), especially for more common diagnoses.
- Be able to recognize key facts that distinguish major diagnoses.
- Questions often describe clinical findings rather than naming eponyms (eg, they cite "audible hip click" instead of "positive Ortolani's sign").
- Questions about acute patient management (eg, trauma) in an emergency setting are common.

The cruel reality of the Step 2 CK is that no matter how much you study, there will still be questions you will not be able to answer with confidence. If you recognize that a question cannot be solved in a reasonable period of time, make an educated guess and move on; you will not be penalized for guessing. Also bear in mind that 10–20% of the USMLE examination questions are "experimental" and will not count toward your score.

HOW LONG WILL I HAVE TO WAIT BEFORE I GET MY SCORES?

The USMLE reports scores 3–4 weeks after the examinee's test date. During peak periods, however, reports may take up to 6 weeks to be scored. Official information concerning the time required for score reporting is posted on the USMLE Web site, www.usmle.org.

HOW ARE THE SCORES REPORTED?

Like the Step 1 score report, your Step 2 CK report includes your pass/fail status, two numeric scores, and a performance profile organized by discipline and disease process (see Figures 1-1A and 1-1B). The first score is a 3-digit scaled score based on a predefined proficiency standard. In 2010, the required passing score was raised to 189. This score requires answering 60–70% of questions correctly. The second score scale, the 2-digit score, defines 75 as the minimum passing score (equivalent to a score of 189 on the first scale). This score is not a percentile. Any adjustments in the required passing score will be available on the USMLE Web site.

Defining Your Goal

The first and most important thing to do in your Step 2 CK preparation is define how well you want to do on the exam, as this will ultimately determine the extent of preparation that will be necessary. The amount of time spent in preparation for this examination varies widely among medical students. Possible goals include the following:

- **Simply passing.** This goal meets the requirements for becoming a licensed physician in the United States. However, if you are taking the Step 2 CK in a time frame in which residency programs will see your score, you should strive to do as well as or better than you did on Step 1.
- **Beating the mean.** This signifies an ability to integrate your clinical and factual knowledge to an extent that is superior to that of your peers (between 200 and 220 for recent examination administrations). Others redefine this goal as achieving a score 1 SD above the mean (usually in the range of 220–240). Highly competitive residency programs may

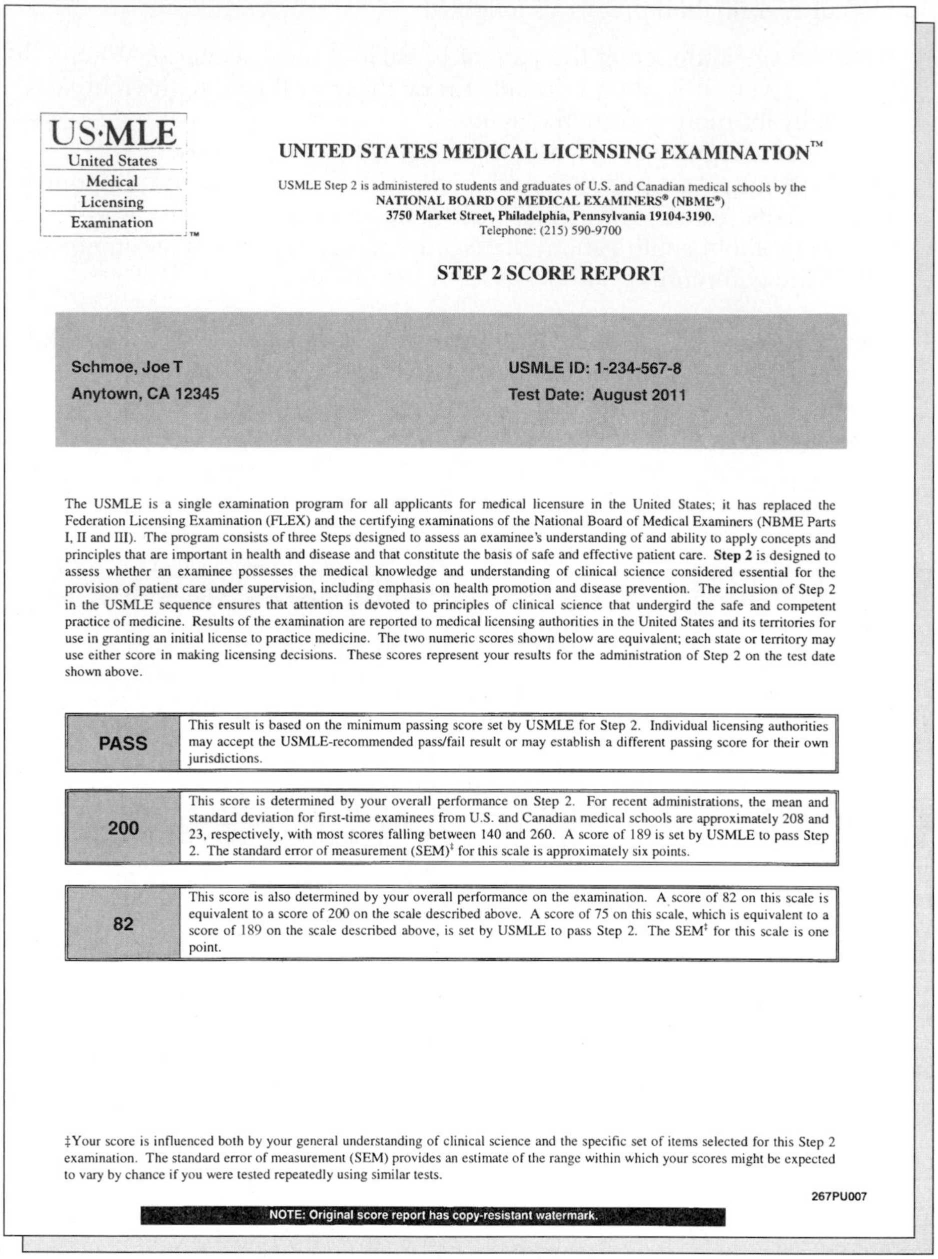

US·MLE
United States
Medical
Licensing
Examination ™

UNITED STATES MEDICAL LICENSING EXAMINATION™

USMLE Step 2 is administered to students and graduates of U.S. and Canadian medical schools by the
NATIONAL BOARD OF MEDICAL EXAMINERS® (NBME®)
3750 Market Street, Philadelphia, Pennsylvania 19104-3190.
Telephone: (215) 590-9700

STEP 2 SCORE REPORT

Schmoe, Joe T   USMLE ID: 1-234-567-8

Anytown, CA 12345   Test Date: August 2011

The USMLE is a single examination program for all applicants for medical licensure in the United States; it has replaced the Federation Licensing Examination (FLEX) and the certifying examinations of the National Board of Medical Examiners (NBME Parts I, II and III). The program consists of three Steps designed to assess an examinee's understanding of and ability to apply concepts and principles that are important in health and disease and that constitute the basis of safe and effective patient care. **Step 2** is designed to assess whether an examinee possesses the medical knowledge and understanding of clinical science considered essential for the provision of patient care under supervision, including emphasis on health promotion and disease prevention. The inclusion of Step 2 in the USMLE sequence ensures that attention is devoted to principles of clinical science that undergird the safe and competent practice of medicine. Results of the examination are reported to medical licensing authorities in the United States and its territories for use in granting an initial license to practice medicine. The two numeric scores shown below are equivalent; each state or territory may use either score in making licensing decisions. These scores represent your results for the administration of Step 2 on the test date shown above.

PASS	This result is based on the minimum passing score set by USMLE for Step 2. Individual licensing authorities may accept the USMLE-recommended pass/fail result or may establish a different passing score for their own jurisdictions.
200	This score is determined by your overall performance on Step 2. For recent administrations, the mean and standard deviation for first-time examinees from U.S. and Canadian medical schools are approximately 208 and 23, respectively, with most scores falling between 140 and 260. A score of 189 is set by USMLE to pass Step 2. The standard error of measurement (SEM)‡ for this scale is approximately six points.
82	This score is also determined by your overall performance on the examination. A score of 82 on this scale is equivalent to a score of 200 on the scale described above. A score of 75 on this scale, which is equivalent to a score of 189 on the scale described above, is set by USMLE to pass Step 2. The SEM‡ for this scale is one point.

‡Your score is influenced both by your general understanding of clinical science and the specific set of items selected for this Step 2 examination. The standard error of measurement (SEM) provides an estimate of the range within which your scores might be expected to vary by chance if you were tested repeatedly using similar tests.

267PU007

NOTE: Original score report has copy-resistant watermark.

FIGURE 1-1A.   Sample Score Report—Front Page

use your Step 1 and Step 2 scores (if available) as a screening tool or as a selection requirement (see Figure 1-2). International medical graduates (IMGs) should aim to beat the mean, as USMLE scores are likely to be a selection factor even for less competitive U.S. residency programs.

- **Acing the exam.** Perhaps you are one of those individuals for whom nothing less than the best will do—and for whom excelling on standardized examinations is a source of pride and satisfaction. A high score on the Step 2 CK might also represent a way to strengthen your application and "make up" for a less-than-satisfactory score on Step 1.
- **Evaluating your clinical knowledge.** In many ways, this goal should serve as the ultimate rationale for taking the Step 2 CK, as it is technically the reason the examination was initially designed. The case-based nature of

INFORMATION PROVIDED FOR EXAMINEE USE ONLY

The Performance Profile below is provided solely for the benefit of the examinee.
These profiles are developed as assessment tools for examinees only and will not be reported or verified to any third party.

USMLE STEP 2 PERFORMANCE PROFILES

PHYSICIAN TASK PROFILE	Lower Performance	Borderline Performance	Higher Performance
Preventive Medicine & Health Maintenance			xxxxxxxxxxxx*
Understanding Mechanisms of Disease			xxxx*
Diagnosis			xxxxx*
Principles of Management			xxxxxxxxxx*

NORMAL CONDITIONS & DISEASE CATEGORY PROFILE

Normal Growth & Development; Principles of Care			xxxxxxxxxxxxxxxxxx*
Immunologic Disorders			xxxxxxxxxxxxx*
Diseases of Blood & Blood Forming Organs			xxxxxxxxxx*
Mental Disorders			xxxxxxxxxxxx*
Diseases of the Nervous System & Special Senses			xxxxxxxxxx*
Cardiovascular Disorders		xxxxxxxxxxxxxxxx	
Diseases of the Respiratory System			xxxxxxxxxxxxxx*
Nutritional & Digestive Disorders			xxxxxxxxxxx*
Gynecologic Disorders			xxxxxxxxxxxxxx*
Renal, Urinary & Male Reproductive Systems			xxxxxxxxxx*
Disorders of Pregnancy, Childbirth & Puerperium		xxxxxxxxxxxxxxxxxxx	
Musculoskeletal, Skin & Connective Tissue Diseases			xxxxxxxxxx*
Endocrine & Metabolic Disorders			xxxxxxxxxxxxxx*

DISCIPLINE PROFILE

Medicine			xxx*
Obstetrics & Gynecology			xxxxxxxxxxxx*
Pediatrics			xxxxxxxx*
Psychiatry			xxxxxxxxxxxx*
Surgery			xx*

The above Performance Profile is provided to aid in self-assessment. The shaded area defines a borderline level of performance for each content area; borderline performance is comparable to a HIGH FAIL / LOW PASS on the total test.

Performance bands indicate areas of relative strength and weakness. Some performance bands are wider than others. The width of a performance band reflects the precision of measurement: narrower bands indicate greater precision. An asterisk indicates that your performance band extends beyond the displayed portion of the scale. Small differences in the location of bands should not be over interpreted. If two bands overlap, the performance in the associated areas should not be interpreted as significantly different.

This profile should not be compared to those from other Step 2 administrations.

Additional information concerning the topics covered in each content area can be found in the *USMLE Step 2 General Instructions, Content Description, and Sample Items.*

007PU267

FIGURE 1-1B.   Sample Score Report—Back Page

the Step 2 CK differs significantly from the more fact-based Step 1 examination in that it more thoroughly assesses your ability to recognize classic clinical presentations, deal with emergent situations, and follow the step-by-step thought processes involved in the treatment of particular diseases.

- **Preparing for internship.** Studying for the USMLE Step 2 CK is an excellent way to review and consolidate all of the information you have learned in preparation for internship.

Matching statistics, including examination scores related to various specialties, are available at the National Resident Matching Program (NRMP) Web site at www.nrmp.org under "Data and Reports."

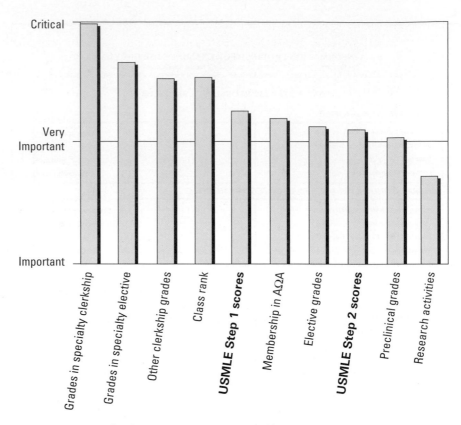

FIGURE 1-2.   Academic Factors Important to Residency Directors

WHEN TO TAKE THE EXAM

The second most important thing to do in your examination preparation is to decide when to take the examination. With the CBT, you now have a wide variety of options regarding when to take the Step 2 CK. Here are a few factors to consider:

- **The nature of your objectives,** as defined above.
- **The specialty to which you are applying.** It is clear that an increasing number of residency programs are viewing the Step 2 CK as an integral part of the residency application process. There are several research publications that demonstrate the increasing importance placed on this examination by residency directors. Some programs are now requiring the Step 2 CK score in order to rank candidates for a residency position. It is therefore in the best interest of candidates to have this examination done in time for scores to be available for the residency application. Taking the examination in June or July ensures that scores will be available for the Match period that begins in September. Some programs, however, will accept scores after the application process starts. Check with programs in your desired specialty to determine when to take the examination.
- **Prerequisite to graduation.** If passing the USMLE Step 2 CK is a prerequisite to graduation at your medical school, you will need to take the examination in the fall or winter at the latest.
- **Proximity to clerkships.** Many students feel that the core clerkship material is fresher in their minds early in the fourth year, making a good argument for taking the Step 2 CK earlier in the fall.
- **The nature of your schedule.**
- **Considerations for MD/PhD students.** The dates of passing the Step 1, Step 2, and Step 3 examinations should occur within a 7-year period.

However, the typical pathway for MD/PhD students consists of 2 years of preclinical work in medical school, 3–4 years of graduate work with research, and finally returning to medical school for clinical work. MD/PhD students typically exceed the 7-year limit. Depending on the state in which licensure is sought, such students may need to petition their licensure body for an exception to this rule.

Study Resources

QUALITY CONSIDERATIONS

Although an ever-increasing number of USMLE Step 2 CK review books and software packages are available on the market, the quality of this material is highly variable (see Section 3). Some common problems include the following:

- Some review books are too detailed to be reviewed in a reasonable amount of time or cover subtopics that are not emphasized on the examination (eg, a 400-page anesthesiology book).
- Many sample question books have not been updated to reflect current trends on the Step 2 CK.
- Many sample question books use poorly written questions, contain factual errors in their explanations, give overly detailed explanations, or offer no explanations at all.
- Software for boards review is of highly variable quality, may be difficult to install, and may be fraught with bugs.

CLINICAL REVIEW BOOKS

Many review books are available, so you must decide which ones to buy by carefully evaluating their relative merits. Toward this goal, you should weigh different opinions from other medical students against each other; read the reviews and ratings in Section 3 of this guide; and examine the various books closely in the bookstore. Do not worry about finding the "perfect" book, as many subjects simply do not have one.

There are two types of review books: those that are stand-alone titles and those that are part of a series. Books in a series generally have the same style, and you must decide if that style is helpful for you and optimal for a given subject.

TEST BANKS

A test bank can serve multiple functions for examinees, including the following:

- Provide information about strengths and weaknesses in your fund of knowledge.
- Add variety to your study schedule.
- Serve as the main form of study.
- Improve test-taking skills.
- Familiarize examinees with the style of the USMLE Step 2 CK examination.

Students report that many test banks have questions that are, on average, shorter and less clinically oriented than those on the current Step 2 CK. Step

2 CK questions demand fast reading skills and the application of clinical facts in a problem-solving format. Approach sample examinations critically, and do not waste time with low-quality questions until you have exhausted better sources.

After you have taken a practice test, try to identify concepts and areas of weakness, not just the facts that you missed. Use this experience to motivate your study and to prioritize the areas in which you need the most work. Analyze the pattern of your responses to questions to determine if you have made systematic errors in answering questions. Common mistakes include reading too much into the question, second-guessing your initial impression, and misinterpreting the question.

KEY FACT

Use test banks to identify concepts and areas of weakness, not just facts that you missed.

TEXTS AND NOTES

Most textbooks are too detailed for high-yield boards review and should be avoided. When using texts or notes, engage in active learning by making tables, diagrams, new mnemonics, and conceptual associations whenever possible. If you already have your own mnemonics, do not bother trying to memorize someone else's. Textbooks are useful, however, to supplement incomplete or unclear material.

COMMERCIAL COURSES

Commercial preparation courses can be helpful for some students, as they offer an effective way to organize study material. However, multiweek courses are costly and require significant time commitment, leaving limited time for independent study. Also note that some commercial courses are designed for first-time test takers, students who are repeating the examination, or IMGs.

NBME/USMLE PUBLICATIONS

We strongly encourage students to use the free materials provided by the testing agencies and to study the following NBME publications:

- **USMLE *Bulletin of Information.*** This publication provides you with nuts-and-bolts details about the examination (included on the Web site www.usmle.org; free to all examinees).
- **USMLE *Step 2 Computer-Based Content and Sample Test Questions.*** This is a hardcopy version of the test questions and test content also found on the CD-ROM or at www.usmle.org.
- **NBME Test Delivery Software (FRED) and Tutorial.** This includes 143 valuable practice questions. The questions are available on the USMLE CD-ROM and on the USMLE Web site. Make sure you are using the new version of FRED and not the older Prometric version.
- **USMLE Web site (www.usmle.org).** In addition to allowing you to become familiar with the CBT format, the sample items on the USMLE Web site provide the only questions that are available directly from the test makers. Student feedback varies as to the similarity of these questions to those on the actual exam, but they are nonetheless worthwhile to know.

Test-Day Checklist

THINGS TO BRING WITH YOU TO THE EXAM

 Be sure to bring your scheduling permit and a photo ID with signature. (You will not be admitted to the examination if you fail to bring your permit, and Prometric will charge a rescheduling fee.)

 Remember to bring lunch, snacks (for a little "sugar rush" on breaks), and fluids.

 Bring clothes to layer to accommodate temperature variations at the testing center.

 Earplugs will be provided at the Prometric center.

Testing Agencies

National Board of Medical Examiners (NBME)
Department of Licensing Examination Services
3750 Market Street
Philadelphia, PA 19104-3102
(215) 590-9500
Fax: (215) 590-9457
www.nbme.org

USMLE Secretariat
3750 Market Street
Philadelphia, PA 19104-3190
(215) 590-9700
Fax: (215) 590-9457
www.usmle.org

Educational Commission for Foreign Medical Graduates (ECFMG)
3624 Market Street
Philadelphia, PA 19104-2685
(215) 386-5900
Fax: (215) 386-9196
www.ecfmg.org
e-mail: info@ecfmg.org

Federation of State Medical Boards (FSMB)
400 Fuller Wiser Road, Suite 300
Euless, TX 76039
(817) 868-4000
Fax: (817) 868-4099
www.fsmb.org
e-mail: usmle@fsmb.org

NOTES

DATABASE OF HIGH-YIELD FACTS

Cardiovascular

Dermatology

Endocrinology

Epidemiology

Ethics and Legal Issues

Gastrointestinal

Hematology/Oncology

Infectious Disease

Musculoskeletal

Neurology

Obstetrics

Gynecology

Pediatrics

Psychiatry

Pulmonary

Renal/Genitourinary

Selected Topics in Emergency Medicine

Rapid Review

How to Use the Database

The eighth edition of *First Aid for the USMLE Step 2 CK* contains a revised and expanded database of clinical material that student authors and faculty have identified as high yield for boards review. The facts are organized according to subject matter, whether medical specialty (eg, Cardiovascular, Renal) or high-yield topic (eg, Ethics). Each subject is then divided into smaller subsections of related facts.

Individual facts are generally presented in a logical fashion, from basic definitions and epidemiology to **History/Physical Exam, Diagnosis,** and **Treatment.** Lists, mnemonics, pull quotes, vignette flash cards, and tables are used when they can help the reader form key associations. In addition, color and black-and-white images are interspersed throughout the text. At the end of Section 2, we also feature a Rapid Review chapter consisting of key facts and classic associations that can be studied a day or two before the exam.

The content contained herein is useful primarily for the purpose of reviewing material already learned. The information presented is not ideal for learning complex or highly conceptual material for the first time.

The Database of High-Yield Facts is not comprehensive. Use it to complement your core study material, not as your primary study source. The facts and notes have been condensed and edited to emphasize essential material. Work with the material, add your own notes and mnemonics, and recognize that not all memory techniques work for all students.

We update Section 2 biannually to keep current with new trends in boards content as well as to expand our database of high-yield information. However, we must note that inevitably many other high-yield entries and topics are not yet included in our database.

We actively encourage medical students and faculty to submit entries and mnemonics so that we may enhance the database for future students. We also solicit recommendations of additional study tools that may be useful in preparing for the examination, such as diagrams, charts, and computer-based tutorials (see How to Contribute, p. xiii).

DISCLAIMER

The entries in this section reflect student opinions of what is high yield. Owing to the diverse sources of material, no attempt has been made to trace or reference the origins of entries individually. We have regarded mnemonics as essentially in the public domain. All errors and omissions will gladly be corrected if brought to the attention of the authors, either through the publisher or directly by e-mail.

CARDIOVASCULAR

Electrocardiogram (ECG)

Methodically assess the ECG for rate, rhythm, axis, intervals, waveforms, and chamber enlargement (see Figure 2.1-1).

RATE

- The normal heart rate (HR) is 60–100 bpm.
- HR < 60 bpm is bradycardia.
- HR > 100 bpm is tachycardia.

RHYTHM

Look for sinus rhythm (P before every QRS and QRS after every P), irregular rhythms, junctional or ventricular rhythms (no P before a QRS), and ectopic beats.

AXIS

- **Normal:** An upright (⊕) QRS in leads I and aVF (0 to +90 degrees).
- **Left-axis deviation:** An upright QRS in lead I and a downward (⊖) QRS in lead aVF. Up to –30 degrees is still considered a normal variant.
- **Right-axis deviation:** A downward QRS in lead I and an upright QRS in lead aVF (up to +105 degrees is considered a normal variant).

INTERVALS

- **Normal:** PR interval between 120 and 200 msec and QRS < 120 msec.
- **Atrioventricular (AV) block:** PR interval > 200 msec, or P with no QRS afterward.
- **Left bundle branch block (LBBB):** QRS duration > 120 msec; no R wave in V_1; wide, tall R waves in I, V_5, and V_6 (see Figure 2.1-2).

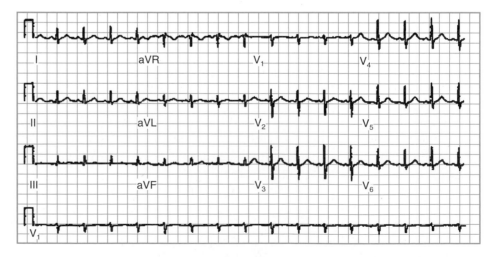

FIGURE 2.1-1. Normal electrocardiogram from a healthy subject. Sinus rhythm is present with a heart rate of 96 bpm. The PR interval is 0.12 sec; the QRS interval (duration) is 0.08 sec; the QT interval is 0.30 sec; QT_c is 0.38 sec; and the mean QRS axis is about +60 degrees. The precordial leads show normal R-wave progression with the transition zone (R wave = S wave) between leads V_2 and V_3. (Adapted with permission from USMLERx.com.)

- **Right bundle branch block (RBBB):** QRS duration > 120 msec; RSR′ complex ("rabbit ears"); qR or R morphology with a wide R wave in V_1; QRS pattern with a wide S wave in I, V_5, and V_6 (see Figure 2.1-3).
- **Long QT syndrome:** QTc > 440 msec. An underdiagnosed congenital disorder that predisposes to ventricular tachyarrhythmias.

ISCHEMIA/INFARCTION

- **Ischemia:** New inverted T waves; poor R-wave progression in precordial leads; ST-segment changes (elevation or depression).
- **Transmural infarct:** Significant Q waves (> 40 msec or more than one-third of the QRS amplitude); ST elevations with T-wave inversions.

CHAMBER ENLARGEMENT

- **Atrial enlargement:**
  - **Right atrial abnormality (P pulmonale):** The P-wave amplitude in lead II is > 2.5 mm.
  - **Left atrial abnormality (P mitrale):** The P-wave width in lead II is > 120 msec, or terminal $\ominus$ deflection in V_1 is > 1 mm in amplitude and > 40 msec in duration. Notched P waves can frequently be seen in lead II.
- **Left ventricular hypertrophy (LVH; see Figure 2.1-4):**
  - **The amplitude of S in V_1 + R in V_5 or V_6 is > 35 mm.**
  - **Alternative criteria:** The amplitude of R in aVL + S in V_3 is > 28 mm in men or > 20 mm in women.
- **Right ventricular hypertrophy (RVH):** Right-axis deviation and an R wave in V_1 > 7 mm.

Cardiac Physical Exam

Key examination findings that can narrow the differential include the following:

- **Jugular venous distention** (JVD, > 7 cm above the sternal angle): Suggests right heart failure, pulmonary hypertension, volume overload, tricuspid regurgitation, or pericardial disease.
- **Hepatojugular reflux:** Fluid overload; impaired right ventricular compliance.
- **Kussmaul's sign** (↑ in JVP with inspiration): Right ventricular infarction, postoperative cardiac tamponade, tricuspid regurgitation, constrictive pericarditis.
- **Systolic murmurs** (see Table 2.1-1 and Figures 2.1-5 and 2.1-6):
  - **Aortic stenosis:** A harsh systolic ejection murmur that radiates to the carotids.

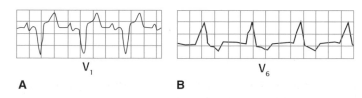

FIGURE 2.1-2.   LBBB. Characteristic ECG findings are seen in leads V_1 (**A**) and V_6 (**B**). (Adapted with permission from USMLERx.com.)

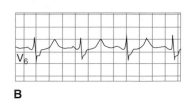

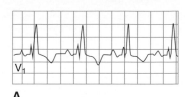

FIGURE 2.1-3. RBBB. Characteristic ECG findings are seen in leads V_1 (**A**) and V_6 (**B**). (Adapted with permission from USMLERx.com.)

> **KEY FACT**

P **P**ulmonale causes **P**eaked P waves.
P **M**itrale causes **M**-shaped P waves.

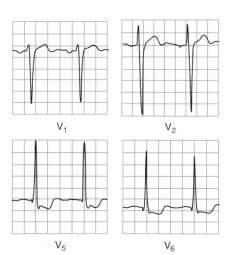

FIGURE 2.1-4. LVH. Shown are leads V_1, V_2, V_5, and V_6. S wave in V_1 + R wave in V_5 = 45 mm. Note ST changes and T-wave inversion in V_5 and V_6, suggesting strain. (Reproduced with permission from Gomella LG, Haist SA. *Clinician's Pocket Reference*, 11th ed. New York: McGraw-Hill, 2007, Fig. 19-27.)

Q

A college-age male "passed out" while playing basketball and had no prodromal symptoms or signs of seizure. His cardiac examination is unremarkable, and an ECG shows a slurred upstroke of the QRS. What are the next best steps?

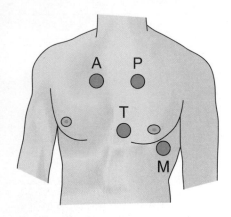

FIGURE 2.1-5. Auscultation locations. Auscultation sites are shown with associated valves. A = aortic valve, P = pulmonic valve, T = tricuspid valve, M = mitral valve.

TABLE 2.1-1. Cardiac Murmurs

SYSTOLIC MURMURS	DIASTOLIC MURMURS
Aortic stenosis	Aortic regurgitation
Mitral regurgitation	Mitral stenosis
Mitral valve prolapse	
Tricuspid regurgitation	

- **Mitral regurgitation:** A holosystolic murmur that radiates to the axilla.
- **Mitral valve prolapse:** A midsystolic or late systolic murmur with a preceding click.
- **Flow murmur:** Very common, and does not imply cardiac disease.
- **Diastolic murmurs** (see Table 2.1-1 and Figures 2.1-5 and 2.1-6): Always abnormal.
  - **Aortic regurgitation:** An early decrescendo murmur.
  - **Mitral stenosis:** A mid- to late, low-pitched murmur.

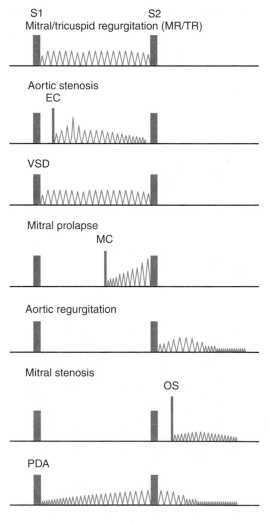

FIGURE 2.1-6. Heart murmurs. Visual representations of common heart murmurs are shown in relation to S1 and S2. EC = ejection click; MC = midsystolic click; OS = opening snap. (Adapted with permission from Le T et al. *First Aid for the USMLE Step 1 2009.* New York: McGraw-Hill, 2009: 250.)

A

This is Wolff-Parkinson-White syndrome (WPW). Advise against vigorous physical activity, treat arrhythmias with procainamide, and refer for an electrophysiology study.

- **Gallops:**
  - **S3 gallop:** Dilated cardiomyopathy (floppy ventricle), mitral valve disease; often normal in younger patients and in high-output states (eg, pregnancy).
  - **S4 gallop:** Hypertension, diastolic dysfunction (stiff ventricle), aortic stenosis; usually pathologic but often normal in younger patients and in athletes.
- **Edema:**
  - **Pulmonary:** Left heart failure (fluid "backs up" into the lungs).
  - **Peripheral:** Right heart failure and biventricular failure (fluid "backs up" into the periphery), peripheral venous disease, constrictive pericarditis, tricuspid regurgitation, hepatic disease, lymphedema. Also nephrotic syndrome, hypoalbuminemia, and drugs.
- **Peripheral pulses:**
  - **Increased:** Compensated aortic regurgitation, coarctation (arms > legs), patent ductus arteriosus.
  - **Decreased:** Peripheral arterial disease; late-stage heart failure.
  - **Pulsus paradoxus** (↓ systolic BP with inspiration): Pericardial tamponade; also asthma and COPD, tension pneumothorax, and foreign body in airway.
  - **Pulsus alternans** (alternating weak and strong pulses): Cardiac tamponade; impaired left ventricular systolic function. Poor prognosis.
  - **Pulsus parvus et tardus** (weak and delayed pulse): Aortic stenosis.

Arrhythmias

BRADYARRHYTHMIAS AND CONDUCTION ABNORMALITIES

Table 2.1-2 outlines the etiologies, clinical presentation, and treatment of common bradyarrhythmias and conduction abnormalities.

TACHYARRHYTHMIAS

Tables 2.1-3 and 2.1-4 outline the etiologies, clinical presentation, and treatment of common supraventricular and ventricular tachyarrhythmias.

Congestive Heart Failure (CHF)

A clinical syndrome caused by inability of the heart to pump enough blood to maintain fluid and metabolic homeostasis. Risk factors include CAD, hypertension, cardiomyopathy, valvular heart disease, and diabetes. The American Heart Association/American College of Cardiology guidelines classify heart failure according to clinical syndromes, but alternative classification systems, including that of the New York Heart Association (NYHA), include functional severity, left-sided vs. right-sided failure, and systolic vs. nonsystolic failure (see Tables 2.1-5 through 2.1-7).

SYSTOLIC DYSFUNCTION

Defined as a ↓ EF (< 50%) and ↑ left ventricular end-diastolic volumes. It is caused by inadequate left ventricular contractility or ↑ afterload. The heart compensates for ↓ EF and ↑ preload through hypertrophy and ventricular dilation (Frank-Starling law), but the compensation ultimately fails, leading to ↑ myocardial work and worsening systolic function.

KEY FACT

Heart auscultation locations: **A**ll (**A**ortic) **P**hysicians (**P**ulmonic) **T**ake (**T**ricuspid) **M**oney (**M**itral).

MNEMONIC

Management options for atrial fibrillation—

ABCD

Anticoagulate
β-blockers to control rate
Cardiovert/**C**alcium channel blockers
Digoxin

KEY FACT

The most common cause of right-sided heart failure is left-sided heart failure.

A man was admitted for a CHF exacerbation with low EF. The patient is now ready for discharge, and his medications include furosemide and metoprolol. What is the next step in management?

TABLE 2.1-2.   **Bradyarrhythmias and Conduction Abnormalities**

TYPE	ETIOLOGY	SIGNS/SYMPTOMS	ECG FINDINGS	TREATMENT
Sinus bradycardia	Normal response to cardiovascular conditioning; can also result from sinus node dysfunction or from β-blocker or calcium channel blocker (CCB) excess.	May be asymptomatic, but may also present with lightheadedness, syncope, chest pain, or hypotension.	Sinus rhythm. Ventricular rate < 60 bpm.	None if asymptomatic; atropine may be used to ↑ heart rate. Pacemaker placement is the definitive treatment in severe cases.
First-degree AV block	Can occur in normal individuals; associated with ↑ vagal tone and with β-blocker or CCB use.	Asymptomatic.	PR interval > 200 msec.	None necessary.
Second-degree AV block **(Mobitz I/ Wenckebach)**	Drug effects (digoxin, β-blockers, CCBs) or ↑ **vagal tone**; right coronary ischemia or infarction.	Usually asymptomatic.	Progressive PR lengthening until a dropped beat occurs; the PR interval then resets.	Stop the offending drug. Atropine as clinically indicated.
Second-degree AV block **(Mobitz II)**	Results from fibrotic disease of the conduction system or from acute, subacute, or prior MI.	Occasionally syncope; **frequent progression to third-degree AV block.**	Unexpected dropped beat(s) without a change in PR interval.	**Pacemaker placement.**
Third-degree AV block (complete)	No electrical communication between the atria and ventricles.	Syncope, dizziness, acute heart failure, hypotension, cannon A waves.	No relationship between P waves and QRS complexes.	**Pacemaker placement.**
Sick sinus syndrome/ tachycardia-bradycardia syndrome	A heterogeneous disorder that leads to intermittent supraventricular tachy- and bradyarrhythmias.	2° to tachycardia or bradycardia; may include syncope, palpitations, dyspnea, chest pain, TIA, and stroke.		**The most common indication for pacemaker placement.**

A

Add an ACEI to this patient's current regimen. ACEIs have been shown to have a ⊕ mortality benefit when used with β-blockers in NYHA class II–IV heart failure patients.

HISTORY/PE

- **Exertional dyspnea is the earliest and most common presenting symptom** and progresses to orthopnea, paroxysmal nocturnal dyspnea (PND), and finally rest dyspnea.
- Patients may report chronic cough, fatigue, peripheral edema, nocturia, and/or abdominal fullness.
- Examination reveals parasternal lift, an elevated and sustained left ventricular impulse, an S3/S4 gallop, JVD, and peripheral edema.
- Look for signs to distinguish left- from right-sided failure (see Table 2.1-6).

TABLE 2.1-3.   **Supraventricular Tachyarrhythmias**

Type	Etiology	Signs/Symptoms	ECG Findings	Treatment
ATRIAL				
Sinus tachycardia	Normal physiologic response to fear, pain, and exercise. Can also be 2° to hyperthyroidism, volume contraction, infection, or pulmonary embolism (PE).	Palpitations, shortness of breath.	Sinus rhythm. Ventricular rate > 100 bpm.	Treat the underlying cause.
Atrial fibrillation (AF)	**Acute AF— PIRATES:** **P**ulmonary disease **I**schemia **R**heumatic heart disease **A**nemia/**A**trial myxoma **T**hyrotoxicosis **E**thanol **S**epsis **Chronic AF—** hypertension, CHF.	Often asymptomatic, but may present with shortness of breath, chest pain, or palpitations. Physical examination reveals an **irregularly irregular pulse.**	No discernible P waves, with variable and irregular QRS response.	**Estimate the risk of stroke using the CHADS2 score. Anticoagulate if ≥ 2.** Anticoagulation if > 48 hours (to prevent CVA); rate control (β-blockers, CCBs, digoxin). Initiate cardioversion only if new onset (< 48 hours) or transesophageal echocardiogram (TEE) shows no left atrial clot, or after 3–6 weeks of warfarin treatment with a satisfactory INR (2–3).
Atrial flutter	Circular movement of electrical activity around the atrium at a rate of approximately 300 times per minute.	Usually asymptomatic, but can present with palpitations, syncope, and lightheadedness.	Regular rhythm; "sawtooth" appearance of P waves can be seen. The atrial rate is usually 240–320 bpm and the ventricular rate ~ 150 bpm.	Anticoagulation, rate control, and cardioversion guidelines as in AF above.
Multifocal atrial tachycardia	Multiple atrial pacemakers or reentrant pathways; COPD, hypoxemia.	May be asymptomatic. At least 3 different P-wave morphologies.	Three or more unique P-wave morphologies; rate > 100 bpm.	Treat the underlying disorder; verapamil or β-blockers for rate control and suppression of atrial pacemakers (not very effective).

(continues)

TABLE 2.1-3. Supraventricular Tachyarrhythmias *(continued)*

TYPE	ETIOLOGY	SIGNS/SYMPTOMS	ECG FINDINGS	TREATMENT
AV JUNCTION				
Atrioventricular nodal reentry tachycardia (AVNRT)	A reentry circuit in the AV node depolarizes the atrium and ventricle nearly simultaneously.	Palpitations, shortness of breath, angina, syncope, lightheadedness.	Rate 150–250 bpm; **P wave is often buried** in QRS or shortly after.	Cardiovert if hemodynamically unstable. Carotid massage, Valsalva, or adenosine can stop the arrhythmia.
Atrioventricular reciprocating tachycardia (AVRT)	An ectopic connection between the atrium and ventricle that causes a reentry circuit. Seen in WPW.	Palpitations, shortness of breath, angina, syncope, lightheadedness.	A retrograde P wave is often seen after a normal QRS. A preexcitation delta wave is characteristically seen in WPW.	Same as that for AVNRT.
Paroxysmal atrial tachycardia	Rapid ectopic pacemaker in the atrium (not sinus node).	Palpitations, shortness of breath, angina, syncope, lightheadedness.	Rate > 100 bpm; P wave with an unusual axis **before** each normal QRS.	Adenosine can be used to unmask underlying atrial activity.

DIAGNOSIS

- **CHF is a clinical syndrome** whose diagnosis is based on signs and symptoms.
- **CXR** may show cardiomegaly, cephalization of pulmonary vessels, pleural effusions, vascular congestion, interstitial edema, and prominent hila (see Figure 2.1-7).
- **Echocardiogram** will show ↓ EF and ventricular dilation.
- **Lab abnormalities** include a BNP > 500 pg/mL, ↑ creatinine (sometimes), and ↓ sodium in later stages.
- **ECG** will usually be nondiagnostic but may help pinpoint an underlying cause, such as AF, an old MI, or LVH as a sign of long-standing hypertension.

TREATMENT

- Acute:
  - Correct underlying causes such as arrhythmias, myocardial ischemia, and drugs (eg, CCBs, antiarrhythmics, NSAIDs, alcohol, thyroid and valvular disease, high-output states).
  - Diurese aggressively with loop and thiazide diuretics (see Table 2.1-8).
  - Give ACEIs to all patients who can tolerate them. Consider an angiotensin receptor blocker (ARB) if the patient cannot tolerate an ACEI.
  - β-blockers should not be used during decompensated CHF but should be started once the patient is euvolemic.
  - Treat acute pulmonary congestion with **LMNOP** (see mnemonic).

KEY FACT

Diuretics and digoxin are for symptomatic relief only and confer no mortality benefit.

MNEMONIC

Acute CHF management—

LMNOP

Lasix
Morphine
Nitrates
Oxygen
Position (upright)

TABLE 2.1-4. **Ventricular Tachyarrhythmias**

TYPE	ETIOLOGY	SIGNS/SYMPTOMS	ECG FINDINGS	TREATMENT
Premature ventricular contraction (PVC)	Ectopic beats arise from ventricular foci. Associated with hypoxia, electrolyte abnormalities, and hyperthyroidism.	Usually asymptomatic, but may lead to palpitations.	Early, wide QRS not preceded by a P wave. PVCs are usually followed by a compensatory pause.	Treat the underlying cause. If symptomatic, give β-blockers or, occasionally, other antiarrhythmics.
Ventricular tachycardia (VT)	Can be associated with CAD, MI, and structural heart disease.	Nonsustained VT is often asymptomatic; sustained VT can lead to palpitations, hypotension, angina, and syncope. Can progress to VF and death.	Three or more consecutive PVCs; wide QRS complexes in a regular rapid rhythm; may see AV dissociation.	Cardioversion and antiarrhythmics (eg, amiodarone, lidocaine, procainamide).
Ventricular fibrillation (VF)	Associated with CAD and structural heart disease. Also associated with cardiac arrest (together with asystole).	Syncope, absence of blood pressure, pulselessness.	Totally erratic wide-complex tracing.	Immediate electrical cardioversion and ACLS protocol.
Torsades de pointes	Associated with long QT syndrome, proarrhythmic response to medications, hypokalemia, congenital deafness, and alcoholism.	Can present with sudden cardiac death; typically associated with palpitations, dizziness, and syncope.	Polymorphous QRS; VT with rates between 150 and 250 bpm.	Give magnesium initially and cardiovert if unstable. Correct hypokalemia; withdraw offending drugs.

TABLE 2.1-5. **NYHA Functional Classification of CHF**

CLASS	DESCRIPTION
I	No limitation of activity; no symptoms with normal activity.
II	Slight limitation of activity; comfortable at rest or with mild exertion.
III	Marked limitation of activity; comfortable only at rest.
IV	Any physical activity brings on discomfort; symptoms present at rest.

TABLE 2.1-6.   Left-Sided vs. Right-Sided Heart Failure

LEFT-SIDED CHF SYMPTOMS	RIGHT-SIDED CHF SYMPTOMS
Dyspnea predominates	**Fluid retention predominates**
Left-sided S3/S4 gallop	Right-sided S3/S4 gallop
Bilateral basilar rales	JVD
Pleural effusions	Hepatojugular reflex
Pulmonary edema	Peripheral edema
Orthopnea, paroxysmal nocturnal dyspnea	Hepatomegaly, ascites

KEY FACT

Loops lose calcium; thiazides take it in.

- Chronic:
  - Control comorbid conditions and limit dietary sodium and fluid intake.
  - Long-term β-blockers and ACEIs/ARBs help prevent remodeling of the heart and ↓ mortality for NYHA class II–IV patients. Avoid CCBs.
  - Daily ASA and a statin are recommended if the underlying cause is a prior MI.
  - Chronic diuretic therapy (loop diuretics +/– a thiazide) can prevent volume overload.
  - Low-dose spironolactone ↓ mortality risk in patients with NYHA class III–IV heart failure.
  - Anticoagulate patients with a history of previous embolic events, AF, or a mobile left ventricular thrombus.
- Consider an implantable biventricular cardiac defibrillator (ICD) in patients with an EF < 35%.
- CHF that is unresponsive to maximal medical therapy may require a mechanical left ventricular assist device or cardiac transplantation.

NONSYSTOLIC DYSFUNCTION

Defined by ↓ ventricular compliance with normal systolic function. The ventricle has either impaired active relaxation (2° to ischemia, aging, and/or hypertrophy) or impaired passive filling (scarring from prior MI; restrictive cardiomyopathy). Left ventricular end-diastolic pressure ↑, cardiac output remains essentially normal, and EF is normal or ↑.

TABLE 2.1-7.   Comparison of Systolic and Diastolic Dysfunction

VARIABLE	SYSTOLIC DYSFUNCTION	NONSYSTOLIC DYSFUNCTION
Patient age	Often < 65 years of age.	Often > 65 years of age.
Comorbidities	Dilated cardiomyopathy, valvular heart disease.	Restrictive or hypertrophic cardiomyopathy; renal disease or hypertension.
Physical examination	Displaced PMI, S3 gallop.	Sustained PMI, S4 gallop.
CXR	Pulmonary congestion, cardiomegaly.	Pulmonary congestion, normal heart size.
ECG/echocardiography	Q waves, ↓ EF (< 40%).	LVH, normal EF (> 55%).

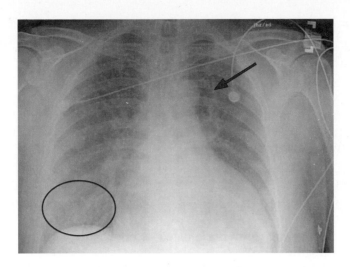

FIGURE 2.1-7. CXR with evidence of CHF. Frontal CXR demonstrates marked cardiomegaly, cephalization of vessels (arrow), interstitial edema (circle), and left-sided pleural effusion that raise concern for CHF. (Reproduced with permission from Tintinalli JE et al. *Tintinalli's Emergency Medicine: A Comprehensive Study Guide*, 7th ed. New York: McGraw-Hill, 2011, Fig. 57-1.)

TABLE 2.1-8. Types of Diuretics

CLASS	EXAMPLES	SITE OF ACTION	MECHANISM OF ACTION	SIDE EFFECTS
Loop diuretics	Furosemide, ethacrynic acid, bumetanide, torsemide	Loop of Henle	↓ $Na^+/K^+/2Cl^-$ cotransporter; ↓ urine concentration; ↑ Ca^{2+} excretion.	Ototoxicity, hypokalemia, hypocalcemia, dehydration, gout.
Thiazide diuretics	HCTZ, chlorothiazide, chlorthalidone	Early distal tubule	↓ NaCl reabsorption leading to ↓ diluting capacity of nephron; ↓ Ca^{2+} excretion.	Hypokalemic metabolic alkalosis, hyponatremia, and hyper**GLUC** (hyper**G**lycemia, hyper**L**ipidemia, hyper**U**ricemia, hyper**C**alcemia).
K^+-sparing agents	Spironolactone, triamterene, amiloride	Cortical collecting tubule	Spironolactone is an aldosterone receptor antagonist; triamterene and amiloride block Na^+ channels.	Hyperkalemia, gynecomastia, sexual dysfunction.
Carbonic anhydrase inhibitors	Acetazolamide	Proximal convoluted tubule	$NaHCO_3$ diuresis ↓ total body $NaHCO_3$.	Hyperchloremic metabolic acidosis, neuropathy, NH_3 toxicity, sulfa allergy.
Osmotic agents	Mannitol	Proximal tubule	Creates ↑ tubular fluid osmolarity, leading to ↑ urine flow.	Pulmonary edema, dehydration. Contraindicated in anuria and CHF.

HISTORY/PE

Associated with stable and unstable angina, shortness of breath, dyspnea on exertion, arrhythmias, MI, heart failure, and sudden death.

TREATMENT

- Diuretics are first-line therapy (see Table 2.1-8).
- Maintain rate and BP control via β-blockers, ACEIs, ARBs, or CCBs.
- Digoxin is not useful in these patients.

Cardiomyopathy

Myocardial disease; categorized as dilated, hypertrophic, or restrictive (see Table 2.1-9 and Figure 2.1-8).

DILATED CARDIOMYOPATHY

The most common cardiomyopathy. Left ventricular dilation and ↓ EF must be present for diagnosis. Most cases are idiopathic, but known 2° causes include alcohol, myocarditis, postpartum status, drugs (doxorubicin, AZT, cocaine), endocrinopathies (thyroid dysfunction, acromegaly, pheochromocytoma), infection (coxsackievirus, HIV, Chagas' disease, parasites), genetic factors, and nutritional disorders (wet beriberi). The most common causes of 2° dilated cardiomyopathy are ischemia and long-standing hypertension.

HISTORY/PE

- Often presents with gradual development of CHF symptoms.
- Examination often reveals displacement of the left ventricular impulse, JVD, an S3/S4 gallop, or mitral/tricuspid regurgitation.

KEY FACT

An S3 gallop signifies rapid ventricular filling in the setting of fluid overload and is associated with dilated cardiomyopathy.

TABLE 2.1-9. Differential Diagnosis of Cardiomyopathies

VARIABLE	TYPE		
	DILATED	HYPERTROPHIC	RESTRICTIVE
Major abnormality	Impaired contractility	Impaired relaxation	Impaired elasticity
Left ventricular cavity size (end diastole)	↑↑	↓	↑
Left ventricular cavity size (end systole)	↑↑	↓↓	↑
EF	↓↓	↑ or ↔	↓ or ↔
Wall thickness	↓, variable	↑↑	↑, variable

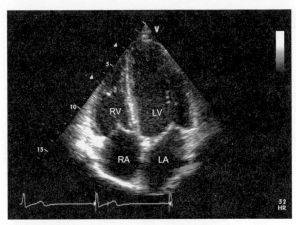
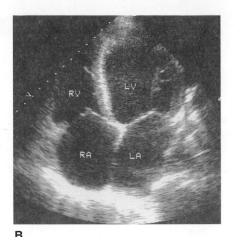

A

B

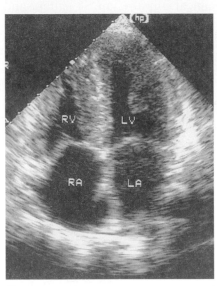

C

FIGURE 2.1-8. **Cardiomyopathies.** Echocardiogram 4-chamber views of (A) a normal heart, (B) dilated cardiomyopathy, and (C) hypertrophic cardiomyopathy. (Reproduced with permission from Fuster V et al. *Hurst's The Heart*, 12th ed. New York: McGraw-Hill, 2008, Figs. 16-17B, 16-108, and 16-109.)

DIAGNOSIS

- Echocardiography is diagnostic.
- ECG may show nonspecific ST-T changes, a low-voltage QRS, sinus tachycardia, and ectopy. LBBB is common.
- CXR shows an enlarged, balloon-like heart and pulmonary congestion.

TREATMENT

- Address the underlying etiology (eg, alcohol use, endocrine disorders).
- Treat symptoms of CHF with diuretics, ACEIs/ARBs, and β-blockers. Digoxin is a second-line agent; **avoid CCBs in heart failure.**
- Consider anticoagulation to ↓ thrombus risk if AF or an intraventricular thrombus is present.
- Consider an ICD if EF is < 35%.

Q

A woman with hypertension and prior MI has an examination notable for a displaced PMI, an S3, a nonelevated JVP, and bibasilar rales. What is the next best step in diagnosis?

HYPERTROPHIC CARDIOMYOPATHY

Defined as impaired left ventricular relaxation and filling (nonsystolic dysfunction) due to thickened ventricular walls. Hypertrophy frequently involves the interventricular septum, leading to left ventricular outflow tract obstruction and impaired ejection of blood. The congenital form, hypertrophic obstructive cardiomyopathy (HOCM), is **inherited as an autosomal dominant trait** in 50% of HOCM patients and is the most common cause of sudden death in young, healthy athletes in the United States. Other causes of marked hypertrophy include hypertension and aortic stenosis.

HISTORY/PE

- Patients may be asymptomatic but may also present with syncope, dyspnea, palpitations, angina, or sudden cardiac death.
- Examination often reveals a sustained apical impulse, an S4 gallop, and a systolic ejection crescendo-decrescendo murmur that ↑ with ↓ preload (eg, Valsalva maneuver, standing) and ↓ with ↑ preload (eg, passive leg raise).

DIAGNOSIS

- Echocardiography is diagnostic and shows an asymmetrically thickened septum and dynamic obstruction of blood flow.
- ECG may show signs of LVH.
- CXR may reveal left atrial enlargement (LAE) 2° to mitral regurgitation.

TREATMENT

- β-blockers are initial therapy for symptomatic relief; CCBs are second-line agents.
- Surgical options for HOCM include dual-chamber pacing, partial excision or alcohol ablation of the myocardial septum, ICD placement, and mitral valve replacement.
- Patients should avoid intense athletic competition and training.

RESTRICTIVE CARDIOMYOPATHY

Defined as ↓ elasticity of myocardium leading to impaired diastolic filling without significant systolic dysfunction (a normal or near-normal EF). It is caused by infiltrative disease (amyloidosis, sarcoidosis, hemochromatosis) or by scarring and fibrosis (2° to radiation).

HISTORY/PE

Signs and symptoms of left-sided and right-sided heart failure occur, but symptoms of right-sided heart failure (JVD, peripheral edema) often predominate.

DIAGNOSIS

- Echocardiography is key for diagnosis, with rapid early filling and a near-normal EF. CXR, MRI, and cardiac catheterization are helpful for characterization (eg, sarcoid, amyloidosis).
- Cardiac biopsy may reveal fibrosis or evidence of infiltration.
- ECG frequently shows LBBB; low voltages are seen in amyloidosis.

TREATMENT

Therapeutic options are limited and are generally palliative only. Medical treatment includes cautious use of diuretics for fluid overload and vasodilators to ↓ filling pressure.

Coronary Artery Disease (CAD)

Clinical manifestations of CAD include stable and unstable angina, shortness of breath, dyspnea on exertion, arrhythmias, MI, heart failure, and sudden death. Risk factors include a family history of premature CAD (males < 55, females < 65), smoking, dyslipidemia, abdominal obesity, hypertension, age (males > 45, females > 55), and male gender. CAD risk equivalents include diabetes mellitus (DM), symptomatic carotid artery disease, peripheral arterial disease, and abdominal aortic aneurysm (AAA).

ANGINA PECTORIS

Defined as substernal chest pain 2° to myocardial ischemia (O_2 supply and demand mismatch). Prinzmetal's (variant) angina mimics angina pectoris but is caused by vasospasm of coronary vessels. It classically affects young women at rest in the early morning and is associated with ST-segment elevation in the absence of cardiac enzyme elevation.

HISTORY/PE

- The **classic triad** consists of **substernal chest pain** that is usually **precipitated by stress** or exertion and is **relieved by rest** or nitrates.
- Pain can radiate and may be associated with shortness of breath, nausea/vomiting, diaphoresis, or lightheadedness.
- Examination of patients experiencing stable angina is generally unremarkable. Look for carotid and peripheral bruits suggesting atherosclerosis and hypertension.

DIAGNOSIS

- Rule out pulmonary, GI, or other cardiac causes of chest pain.
- Significant ST-segment changes on exercise stress test with ECG monitoring are diagnostic of CAD.
- Maintain a high index of suspicion in patient populations such as women and diabetics in view of their propensity for "silent" events.

TREATMENT

- Treat acute symptoms with ASA, O_2, IV nitroglycerin, and IV morphine, and consider IV β-blockers. The efficacy of nondihydropyridine CCBs (diltiazem, verapamil) and ACEIs has also been validated.
- Admit to the hospital and monitor until acute MI has been ruled out by serial cardiac enzymes.
- Treat chronic symptoms with nitrates, ASA, and β-blockers; CCBs are second-line agents for symptomatic control only.
- Initiate risk factor reduction (eg, smoking, cholesterol, hypertension). Hormone replacement therapy is not protective in postmenopausal women.

KEY FACT

Major risk factors for CAD include age, male gender, ↑ LDL, ↓ HDL, DM, hypertension, a family history, smoking, and peripheral arterial disease.

KEY FACT

Prinz**metal's** angina doesn't **meddle** with enzymes.

KEY FACT

Women, diabetics, the elderly, and post–heart transplant patients may have atypical, clinically silent MIs.

KEY FACT

Only ASA and β-blockers have been shown to have a mortality benefit in the treatment of angina.

Acute Coronary Syndromes

A spectrum of clinical syndromes caused by plaque disruption or vasospasm that leads to acute myocardial ischemia.

UNSTABLE ANGINA/NON-ST-ELEVATION MYOCARDIAL INFARCTION (NSTEMI)

Unstable angina is defined as chest pain that is new onset, is accelerating (ie, occurs with less exertion, lasts longer, or is less responsive to medications), or occurs at rest; it is distinguished from stable angina pectoris by patient history. It signals the presence of possible **impending infarction** based on plaque instability. In contrast, **NSTEMI** indicates myocardial necrosis marked by elevations in **troponin I and CK-MB** without ST-segment elevations seen on ECG.

KEY FACT

U Ain't got enzymes with **U**nstable **A**ngina.

Diagnosis

- Patients should be risk stratified according to the Thrombolysis in Myocardial Infarction (TIMI) study criteria to determine the likelihood of adverse cardiac events (see Table 2.1-10).
- Unstable angina is not associated with elevated cardiac markers, but ST changes may be seen on ECG.
- NSTEMI is diagnosed by serial cardiac enzymes and ECG.

Treatment

- Acute treatment of symptoms is the same as that for stable angina and consists of clopidogrel, unfractionated heparin, or enoxaparin.
- Patients with chest pain refractory to medical therapy, a TIMI score of ≥ 3, a troponin elevation, or ST changes > 1 mm should be given IV heparin and scheduled for angiography and possible revascularization (percutaneous coronary intervention [PCI] or CABG).

TABLE 2.1-10. TIMI Risk Score for Unstable Angina/NSTEMI

CHARACTERISTICS	POINT
History	
Age ≥ 65 years	1
≥ 3 CAD risk factors (premature family history, DM, smoking, hypertension, ↑ cholesterol)	1
Known CAD (stenosis > 50%)	1
ASA use in past 7 days	1
Presentation	
Severe angina (≥ 2 episodes within 24 hours)	1
ST deviation ≥ 0.5 mm	1
+ cardiac marker	1
Risk score—total points[a]	(0–7)

[a] Higher-risk patients (risk score ≥ 3) benefit more from enoxaparin (vs. unfractionated heparin), glycoprotein IIb/IIIa inhibitors, and early angiography.

ST-ELEVATION MYOCARDIAL INFARCTION (STEMI)

Defined as ST-segment elevations and cardiac enzyme release 2° to prolonged cardiac ischemia and necrosis.

HISTORY/PE

- Presents with acute-onset substernal chest pain, commonly described as a pressure or tightness that can radiate to the left arm, neck, or jaw.
- Associated symptoms may include diaphoresis, shortness of breath, lightheadedness, anxiety, nausea/vomiting, and syncope.
- Physical examination may reveal arrhythmias, hypotension (cardiogenic shock), and evidence of new CHF.
- **The best predictor of survival is left ventricular EF.**

DIAGNOSIS

- **ECG** will show ST-segment elevations or new LBBB. ST-segment depressions and dominant R waves in leads V_1–V_2 can also be reciprocal change indicating posterior wall infarct.
- **Sequence of ECG changes:** Peaked T waves → ST-segment elevation → Q waves → T-wave inversion → ST-segment normalization → T-wave normalization over several hours to days.
- **Cardiac enzymes:** Troponin I is the most sensitive and specific cardiac enzyme; CK-MB and the CK-MB/total CK ratio (CK index) are also regularly checked. Both troponin I and CK-MB can take up to 6 hours to rise following the onset of chest pain (see Figure 2.1-9).
- **ST-segment abnormalities:**
  - ST-segment elevation in leads **II, III,** and **aVF** is consistent with an **inferior MI involving the RCA/PDA and LCA** (see Figure 2.1-10). Obtain a right-sided ECG to look for ST elevations in the right ventricle.
  - ST-segment elevation in leads V_1–V_4 usually indicates an **anterior MI** involving the LAD and diagonal branches (see Figure 2.1-11).
  - ST-segment elevation in leads **I, aVL,** and V_5–V_6 points to a **lateral MI** involving the LCA.
  - ST-segment depression in leads V_1–V_2 (anterior leads) can be indicative of an acute transmural infarct in the posterior wall. Obtain posterior ECG leads V_7–V_9 to assess for ST-segment elevations.

MNEMONIC

When your patient is MOANing from an MI, remember–

MONA

Morphine
Oxygen
Nitrogen
Aspirin

KEY FACT

Common causes of chest pain include GERD, angina, esophageal pain, musculoskeletal disorders (costochondritis, trauma), and pneumonia.

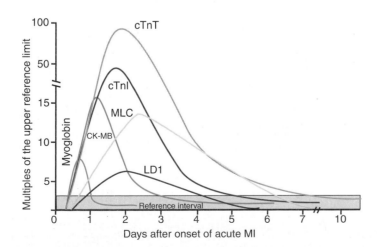

FIGURE 2.1-9. **Typical pattern of serum marker elevation after an acute MI.** CK-MB = creatine kinase, MB isoenzyme; cTnI = cardiac troponin I; cTnT = cardiac troponin T; LD1 = lactate dehydrogenase isoenzyme 1; MLC = myosin light chain. (Reproduced with permission from Tintinalli JE et al. *Tintinalli's Emergency Medicine: A Comprehensive Study Guide,* 6th ed. New York: McGraw-Hill, 2004, Fig. 49-1.)

A woman is found with pulseless electrical activity on hospital day 7 after suffering a lateral wall STEMI. The ACLS protocol is initiated. What is the next best step?

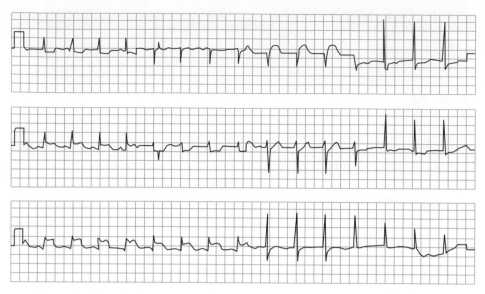

FIGURE 2.1-10. **Inferior wall MI.** In this patient with acute chest pain, the ECG demonstrated acute ST-segment elevation in leads II, III, and aVF with reciprocal ST-segment depression and T-wave flattening in leads I, aVL, and V_4–V_6.

TREATMENT

- Six key medications should be considered: ASA, β-blockers, clopidogrel, morphine, nitrates, and O_2.
- If the patient is in heart failure or in cardiogenic shock, do not give β-blockers; instead, give ACEIs provided that the patient is not hypotensive.
- **Emergent angiography and PCI** should be performed; if possible, the patient should undergo PCI for the lesion thought to be responsible for the STEMI.
- If PCI cannot be performed within 90 minutes, there are no contraindications to thrombolysis (eg, a history of hemorrhagic stroke or recent ischemic stroke, severe heart failure, or cardiogenic shock), and the patient presents within 3 hours of chest pain onset, thrombolysis with tPA, reteplase, or streptokinase should be performed instead of PCI.

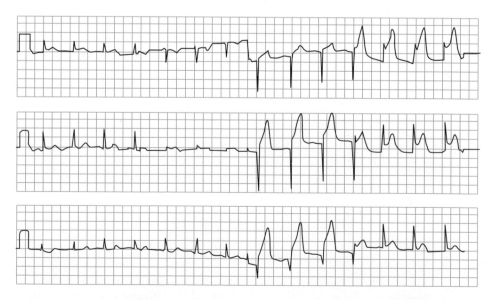

A

This patient has likely suffered a left ventricular free-wall rupture with acute cardiac tamponade. Emergent pericardiocentesis is the next best therapeutic and diagnostic step.

FIGURE 2.1-11. **Anterior wall MI.** This patient presented with acute chest pain. The ECG showed acute ST-segment elevation in leads aVL and V_1–V_6, and hyperacute T waves.

- **PCI should be attempted immediately** for the lesion thought to be responsible for STEMI; the patient is a candidate for CABG afterward.
- Long-term treatment includes ASA, ACEIs, β-blockers, high-dose statins, and clopidogrel (if PCI was performed). Modify risk factors with dietary changes, exercise, and tobacco cessation.

COMPLICATIONS

- Arrhythmia is the most common complication following acute MI; lethal arrhythmia is the most frequent cause of death.
- Less common complications include reinfarction, left ventricular wall rupture, VSD, pericarditis, papillary muscle rupture (with mitral regurgitation), left ventricular aneurysm or pseudoaneurysm, and mural thrombi.
- Dressler's syndrome, an autoimmune process occurring 2–10 weeks post-MI, presents with fever, pericarditis, pleural effusion, leukocytosis, and ↑ ESR.
- A timeline of common post-MI complications is as follows:
    - **First day:** Heart failure.
    - **2–4 days:** Arrhythmia, pericarditis.
    - **5–10 days:** Left ventricular wall rupture (acute pericardial tamponade causing electrical alternans, pulseless electrical activity), papillary muscle rupture (severe mitral regurgitation).
    - **Weeks to months:** Ventricular aneurysm (CHF, arrhythmia, persistent ST-segment elevation, mitral regurgitation, thrombus formation).

MNEMONIC

Indications for CABG are UnLimiTeD:

Unable to perform PCI (diffuse disease)
Left main coronary artery disease
Triple-vessel disease
Depressed ventricular function

Dyslipidemia

Defined as a total cholesterol level > 200 mg/dL, LDL > 130 mg/dL, triglycerides > 150 mg/dL, and HDL < 40 mg/dL, all of which are risk factors for CAD. Etiologies include obesity, DM, alcoholism, hypothyroidism, nephrotic syndrome, hepatic disease, Cushing's syndrome, OCP use, high-dose diuretic use, and familial hypercholesterolemia.

HISTORY/PE

- Most patients have **no specific signs or symptoms.**
- Patients with extremely high triglyceride or LDL levels may have xanthomas (eruptive nodules in the skin over the tendons), xanthelasmas (yellow fatty deposits in the skin around the eyes), and lipemia retinalis (creamy appearance of retinal vessels).

DIAGNOSIS

- Conduct a fasting lipid profile for patients ≥ 35 years of age or in those ≥ 20 **years of age with CAD risk factors,** and repeat **every 5 years** or sooner if lipid levels are elevated.
- Total serum cholesterol > 200 mg/dL on 2 different occasions is diagnostic of hypercholesterolemia.
- LDL > 130 mg/dL or HDL < 40 mg/dL is diagnostic of dyslipidemia even if total serum cholesterol is < 200 mg/dL.

TREATMENT

- Based on risk stratification (see Table 2.1-11).
- The **first intervention** should be a **12-week trial of diet and exercise** in a patient with no known atherosclerotic vascular disease. Commonly used lipid-lowering agents are listed in Table 2.1-12.

KEY FACT

Dyslipidemia:
- LDL > 130 mg/dL or
- HDL < 40 mg/dL

TABLE 2.1-11. ATP III Guidelines for Risk Stratification of Dyslipidemia

RISK CATEGORY	LDL GOAL	LDL TO START LIFESTYLE MODIFICATION	LDL TO CONSIDER DRUG THERAPY
CAD or CAD risk equivalents[a]	< 100 mg/dL (or < 70)	≥ 100 mg/dL	≥ 130 mg/dL
2+ risk factors[b]	< 130 mg/dL	≥ 130 mg/dL	≥ 160 mg/dL
0–1 risk factor[b]	< 160 mg/dL	≥ 160 mg/dL	≥ 190 mg/dL

[a] CAD risk equivalents include symptomatic carotid artery disease, peripheral arterial disease, AAA, and diabetes.

[b] Risk factors include cigarette smoking, hypertension, low HDL (< 40 mg/dL), a family history of premature CAD, and age (men > 45 years; women > 55 years). An HDL > 60 mg/dL counts as a "negative" risk factor and removes 1 risk factor from the total score.

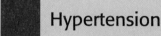

Hypertension

Defined as a systolic BP > 140 mm Hg and/or a diastolic BP > 90 mm Hg based on 3 measurements separated in time (see Table 2.1-13). Classified as 1° or 2°.

KEY FACT

The BP goal in uncomplicated hypertension is < 140/< 90 mm Hg. For diabetics or patients with renal disease, the goal is < 130/< 80 mm Hg.

1° (ESSENTIAL) HYPERTENSION

Hypertension with no identifiable cause. Represents 95% of cases of hypertension. Risk factors include a family history of hypertension or heart disease, a

TABLE 2.1-12. Lipid-Lowering Agents

CLASS	EXAMPLES	MECHANISM OF ACTION	EFFECT ON LIPID PROFILE	SIDE EFFECTS
HMG-CoA reductase inhibitors (statins)	Atorvastatin, simvastatin, lovastatin, pravastatin, rosuvastatin	Inhibit the rate-limiting step in cholesterol synthesis.	↓ LDL, ↓ triglycerides	↑ LFTs, myositis, warfarin potentiation.
Lipoprotein lipase stimulators (fibrates)	Gemfibrozil	↑ lipoprotein lipase, leading to ↑ VLDL and triglyceride catabolism.	↓ triglycerides, ↑ HDL	GI upset, cholelithiasis, myositis, ↑ LFTs.
Cholesterol absorption inhibitors	Ezetimibe (Zetia)	↓ absorption of cholesterol at the small intestine brush border.	↓ LDL	Diarrhea, abdominal pain. Can cause angioedema.
Niacin	Niaspan	↓ fatty acid release from adipose tissue; ↓ hepatic synthesis of LDL.	↑ HDL, ↓ LDL	Skin flushing (can be prevented with ASA), paresthesias, pruritus, GI upset, ↑ LFTs.
Bile acid resins	Cholestyramine, colestipol, colesevelam	Bind intestinal bile acids, leading to ↓ bile acid stores and ↑ catabolism of LDL from plasma.	↓ LDL	Constipation, GI upset, LFT abnormalities, myalgias. Can ↓ absorption of other drugs from the small intestine.

high-sodium diet, smoking, obesity, ethnicity (blacks > whites), and advanced age.

HISTORY/PE

- Hypertension is asymptomatic until complications develop.
- Patients should be evaluated for end-organ damage to the brain (stroke, dementia), eye (cotton-wool exudates, hemorrhage), heart (LVH), and kidney (proteinuria, chronic kidney disease). Renal bruits may signify renal artery stenosis as the cause of hypertension.

DIAGNOSIS

Obtain a UA, BUN/creatinine, a CBC, and electrolytes to assess the extent of end-organ damage and possible 2° causes.

TREATMENT

- Rule out 2° causes of hypertension, particularly in patients with new-onset hypertension at extremes of age.
- Begin with lifestyle modifications. Weight loss is the single most effective lifestyle modification.
- The BP goal in otherwise healthy patients is < 140/< 90 mm Hg. The goal in diabetics or patients with renal disease with proteinuria is < 130/< 80 mm Hg.
- Diuretics, ACEIs, and β-blockers have been shown to ↓ mortality in uncomplicated hypertension. They are first-line agents unless a comorbid condition requires another medication (see Table 2.1-14).
- Periodically test for end-organ complications, including renal complications (BUN, creatinine, urine protein-to-creatinine ratio) and cardiac complications (ECG evidence of hypertrophy).

2° HYPERTENSION

Hypertension 2° to an identifiable organic cause. See Table 2.1-15 for the diagnosis and treatment of common causes.

Q

A 40-year-old male presents for a routine examination. His examination is significant for a BP of 145/75 mm Hg but is otherwise unremarkable, as are his labs. What is the next best step?

MNEMONIC

Treatment of hypertension—

ABCD

ACEIs/**A**RBs
β-blockers
CCBs
Diuretics

MNEMONIC

Causes of 2° hypertension—

CHAPS

Cushing's syndrome
Hyperaldosteronism (Conn's syndrome)
Aortic coarctation
Pheochromocytoma
Stenosis of renal arteries

TABLE 2.1-13. JNC-7 Classification and Management of Hypertension

BP CLASSIFICATION	SYSTOLIC BP (mm Hg)		DIASTOLIC BP (mm Hg)	LIFESTYLE MODIFICATION	DRUG THERAPY WITH NO COMORBIDITIES
Normal	< 120	and	< 80	Encourage	
Prehypertension	120–139	or	80–89	Yes	No antihypertensive drug indicated.
Stage 1 hypertension	140–159	or	90–99	Yes	**Thiazide diuretics** for most patients; ACEIs, ARBs, β-blockers, CCBs, or a combination may be considered.
Stage 2 hypertension	≥ 160	or	≥ 100	Yes	**Two-drug combination** for most patients (usually a thiazide diuretic plus an ACEI, an ARB, a β-blocker, or a CCB).

With a single BP recording and no evidence of end-organ damage, the next best step should consist of a repeat BP measurement at the end of the examination with a return visit if BP is still high.

TABLE 2.1-14. Treatment of 1° Hypertension in Specific Populations

Population	Agents
Uncomplicated	Diuretics, β-blockers, ACEIs.
CHF	Diuretics, β-blockers, ACEIs, ARBs, aldosterone antagonists.
Diabetes	Diuretics, β-blockers, ACEIs, ARBs, CCBs.
Post-MI	β-blockers, ACEIs, ARBs, aldosterone antagonists.
Chronic kidney disease	ACEIs, ARBs.
BPH	Diuretics, α_1-adrenergic blockers.
Isolated systolic hypertension	Diuretics, ACEIs, CCBs (dihydropyridines).

TABLE 2.1-15. Common Causes of 2° Hypertension

Etiology	Description	Management
1° renal disease	Often unilateral renal parenchymal disease.	Treat with ACEIs, which slow the progression of renal disease.
Renal artery stenosis	Especially common in patients < 25 and > 50 years of age with recent-onset hypertension. Etiologies include fibromuscular dysplasia (younger patients) and atherosclerosis (older patients).	Diagnose with MRA or renal artery Doppler ultrasound. May be treated with angioplasty or stenting. Consider ACEIs in unilateral disease. (In bilateral disease, ACEIs can accelerate kidney failure by preferential vasodilation of the efferent arteriole.) Open surgery is a second option if angioplasty is not effective or feasible.
OCP use	Common in women > 35 years of age, obese women, and those with long-standing use.	Discontinue OCPs (effect may be delayed).
Pheochromocytoma	An adrenal gland tumor that secretes epinephrine and norepinephrine, leading to **episodic headache, sweating, and tachycardia.**	Diagnose with urinary metanephrines and catecholamine levels or plasma metanephrine. Surgical removal of tumor after **treatment with both α-blockers and β-blockers.**
Conn's syndrome (hyperaldosteronism)	Most often 2° to an aldosterone-producing adrenal adenoma. Causes the **triad of hypertension, unexplained hypokalemia, and metabolic alkalosis.**	Metabolic workup with plasma aldosterone and renin level; ↑ aldosterone and ↓ renin levels suggest 1° hyperaldosteronism. Surgical removal of tumor.
Cushing's syndrome	Due to an ACTH-producing pituitary tumor, an ectopic ACTH-secreting tumor, or cortisol secretion by an adrenal adenoma or carcinoma. Also due to exogenous steroid exposure. (See the Endocrinology chapter for more details.)	Surgical removal of tumor; removal of exogenous steroids.
Coarctation of the aorta	See the Pediatrics chapter.	Surgical repair.

HYPERTENSIVE CRISES

A spectrum of clinical presentations in which elevated BPs lead to end-organ damage.

HISTORY/PE

Present with end-organ damage revealed by renal disease, chest pain (ischemia or MI), back pain (aortic dissection), or changes in mental status (hypertensive encephalopathy).

DIAGNOSIS

- **Hypertensive urgency:** Elevated BP with mild to moderate symptoms (headache, chest pain) without end-organ damage.
- **Hypertensive emergency:** Elevated BP with signs or symptoms of impending end-organ damage such as acute kidney injury, intracranial hemorrhage, papilledema, or ECG changes suggestive of ischemia or pulmonary edema.
- **Malignant hypertension:** Diagnosed on the basis of progressive renal failure and/or encephalopathy with papilledema.

TREATMENT

- **Hypertensive urgencies:** Can be treated with oral antihypertensives (eg, β-blockers, clonidine, ACEIs) with the goal of gradually lowering BP over 24–48 hours (see Table 2.1-16).
- **Hypertensive emergencies:** Treat with IV medications (labetalol, nitroprusside, nicardipine) with the goal of lowering mean arterial pressure by no more than 25% over the first 2 hours to prevent cerebral hypoperfusion or coronary insufficiency.

KEY FACT

Hypertensive crises are diagnosed on the basis of the extent of end-organ damage, not BP measurement.

Pericardial Disease

Results from acute or chronic pericardial insults; may lead to pericardial effusion.

PERICARDITIS

Defined as inflammation of the pericardial sac. It can compromise cardiac output via tamponade or constrictive pericarditis. Most commonly idiopathic, although known etiologies include viral infection, TB, SLE, uremia, drugs, radiation, and neoplasms. May also occur after MI (either within days after MI or as a delayed phenomenon, ie, Dressler's syndrome) or open heart surgery.

HISTORY/PE

- May present with pleuritic chest pain, dyspnea, cough, and fever.
- Chest pain tends to worsen in the supine position and with inspiration.
- Examination may reveal a pericardial friction rub. Elevated JVP and pulsus paradoxus (a ↓ in systolic BP > 10 mm Hg on inspiration) can be present with tamponade.

DIAGNOSIS

- CXR, ECG, and echocardiogram to rule out MI and pneumonia.
- ECG changes include **diffuse ST-segment elevation and PR-segment depressions** followed by T-wave inversions (see Figure 2.1-12).
- Pericardial thickening or effusion may be evident on echocardiography.

MNEMONIC

Causes of pericarditis—

CARDIAC RIND

Collagen vascular disease
Aortic dissection
Radiation
Drugs
Infections
Acute renal failure
Cardiac (MI)
Rheumatic fever
Injury
Neoplasms
Dressler's syndrome

Q

A 20-year-old male presents with an initial BP of 150/85 mm Hg, and repeat measurement yields 147/85 mm Hg. The patient's potassium level is 3.2 mg/dL. What is the next appropriate diagnostic step?

TABLE 2.1-16.   Major Classes of Antihypertensive Agents

CLASS	AGENTS	MECHANISM OF ACTION	SIDE EFFECTS
Diuretics	Thiazide, loop, K+ sparing	↓ extracellular fluid volume and thereby ↓ vascular resistance.	Hypokalemia (not with K+ sparing), hyperglycemia, hyperlipidemia, hyperuricemia, azotemia.
β-blockers	Propranolol, metoprolol, nadolol, atenolol, timolol, carvedilol, labetalol	↓ cardiac contractility and renin release.	Bronchospasm (in severe active asthma), bradycardia, CHF exacerbation, impotence, fatigue, depression.
ACEIs	Captopril, enalapril, fosinopril, benazepril, lisinopril	Block aldosterone formation, reducing peripheral resistance and salt/water retention.	Cough, rashes, leukopenia, hyperkalemia.
ARBs	Losartan, valsartan, irbesartan	Block aldosterone effects, reducing peripheral resistance and salt/water retention.	Rashes, leukopenia, and hyperkalemia but no cough.
CCBs	Dihydropyridines (nifedipine, felodipine, amlodipine), nondihydropyridines (diltiazem, verapamil)	↓ smooth muscle tone and cause vasodilation; may also ↓ cardiac output.	**Dihydropyridines:** Headache, flushing, peripheral edema. **Nondihydropyridines:** ↓ contractility.
Vasodilators	Hydralazine, minoxidil	↓ peripheral resistance by dilating arteries/arterioles.	**Hydralazine:** Headache, lupus-like syndrome. **Minoxidil:** Orthostasis, hirsutism.
α_1-adrenergic blockers	Prazosin, terazosin, phenoxybenzamine	Cause vasodilation by blocking actions of norepinephrine on vascular smooth muscle.	Orthostatic hypotension.
Centrally acting adrenergic agonists	Methyldopa, clonidine	Inhibit the sympathetic nervous system via central α_2-adrenergic receptors.	Somnolence, orthostatic hypotension, impotence, rebound hypertension.

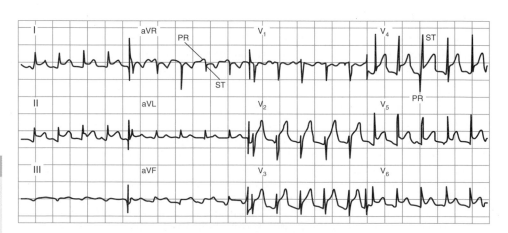

A hyperaldosteronism workup with serum aldosterone and renin levels is an appropriate next diagnostic step.

FIGURE 2.1-12.   Acute pericarditis. Diffuse ST-segment elevations in multiple leads not consistent with any discrete coronary vascular territory and PR-segment depressions. (Reproduced with permission from Fauci AS et al. *Harrison's Principles of Internal Medicine,* 17th ed. New York: McGraw-Hill, 2008, Fig. 232-1.)

TREATMENT

- Address the underlying cause (eg, corticosteroids/immunosuppressants for SLE, dialysis for uremia) or symptoms (eg, ASA for post-MI pericarditis, ASA/NSAIDs for viral pericarditis). Avoid corticosteroids within a few days after MI, as they can predispose to ventricular wall rupture.
- Pericardial effusions without symptoms can be monitored, but evidence of tamponade requires pericardiocentesis with continuous drainage as needed.

CARDIAC TAMPONADE

Defined as excess fluid in the pericardial sac, leading to compromised ventricular filling and ↓ cardiac output. The rate of fluid formation is more important than the size of the effusion. Risk factors include pericarditis, malignancy, SLE, TB, and trauma (commonly stab wounds medial to the left nipple).

HISTORY/PE

- Presents with fatigue, dyspnea, anxiety, tachycardia, and tachypnea that can rapidly progress to shock and death.
- Examination of a patient with acute tamponade may reveal Beck's triad (hypotension, distant heart sounds, and JVD), a narrow pulse pressure, pulsus paradoxus, and Kussmaul's sign (JVD on inspiration).

DIAGNOSIS

- Echocardiogram shows right atrial and right ventricular diastolic collapse.
- CXR may show an enlarged, globular, water-bottle-shaped heart with a large effusion (see Figure 2.1-13).
- If present on ECG, electrical alternans is diagnostic of a large pericardial effusion.

TREATMENT

- Aggressive volume expansion with IV fluids.
- Urgent pericardiocentesis (aspirate will be nonclotting blood).
- Decompensation may warrant pericardial window.

Valvular Heart Disease

Until recently, rheumatic fever (which affects the mitral valve more often than the aortic valve) was the most common cause of valvular heart disease in U.S. adults; the leading cause is now mechanical degeneration. Subtypes are listed in Table 2.1-17 along with their etiologies, presentation, diagnosis, and treatment.

Vascular Disease

AORTIC ANEURYSM

Defined as > 50% dilatation of all 3 layers of the aortic wall. Aortic aneurysms are most commonly **associated with atherosclerosis**. Most are abdominal, and > 90% originate below the renal arteries.

KEY FACT

Beck's triad can diagnose acute cardiac tamponade:
- JVD
- Hypotension
- Distant heart sounds

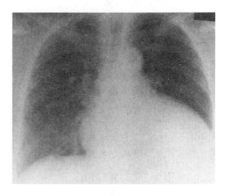

FIGURE 2.1-13. Water-bottle-shaped heart seen on CXR with pericardial effusion. (Reproduced with permission from Chen MY et al. *Basic Radiology,* 2nd ed. New York: McGraw-Hill, 2011, Fig. 3-26.)

TABLE 2.1-17. **Types of Valvular Heart Disease**

Type	Etiology	History	Exam/Diagnosis	Treatment
Aortic stenosis	Most often seen in the elderly. Unicuspid and bicuspid valves can lead to symptoms in childhood and adolescence.	May be asymptomatic for years despite significant stenosis. Once symptomatic, usually progresses from angina to syncope to CHF to death within 5 years. **Sx** (also indications for valve replacements): **ACS**—**A**ngina, **C**HF, **S**yncope.	**PE:** Pulsus parvus et tardus (weak, delayed carotid upstroke) and a single or paradoxically split S2 sound; systolic murmur radiating to the carotids. **Dx:** Echocardiography.	Aortic valve replacement.
Aortic regurgitation	**Acute:** Infective endocarditis, aortic dissection, chest trauma. **Chronic:** Valve malformations, rheumatic fever, connective tissue disorders.	**Acute:** Rapid onset of pulmonary congestion, cardiogenic shock, and severe dyspnea. **Chronic:** Slowly progressive onset of dyspnea on exertion, orthopnea, and PND.	**PE:** Blowing diastolic murmur at the left sternal border, mid-diastolic rumble (Austin Flint murmur), and midsystolic apical murmur. Widened pulse pressure causes de Musset's sign (head bob with heartbeat), Corrigan's sign (water-hammer pulse), and Duroziez's sign (femoral bruit). **Dx:** Echocardiography.	Vasodilator therapy (dihydropyridines or ACEIs) for isolated aortic regurgitation until symptoms become severe enough to warrant valve replacement.
Mitral valve stenosis	The most common etiology continues to be rheumatic fever.	Symptoms range from dyspnea, orthopnea, and PND to infective endocarditis and arrhythmias.	**PE:** Opening snap and mid-diastolic murmur at the apex; pulmonary edema. **Dx:** Echocardiography.	Antiarrhythmics (β-blockers, digoxin) for symptomatic relief; mitral balloon valvotomy and valve replacement are effective for severe cases.
Mitral valve regurgitation	Primarily 2° to rheumatic fever or chordae tendineae rupture after MI. Infective endocarditis.	Patients present with dyspnea, orthopnea, and fatigue.	**PE:** Holosystolic murmur radiating to the axilla. **Dx:** Echocardiography will demonstrate regurgitant flow; angiography can assess the severity of disease.	Antiarrhythmics if necessary (AF is common with LAE; nitrates and diuretics to ↓ preload). Valve repair or replacement for severe cases.

History/PE

- **Usually asymptomatic** and discovered incidentally on examination or radiologic study.
- Risk factors include hypertension, high cholesterol, other vascular disease, a ⊕ family history, smoking, gender (males > females), and age.

- Examination demonstrates a **pulsatile abdominal mass or abdominal bruits.**
- Ruptured aneurysm leads to hypotension and severe, tearing abdominal pain that radiates to the back.

DIAGNOSIS

- All men 65–75 years of age with a history of smoking should be screened once by ultrasound for AAA (see Figure 2.1-14).
- Abdominal ultrasound is used for diagnosis or to follow an aneurysm over time.
- CT with contrast may be useful to determine the precise anatomy.

TREATMENT

- In asymptomatic patients, monitoring is appropriate for lesions < 5 cm.
- Surgical repair is indicated if the lesion is > 5.5 cm (abdominal), > 6 cm (thoracic), or smaller but rapidly enlarging.
- Emergent surgery for symptomatic or ruptured aneurysms.

AORTIC DISSECTION

Defined as a transverse tear in the intima of a vessel that results in blood entering the media, creating a false lumen and leading to a hematoma that propagates longitudinally. **Most commonly 2° to hypertension.** The most common sites of origin are above the aortic valve and distal to the left subclavian artery. Most often occurs at 40–60 years of age, with a greater frequency in males than in females.

HISTORY/PE

- Presents with sudden tearing/ripping pain in the anterior chest (ascending) or back (descending).
- Patients are typically hypertensive. If a patient is hypotensive, consider pericardial tamponade, hypovolemia from blood loss, or other cardiopulmonary etiologies.

Q

A 70-year-old male with hypertension presents for a routine appointment. He quit smoking 20 years ago but has a 20-pack-year history. What screening, if any, is indicated?

KEY FACT

Aortic aneurysm is most often associated with atherosclerosis, whereas aortic dissection is commonly linked to hypertension.

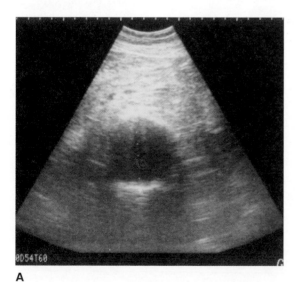
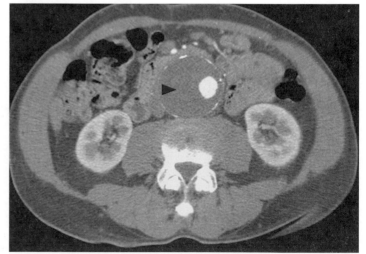

A   **B**

FIGURE 2.1-14. **Abdominal aortic aneurysm. (A)** Ultrasound image of an AAA (Ao = aorta). **(B)** Transaxial image from a contrast-enhanced CT showing an aneurysm with extensive mural thrombus (arrowhead). (Image A reproduced with permission from Tintinalli JE et al. *Tintinalli's Emergency Medicine: A Comprehensive Study Guide*, 6th ed. New York: McGraw-Hill, 2004, Fig. 58-2. Image B reproduced with permission from Doherty GM. *Current Diagnosis & Treatment: Surgery*, 13th ed. New York: McGraw-Hill, 2010, Fig. 34-16.)

The United States Preventive Services Task Force (USPSTF) guidelines recommend one-time screening for AAA by ultrasound in males ages 65–75 who have ever smoked.

KEY FACT

Ascending aortic dissections are surgical emergencies; descending dissections are still emergencies but can often be treated medically.

KEY FACT

Virchow's triad: (1) hemostasis, (2) trauma (endothelial damage), (3) hypercoagulability.

- Signs of pericarditis or pericardial tamponade may be seen.
- **Asymmetric pulses and BP measurements** are indicative of aortic dissection.
- A murmur of aortic regurgitation may be heard if the aortic valve is involved with a proximal dissection.
- **Neurologic deficits** may be seen if the **aortic arch or spinal arteries** are involved.

DIAGNOSIS

- CT angiography is the gold standard of imaging. MRA can be used if contrast CT is contraindicated.
- TEE can provide details of the thoracic aorta, the proximal coronary arteries, the origins of arch vessels, the presence of a pericardial effusion, and aortic valve integrity.
- The **Stanford system** classifies any dissection proximal to the left subclavian artery as type A and all others as type B (see Figure 2.1-15).

TREATMENT

- Monitor and medically manage BP and heart rate as necessary. Avoid thrombolytics. Begin β-blockade before starting vasodilators to prevent reflex tachycardia.
- If the dissection involves the ascending aorta, it is a surgical emergency; descending dissections can often be managed with BP and heart rate control.

DEEP VENOUS THROMBOSIS (DVT)

Clot formation in the large veins of the extremities or pelvis. The classic **Virchow's triad** of risk factors includes venous stasis (eg, from plane flights, bed rest, or incompetent venous valves in the lower extremities), endothelial

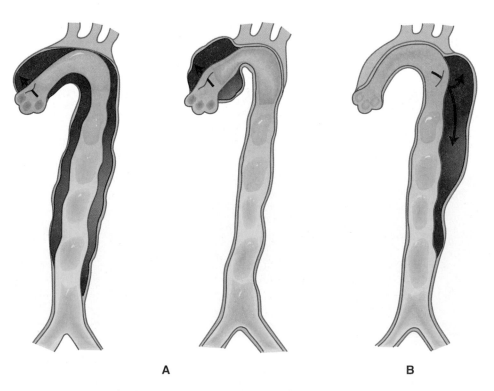

A   B

FIGURE 2.1-15. **Aortic dissection.** Stanford classification of aortic dissections. Shown are **(A)** proximal or ascending types and **(B)** descending type. (Reproduced with permission from Doherty GM. *Current Diagnosis & Treatment: Surgery*, 13th ed. New York: McGraw-Hill, 2010, Fig. 19-16.)

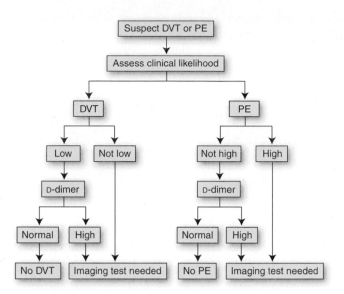

FIGURE 2.1-16. **Algorithm for diagnostic imaging of DVT and PE.** (Reproduced with permission from Fauci AS et al. *Harrison's Principles of Internal Medicine*, 17th ed. New York: McGraw-Hill, 2008, Fig. 256-1.)

trauma (eg, surgery, injury to the lower extremities), and hypercoagulable states (eg, malignancy, pregnancy, OCP use).

HISTORY/PE

- Presents with unilateral lower extremity pain and swelling.
- **Homans' sign** is calf tenderness with passive foot dorsiflexion (poor sensitivity and specificity for DVT).

DIAGNOSIS

Doppler ultrasound; a spiral CT or V/Q scan may be used to evaluate for PE (see Figure 2.1-16).

TREATMENT

- Anticoagulate with IV unfractionated heparin or SQ low-molecular-weight heparin (LMWH) followed by PO warfarin for a total of 3–6 months.
- In patients with contraindications for anticoagulation, IVC filters should be placed.
- Hospitalized patients should receive DVT prophylaxis consisting of exercise as tolerated, anti-thromboembolic stockings, and SQ unfractionated heparin or LMWH.

KEY FACT

A ⊖ D-dimer test can be used to rule out the possibility of PE in low-risk patients.

PERIPHERAL ARTERIAL DISEASE

Defined as a restriction of the blood supply to the extremities by atherosclerotic plaque. The lower extremities are most commonly affected. Clinical manifestations depend on the vessels involved, the extent and rate of obstruction, and the presence of collateral blood flow.

HISTORY/PE

- Presents with intermittent claudication (reproducible leg pain that occurs with walking and is relieved with rest). As the disease progresses, pain occurs at rest and affects the distal extremities. Dorsal foot ulcerations may develop 2° to poor perfusion. A painful, cold, numb foot is characteristic of critical limb ischemia.

MNEMONIC

The 6 P's of acute ischemia:

Pain
Pallor
Paralysis
Pulse deficit
Paresthesias
Poikilothermia

KEY FACT

$ABI = P_{leg} / P_{arm}$.
ABI < 0.4 with rest pain.

- **Aortoiliac disease:** Buttock claudication, ↓ femoral pulses, male impotence (Leriche's syndrome).
- **Femoropopliteal disease:** Calf claudication; ↓ pulses below the femoral artery.
- **Acute ischemia:**
  - Most often caused by embolization from the heart; acute occlusions commonly occur at bifurcations distal to the last palpable pulse (see mnemonic).
  - May also be 2° to cholesterol atheroembolism ("blue toe syndrome").
- **Chronic ischemia:** Lack of blood perfusion leads to muscle atrophy, pallor, cyanosis, hair loss, and gangrene/necrosis.

DIAGNOSIS

- Measurement of ankle and brachial systolic BP (ankle-brachial index, or ABI) can provide objective evidence of atherosclerosis (rest pain usually occurs with an ABI < 0.4). A very high ABI can indicate calcification of the arteries.
- Doppler ultrasound helps identify stenosis and occlusion. Normal ankle Doppler readings are > 90% of brachial readings.
- Arteriography and digital subtraction angiography are necessary for surgical evaluation.

TREATMENT

- Control underlying conditions (DM, tobacco) and institute careful hygiene and foot care. **Exercise helps develop collateral circulation.**
- ASA, cilostazol, and thromboxane inhibitors may improve symptoms; anticoagulants may prevent clot formation.
- Angioplasty and stenting have a variable success rate that is dependent on the area of occlusion.
- Surgery (arterial bypass) or amputation can be employed when conservative treatment fails.

LYMPHEDEMA

A disruption of the lymphatic circulation that results in peripheral edema and chronic infection of the extremities. It is often a complication of surgery involving lymph node dissection. In underdeveloped countries, parasitic infection can lead to lymphatic obstruction. Congenital malformations of the lymphatic system (eg, Milroy's disease) can present with lymphedema in childhood.

HISTORY/PE

- Postmastectomy patients present with unexplained swelling of the upper extremity.
- Immigrants present with progressive swelling of the lower extremities bilaterally with no cardiac abnormalities (ie, filariasis).
- Children present with progressive, bilateral swelling of the extremities.

DIAGNOSIS

Diagnosis is clinical. Rule out other causes of edema, such as cardiac and metabolic disorders.

TREATMENT

- Directed at symptom management, including exercise, massage therapy, and pressure garments to mobilize and limit fluid accumulation.

- Diuretics are ineffective and relatively contraindicated.
- Maintain vigilance for cellulitis with prompt gram-⊕ antibiotic coverage for infection.

Syncope

A sudden, temporary loss of consciousness and postural tone 2° to cerebral hypoperfusion. Etiologies are either cardiac or noncardiac:

- **Cardiac:** Valvular lesions, arrhythmias, PE, cardiac tamponade, aortic dissection.
- **Noncardiac:** Orthostatic/hypovolemic hypotension, neurologic (TIA, stroke), metabolic abnormalities, neurocardiogenic syndromes (eg, vasovagal/micturition syncope), psychiatric.

History/PE

- Triggers, prodromal symptoms, and associated symptoms should be investigated.
- Cardiac causes of syncope are typically associated with very brief or absent prodromal symptoms, a history of exertion, lack of association with changes in position, and/or a history of cardiac disease.

Diagnosis

Depending on the suspected etiology, Holter monitors or event recorders (arrhythmias), echocardiograms (structural abnormalities), stress tests (ischemia), and tilt-table testing (neurally mediated syncope) can be useful.

Treatment

Tailored to the etiology; commonly β-blockers for rate control.

KEY FACT

Cardiac syncope is associated with 1-year sudden cardiac death rates of up to 40%.

NOTES

DERMATOLOGY

Layers of the Skin

The skin consists of 3 layers: the epidermis, the dermis, and subcutaneous tissue (see Figure 2.2-1).

Common Terminology

Table 2.2-1 outlines terms frequently used to describe common manifestations of dermatologic disease.

Allergic and Immune-Mediated Disorders

HYPERSENSITIVITY REACTIONS

Table 2.2-2 outlines the types and mechanisms of hypersensitivity reactions.

ATOPIC DERMATITIS (ECZEMA)

A relapsing inflammatory skin disorder that is common in infancy and presents differently in different age groups. It is characterized by **pruritus leading to lichenification** (see Figure 2.2-2).

HISTORY/PE

- Patients are at ↑ risk of 2° bacterial (*S aureus*) and viral (HSV or molluscum) infection.
- Triggers include climate, food, contact with allergens or physical or chemical irritants, and emotional factors.

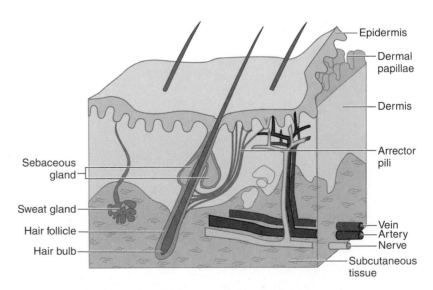

FIGURE 2.2-1.   Layers of the skin. (Adapted with permission from Hardman JG et al. *Goodman and Gilman's The Pharmacological Basis of Therapeutics,* 10th ed. New York: McGraw-Hill, 2001: 1805.)

TABLE 2.2-1.   Common Terms Used to Describe Skin Lesions

TERM	DEFINITION	APPEARANCE
Macule	A flat lesion that differs in color from surrounding skin (< 1 cm in diameter).	
Papule	An elevated solid lesion that is generally small (< 5 mm in diameter).	
Patch	A small, circumscribed area differing in color from the surrounding surface (> 1 cm in diameter).	See Macule above.
Plaque	An elevated solid lesion (> 5 mm in diameter).	See Papule above.
Cyst	An epithelial-lined sac containing fluid or semisolid material.	
Vesicle	A fluid-filled, very small (< 5 mm), elevated lesion.	
Bulla	A large vesicle (> 5 mm).	See Vesicle above.
Wheal (or hive)	An area of localized edema that follows vascular leakage and usually disappears within hours.	
Erosion	A circumscribed, superficial depression resulting from the loss of some or all of the epidermis.	

(continues)

TABLE 2.2-1. **Common Terms Used to Describe Skin Lesions** *(continued)*

TERM	DEFINITION	APPEARANCE
Ulcer	A deeper depression resulting from destruction of the epidermis and upper dermis.	
Scale	Abnormal shedding or accumulation of stratum corneum in flakes.	
Crust	A hardened deposit of dried serum, blood, or purulent exudates.	
Lichenification	Thickening and hardening of the skin with accentuation of normal skin markings.	
Scar	A healing defect of the dermis (the epidermis alone heals without a scar).	

(Images adapted with permission from LeBlond RF et al. *DeGowin's Diagnostic Examination,* 9th ed. New York: McGraw-Hill, 2009, Figs. 6-5 through 6-11.)

KEY FACT

Atopic dermatitis is commonly associated with asthma and allergic rhinitis.

KEY FACT

Erythema toxicum neonatorum typically begins 1–3 days after delivery and resembles eczema, presenting with red papules, pustules, and/or vesicles with surrounding erythematous halos. ↑ eosinophils are present in the pustules or vesicles. This benign rash usually resolves in 1–2 weeks with no treatment.

- Clinical manifestations by age group are as follows:
  - **Infants:** Erythematous, edematous, weeping, pruritic papules and plaques on the face, scalp, and extensor surfaces of the extremities. The diaper area is often spared.
  - **Children:** Dry, scaly, pruritic, excoriated papules and plaques in the flexural areas and neck.
  - **Adults:** Lichenification and dry, fissured skin in a flexural distribution. Often there is hand or eyelid involvement.

DIAGNOSIS

Diagnosis is clinical. Patients may have **mild eosinophilia and ↑ IgE.**

TREATMENT

- Prophylactic measures include use of nondrying soaps, application of moisturizers, and avoidance of known triggers.
- Topical corticosteroids are the first-line therapy. Topical immunomodulators (eg, tacrolimus, pimecrolimus) are useful for moderate to severe eczema if the patient is > 2 years of age.
- **Topical corticosteroids should not be used for longer than 2–3 weeks** to avoid decreasing the integrity of the skin.

TABLE 2.2-2. Types and Mechanisms of Hypersensitivity Reactions

DESCRIPTION	MECHANISM	COMMENTS	EXAMPLES
TYPE I			
Anaphylactic and atopic	Antigen cross-links **IgE** on presensitized mast cells and basophils, triggering the release of vasoactive amines like histamine. Reaction develops rapidly as a result of preformed antibody.	First and Fast (like anaphylaxis). Types I, II, and III are all antibody mediated.	Anaphylaxis, asthma, urticarial drug reactions, local wheal and flare.
TYPE II			
Cytotoxic	**IgM** and **IgG** bind to antigen on an "enemy" cell, leading to lysis by complement or phagocytosis.	Cy-2-toxic. Antibody and complement lead to membrane attack complex (MAC).	Autoimmune hemolytic anemia, erythroblastosis fetalis, Goodpasture's syndrome, rheumatic fever.
TYPE III			
Immune complex	Antigen-antibody complexes activate complement, which attracts PMNs; PMNs release lysosomal enzymes.	Imagine an immune complex as 3 things stuck together: antigen-antibody-complement. Includes many glomerulonephritides and vasculitides.	Polyarteritis nodosa, immune complex glomerulonephritis, SLE, rheumatoid arthritis.
Serum sickness	Antibodies to the foreign proteins are produced in ~ 5 days. Immune complexes form and are deposited in membranes, where they lead to tissue damage by fixing complement.	Most serum sickness is now caused by drugs (not serum). Fever, urticaria, arthralgias, proteinuria, and lymphadenopathy occur 5–10 days after antigen exposure. More common than Arthus reaction.	Drug reaction.
Arthus reaction	A local reaction to antigen by **preformed antibodies** characterized by vascular necrosis and thrombosis.	Arthus reaction occurs rarely 4–12 hours after vaccination.	Hypersensitivity pneumonitis.
TYPE IV			
Delayed (cell-mediated) type	**Sensitized T lymphocytes** encounter antigen and then release lymphokines (leading to macrophage activation).	**4th** and last—**delayed. Cell mediated,** not antibody mediated; therefore, it is not transferable by serum.	TB skin tests, transplant rejection, contact dermatitis.

CONTACT DERMATITIS

A **type IV hypersensitivity reaction** that results from contact with an allergen to which the patient has **previously been exposed and sensitized.** More common in adults than in children.

An infant with a history of eczema treated with corticosteroids is brought in for a new-onset rash and fever. Physical examination reveals grouped vesicles involving eczematous areas of the infant's extremities and face. What is the appropriate therapy?

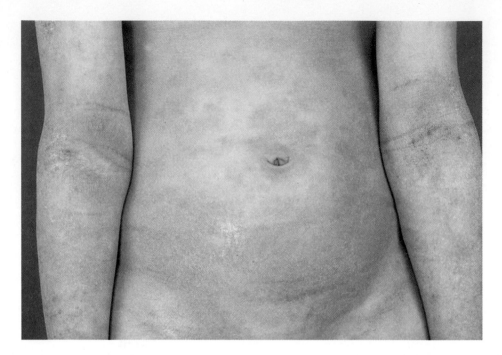

FIGURE 2.2-2. Atopic dermatitis. Lichenification, excoriations, and ill-defined, scaling erythema are characteristic. (Reproduced with permission from Tintinalli JE et al. *Tintinalli's Emergency Medicine: A Comprehensive Study Guide,* 7th ed. New York: McGraw-Hill, 2011, Fig. 249-10.)

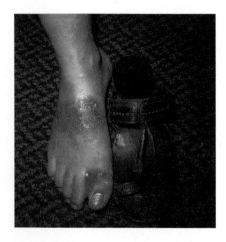

FIGURE 2.2-3. Contact dermatitis. Shown are erythematous papules and vesicles with serous weeping localized to areas of contact with the offending agent. (Reproduced with permission from Hurwitz RM. *Pathology of the Skin: Atlas of Clinical-Pathological Correlation,* 2nd ed. Stamford, CT: Appleton & Lange, 1998: 3.)

A

This infant has eczema herpeticum, a medical emergency that is due to the propensity for HSV infection to spread systemically, potentially affecting the brain. IV acyclovir must be started immediately!

HISTORY/PE

- Commonly presents with pruritus and rash, but can also present with edema, fever, and lymphadenopathy.
- Frequently implicated allergens include poison ivy, poison oak, nickel, soaps, detergents, cosmetics, and rubber products containing latex (eg, gloves and elastic bands in clothing).
- The overall shape of the rash often mimics that of the exposing object (see Figure 2.2-3), and characteristic distributions of involvement are often seen where makeup, clothing, perfume, nickel jewelry, and plants come into contact with the skin. The rash can spread over the body via transfer of allergen by the hands or via circulating T lymphocytes.
- Patients are at ↑ risk of 2° infection.

DIAGNOSIS

Diagnosed by clinical impression. **Patch testing** can be used to establish the causative allergen after the acute-phase rash has been treated.

TREATMENT

- Prophylaxis consists of avoidance of the offending allergen.
- Treat with topical or systemic corticosteroids as needed and with cool, wet compresses to soothe crusted lesions of the skin.

SEBORRHEIC DERMATITIS

A common disease that may be caused by *Pityrosporum ovale,* a generally harmless yeast found in sebum and hair follicles. It has a predilection for **areas with oily skin.**

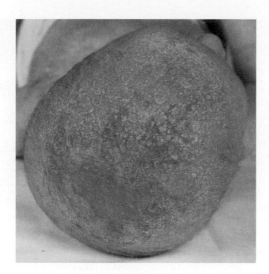

FIGURE 2.2-4. **Seborrheic dermatitis (cradle cap) in an infant.** Note the yellow, scaly crust present on the infant's scalp with an area of erosion. (Reproduced with permission from Tintinalli JE et al. *Tintinalli's Emergency Medicine: A Comprehensive Study Guide,* 7th ed. New York: McGraw-Hill, 2011, Fig. 134-25.)

HISTORY/PE

- The appearance of the rash varies with age:
  - **Infants:** Presents as a severe, red diaper rash with yellow scale, erosions, and blisters. A thick crust (**"cradle cap"**) may be seen on the scalp (see Figure 2.2-4).
  - **Children/adults:** Red, scaly patches are seen around the ears, eyebrows, nasolabial fold, midchest, and scalp. The rash is more localized and less dramatic than that seen in infants.
- Patients with **HIV/AIDS and Parkinson's disease can develop severe seborrheic dermatitis.**

DIAGNOSIS

Diagnosed by clinical impression. Rule out contact dermatitis and psoriasis.

TREATMENT

Treatment consists of **selenium sulfide or zinc pyrithione shampoos** for the scalp, and topical antifungals and/or topical corticosteroids for other areas in adults. Cradle cap often resolves with routine bathing and application of emollients in infants.

PSORIASIS

A T-cell-mediated inflammatory dermatosis characterized by **erythematous plaques with silvery scales** (see Figure 2.2-5A) due to dermal inflammation and epidermal hyperplasia. The condition usually starts in puberty or young adulthood.

HISTORY/PE

- Lesions are classically found on the **extensor surfaces,** including the elbows, knees, scalp, and lumbosacral regions.
- Lesions may initially appear very small but may become confluent. The patient's nails are frequently affected as well; psoriatic nails feature pitting, "oil spots," and onycholysis, or lifting of the nail plate (see Figure 2.2-5B).

Q

A 23-year-old female is seen for an itchy, linear rash on her right leg. She returned from a camping trip 4 days ago and denies using any new makeup, clothing, or jewelry. What features of this presentation favor a contact dermatitis?

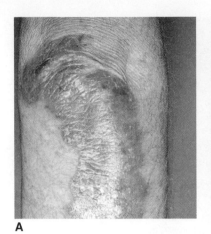
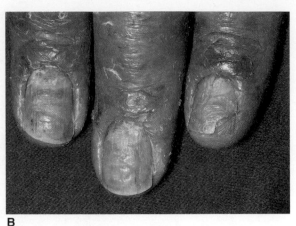

A　　　　　　　**B**

FIGURE 2.2-5. **Psoriasis.** (A) **Skin changes.** The classic sharply demarcated plaques with silvery scales are commonly located on the extensor surfaces (eg, elbows, knees). (B) **Nail changes.** Note the pitting, onycholysis, and "oil spots." (Reproduced with permission from Hurwitz RM. *Pathology of the Skin: Atlas of Clinical-Pathological Correlation,* 2nd ed. Stamford, CT: Appleton & Lange, 1998: 15, 18.)

KEY FACT

A rash commonly involving the extensor surfaces? Think psoriasis. A rash commonly involving the flexor surfaces? Think atopic dermatitis.

KEY FACT

Five percent of patients with psoriasis also have a seronegative arthritis.

■ Psoriatic lesions can be provoked by local irritation or by trauma (**Koebner's phenomenon**). Some medications, such as β-blockers, lithium, and ACEIs, can also induce psoriasis.

DIAGNOSIS

■ Classically presents with the **Auspitz sign (bleeding when scale is scraped).**
■ Biopsy can be useful. Histology classically shows a thickened epidermis, elongated rete ridges, an absent granular cell layer, preservation of nuclei in the stratum corneum (parakeratosis), and a sterile neutrophilic infiltrate in the stratum corneum (**Munro's microabscess**).

TREATMENT

Treat with topical steroids combined with keratolytic agents, tar, or anthralin along with UV therapy. Methotrexate may be used for severe cases. Retinoids (vitamin A derivatives) and vitamin D₃ analogs may also be used.

URTICARIA (HIVES)

Urticaria is characterized by superficial, intense erythema and edema in a localized area. It is usually acute but can also be chronic (lasting > 6 weeks). The condition results from the release of **histamine and prostaglandins from mast cells in a type I hypersensitivity response.**

HISTORY/PE

■ The typical lesion is an elevated papule or plaque that is reddish or white and variable in size. Lesions are widespread and last a few hours.
■ In severe allergic reactions, **extracutaneous manifestations** can include tongue swelling, angioedema (deeper, more diffuse swelling), asthma, GI symptoms, joint swelling, and fever.
■ Acute urticaria is a response to a trigger that may be a food, drug, virus, insect bite, or physical stimulus. Chronic urticaria is usually idiopathic.

DIAGNOSIS

Diagnosed by clinical impression and patient report. It can often be difficult to determine the cause.

A

The asymmetric involvement of the rash, its linear arrangement (possibly from contact with a plant during the camping trip), and the time from exposure to rash presentation all point to contact dermatitis.

TREATMENT

Treat urticaria with **systemic antihistamines;** anaphylaxis requires epinephrine IM, antihistamines, IV fluids, and airway maintenance.

DRUG ERUPTION

Maintain a high suspicion for a cutaneous drug reaction in patients who are hospitalized and develop rashes. Such reactions can take many forms. Drugs can cause **all 4 types of hypersensitivity reactions,** and sometimes the same drug may cause different types of reactions in different patients.

HISTORY/PE

- Eruptions usually occur 7–14 days after exposure, so **if a patient reacts within 1–2 days of starting a new drug, that drug is probably not the causative agent.**
- Eruptions are generally **widespread, relatively symmetrical,** and **pruritic.** Most are relatively short-lived, disappearing within 1–2 weeks following removal of the offending agent.
- Extreme complications of drug eruptions include erythroderma, Stevens-Johnson syndrome (SJS), and toxic epidermal necrolysis (TEN).

DIAGNOSIS

Diagnosed by clinical impression.

TREATMENT

Discontinue the offending agent; treat symptoms with antihistamines and topical steroids to relieve pruritus.

ERYTHEMA MULTIFORME (EM)

A cutaneous reaction pattern with classic **targetoid lesions** (see Figure 2.2-6) that has many triggers and is often recurrent.

HISTORY/PE

- The disease can occur on mucous membranes, where erosions are seen. Typically, lesions start as erythematous macules that become centrally clear and then develop a blister. The **palms and soles are often affected.**
- May be associated with systemic symptoms, including fever, myalgias, headache, and arthralgias.
- In its minor form, the disease is uncomplicated and localized to the skin. However, **EM major can lead to TEN or SJS.**

DIAGNOSIS

Diagnosed by clinical impression.

TREATMENT

- Symptomatic treatment is all that is necessary; systemic corticosteroids are of no benefit.
- Minor cases can be treated with antipruritics; major cases should be treated as burns.

KEY FACT

Patients with drug eruptions often have eosinophilia and eosinophils on histopathology.

KEY FACT

EM is often triggered by recurrent HSV infection of the lip. Other common triggers are drugs and mycoplasmal infections.

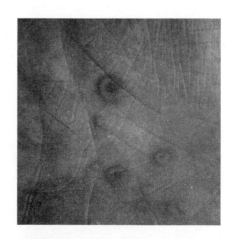

FIGURE 2.2-6. Erythema multiforme. Evolving erythematous plaques and papules are seen with a target appearance consisting of a dull red center, a pale zone, and a darker outer ring. (Reproduced with permission from Hurwitz RM. *Pathology of the Skin: Atlas of Clinical-Pathological Correlation,* 2nd ed. Stamford, CT: Appleton & Lange, 1998: 24.)

STEVENS-JOHNSON SYNDROME (SJS)/TOXIC EPIDERMAL NECROLYSIS (TEN)

SJS and TEN constitute 2 different points on the spectrum of **life-threatening exfoliative mucocutaneous diseases** that are often caused by a drug-induced immunologic reaction. **The epidermal separation of SJS involves < 10% of body surface area (BSA), whereas TEN involves > 30% of BSA.**

HISTORY/PE

- May be preceded by EM, a flulike prodrome, skin tenderness, a maculopapular drug rash, or painful mouth lesions.
- Often associated with a history of exposure to new drugs, such as sulfonamides, penicillin, seizure medications (eg, phenytoin, carbamazepine), quinolones, cephalosporins, allopurinol, corticosteroids, or NSAIDs.
- Examination reveals severe mucosal erosions with widespread erythematous, dusky red or purpuric macules or atypical targetoid lesions (see Figure 2.2-7). The epidermal lesions often become confluent and show a ⊕ **Nikolsky's sign (separation of the superficial skin layers with slight rubbing)** and epidermal detachment.
- The mucous membranes of the eyes, mouth, and genitals often become eroded and hemorrhagic as well.

DIAGNOSIS

- **SJS:** Biopsy shows **degeneration of the basal layer of the epidermis.**
- **TEN:** Biopsy shows **full-thickness eosinophilic epidermal necrosis.**
- The differential also includes staphylococcal scalded-skin syndrome (SSSS), graft-versus-host reaction (usually after bone marrow transplant), radiation therapy, and burns.

TREATMENT

- Patients have the **same complications as burn victims,** including thermoregulatory difficulties, electrolyte disturbances, and 2° infections.

KEY FACT

Always include SJS and TEN in your differential diagnosis if a ⊕ Nikolsky's sign is present.

KEY FACT

Don't confuse SJS and TEN with SSSS. SSSS is usually seen in children < 6 years of age and has an infectious etiology. SJS/TEN is generally seen in adults and is usually caused by a drug reaction.

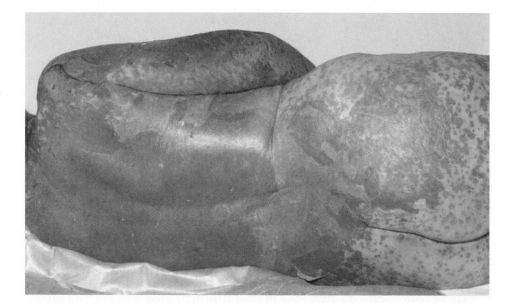

FIGURE 2.2-7. **Toxic epidermal necrolysis.** Note the diffuse erythematous bullae and areas of sloughing 2° to the full-thickness necrosis of the epidermis. (Reproduced with permission from Tintinalli JE et al. *Tintinalli's Emergency Medicine: A Comprehensive Study Guide,* 7th ed. New York: McGraw-Hill, 2011, Fig. 245-5.)

- Treatment includes skin coverage and maintenance of fluid and electrolyte balance. Pharmacologic therapy includes systemic corticosteroids in the early stages of SJS/ TEN and IVIG. There is a high risk of mortality.

ERYTHEMA NODOSUM

A **panniculitis** (or an inflammatory process of the subcutaneous adipose tissue) whose triggers include infection (eg, *Streptococcus*, *Coccidioides*, *Yersinia*, TB), drug reactions (eg, sulfonamides, various antibiotics, OCPs), and chronic inflammatory diseases (eg, sarcoidosis, Crohn's disease, ulcerative colitis, Behçet's disease).

HISTORY/PE

- **Painful, erythematous nodules** appear on the patient's **lower legs** (see Figure 2.2-8) and slowly spread, turning brown or gray. Patients may present with fever and joint pain.
- Patients with erythema nodosum may have a false-⊕ VDRL (as in SLE).

DIAGNOSIS

- Diagnosed by clinical impression.
- Workup can include an ASO titer, a PPD test in high-risk patients, a CXR to rule out sarcoidosis, or a small bowel series to rule out IBD based on the patient's complaints.

TREATMENT

Remove the triggering factor and treat the underlying disease where possible. NSAIDs can be used.

BULLOUS PEMPHIGOID/PEMPHIGUS VULGARIS

Table 2.2-3 contrasts the clinical features of bullous pemphigoid with those of pemphigus vulgaris.

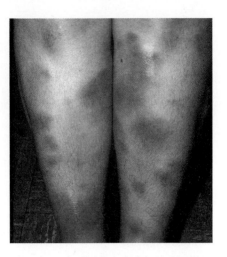

FIGURE 2.2-8. Erythema nodosum. Erythematous plaques and nodules are commonly located on pretibial areas. Lesions are painful and indurated but heal spontaneously without ulceration. (Reproduced with permission from Hurwitz RM. *Pathology of the Skin: Atlas of Clinical-Pathological Correlation*, 2nd ed. Stamford, CT: Appleton & Lange, 1998: 132.)

Infectious Disease Manifestations

VIRAL DISEASES

Herpes Simplex

A painful, recurrent vesicular eruption of the mucocutaneous surfaces due to infection with HSV. **HSV-1 usually produces oral-labial lesions, whereas HSV-2 usually causes genital lesions.** The virus spreads through epidermal cells, causing them to fuse into **giant cells.** The local host inflammatory response leads to erythema and swelling.

HISTORY/PE

- The initial infection is passed by direct contact, after which the herpesvirus remains dormant in local nerve ganglia. **1° episodes are generally longer and more severe** than recurrences.
- Onset is preceded by prodromal tingling, burning, or pain but can also present with lymphadenopathy, fever, discomfort, malaise, and edema of involved tissue.

 KEY FACT

Dermatitis herpetiformis (DH) looks like herpes but is not caused by HSV. DH consists of pruritic papules and vesicles on the elbows, knees, buttocks, neck, and scalp, and **it is associated with celiac disease** (15–25%). Treat with dapsone and a gluten-free diet.

 Q

A 28-year-old African American female is seen by her physician for a new-onset, painful rash. She noticed the erythematous nodules on both lower legs 3 days ago. She has a history of uveitis. What is the next best step to identify the underlying cause of this rash?

TABLE 2.2-3. Acquired, Autoimmune Blistering Dermatoses

VARIABLE	BULLOUS PEMPHIGOID	PEMPHIGUS VULGARIS
Anatomic location of blisters	Basement membrane zone.	Intraepidermal.
Autoantibodies	Anti–bullous pemphigoid antigen.	Anti-desmoglein; desmoglein is responsible for keratinocyte adhesion.
Blister appearance	Firm, stable blisters; may be preceded by urticaria (see Figure 2.2-9).	Erosions are more common than intact blisters owing to the lack of keratinocyte adherence (see Figure 2.2-10).
Nikolsky's sign	⊖	⊕
Mucosal involvement	Rare.	Common.
Patient age	Usually > 60 years of age.	Usually 40–60 years of age.
Associated medication triggers	Generally idiopathic.	ACEIs, penicillamine, phenobarbital, penicillin.
Mortality	Rare and milder course.	Possible.
Diagnosis	Clinical features, skin biopsy with immunofluorescence, and/or ELISA.	Same as that for bullous pemphigoid.
Treatment	Steroids (prednisone).	High-dose steroids (prednisone) + immunomodulatory therapy (IVIG, MMF, rituximab).

KEY FACT

No multinucleated giant cells on Tzanck smear? Tzanck goodness it's not herpes!

A CXR to look for bilateral hilar adenopathy, which is suggestive of sarcoidosis. Erythema nodosum is the most common nonspecific cutaneous manifestation of sarcoidosis, after cutaneous sarcoidosis.

- Recurrences are limited to mucocutaneous areas innervated by the involved nerve.
  - **Recurrent oral herpes (HSV-1):** Typically consists of the common "cold sore," which presents as a cluster of crusted vesicles on an erythematous base (see Figure 2.2-11A). It is often triggered by sun and fever.
  - **Recurrent genital herpes (HSV-2):** Unilateral and characterized by a cluster of blisters on an erythematous base, but with less pain and systemic involvement than the 1° infection.

DIAGNOSIS

Diagnosed primarily by the clinical picture. **Multinucleated giant cells on Tzanck smear** (see Figure 2.2-11B) yield a presumptive diagnosis.

TREATMENT

- Oral or IV acyclovir (IV for severe cases or for immunocompromised patients) ↓ both the frequency and the severity of recurrences. Daily acyclovir, valacyclovir, or famciclovir suppressive therapy may be used in patients with > 6 outbreaks per year or for those with EM.
- Acyclovir ointment is somewhat effective in reducing the duration of viral shedding but does not prevent recurrence.

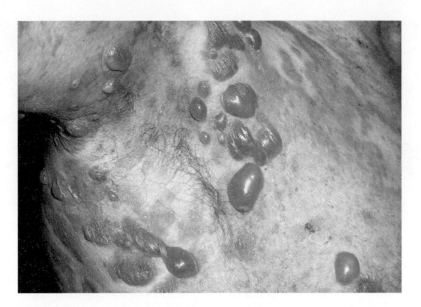

FIGURE 2.2-9.   Bullous pemphigoid. Multiple tense vesicles and bullae can be seen. (Reproduced with permission from Wolff K, Johnson RA. *Fitzpatrick's Color Atlas & Synopsis of Clinical Dermatology,* 6th ed. New York: McGraw-Hill, 2009, Fig. 6-13.)

- In AIDS patients, HSV can persist, with ulcers remaining resistant to antiviral therapy. Symptomatic HSV infection lasting > 1 month can be considered an AIDS-defining illness.

Varicella-Zoster Virus (VZV)

VZV causes 2 different diseases, varicella and herpes zoster—with transmission occurring via respiratory droplet or by direct contact. VZV has an incubation period of 10–20 days, with contagion beginning 24 hours before the eruption appears and lasting until lesions have crusted.

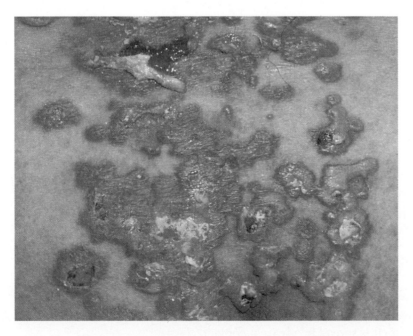

FIGURE 2.2-10.   Pemphigus vulgaris. Note the confluent, flaccid blisters and erosions, which are extremely painful. Mucous involvement is common. (Reproduced with permission from Wolff K, Johnson RA. *Fitzpatrick's Color Atlas & Synopsis of Clinical Dermatology,* 6th ed. New York: McGraw-Hill, 2009, Fig. 6-10.)

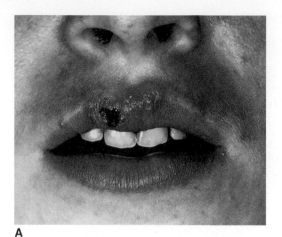
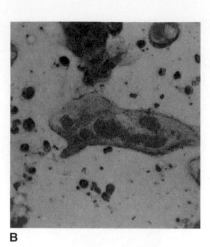

A

B

FIGURE 2.2-11. **Herpes simplex.** (A) 1° infection. Grouped vesicles on an erythematous base on the patient's lips and oral mucosa may progress to pustules before resolving. (B) **Tzanck smear.** The multinucleated giant cells from vesicular fluid provide a presumptive diagnosis of HSV infection. The Tzanck smear cannot distinguish between HSV and VZV infection. (Reproduced with permission from Hurwitz RM. *Pathology of the Skin: Atlas of Clinical-Pathological Correlation,* 2nd ed. Stamford, CT: Appleton & Lange, 1998: 145.)

> **KEY FACT**
>
> Immunocompromised patients, cancer patients (especially those undergoing chemotherapy), the elderly, and severely stressed individuals are more susceptible to zoster infection.

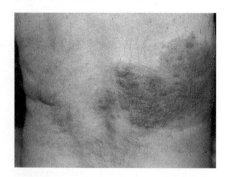

FIGURE 2.2-12. **Varicella zoster.** The unilateral dermatomal distribution of the grouped vesicles on an erythematous base is characteristic. (Reproduced with permission from Wolff K et al. *Fitzpatrick's Color Atlas & Synopsis of Clinical Dermatology,* 5th ed. New York, McGraw-Hill, 2005: 823.)

> **KEY FACT**
>
> If you see giant molluscum contagiosum, think HIV or ↓ cellular immunity.

History/PE

- Varicella:
    - A prodrome consisting of malaise, fever, headache, and myalgia occurs 24 hours before the onset of the rash.
    - Pruritic lesions appear in crops over a period of 2–3 days, evolving from red macules to vesicles that then crust over.
    - At any given time, patients have **all stages of lesions over their entire body.** The trunk, face, scalp, and mucous membranes are involved, but the **palms and soles are spared.**
    - In adults, chickenpox is often more severe, with **systemic complications** such as **pneumonia** and **encephalitis.**
- Zoster:
    - Herpes zoster, also called shingles, represents the recurrence of VZV in a specific nerve, with lesions cropping up along the nerve's **dermatomal** distribution. Outbreaks are usually preceded by intense local pain and then arise as grouped blisters on an erythematous base (see Figure 2.2-12).
    - Older patients with severe zoster may develop **postherpetic neuralgia.**

Diagnosis

Diagnosed by the clinical picture.

Treatment

- Varicella is self-limited in healthy children. A vaccine is available.
- Adults should be treated with systemic acyclovir. Although acyclovir may speed the cutaneous course of zoster, **pain control** is most important for patients with this disease.

Molluscum Contagiosum

A **poxvirus infection** that is most common in young children and in **AIDS patients.** It is spread by physical contact.

HISTORY/PE

- The rash is composed of **tiny waxy papules,** frequently with **central umbilication.** In children, lesions are found on the trunk, extremities, or face (see Figure 2.2-13). In adults, they are commonly found on the genitalia and in the perineal region.
- **Lesions are asymptomatic** unless they become inflamed or irritated.

DIAGNOSIS

Diagnosed by the clinical picture, and confirmed by expressing and staining the contents of the papules for **large inclusion or molluscum bodies.**

TREATMENT

Any local destructive method is effective, including curetting, freezing, or applying trichloroacetic acid to the lesions. Lesions resolve spontaneously over months to years and are often left untreated in children.

Verrucae (Warts)

Warts are caused by many different types of HPV and can occur on skin, mucous membranes, and other epithelia. Although usually benign, **some subtypes of HPV (especially 16 and 18)** lead to **squamous malignancies.** Spread is by direct contact.

HISTORY/PE

- Common warts are the most prevalent HPV infection. Although most often seen on the hands, they can occur anywhere.
- The classic genital wart is a **cauliflower-like papule or nodule** appearing on the glans penis, the vulva, or the perianal region. Warts on mucous membranes are generally velvety and white. Mothers with genital HPV can transmit laryngeal warts to the infant by aspiration during delivery.

DIAGNOSIS

- Diagnosed by the clinical picture. Acetowhitening can be helpful in visualizing mucosal lesions.
- There is a long latency period, with children sometimes acquiring HPV at birth and not manifesting any lesions until years later.

TREATMENT

Genital warts are treated locally with cryotherapy, podophyllin, trichloroacetic acid, imiquimod, or 5-FU. HPV lesions on the cervix must be monitored cytologically and histologically for evidence of malignancy.

BACTERIAL INFECTIONS

Impetigo

A superficial, weeping local infection that primarily occurs in children and is caused by both **group A streptococcal and staphylococcal** organisms. It is transmitted by direct contact. **Streptococcal impetigo can be complicated by acute streptococcal glomerulonephritis.**

HISTORY/PE

- **Common type:** Characterized by pustules and **honey-colored crusts** on an erythematous base; generally appears on the face (see Figure 2.2-14).

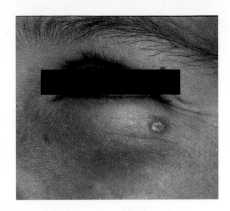

FIGURE 2.2-13. **Molluscum contagiosum.** The dome-shaped, fleshy, umbilicated papule on the child's eyelid is characteristic. (Reproduced with permission from Hurwitz RM. *Pathology of the Skin: Atlas of Clinical-Pathological Correlation,* 2nd ed. Stamford, CT: Appleton & Lange, 1998: 149.)

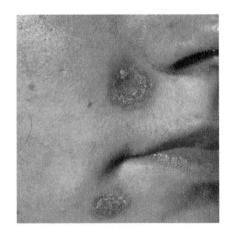

FIGURE 2.2-14. **Impetigo.** Dried pustules with a superficial golden-brown crust are most commonly found around the nose and mouth. (Reproduced with permission from Bondi EE. *Dermatology: Diagnosis and Therapy,* 1st ed. Stamford, CT: Appleton & Lange, 1991: 390.)

Q

A 7-year-old female presents with fever, sore throat, and a facial rash. Physical examination reveals an erythematous pharynx without exudates and a red, painful patch on the child's cheek that the mother notes has been expanding. What is the appropriate therapy?

- **Bullous type:** Characterized by large stable blisters that frequently involve the acral surfaces. **Bullous impetigo is almost always caused by *S aureus*** and can evolve into SSSS.

DIAGNOSIS

Diagnosed by the clinical picture.

TREATMENT

Treat with antibiotics with antistaphylococcal activity. Topical antibiotics are often sufficient, but systemic agents can hasten recovery and prevent spread to other patients.

Cellulitis

A deep, local infection involving the connective tissue, subcutaneous tissue, or muscle in addition to the skin. It is commonly caused by **staphylococci** or **group A streptococci** originating from an area of damaged skin or from a systemic source of infection. **Community-acquired MRSA** is an increasingly common cause. Risk factors include diabetes, IV drug use, venous stasis, and immune compromise.

HISTORY/PE

Presents with **red, hot, swollen, tender skin.** Fever and chills are also common.

DIAGNOSIS

- Diagnosed by the clinical picture; wound culture may aid in diagnosis and help determine antibiotic sensitivities for treatment.
- Blood cultures should be obtained when bacteremia is suspected. Culture and sensitivities are important in ruling out MRSA. Rule out abscess, osteomyelitis, and necrotizing fasciitis.

TREATMENT

Treat with 7–10 days of oral antibiotics for mild cases or with IV antibiotics if there is evidence of systemic toxicity, comorbid conditions, diabetes mellitus (DM), extremes of age, hand or orbital involvement, or other concerns.

Necrotizing Fasciitis

Deep infection along a fascial plane causing severe pain followed by anesthesia. Infection is caused by ***S pyogenes* (10% of cases) or, commonly, by a mixed infection of anaerobic and aerobic bacteria that includes *S aureus*, *E coli*, and *Clostridium perfringens*.** A history of trauma or a recent surgery to the affected area is often but not always elicited.

HISTORY/PE

- Presents with sudden onset of pain and swelling at the site of trauma or recent surgery. Pain often progresses to anesthesia.
- An area of **erythema quickly spreads over the course of hours to days.** Margins move out into normal skin, and skin becomes dusky or purplish near the site of insult, ultimately leading to necrosis.
- Necrosis can initially have the appearance of undermining of the skin and subcutaneous layer; if the skin is open, gloved fingers can easily pass

between the 2 layers to reveal yellow-green necrotic fascia (infection spreads quickly in deep fascia).

- The most important signs are **tissue necrosis, a putrid discharge, bullae, severe pain, gas production,** rapid burrowing through fascial planes, lack of classical tissue inflammatory signs, and intravascular volume loss.

DIAGNOSIS

Local radiographs or CT scans show air in tissue. Biopsy from the edge of the lesion can be diagnostic.

TREATMENT

- A **surgical emergency.** Early and aggressive surgical debridement is critical.
- If *Streptococcus* is the principal organism involved, penicillin G is the drug of choice. Clindamycin is second line. For anaerobic coverage, give metronidazole or a third-generation cephalosporin. In most cases, broad-spectrum coverage is necessary.

Folliculitis

Inflammation of the hair follicle. Although typically caused by infection with *Staphylococcus, Streptococcus,* and gram-$\ominus$ bacteria, folliculitis may occasionally be caused by yeast such as *Candida albicans,* or it may arise from ingrown hairs.

HISTORY/PE

- Presents as a tiny pustule that appears at the opening of a hair follicle and usually has a hair penetrating it. When the infection is deeper, a **furuncle,** or hair follicle abscess, develops. Furuncles may disseminate to adjacent follicles to form a **carbuncle.**
- Patients with diabetes or immunosuppression are at ↑ risk. Folliculitis can also be a critical problem in AIDS patients, in whom the disease is intensely pruritic and resistant to therapy.

DIAGNOSIS

Diagnosed by the clinical picture.

TREATMENT

Topical antibiotics can be used to treat mild disease, but severe cases require systemic antibiotics. Large lesions must be incised, drained, and cultured to rule out MRSA.

Acne Vulgaris

An endogenous skin disease that is common among adolescents. The pathogenesis involves **hormonal activation of sebaceous glands,** the development of the comedo or **plugged sebaceous follicle,** and involvement of *Propionibacterium acnes* in the follicle, causing inflammation. Acne lesions may be caused by medications (eg, lithium, corticosteroids) or by topical occlusion (eg, cosmetics).

HISTORY/PE

- There are 3 stages of acne lesions:
  - **Comedo:** May be open ("**blackheads**") or closed ("**whiteheads**"); present in large quantities but with little inflammation.
  - **Inflammatory:** The comedo ruptures, creating a pustule that can be large and nodular.

Q   **1**

A 42-year-old male is admitted for cellulitis after injuring his leg while swimming. He is febrile and has a well-demarcated area of erythema on the anterior aspect of his right knee. Antibiotics are started. Six hours later, the patient is in excruciating pain. The erythema has spread circumferentially around the knee, and the anterior aspect of the knee now has a purplish hue. What is the next best step?

Q   **2**

A 17-year-old female has been followed by a dermatologist for severe cystic acne that has been refractory to both topical and systemic antibiotics. She inquires about isotretinoin (Accutane). Given this drug's potentially hazardous side effects, what laboratory tests would have to be performed monthly if this patient were to be placed on isotretinoin?

1 **A**

Emergent surgical consult for debridement given the clinical suspicion for necrotizing fasciitis, a surgical emergency.

2 **A**

Serum β-hCG (to rule out pregnancy), LFTs, cholesterol, and triglycerides.

- **Scar:** As the inflammation heals, scars may develop. Picking at papules exacerbates scarring.
- Acne first develops at puberty and typically persists for several years. Males are more likely to have severe cystic acne than are females. Women in their 20s tend to have a variant that **flares cyclically with menstruation,** featuring fewer comedones and more painful lesions on the chin. Androgenic stimulation may contribute to these lesions.

DIAGNOSIS

Diagnosed by the clinical picture.

TREATMENT

- **Comedonal acne:** Topical tretinoin (Retin-A) and benzoyl peroxide.
- **Pustulocystic, or inflammatory, acne:** Benzoyl peroxide plus topical antibiotics (eg, erythromycin, clindamycin). Systemic antibiotics (eg, tetracycline, erythromycin) are used for acne refractory to topical antibiotics.
- **Severe cystic acne:** Isotretinoin (Accutane) leads to marked improvement in > 90% of acne patients.
  - Isotretinoin is, however, a **teratogen** and may **cause transient elevations in cholesterol, triglycerides, and LFTs,** and it may also be associated with **depression.**
  - Patients on isotretinoin thus require monthly blood tests to check quantitative serum β-hCG (to rule out pregnancy), LFTs, cholesterol, and triglycerides. Monthly refills are contingent on the completion of blood testing and evaluation by a dermatologist.

Pilonidal Cysts

Abscesses in the sacrococcygeal region that usually occur near the top of the natal cleft. Their name may not be appropriate, as not all contain hair or are true cysts. Repetitive trauma to the region plays a role. The condition is thought to start as a folliculitis that becomes an abscess complicated by perineal microbes, especially *Bacteroides.* It most commonly occurs between the ages of 20 and 40, affecting males more often than females.

HISTORY/PE

- Patients present with an abscess at the natal cleft that can be tender, fluctuant, warm, and indurated and is sometimes associated with purulent drainage or cellulitis. Systemic symptoms are uncommon, but cysts may develop into perianal fistulas.
- Risk factors include deep and hairy natal clefts, obesity, and a sedentary lifestyle.

DIAGNOSIS

Diagnosed by the clinical picture. Rule out perirectal and anal abscess.

TREATMENT

- Treatment consists of **incision and drainage** of the abscess under local anesthesia followed by sterile packing of the wound.
- Good local hygiene and shaving of the sacrococcygeal skin can help prevent recurrence. Patients should follow up with a surgeon.

FUNGAL INFECTIONS

Tinea Versicolor

Caused by *Malassezia furfur,* a yeast that is part of the normal skin flora. It is unclear what leads the organism to become a pathogen, but humid and sweaty conditions as well as host factors such as oily skin can contribute. Cushing's syndrome and immunosuppression are also risk factors.

HISTORY/PE

- Patients present with small, scaly patches of varying color, usually on the chest or back (see Figure 2.2-15A).
- Lesions may be **hypopigmented** as a result of interference with melanin production, or they may be **hyperpigmented** by virtue of thickened scale.

DIAGNOSIS

Diagnosed by clinical impression, and confirmed by KOH preparation of scale that reveals a "**spaghetti and meatballs**" pattern of hyphae and spores (see Figure 2.2-15B).

TREATMENT

Treat lesions with topical **ketoconazole or selenium sulfide.**

Candidiasis

Commonly called "yeast infection" or "thrush," candidiasis can be caused by any *Candida* species but is most commonly caused by *C albicans.* In immune-competent patients, it typically presents as a superficial infection of the skin or mucous membranes in moist areas such as skin folds, armpits, the vagina, and below the breasts. Oral thrush is not uncommon among children, but in adults it is often a sign of a weakened immune system.

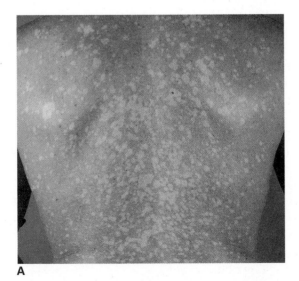

A

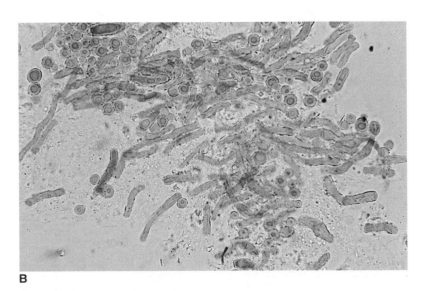

B

FIGURE 2.2-15. **Tinea versicolor.** (A) Note the discrete, hypopigmented patches extensively involving the patient's back. Tinea versicolor may also present as hyperpigmented macules or patches in some individuals. (B) KOH preparation shows the characteristic "spaghetti and meatballs" pattern. (Image A reproduced with permission from Tintinalli JE et al. *Tintinalli's Emergency Medicine: A Comprehensive Study Guide,* 7th ed. New York: McGraw-Hill, 2011, Fig. 249-8. Image B reproduced with permission from Wolff K et al. *Fitzpatrick's Dermatology in General Medicine,* 7th ed. New York: McGraw-Hill, 2008, Fig. 189-11.)

HISTORY/PE

- Patients often have a **history of antibiotic use, steroid use, or diabetes.**
- **Oral candidiasis:** Presents with painless white plaques that can easily be scraped off.
- **Candidiasis of the skin:** Presents as markedly erythematous patches with occasional erosions and smaller satellite lesions seen nearby, often in skin folds. In infants, infection can often be seen in the diaper area and along the inguinal folds.

DIAGNOSIS

Diagnosed by the clinical picture; confirmed by KOH preparation of a scraping or swab of the affected area. KOH dissolves the skin cells but leaves the *Candida* untouched such that **candidal hyphae and pseudospores** become visible.

TREATMENT

- **Oral candidiasis:** Oral fluconazole; nystatin swish and swallow.
- **Superficial (skin) candidiasis:** Topical antifungals; keep skin clean and dry.
- **Diaper rash:** Topical nystatin.

Dermatophyte Infections

Dermatophytes live only in tissues with keratin (ie, the skin, nails, and hair) and are a common cause of infection. **Causative organisms include *Microsporum, Trichophyton,* and *Epidermophyton.* *Trichophyton rubrum* is the most common dermatophyte worldwide. Risk factors include diabetes, ↓ peripheral circulation, immune compromise, and chronic maceration of skin (eg, from athletic activities).

HISTORY/PE

Presentation varies according to subtype:

- **Tinea corporis:** Presents as a scaly, pruritic eruption with a sharp, irregular border, often with central clearing (see Figure 2.2-16). May be seen in immunocompromised patients or in children following contact with infected pets.
- **Tinea pedis/manuum:** Presents as chronic interdigital scaling with erosions between the toes (**"athlete's foot"**) or as a thickened, scaly skin on the soles and interdigital web spaces. Asymmetric involvement of the hands is typical.
- **Tinea cruris ("jock itch"):** A chronic infection of the groin (typically sparing the scrotum) that is usually associated with tinea pedis.
- **Tinea capitis:** A diffuse, scaly scalp eruption similar to seborrheic dermatitis.

DIAGNOSIS

Diagnosed by the clinical picture; confirmed by scales prepared in **KOH showing hyphae.**

TREATMENT

Patients can be treated with topical or systemic antifungals. Tinea capitis must be treated with systemic drugs; systemic treatment should also be considered in immunocompromised patients.

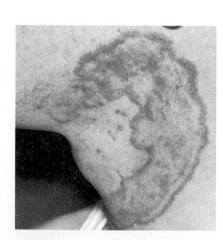

FIGURE 2.2-16. Tinea corporis. Note the "ringworm-like" rash with a scaly, erythematous, distinct border and central clearing. (Reproduced with permission from Wolff K et al. *Fitzpatrick's Dermatology in General Medicine,* 7th ed. New York: McGraw-Hill, 2008, Fig. 188-11.)

PARASITIC INFECTIONS

Lice

Lice live off blood and on specific parts of the body, depending on their species (head lice, body lice, pubic lice). Lice are spread through body contact or by the sharing of bedclothes and other garments or hair accessories. They secrete local toxins that lead to pruritus.

HISTORY/PE

- Patients with lice often experience severe pruritus, and 2° bacterial infection of the excoriations is a risk. **Classroom epidemics** of head lice are common.
- Body lice are seen in people with inadequate hygiene or in those with crowded living conditions. Pubic lice (called "crabs" because of their squat, crablike body shape) contain anticoagulant in their saliva, so their bites often turn blue.

DIAGNOSIS

Lice can be seen on hairs or in clothes.

TREATMENT

- **Head lice:** Treat with OTC pyrethrin (RID), benzyl alcohol, and mechanical removal of nits.
- **Body lice:** Wash body, clothes, and bedding thoroughly. Treating the body with topical permethrin or pyrethrin may also be required.
- **Pubic lice:** Treat with RID.

Scabies

Caused by *Sarcoptes scabiei*. The burrowing of this arthropod into the epidermis leads to **pruritus** that ↑ in intensity once an allergy to the mite or its products develops. Scabies mites are spread through close contact.

HISTORY/PE

- Patients present with intense pruritus, especially at **night and after hot showers,** and erythematous, pimple-like papules with **linear tracks, representing the burrows** of the mite.
- The most commonly affected sites are the hands (often includes the **spaces between knuckles**), axillae, and genitals.
- 2° bacterial infection is common.

DIAGNOSIS

A history of pruritus in several family members is suggestive. The mite may be identifiable by scraping an intact tunnel and looking under the microscope.

TREATMENT

- Patients should be treated overnight with 1–2 applications of 5% **permethrin from the neck down,** and their contacts should be treated as well. Oral **ivermectin** is also effective.
- Pruritus may persist for 2 weeks after treatment, so symptomatic treatment should be provided.

KEY FACT

Get **rid** of lice with **RID.**

Ischemic Disorders

DECUBITUS ULCERS

Result from ischemic necrosis following continuous pressure on an area of skin that restricts microcirculation to the area.

HISTORY/PE

Ulcers are most commonly seen in **bedridden patients** who lie in the same spot for too long. An underlying bony prominence or lack of fat ↑ the likelihood of ulcer formation. Patients who lack mobility or cutaneous sensation are also at ↑ risk. Incontinence of urine or stool may macerate the skin, facilitating ulceration.

DIAGNOSIS

Diagnosed by the history and clinical appearance.

TREATMENT

- Prevention is key and involves routinely moving bedridden patients and using special beds that distribute pressure.
- Once an ulcer has developed, low-grade lesions can be treated with routine wound care, including hydrocolloid dressings. High-grade lesions require **surgical debridement.**

GANGRENE

Defined as necrosis of body tissue. There are 3 subtypes: **dry, wet,** and **gas.** Etiologies are as follows:

- **Dry gangrene:** Due to insufficient blood flow to tissue, typically from atherosclerosis.
- **Wet gangrene:** Involves bacterial infection, usually with skin flora.
- **Gas gangrene:** Due to *C perfringens* infection.

HISTORY/PE

- **Dry gangrene:** Early signs are a dull ache, cold, and pallor of the flesh. As necrosis sets in, the tissue (usually a toe) becomes bluish-black, dry, and shriveled. Diabetes, vasculopathy, and smoking are risk factors.
- **Wet gangrene:** The tissue appears bruised, swollen, or blistered with pus.
- **Gas gangrene:** Typically occurs at a site of recent injury or surgery, presenting with swelling around the injury and with skin that turns pale and then dark red. Bacteria are rapidly destructive of tissue, producing gas that separates healthy tissue and exposes it to infection. **A medical emergency.**

DIAGNOSIS

Diagnosed by clinical impression.

TREATMENT

- Surgical **debridement,** with amputation if necessary, is the mainstay of treatment. **Antibiotics alone do not suffice** by virtue of inadequate blood flow, but they should be given as an adjuvant to surgery.
- Gas gangrene can be treated with hyperbaric oxygen, which is toxic to the anaerobic *C perfringens.* Susceptible patients should maintain careful foot care and should avoid trauma.

Miscellaneous Skin Disorders

ACANTHOSIS NIGRICANS

- A condition in which the skin in the **intertriginous zones** (genital and axillary regions, and especially the nape of the neck) is hyperkeratotic and **hyperpigmented with a velvety appearance** (see Figure 2.2-17).
- Associated with DM, Cushing's disease, polycystic ovarian syndrome, and obesity. May also be a paraneoplastic sign of underlying adenocarcinoma (usually GI).
- **Tx:** Typically not treated. Patients should be encouraged to lose weight.

LICHEN PLANUS

- A chronic inflammatory dermatosis involving the skin and mucous membranes. The condition is intensely pruritic, can be induced by drugs, and can be associated with HCV infection.
- **Hx/PE:** Presents with **violaceous, flat-topped, polygonal papules** (see Figure 2.2-18). Lesions may have prominent **Koebner's phenomena** (lesions that appear at the site of trauma). The initial lesions often appear on the genitalia, where they are erosive.
- **Tx:** Mild cases are treated with topical corticosteroids. For severe disease, systemic corticosteroids and phototherapy may be used.

ROSACEA

- A chronic disorder of pilosebaceous units whose etiology is unclear. Early in the disease, **central facial erythema** is seen with **telangiectasias.** Later, papules and pustules may develop.
- **Hx/PE:**
    - Patients are generally **middle-aged persons with fair skin** and often have an **abnormal flushing** response to various substances. There is a female predominance.
    - Rosacea can be confused with acne but is not follicular in origin and involves an older age group.
- **Tx:** Treat with topical **metronidazole.** For more severe disease, systemic antibiotics may be used.

PITYRIASIS ROSEA

- An acute dermatitis whose etiology is unknown but has been hypothesized to represent a reaction to a **viral infection with human herpesvirus (HHV) 6 or 7** because it tends to occur in mini-epidemics among young adults.
- **Hx/PE:**
    - The initial lesion is a **herald patch** that is erythematous with a peripheral scale.
    - Days to weeks later, a 2° exanthem appears, presenting with multiple tiny, symmetric papules with a fine **"cigarette paper"** scale (see Figure 2.2-19). Papules are arranged along skin lines, giving a classic **"Christmas tree" pattern** on the patient's back.
- **Dx:** Diagnosed by clinical impression and confirmed by KOH exam to rule out fungus (the herald patch may be mistaken for tinea corporis). Syphilis should also be ruled out with RPR.

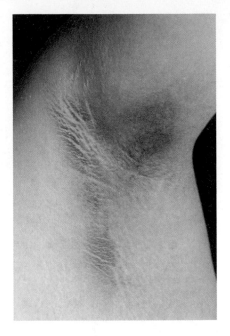

FIGURE 2.2-17. Acanthosis nigricans. Velvety, dark brown epidermal thickening of the armpit is seen with prominent skin fold and feathered edges. (Reproduced with permission from Wolff K, Johnson RA. *Fitzpatrick's Color Atlas & Synopsis of Clinical Dermatology,* 6th ed. New York: McGraw-Hill, 2009, Fig. 5-1.)

 KEY FACT

Lichen planus is the "P" disease: **P**lanar, **P**urple, **P**ruritic, **P**ersistent, **P**olygonal, **P**enile, **P**erioral, **P**uzzling, and Koebner's **P**henomenon.

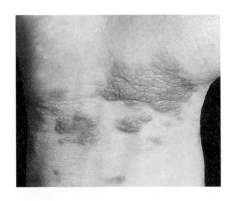

FIGURE 2.2-18. Lichen planus. Flat-topped, polygonal, sharply defined papules of violaceous color are grouped and confluent. The surface is shiny and reveals fine white lines (Wickham's striae). (Reproduced with permission from Wolff K et al. *Fitzpatrick's Dermatology in General Medicine,* 7th ed. New York: McGraw-Hill, 2008, Fig. 26-1.)

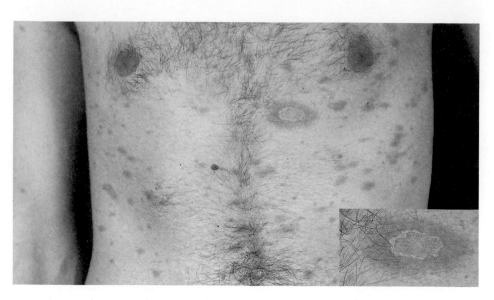

FIGURE 2.2-19. **Pityriasis rosea.** The round to oval erythematous plaques are often covered with a fine white scale ("cigarette paper") and are often found on the trunk and proximal extremities. Plaques are often preceded by a larger herald patch (inset). (Reproduced with permission from Tintinalli JE et al. *Tintinalli's Emergency Medicine: A Comprehensive Study Guide,* 7th ed. New York: McGraw-Hill, 2011, Fig. 249-6.)

- **Tx:** Patients usually heal without treatment in 6–8 weeks, but skin lubrication, topical antipruritics, and systemic antihistamines are supportive therapies.

VITILIGO

- A disease of depigmentation 2° to the absence of functional melanocytes. Its pathogenesis is unknown.
- **Hx/PE:** Patients develop **small, sharply demarcated, depigmented macules or patches** on otherwise normal skin, often on the hands, face, or genitalia. These spots then expand to include large segments of skin. The disease is usually **chronic and progressive,** with some patients becoming completely depigmented.
- **Dx:** Many patients have **serologic markers of autoimmune disease** (eg, antithyroid antibodies, DM, pernicious anemia) but seldom present with these diseases.
- **Tx:** Topical or systemic psoralens and exposure to sunlight or PUVA may be helpful. Patients must wear **sunscreen** because depigmented skin lacks inherent sun protection. Dyes and makeup may be used to color the skin, or the skin may be chemically bleached to produce a uniformly white color.

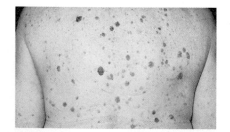

FIGURE 2.2-20. **Seborrheic keratoses.** Multiple brown, warty papules and nodules are seen on the back and are characterized by a "stuck-on" appearance. (Reproduced with permission from Wolff K, Johnson RA. *Fitzpatrick's Color Atlas & Synopsis of Clinical Dermatology,* 6th ed. New York: McGraw-Hill, 2009, Fig. 9-41.)

Neoplasms

SEBORRHEIC KERATOSIS

A very common skin tumor that appears in almost all patients after age 40. The etiology is unknown. Lesions have no malignant potential but may be a cosmetic problem (see Figure 2.2-20).

HISTORY/PE

- Present as exophytic, waxy brown papules and plaques with prominent follicle openings (see Figure 2.2-20). Lesions often appear in great numbers and **have a "stuck-on" appearance.**
- Lesions may become irritated either spontaneously or by external trauma, especially in the groin, breast, or axillae.

DIAGNOSIS

Diagnosed by the clinical picture.

TREATMENT

Cryotherapy or curettage is curative.

ACTINIC KERATOSIS

A precursor of squamous cell carcinoma in situ. Lesions are caused by exposure to sunlight.

HISTORY/PE

Lesions appear on sun-exposed areas (especially the face and arms) and primarily affect older patients, who rarely have a solitary lesion. They are erythematous with a light scale that can become thick and crusted (see Figure 2.2-21).

DIAGNOSIS

Diagnosed by clinical impression.

TREATMENT

Cryosurgery, topical 5-FU, or topical imiquimod can be used to destroy the lesion. If carcinoma is suspected, biopsy followed by excision or curettage is appropriate. Patients should be advised to use sun protection.

SQUAMOUS CELL CARCINOMA (SCC)

The second most common skin cancer, with locally destructive effects as well as the potential for **metastasis and death. UV light** is the most common causative factor, but exposure to **chemical carcinogens,** prior **radiation** therapy, and sites of **chronic trauma** (as in draining infectious sinuses in osteomyelitis) also predispose patients to developing SCC. Most SCCs occur in older adults with sun-damaged skin, arising from actinic keratoses. **Arsenic exposure** is a well-defined cause of multiple SCCs in a palmoplantar distribution.

HISTORY/PE

- SCCs have a variety of forms, and a single patient will often have multiple variants (see Figure 2.2-22). **Bowen's disease** is a form of SCC in situ.
- SCCs that arise from actinic keratoses rarely metastasize, but those that arise on the lips and on ulcers are more likely to do so. SCC occurs on the lip far more commonly than does basal cell carcinoma (BCC).

DIAGNOSIS

Diagnosed by clinical suspicion and confirmed by biopsy, which is necessary for accurate diagnosis and appropriate therapeutic planning.

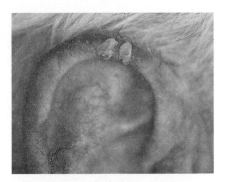

FIGURE 2.2-21. Actinic keratosis. The discrete patch above has an erythematous base and a rough white scale. (Reproduced with permission from Hurwitz RM. *Pathology of the Skin: Atlas of Clinical-Pathological Correlation,* 2nd ed. Stamford, CT: Appleton & Lange, 1998: 359.)

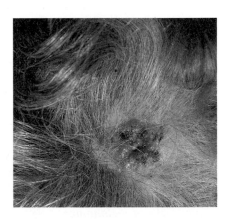

FIGURE 2.2-22. Squamous cell carcinoma. Note the crusting and ulceration of this erythematous plaque. Most lesions are exophytic nodules with erosion or ulceration. (Reproduced with permission from Hurwitz RM. *Pathology of the Skin: Atlas of Clinical-Pathological Correlation,* 2nd ed. Stamford, CT: Appleton & Lange, 1998: 360.)

Q

A 72-year-old male presents to a new internist after moving to Florida. The internist notes a chronic wound on the patient's right lower leg. The patient states that the wound followed an episode of cellulitis and has been present for 3 years. What is the next best step?

TREATMENT

Surgical excision or Mohs' surgery (microscopic surgery for close excision and identification of clear tumor margins). Lesions with high metastatic potential may require additional radiation or chemotherapy.

BASAL CELL CARCINOMA (BCC)

The most common malignant skin cancer, BCC is slow growing and locally destructive but has **virtually no metastatic potential. Chronic UV light** exposure is the main risk factor. Multiple lesions on non-sun-exposed areas are suggestive of **inherited basal cell nevus syndrome.** Most lesions appear on the face and on other sun-exposed areas.

HISTORY/PE

There are many types of BCC with varying degrees of pigmentation, ulceration, and depth of growth (see Figure 2.2-23).

DIAGNOSIS

Diagnosed by clinical impression.

TREATMENT

Options include excision, curettage and electrodesiccation/cautery, deep cryotherapy, superficial radiation therapy, and Mohs' surgery.

MELANOMA

The most common life-threatening dermatologic disease. Risk factors include **fair skin and a tendency to burn; intense bursts of sun exposure** (especially in childhood and with intermittent exposure); and the presence of **large congenital melanocytic nevi, an ↑ number of nevi, or dysplastic nevi.** Immunosuppression also ↑ risk. Some patients inherit a predisposition to melanoma with the **familial atypical mole and melanoma (FAM-M) syndrome.** There are several subtypes (see Table 2.2-4).

HISTORY/PE

- Malignant melanomas usually begin in the epidermal basal layer, where melanocytes are normally found.
- Malignant melanomas may metastasize, and 3–5% of patients with metastatic melanoma have no known 1° lesion.

DIAGNOSIS

- Early recognition and treatment are essential. All adults should be examined for lesions that are suspicious for melanoma according to the **ABCDE criteria,** which identify dysplastic nevi and superficial spreading melanoma (see mnemonic and Figure 2.2-24).
- The onset of **pruritus** is also an early sign of malignant change. An **excisional biopsy** should be performed on any suspicious lesion. **Malignancy is determined histologically.**
- Malignant melanomas are staged by Breslow's thickness (depth of invasion measured in millimeters) and by tumor-node-metastasis **(TNM) staging.** Ulceration is a poor prognostic sign.

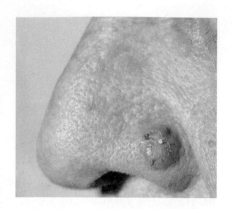

FIGURE 2.2-23. Nodular basal cell carcinoma. A smooth, pearly nodule with telangiectasias. (Reproduced with permission from Wolff K et al. *Fitzpatrick's Color Atlas & Synopsis of Clinical Dermatology,* 5th ed. New York: McGraw-Hill, 2005: 283.)

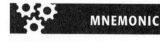

MNEMONIC

The ABCDEs of melanoma:

Asymmetric
Irregular **B**order
Irregular **C**olor
Diameter > 6 mm
Evolution: changing or new lesions

Biopsy the lesion to rule out SCC.

TREATMENT

- Lesions confined to the skin are treated by **excision with margins.** Sentinel lymph node biopsy is useful for staging but does not ↑ survival. Chemotherapy (including interferon) and radiation therapy may be used but are not likely to be successful.
- Malignant melanoma has the potential to **relapse after several years and is known for its tendency to bleed;** patients with early melanoma are at low risk for relapse but are at high risk for the development of **subsequent melanomas. Patient surveillance** is thus essential.

KAPOSI'S SARCOMA (KS)

A vascular proliferative disease that has been attributed to a herpesvirus, HHV-8, which is also called Kaposi's sarcoma–associated herpesvirus (KSHV).

HISTORY/PE

- Patients present with multiple red to violaceous macules, papules, or nodules that can progress to plaques on the lower limbs, back, face, mouth, and genitalia (see Figure 2.2-25).
- **Epidemic HIV-associated KS** is an aggressive form of the disease, and although less common since the advent of HAART, it remains the **most common HIV-associated malignancy.**

DIAGNOSIS

Diagnosed by history, clinical impression, and histology.

TREATMENT

Treatment is technically palliative. Local lesions may be treated with radiation or cryotherapy; surgery is not recommended. Widespread or internal disease is treated with systemic chemotherapy (anthracyclines, paclitaxil, or IFN-α).

MYCOSIS FUNGOIDES (CUTANEOUS T-CELL LYMPHOMA)

Not a fungus, but rather a slow, progressive neoplastic proliferation of T cells. The disease is chronic and is more common in males than in females.

HISTORY/PE

- The early lesion is a nonspecific, psoriatic-appearing plaque that is palpable and often pruritic with a predilection for the buttocks. A later lesion is characterized by limited or generalized skin involvement with palpable lymph nodes or 1 or more skin tumors with multicentric, often confluent reddish-brown nodules (see Figure 2.2-26).
- Patients may have dermatopathic lymphadenopathy without actual tumor involvement of the node. However, the **internal organs can be involved,** including the lymph nodes, liver, and spleen.
- **Sézary's syndrome** is the leukemic phase of cutaneous T-cell lymphoma and is characterized by circulating Sézary cells in the peripheral blood, erythroderma, and lymphadenopathy.

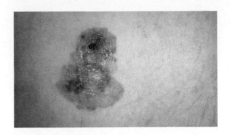

FIGURE 2.2-24. Melanoma. Note the asymmetry, border irregularity, color variation, and large diameter of this plaque. (Reproduced with permission from Hurwitz RM. *Pathology of the Skin: Atlas of Clinical-Pathological Correlation,* 2nd ed. Stamford, CT: Appleton & Lange, 1998: 432.)

KEY FACT

Bacillary angiomatosis, caused by *Bartonella henselae* and *Bartonella quintana,* can mimic KS and should be excluded in suspected KS patients; erythromycin is the treatment of choice.

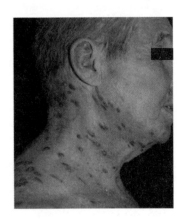

FIGURE 2.2-25. Kaposi's sarcoma. Note the multiple violaceous papules on the neck, back, and face. (Reproduced with permission from Wolff K et al. *Fitzpatrick's Color Atlas & Synopsis of Clinical Dermatology,* 5th ed. New York: McGraw-Hill, 2005, Fig. 1e-HIV7.)

TABLE 2.2-4. **Types of Melanoma**

TYPE	PRESENTATION
Lentigo maligna	Arises in a lentigo. Usually found on sun-damaged skin of the face.
Superficial spreading	Typically affects younger adults, presenting on the trunk in men and on the legs in women. A relatively prolonged horizontal growth phase helps identify the disease early, when it is still confined to the epidermis.
Nodular	Lesions have a rapid vertical growth phase and appear as a rapidly growing reddish-brown nodule with ulceration or hemorrhage.
Acral lentiginous	Begins on the hands and feet as a slowly spreading, pigmented patch. Most commonly seen in Asians and African Americans.
Amelanotic	Presents as a lesion without clinical pigmentation. Extremely difficult to identify. This variant of melanoma can be further classified into any of the above types.

DIAGNOSIS

- Diagnosed by clinical features and histology, with immunologic characterization and electron microscopy showing the typical **Sézary or Lutzner cells (cerebriform lymphocytes).**
- The early lesion is clinically indistinguishable from dermatitis, **so histologic diagnosis is indicated for any dermatitis that is chronic and resistant to treatment.**

TREATMENT

Phototherapy is the mainstay of treatment for many patients. For more extensive or advanced disease, radiation therapy is an effective option. Treatment modalities, including steroids, chemotherapy, retinoids, monoclonal antibodies, and interferon, are often combined.

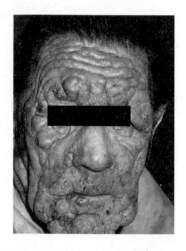

FIGURE 2.2-26. Mycosis fungoides. Massive nodular infiltration of the face leads to a leonine facies. (Reproduced with permission from Wolff K et al. *Fitzpatrick's Dermatology in General Medicine,* 7th ed. New York: McGraw-Hill, 2008, Fig. 146-7.)

ENDOCRINOLOGY

Disorders of Glucose Metabolism

TYPE 1 DIABETES MELLITUS (TYPE 1 DM)

Due to autoimmune **pancreatic β-cell destruction,** leading to insulin deficiency and abnormal glucose metabolism.

HISTORY/PE

- Classically presents with **polyuria, polydipsia,** polyphagia, and rapid, unexplained weight loss. Patients may also present with **ketoacidosis** (see Table 2.3-2).
- Usually affects nonobese children or young adults.
- Associated with HLA-DR3 and -DR4.
- Type I DM in adults is known as latent autoimmune diabetes of adults (LADA).

DIAGNOSIS

- At disease onset, **anti–islet cell** and **anti–glutamic acid decarboxylase (anti-GAD) antibodies** may be present in serum.
- At least 1 of the following is required to make the diagnosis:
    - A fasting (> 8-hour) plasma glucose level ≥ 126 mg/dL on 2 separate occasions.
    - A random plasma glucose level ≥ 200 mg/dL plus symptoms.
    - A 2-hour postprandial glucose level ≥ 200 mg/dL following an oral glucose tolerance test on 2 separate occasions if the results of initial testing are equivocal.
    - Hemoglobin A_{1c} (HbA_{1c}) > 6.5%.

TREATMENT

- Insulin injections (see Table 2.3-1 and Figure 2.3-1) to maintain blood glucose in the normal range (80–120 mg/dL). Higher blood glucose levels (≥ 200 mg/dL) can be tolerated, particularly in the very young, in light of the ↑ risk of hypoglycemia.
- Consider the use of an insulin pump, which provides continuous, short-acting insulin infusion.

TABLE 2.3-1. **Types of Insulin**

INSULIN[a]	ONSET	PEAK EFFECT	DURATION
Regular	30–60 minutes	2–4 hours	5–8 hours
Short acting (lispro, aspart, glulisine)	5–20 minutes	0.5–3.0 hours	3–8 hours
NPH	2–4 hours	6–10 hours	18–28 hours
Long acting (detemir, glargine)	1–3 hours	No discernible peak	20–24 hours

[a] Combination preparations mix longer-acting and shorter-acting types of insulin together to provide immediate and extended coverage in the same injection (eg, 70 NPH/30 regular = 70% NPH + 30% regular).

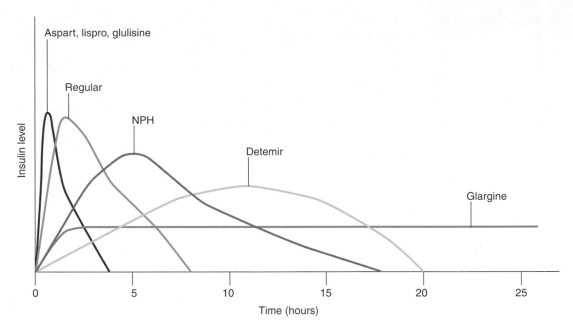

FIGURE 2.3-1. Pharmacokinetics of insulin preparations.

- Encourage routine HbA_{1c} testing every 3 months (with a goal $HbA_{1c} < 8\%$ in children and $< 7\%$ in adults), frequent BP checks, a cardiac review of systems in adults at each clinic visit, monofilament foot exams, annual dilated-eye exams, annual urine microalbuminuria screening, and a fasting lipid profile every 2–5 years.

COMPLICATIONS

Table 2.3-2 outlines the acute, chronic, and treatment-related complications of DM.

TYPE 2 DIABETES MELLITUS (TYPE 2 DM)

A dysfunction in glucose metabolism due to varying degrees of **insulin resistance in peripheral tissues** that may ultimately lead to β-cell failure and complete insulin dependence.

HISTORY/PE

- Patients typically present with symptoms of hyperglycemia (polyuria, polydipsia, polyphagia, blurred vision, fatigue).
- Onset is more **insidious** than that of type 1 DM, and patients often present with complications.
- **Nonketotic hyperosmolar hyperglycemia** may be seen in the setting of poor glycemic control.
- Usually occurs in older adults with obesity (often truncal) and has a strong genetic predisposition; diagnosed increasingly in obese children.
- Risk factors include obesity, rapid weight gain, a ⊕ family history, a sedentary lifestyle, increasing age, and other components of metabolic syndrome (see below).

DIAGNOSIS

- Diagnostic criteria are the **same as those for type 1 DM.**
- Anti–islet cell and anti-GAD antibodies will be ⊖.

TABLE 2.3-2. Complications of DM

COMPLICATION	DESCRIPTION
TREATMENT COMPLICATIONS	
Dawn phenomenon	Morning hyperglycemia due to the normal nocturnal release of counterregulatory hormones (eg, glucagon, epinephrine, cortisol), which ↑ insulin resistance and blood glucose levels (see Figure 2.3-2). ↑ P.M. **NPH insulin.**
Somogyi effect	**Rebound hyperglycemia.** Results from excess exogenous insulin, which causes hypoglycemia overnight and stimulates the release of counterregulatory hormones that in turn ↑ blood glucose levels (see Figure 2.3-2). ↓ P.M. **NPH insulin.**
ACUTE COMPLICATIONS	
DKA	Hyperglycemia-induced crisis that most commonly occurs in **type 1 DM.** Often precipitated by stress (including infections, MI, trauma, or alcohol) or by noncompliance with insulin therapy. May present with **abdominal pain, vomiting, Kussmaul respirations,** and a **fruity, acetone breath odor.** Patients are severely dehydrated with electrolyte abnormalities and may also develop **mental status changes.** Treatment includes fluids, potassium, **insulin,** bicarbonate (if pH is < 7), and treatment of the initiating event or underlying disease process.
Hyperosmolar hyperglycemic state	Presents with profound dehydration, mental status changes, hyperosmolarity, and extremely high plasma glucose (> 600 mg/dL) **without acidosis and with small or absent ketones.** Occurs in **type 2 DM;** precipitated by acute stress (dehydration, infections) and can often be fatal. Treatment includes aggressive fluid, electrolyte replacement, and insulin. Treat the initiating event.
CHRONIC COMPLICATIONS	
Retinopathy (nonproliferative, proliferative)	Appears when diabetes has been present for **at least 3–5 years** (see Figure 2.3-3). Preventive measures include control of hyperglycemia and hypertension, annual eye exams, and **laser photocoagulation therapy for retinal neovascularization.**
Diabetic nephropathy	Characterized by glomerular hyperfiltration followed by **microalbuminuria.** Preventive measures include **ACEIs** or angiotensin receptor blockers (ARBs) and BP/glucose control.
Neuropathy	Peripheral, symmetric sensorimotor neuropathy leading to burning pain, foot trauma, infections, and diabetic ulcers. Treat with preventive **foot care** and **analgesics.** Late complications due to autonomic dysfunction include delayed gastric emptying, esophageal dysmotility, impotence, and orthostatic hypotension.
Macrovascular complications	Cardiovascular, cerebrovascular, and peripheral vascular disease. **Cardiovascular disease is the most common cause of death in diabetic patients.** The goal BP is < 130/< 80 mm Hg; ↓ LDL to < 100 mg/dL and ↓ triglycerides to < 150 mg/dL. Patients should also be started on low-dose ASA.

- Screening recommendations:
    - **Patients with no risk factors:** Test HbA_{1c} at age 45; retest every 3 years if HbA_{1c} is < 5.7% and no other risk factors develop.
    - **Patients with impaired fasting glucose (> 110 mg/dL but < 126 mg/dL) or impaired glucose tolerance:** Follow up with frequent retesting.

TREATMENT

The goal of treatment is tight glucose control (see Table 2.3-3)—ie, blood glucose levels ranging from 80 to 120 mg/dL and HbA_{1c} levels < 7%. Treatment measures are outlined in Table 2.3-3.

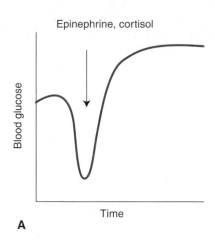
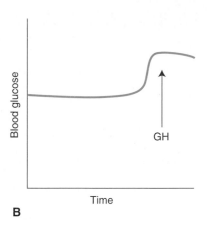

FIGURE 2.3-2. Mechanisms of morning hyperglycemia in diabetes. (A) Somogyi effect. (B) Dawn phenomenon.

COMPLICATIONS

See Table 2.3-2 for an outline of the complications of DM.

METABOLIC SYNDROME

Also known as insulin resistance syndrome or syndrome X. Associated with an ↑ risk of CAD and mortality from a cardiovascular event.

HISTORY/PE

Presents with abdominal obesity, high BP, impaired glycemic control, and dyslipidemia.

DIAGNOSIS

Three out of five of the following criteria must be met:

- Abdominal obesity (↑ waist girth): > 40 inches in men and > 35 inches in women.
- Triglycerides ≥ 150 mg/dL.
- HDL < 40 mg/dL in men and < 50 mg/dL in women.
- BP ≥ 130/85 mm Hg or a requirement for antihypertensive drugs.
- Fasting glucose ≥ 100 mg/dL.

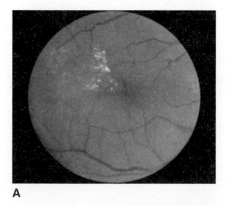
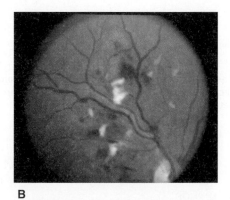

FIGURE 2.3-3.   Diabetic retinopathy. (A) **Nonproliferative retinopathy** presents with exudates, dot-blot hemorrhages, and microaneurysms. (B) **Proliferative retinopathy** presents with macular edema, vitreous traction, and neovascularization of the retinal vasculature. (Reproduced with permission from USMLERx.com.)

TABLE 2.3-3. Treatment of Type 2 DM

TREATMENT	DESCRIPTION
LIFESTYLE MODIFICATIONS	
Diet	Low-fat, moderate-carbohydrate, low-calorie personalized diet.
Weight loss	Goal: 5–10% body weight loss with a combination of diet and exercise.
Exercise	Moderate-intensity exercise for 30 minutes 5 days per week.
PHARMACOTHERAPY (MONOTHERAPY OR COMBINATION THERAPY IF POOR GLYCEMIC CONTROL)	
Sulfonylureas (glipizide, glyburide, glimepiride)	↑ endogenous insulin secretion. Side effects include hypoglycemia and weight gain.
Metformin	Inhibits hepatic gluconeogenesis and ↑ peripheral sensitivity to insulin. Side effects include weight loss, GI upset, and, rarely, lactic acidosis. Contraindicated in the elderly (> 80 years of age) and in renal insufficiency, hepatic failure, or heart failure.
Thiazolidinediones (rosiglitazone, pioglitazone)[a]	↑ insulin sensitivity. Side effects include weight gain, edema, hepatotoxicity, and bone loss. Contraindicated in patients with heart failure.
α-glucosidase inhibitors	↓ intestinal absorption of carbohydrates. Side effects include flatulence and hypoglycemia.
DPP-4 inhibitors (sitagliptin)	Inhibit the degradation of glucagon-like peptide 1 (GLP-1).
Incretins (exenatide)	GLP-1 agonists. Injected subcutaneously. Delay absorption of food; ↑ insulin secretion and ↓ glucagon secretion. Side effects include nausea and, rarely, pancreatitis.
Insulin	Given alone or in conjunction with oral agents.
GENERAL HEALTH MAINTENANCE	
Cardiovascular risk modification	**The presence of diabetes is equivalent to the highest risk for cardiovascular disease regardless of all other risk factors.** ASA for patients at risk of cardiovascular disease or for those > 40 years of age. Statins for hypercholesterolemia (goal LDL < 100 mg/dL; optimal goal LDL < 70 mg/dL for persons with cardiac disease).
BP management	Strict BP control to < 130/80 mm Hg; ACEIs/ARBs are first-line agents.
Screening exams	Annual physical examination to screen for cardiovascular disease, nephropathy, retinopathy, and neuropathy.

[a] In September 2010, the FDA restricted access to rosiglitazone because of concern for ↑ cardiovascular risks. The drug is still available but is restricted to patients currently on the medication who acknowledge that they understand the risks and to patients who cannot achieve adequate glycemic control with other medications.

TREATMENT

Intensive weight loss, aggressive cholesterol management, and BP control. Metformin has been shown to slow the onset of diabetes in this high-risk population.

TABLE 2.3-4.   TFTs in Thyroid Disease

DIAGNOSIS	TSH	T₄	T₃	CAUSES
1° hyperthyroidism	↓	↑	↑	Graves' disease, toxic multinodular goiter, toxic adenoma, amiodarone, postpartum thyrotoxicosis, postviral thyroiditis.
1° hypothyroidism	↑	↓	↓	Hashimoto's thyroiditis, iatrogenic (radioactive ablation, excision), drugs (lithium, amiodarone).

Thyroid Disorders

TESTING OF THYROID FUNCTION

Thyroid function tests (TFTs) include the following (see also Table 2.3-4):

- **TSH measurement: The single best test for the screening of thyroid disease and for the assessment of thyroid function.** High TSH levels are associated with 1° hypothyroidism; low TSH levels are associated with hyperthyroidism.
- **Radioactive iodine uptake (RAI) and scan:** Determines the level and distribution of iodine uptake by the thyroid. Useful for the differentiation of hyperthyroid states, but has a limited role in determining malignancy.
- **Total T₄ measurement:** Not an adequate screening test. Ninety-nine percent of circulating T₄ is bound to thyroxine-binding globulin (TBG). Total T₄ levels can be altered by changes in levels of binding proteins.
- **Free T₄ measurement:** The **preferred screening test for thyroid hormone levels.**

HYPERTHYROIDISM

A state involving ↑ levels of T₃/T₄. Most commonly due to **Graves' disease**, but can also result from other causes (see Table 2.3-4).

- **Graves' disease:** The **autoimmune** form of hyperthyroidism. **Thyroid-stimulating antibodies** ↑ T₃/T₄. RAI percent uptake will be high, and RAI scan will show diffuse iodine uptake.
- **Toxic adenoma/toxic multinodular goiter:** Result in hyperthyroidism due to autonomous hyperactive thyroid nodules. RAI percent uptake will be normal to high, and RAI scan will show nodules/regions of ↑ uptake only.
- **Thyroiditis (postpartum, postviral, subacute):** Due to transient inflammation of the thyroid gland with release of previously synthesized thyroid hormone; causes a temporary ↑ in circulating T₃/T₄. RAI percent uptake will be low, and RAI scan will show low iodine uptake. A hypothyroid phase may follow the hyperthyroid phase (see below).

HISTORY/PE

- Presents with **weight loss, heat intolerance, anxiety, palpitations, ↑ bowel frequency,** insomnia, and menstrual abnormalities.

KEY FACT

↑ TBG can be found in pregnancy, estrogen administration, infection, and nephritic syndrome. You do not need to treat.

KEY FACT

In 1° endocrine disturbances, the gland itself is abnormal. In 2° endocrine disturbances, the pituitary gland is the source. In 3° endocrine disturbances, the hypothalamus malfunctions (see Figure 2.3-4).

KEY FACT

Exophthalmos, pretibial myxedema, and thyroid bruits are specific for Graves' disease.

A 10-year-old male presents to the ER with 2 weeks of polyuria and polydipsia together with new-onset lethargy. Physical examination reveals signs of severe dehydration, and labs reveal a blood glucose level of 800 mg/dL. The diagnosis of diabetic ketoacidosis (DKA) is made, and the patient is started on insulin and IV fluids. What is the next best step in management?

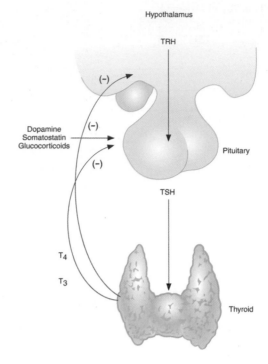

FIGURE 2.3-4.   The hypothalamic-pituitary-thyroid axis. (Reproduced with permission from Molina PE. *Endocrine Physiology,* 3rd ed. New York: McGraw-Hill, 2009, Fig. 4-1.)

KEY FACT

TSH receptor-stimulating antibodies are found in patients with Graves' disease.

KEY FACT

Thyroid storm is an acute, life-threatening form of thyrotoxicosis that may present with AF, fever, and delirium. Administer IV propranolol and steroids, and admit to the ICU.

Add 5% dextrose to the IV fluids. In the management of DKA, it is important to start IV fluids and insulin immediately. Initially, the goal is to rehydrate the patient and lower blood glucose, but as blood glucose reaches 250–300 mg/dL, it is important to add 5% dextrose to ↓ the risk of hypoglycemia.

■ Examination reveals warm, moist skin, goiter, sinus **tachycardia** or **atrial fibrillation (AF)**, fine **tremor, lid lag,** and hyperactive reflexes. **Exophthalmos,** pretibial myxedema, and thyroid bruits are seen only in Graves' disease (see Figure 2.3-5).

Diagnosis

The initial test of choice is a serum TSH level, followed by T_4 levels and, rarely, T_3 (unless TSH is low and free T_4 is not elevated). See Table 2.3-4.

Treatment

■ **Symptomatic treatment: Propranolol** to manage adrenergic symptoms.
■ **Pharmacologic treatment:** Antithyroid drugs (methimazole or propylthiouracil).
■ **Definitive treatment:** Radioactive ^{131}I thyroid ablation or total thyroidectomy (less common in the United States).
■ Administer levothyroxine (oral T_4 replacement) to prevent hypothyroidism in patients who have undergone ablation or surgery.

Complications

Thyroid storm, an acute, life-threatening form of thyrotoxicosis. Treat urgently with IV propranolol, propylthiouracil, and corticosteroids. High-dose potassium iodide (SSKI) is also effective.

HYPOTHYROIDISM

A state involving ↓ levels of T_3/T_4. Most commonly due to **Hashimoto's thyroiditis,** but can result from other causes (see Table 2.3-4).

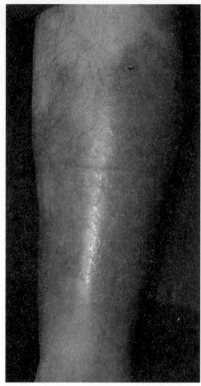

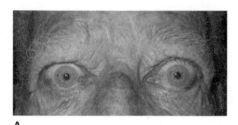

A   **B**

FIGURE 2.3-5. **Physical signs of Graves' disease**. (A) Graves' ophthalmopathy. (B) Pretibial myxedema. (Reproduced with permission from USMLERx.com.)

- **Hashimoto's thyroiditis (autoimmune hypothyroidism):** Associated with ⊕ **antithyroglobulin and antimicrosomal (anti-TPO) antibodies** that precipitate thyroid destruction.
- **Thyroiditis (postpartum, postviral, subacute):** Can have a hypothyroid phase that follows the hyperthyroid phase. Hypothyroidism can be permanent.

HISTORY/PE

- Presents with weakness, fatigue, **cold intolerance, constipation,** weight gain, **depression,** hair loss, menstrual irregularities, and **hoarseness.**
- Examination reveals **dry, cold, puffy skin** accompanied by edema, **bradycardia,** and delayed relaxation of DTRs.

DIAGNOSIS

The initial test of choice is serum TSH level, followed by free T_4 levels. See Table 2.3-4.

TREATMENT

For uncomplicated hypothyroidism (eg, Hashimoto's disease), administer levothyroxine.

COMPLICATIONS

Myxedema coma: severe hypothyroidism with ↓ mental status, hypothermia, and other parasympathetic symptoms. Mortality is 30–60%. Admit to the ICU and treat urgently with IV levothyroxine and IV hydrocortisone (if adrenal insufficiency has not been excluded).

THYROIDITIS

Inflammation of the thyroid gland. Common subtypes include subacute granulomatous, radiation-induced, autoimmune, postpartum, and drug-induced (eg, amiodarone) thyroiditis.

HISTORY/PE

- The **subacute form presents with a tender thyroid,** malaise, and URI symptoms.
- All other forms are associated with painless goiter.

DIAGNOSIS

Thyroid dysfunction (typically thyrotoxicosis followed by hypothyroidism), with ↓ uptake on RAI and scan during the hyperthyroid phase.

TREATMENT

- β-blockers for hyperthyroidism; levothyroxine for hypothyroidism.
- Subacute thyroiditis is usually self-limited; for severe cases, treat with NSAIDs or with oral corticosteroids.

THYROID NEOPLASMS

Thyroid nodules are very common and show an ↑ incidence with age. Most (~ 95%) are benign.

HISTORY/PE

- Usually asymptomatic on initial presentation; discovered incidentally with imaging for other purposes (eg, carotid ultrasound) or on examination.
- Hyperfunctioning nodules present with hyperthyroidism.
- Large nodules adjacent to the trachea/esophagus present with local symptoms (dysphagia, dyspnea, cough, choking sensation) and are associated with a ⊕ family history (especially medullary thyroid cancer).
- An ↑ risk of malignancy is associated with a **history of childhood neck irradiation, "cold" nodules** (minimal uptake on RAI scan), female sex, age < 20 or > 70, firm and fixed solitary nodules, a ⊕ family history (especially medullary thyroid cancer), and **rapidly growing nodules with hoarseness.**
- Check for anterior cervical lymphadenopathy. Carcinoma (see Table 2.3-5) may be **firm and fixed.**
- Medullary thyroid carcinoma is associated with multiple endocrine neoplasia (MEN) type 2.

DIAGNOSIS

- **TFTs** to detect hyperfunctioning nodules, followed by RAI scan, which will show a "hot" nodule. Hot nodules are not cancerous and should not be biopsied.
- **Ultrasound** to determine if the nodule is solid or cystic. Cystic nodules are more likely to be benign.
- The best method to assess a nodule for malignancy is **fine-needle aspiration** (FNA), which has high sensitivity and moderate specificity. "Cold" nodules on RAI scan should be biopsied.

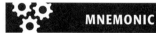

TABLE 2.3-5.   Types of Thyroid Carcinoma

TYPE[a]	CHARACTERISTICS	PROGNOSIS
Papillary	Represents **75–80% of thyroid cancers.** The female-to-male ratio is 3:1. Slow growing; found in thyroid hormone–producing follicular cells.	Ninety percent of patients survive 10 years or more after diagnosis; the prognosis is worse in elderly patients or those with large tumors.
Follicular	Accounts for 17% of thyroid cancers; found in thyroid hormone–producing follicular cells.	Same as above.
Medullary	Responsible for 6–8% of thyroid cancers. Found in calcitonin-producing C cells; the prognosis is related to degree of vascular invasion.	Eighty percent of patients survive at least 10 years after surgery. Consider MEN 2A or 2B based on family history.
Anaplastic	Accounts for < 2% of thyroid cancers; rapidly enlarges and metastasizes.	Ten percent of patients survive for > 3 years.

[a] Tumors may contain mixed papillary and follicular pathologies.

TREATMENT

- **Benign FNA:** Follow with physical examination/ultrasound to assess for continued nodule growth or for the development of suspicious characteristics (eg, calcification, ↑ vascular flow).
- **Malignant FNA:** Surgical resection with hemi- or total thyroidectomy is first-line treatment; adjunctive radioiodine ablation following excision is appropriate for some follicular lesions.
- **Indeterminate FNA:** Watchful waiting vs. hemithyroidectomy (10–30% chance of malignancy). If resected, await final pathology to guide further treatment.

Bone and Mineral Disorders

OSTEOPOROSIS

A common metabolic bone disease characterized by low bone mass and microarchitectural disruption, with **bone mineral density (BMD) < 2.5 SDs from normal peak bone mass** (at 30 years of age). It most often affects thin, postmenopausal women (17%), especially Caucasians and Asians, with risk doubling after age 65. Males are also at risk for osteoporosis, but the diagnosis is often overlooked.

HISTORY/PE

- Commonly asymptomatic even in the presence of a vertebral fracture.
- Examination may reveal **hip fractures, vertebral compression fractures** (loss of height and progressive thoracic kyphosis), and/or distal radius fractures (Colles' fracture) following minimal trauma (see Figure 2.3-6).

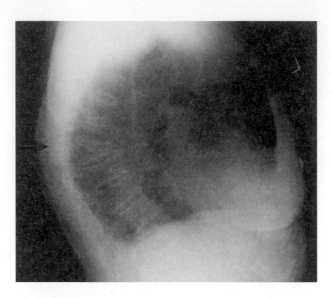

FIGURE 2.3-6. **Radiographic findings in osteoporosis.** Lateral thoracic spine radiograph shows osteoporosis and an anterior wedge deformity of a lower thoracic vertebral body with associated kyphosis. This is a typical insufficiency fracture in osteoporotic patients. (Reproduced with permission from Fauci AS et al. *Harrison's Principles of Internal Medicine,* 17th ed. New York: McGraw-Hill, 2008, Fig. 348-2.)

KEY FACT

Osteoporosis is the most common cause of pathologic fractures in thin, elderly women and men.

- Bone pain (especially anterior tibial pain) unrelated to fracture is most likely osteomalacia, a mineralization defect, rather than osteoporosis.
- **Smoking, age,** excessive caffeine or alcohol intake, a history of estrogen-depleting conditions in women (eg, amenorrhea, eating disorders) or hypogonadism in men, uncontrolled hyperthyroidism, chronic inflammatory disease, and **corticosteroid use** are all associated with an ↑ risk.

Diagnosis

- **Dual-energy x-ray absorptiometry (DEXA):** The standard imaging technique for diagnosing osteoporosis; reveals BMD < 2.5 SDs from the normal peak level, with sites reported including the vertebral bodies, proximal femur, and distal radius.
- **Labs:** Rule out 2° causes with TFTs, CMP, 24-hour urine calcium, serum 25-hydroxyvitamin D, CBC, testosterone (in men), and SPEP/UPEP (to rule out multiple myeloma).
- **X-rays:** Global demineralization is apparent only after > 30% of bone density is lost.

Treatment

- Prevention and treatment with **calcium** and **vitamin D supplementation.**
- Smoking cessation and weight-bearing exercises help maintain and even restore some bone density.
- Antiresorptive agents that can prevent further bone loss include bisphosphonates (eg, alendronate, risedronate, ibandronate, zoledronic acid), selective estrogen receptor modulators (eg, raloxifene), intranasal calcitonin, and denosumab (a monoclonal antibody to RANK-L).

Complications

Fracture is the most devastating consequence of low BMD/osteoporosis, carrying a 50% chance of mortality in the year following hip fracture.

PAGET'S DISEASE

Characterized by an ↑ rate of bone turnover with both excessive resorption and formation of bone, leading to a **"mosaic" lamellar bone pattern** on x-ray. Suspected to be due to the effects of a latent viral infection in genetically susceptible individuals. Occurs in roughly 4% of men and women > 40 years of age. Associated with 1° hyperparathyroidism in up to one-fifth of patients.

HISTORY/PE

- Usually asymptomatic, but may present with aching bone or joint pain, headaches (if the skull is involved), bony deformities, fracture at a pagetoid site, or nerve entrapment (leads to loss of hearing in 30–40% of cases involving the skull).
- The disease can affect 1 (monostotic) or many (polyostotic) bones, with the skull, vertebral bodies, pelvis, and long bones most commonly affected.

DIAGNOSIS

Based on clinical history, characteristic radiographic changes (see Figure 2.3-7), and lab findings.

- **Labs:** Abnormalities include ↑ **serum alkaline phosphatase with normal calcium and phosphate levels.** Must be distinguished from metastatic bone disease.
- **Imaging:** Radionuclide bone scan is the most sensitive test in early Paget's disease, but plain films are critical to diagnosis.

TREATMENT

- **Most patients are asymptomatic and require no treatment.**
- There is no cure for Paget's disease. In the setting of severe pain, involvement of a vulnerable site (femoral neck), or fracture, bisphosphonates and calcitonin can be used to slow osteoclastic bone resorption; NSAIDs and acetaminophen can be given for pain management.

COMPLICATIONS

Pathologic fractures, high-output cardiac failure, osteosarcoma (up to 1%).

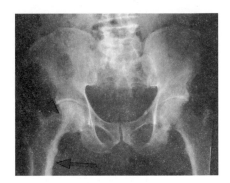

FIGURE 2.3-7.   Radiographic findings in Paget's disease. Pelvic radiograph demonstrates a thickened cortex (arrow), thickened trabeculae (arrowhead), and expansion of the right femoral head, classic signs of Paget's disease. (Reproduced with permission from Fauci AS et al. *Harrison's Principles of Internal Medicine*, 17th ed. New York: McGraw-Hill, 2008, Fig. 349-3.)

HYPERPARATHYROIDISM

The parathyroid glands make parathyroid hormone (PTH) and are responsible for calcium and phosphate regulation in the body. Hyperparathyroidism is defined as an ↑ serum PTH level with variable effects on calcium and phosphate, depending on the specific cause.

- **1° hyperparathyroidism:** Most cases (80%) are due to a single hyperfunctioning adenoma, with the rest (15%) resulting from parathyroid hyperplasia and, rarely (5%), parathyroid carcinoma.
- **2° hyperparathyroidism:** A physiologic ↑ of PTH in response to **renal insufficiency,** calcium deficiency, or vitamin D deficiency.
- **3° hyperparathyroidism:** Seen in **dialysis patients** with long-standing 2° hyperparathyroidism that leads to hyperplasia of the parathyroid glands. When 1 or more of the glands become autonomous, 3° hyperparathyroidism results.

Q

An asymptomatic 36-year-old male presents for his annual physical. The patient has no past medical history and takes no medications. His physical examination is unremarkable. Routine labs reveal a serum calcium level of 11.3 mg/dL. He returns in 2 weeks, and his serum calcium level remains persistently elevated. Further workup is initiated, and additional studies show a normal serum PTH level and a low 24-hour urinary calcium level. What is the most likely diagnosis?

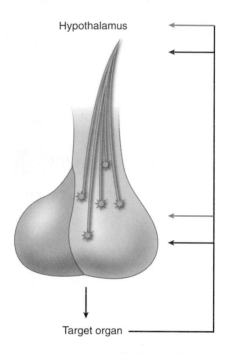

Hypothalamus

Target organ

FIGURE 2.3-8.   The hypothalamic-pituitary axis.

HISTORY/PE

Most cases of 1° hyperparathyroidism are **asymptomatic,** but signs and symptoms of **hypercalcemia** may be mild and include **stones** (nephrolithiasis), **bones** (bone pain, myalgias, arthralgias, fractures), abdominal **groans** (abdominal pain, nausea, vomiting, PUD, pancreatitis), and **psychiatric overtones** (fatigue, depression, anxiety, sleep disturbances).

DIAGNOSIS

- Labs in 1° hyperparathyroidism reveal **hypercalcemia, hypophosphatemia,** and hypercalciuria. Intact PTH is inappropriately ↑ relative to total and ionized calcium (see Table 2.3-6).
- DEXA may reveal low bone density or frank osteoporosis in the distal radius or other sites.
- A ^{99m}Tc sestamibi scan, in conjunction with thyroid ultrasound, can help localize a solitary adenoma.

TREATMENT

- **Parathyroidectomy** if the patient is symptomatic or if certain criteria are met. In the case of a solitary adenoma, 1 gland may be removed. In the setting of hyperplasia, 3.5 glands must be removed.
- For acute hypercalcemia, give **IV fluids, loop diuretics, and an IV bisphosphonate.**
- In patients with renal insufficiency, administer oral phosphate binders (calcium salts, sevelamer hydrochloride, and lanthanum carbonate) and restrict dietary phosphate intake to prevent 2° hyperparathyroidism.
- Cinacalcet is a calcimimetic that acts to lower serum PTH levels and is approved for use in hyperparathyroidism due to renal failure.

COMPLICATIONS

Hypercalcemia is the most severe complication of 1° hyperparathyroidism, presenting acutely with coma or altered mental status, bone disease, nephrolithiasis, and abdominal pain with nausea and vomiting.

TABLE 2.3-6.   Lab Values in Hyperparathyroidism

	PTH	**CALCIUM**	**PO$_4$**
1°	↑	↑	↓
2°	↑	Nl/↓	↑
3°	↑	↑	↑
Ectopic PTHrP[a]	↓	↑	↓

[a] PTH-releasing peptide (PTHrP) is a member of the PTH family and acts on the same PTH receptors. Some tumors (eg, breast, lung) produce PTHrP, causing hypercalcemia of malignancy.

Pituitary and Hypothalamic Disorders

Figure 2.3-8 illustrates the hypothalamic-pituitary axis. The sections that follow outline the manner in which the components of this axis interact with target organs in various pathologic states.

CUSHING'S SYNDROME

The result of elevated serum cortisol levels, Cushing's syndrome is most frequently iatrogenic, resulting from prolonged treatment with exogenous corticosteroids. The most common endogenous cause is hypersecretion of ACTH from a pituitary adenoma (known as Cushing's disease; see Figure 2.3-9). Other endogenous causes include excess adrenal secretion of cortisol (eg, bilateral adrenal hyperplasia, adenoma, adrenal cancer) and ectopic ACTH production from an occult neoplasm (eg, carcinoid tumor, medullary thyroid cancer, small cell lung cancer).

HISTORY/PE

- Presents with **hypertension, type 2 DM, depression, weight gain,** muscle weakness, easy bruisability, ↑ susceptibility to infection, psychological disturbances, oligomenorrhea, and **hirsutism.**
- Examination reveals **central obesity,** growth retardation, proximal muscle wasting and weakness, acne, **excessive hair growth,** wide purple **striae, moon facies,** and supraclavicular or retrocervical fat pads ("**buffalo hump**").
- **Headache** or cranial nerve deficits (bitemporal hemianopsia, impaired extraocular movements) can occur with increasing size of the pituitary mass.

DIAGNOSIS

Diagnosis is as follows (see also Table 2.3-7):

- **Begin with a screen:** Pick 2 of 3 tests: (1) an elevated 24-hour free urine cortisol; (2) an elevated midnight salivary cortisol level on 2 separate nights; or (3) a 1-mg dexamethasone suppression test (⊕ if A.M. **cortisol is persistently elevated the morning after administration of dexamethasone**).
- **Distinguish ACTH-dependent (pituitary/ectopic) from ACTH-independent causes (adrenal):** Measure morning (8:00 A.M.) cortisol and ACTH levels. If ACTH is elevated, Cushing's disease or ectopic ACTH is likely.
- A pituitary MRI should be ordered only if laboratory testing suggests Cushing's disease (associated with a high risk of pituitary incidentalomas).
- Adrenal imaging should be ordered only if the workup suggests an ACTH-independent etiology (associated with a high risk of adrenal incidentalomas).
- Hyperglycemia, glycosuria, and hypokalemia may also be present.

TREATMENT

- **Surgical resection** of the source (pituitary, adrenal, neoplasm).
- Inhibitors of adrenal steroidogenesis (eg, spironolactone, eplerenone) are helpful in cases of bilateral adrenal hyperplasia.
- Permanent hormone replacement therapy to correct deficiencies after treatment of the 1° lesion.

> **KEY FACT**
>
> **Cushing's syndrome** = too much cortisol. **Cushing's disease** = too much cortisol from an ACTH-producing pituitary adenoma.

> **KEY FACT**
>
> In Cushing's disease, cortisol secretion remains elevated with the low-dose dexamethasone test but is suppressed with the high-dose dexamethasone test.

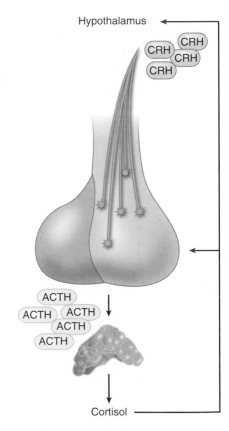

FIGURE 2.3-9.   The hypothalamic-pituitary axis: Cushing's disease.

TABLE 2.3-7. Laboratory Findings in Cushing's Syndrome

	Cushing's Disease (Pituitary Hypersecretion)	Exogenous Steroid Use	Ectopic ACTH Secretion	Adrenal Cortisol Hypersecretion
24-hour urinary free cortisol	↑	↑	↑	↑
Salivary cortisol	↑	↑	↑	↑
ACTH	↑	↓	↑	↓
Dexamethasone suppression test morning cortisol level:				
Low dose	↑	↑	↑	↑
High dose	↓	↑	↑	N/A[a]

[a] A high-dose dexamethasone suppression test is not required once the diagnosis of ACTH-independent Cushing's syndrome is made.

ACROMEGALY

Elevated growth hormone (GH) levels in adults, most commonly due to a benign pituitary GH-secreting adenoma (see Figure 2.3-10). Children with excess GH production present with **gigantism.**

HISTORY/PE

- Presents with **enlargement of the skull, hands, and feet and coarsening of facial features.** Associated with an ↑ risk of carpal tunnel syndrome, obstructive sleep apnea, type 2 DM, heart disease (diastolic dysfunction), hypertension, and arthritis.
- **Bitemporal hemianopsia** may result from compression of the optic chiasm by a pituitary adenoma.
- Excess GH may also lead to **glucose intolerance** or **diabetes.**

DIAGNOSIS

- **Labs:** Measure insulin-like growth factor 1 (IGF-1) levels (↑ with acromegaly); confirm the diagnosis with an oral glucose suppression test (GH levels will remain elevated despite glucose administration). Baseline GH is not a reliable test.
- **Imaging:** MRI shows a sellar lesion.

TREATMENT

- Transsphenoidal surgical resection or external beam radiation of the tumor.
- Octreotide (a somatostatin analog) can be used to suppress GH secretion; pegvisomant (a GH receptor antagonist) can be used to block the peripheral actions of GH.

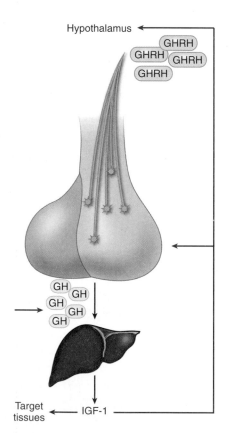

FIGURE 2.3-10. The hypothalamic-pituitary axis: acromegaly.

HYPERPROLACTINEMIA

Elevated prolactin levels, most commonly due to a pituitary adenoma (see Figure 2.3-11). **Prolactinoma is the most common functioning pituitary tumor.** Other causes include pituitary stalk compression from other masses (eg, craniopharyngioma, meningioma), drugs (eg, dopamine antagonists), renal failure, and cirrhosis.

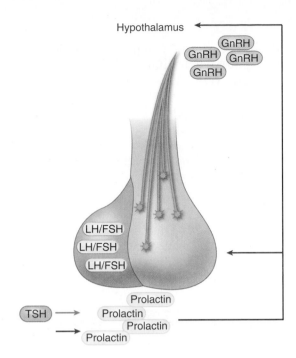

FIGURE 2.3-11. **The hypothalamic-pituitary axis: prolactinoma.**

HISTORY/PE

Elevated prolactin inhibits GnRH secretion and consequently lowers LH and FSH secretion, manifesting as **infertility, galactorrhea, and amenorrhea.** Bitemporal hemianopsia may also be present.

DIAGNOSIS

- The serum **prolactin level is typically > 200 ng/mL.**
- MRI shows a sellar lesion.

TREATMENT

- **First line:** Dopamine agonists (eg, cabergoline, bromocriptine).
- **Surgery:** Indicated in adenomas refractory to medical management or with compressive effects (eg, visual loss).

DIABETES INSIPIDUS (DI)

Inability to produce concentrated urine as a result of ADH dysfunction. The 2 subtypes are as follows:

- **Central DI (ADH deficiency):** The posterior pituitary fails to secrete ADH. Causes include tumor, ischemia (Sheehan's syndrome), pituitary hemorrhage, traumatic brain injury, infection, metastatic disease, and autoimmune disorders (see Figure 2.3-12).
- **Nephrogenic DI (ADH resistance):** The kidneys fail to respond to circulating ADH. Causes include renal disease and drugs (eg, **lithium,** demeclocycline).

HISTORY/PE

- Presents with **polydipsia, polyuria,** and **persistent thirst** with dilute urine. Most cases are normonatremic.
- If access to water is limited (eg, in the institutionalized or elderly), patients may present with dehydration and severe hypernatremia leading to altered mental status, lethargy, seizures, and coma.

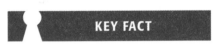

KEY FACT

Rule out pregnancy in all cases of hyperprolactinemia.

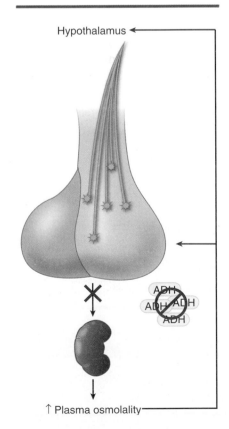

FIGURE 2.3-12. **The hypothalamic-pituitary axis: DI.**

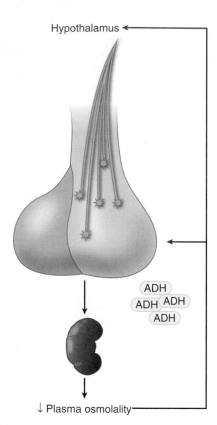

Hypothalamus

ADH
ADH   ADH
ADH

↓ Plasma osmolality

FIGURE 2.3-13. **The hypothalamic-pituitary axis: SIADH.**

DIAGNOSIS

- **Water deprivation test:** In central and nephrogenic DI, patients excrete a high volume of inappropriately dilute urine.
- **Desmopressin acetate (DDAVP, a synthetic analog of ADH) replacement test:**
  - **Central DI:** ↓ urine output and ↑ urine osmolarity.
  - **Nephrogenic DI:** No effect is seen on urine output or urine osmolarity.
- MRI may show a pituitary or hypothalamic mass in central DI.

TREATMENT

- Treat the underlying cause.
- **Central DI:** Administer DDAVP intranasally or orally.
- **Nephrogenic DI:** First-line treatment consists of salt restriction and water intake. Thiazide diuretics can be used to promote mild volume depletion and to stimulate ↑ water reabsorption.

SIADH

A common cause of euvolemic hyponatremia that results from **persistent ADH release independent of serum osmolality** (see Figure 2.3-13).

HISTORY/PE

Associated with **CNS disease** (eg, head injury, tumor), **pulmonary disease** (eg, sarcoid, COPD, pneumonia), ectopic tumor production/paraneoplastic syndrome (eg, small cell lung carcinoma), and drugs (eg, antipsychotics, antidepressants).

DIAGNOSIS

- Urine osmolality is > 50–100 mOsm/kg in the setting of serum hypoosmolarity without a physiologic reason for ↑ ADH (eg, CHF, cirrhosis, hypovolemia).
- **A urinary sodium level ≥ 20 mEq/L** demonstrates that the patient is not hypovolemic.
- Serum uric acid is < 4 mg/dL.

TREATMENT

- **Restrict fluid** and address the underlying cause.
- If hyponatremia is severe (< 110 mEq/L) or if the patient is significantly symptomatic (eg, comatose, seizing), **cautiously give hypertonic saline.** Patients must be monitored in the ICU to prevent **central pontine myelinolysis.**
- Demeclocycline, an ADH receptor antagonist, can help normalize serum sodium.

Adrenal Gland Disorders

ADRENAL INSUFFICIENCY (AI)

Inadequate production of adrenal hormones, including glucocorticoids and/or mineralocorticoids. May be 1° or 2°/3°. Etiologies are as follows:

- 1°: In the United States, most commonly due to autoimmune adrenal cortical destruction (**Addison's disease**), leading to deficiencies of mineralocorticoids and glucocorticoids. Other causes include congenital enzyme deficiencies, adrenal hemorrhage, and infections (*Neisseria meningitidis*, HIV, histoplasmosis, TB). TB is the most common cause of AI worldwide.
- 2°/3°: Caused by ↓ ACTH production by the pituitary; **most often due to cessation of long-term glucocorticoid treatment.**

HISTORY/PE

- Most symptoms are nonspecific.
- **Weakness, fatigue,** and **anorexia with weight loss** are common. GI manifestations, hypoglycemia, hypotension, and salt craving are also seen.
- **Hyperpigmentation** (due to ↑ ACTH secretion) is seen in Addison's disease, especially in areas of sun exposure or friction.

DIAGNOSIS

- Labs show **hyponatremia** and **eosinophilia** (1° or 2°).
- **Hyperkalemia is specific to 1° AI.**
- Hypercalcemia is seen in up to one-third of cases.
- Confirm with 8 A.M. plasma cortisol levels and a synthetic ACTH stimulation test:
    - An 8 A.M. plasma cortisol level < 3 µg/dL in the absence of exogenous glucocorticoid administration is diagnostic of AI.
    - Failure of cortisol to rise > 18 µg/dL following ACTH administration confirms the diagnosis.
    - A random plasma cortisol level > 18 µg/dL excludes the diagnosis.

TREATMENT

- 1°: Glucocorticoid and mineralocorticoid replacement.
- 2°/3°: Only glucocorticoid replacement is necessary (mineralocorticoid production is not ACTH dependent).
- In adrenal crisis, provide IV steroids; correct electrolyte abnormalities as needed; provide 50% dextrose to correct hypoglycemia; and initiate aggressive volume resuscitation.
- ↑ steroids during periods of stress (eg, major surgery, trauma, infection).
- In patients on chronic steroid therapy, taper slowly to prevent 2°/3° AI.

PHEOCHROMOCYTOMA

A tumor of chromaffin tissue that secretes catecholamines and is found either in the adrenal medulla or in extra-adrenal sites. Most commonly associated with MEN 2A and 2B.

HISTORY/PE

- Presents with **paroxysmal** tachycardia, palpitations, chest pain, diaphoresis, hypertension, headache, tremor, and anxiety.
- It is important to obtain a family history in order to rule out genetic causes of pheochromocytoma (eg, MEN 2A/2B, von Hippel–Lindau disease, neurofibromatosis).

DIAGNOSIS

- CT and MRI are both sensitive for pheochromocytomas. A nuclear MIBG scan can localize extra-adrenal lesions and metastatic disease.

MNEMONIC

The 4 S's of adrenal crisis management:

Salt: 0.9% saline
Steroids: IV hydrocortisone 100 mg q 8 h
Support
Search for the underlying illness

KEY FACT

Do not delay the administration of steroids in a patient with suspected AI.

MNEMONIC

Pheochromocytoma rule of 10's:

10% extra-adrenal
10% bilateral
10% malignant
10% occur in children
10% familial

Q   1

A 23-year-old male with a history of schizophrenia presents with complaints of fatigue, weakness, cramps, and headache for the past several days. He denies any other symptoms, although he had to urinate several times while in the office. Routine labs reveal hyponatremia. With water deprivation, his urine osmolality ↑. What is the most likely diagnosis?

Q   2

An asymptomatic 36-year-old female presents with a 2-cm thyroid mass. TFTs are unremarkable, but FNA reveals medullary carcinoma. Total thyroidectomy with thyroid hormone replacement is recommended. What is the most important screening test to perform prior to surgery?

MNEMONIC

The 5 P's of pheochromocytoma:

Pressure (BP)
Pain (headache)
Perspiration
Palpitations
Pallor

KEY FACT

In pheochromocytoma, administer α-blockers before β-blockers to prevent hypertensive crisis.

---

1 **A**

1° (psychogenic) polydipsia, a condition in which patients consume large volumes of fluid, resulting in polyuria. It most often occurs in patients with psychiatric disorders. Patients present with symptoms similar to DI, but following a water deprivation test, urine osmolality ↑ (vs. DI, in which urine remains dilute).

---

2 **A**

VMA and metanephrines. Medullary carcinoma of the thyroid is associated with MEN type 2A/2B, an autosomal dominant condition that predisposes patients not only to medullary carcinoma but also to parathyroid adenomas and pheochromocytomas. Screening for pheochromocytoma with urine VMA and metanephrines prior to surgery can prevent potentially life-threatening hypertensive crises during thyroidectomy.

- Look for elevated plasma-free metanephrines (metanephrine and normetanephrine) or 24-hour urine metanephrines and catecholamines.

TREATMENT

- Surgical resection.
- Preoperatively, use α-adrenergic blockade first to control hypertension, followed by β-blockade to control tachycardia. **Never give β-blockade first,** as unopposed α-adrenergic stimulation will lead to refractory hypertension.

HYPERALDOSTERONISM

Results from excessive secretion of aldosterone from the zona glomerulosa of the adrenal cortex. It is usually due to adrenocortical hyperplasia (70%) but can also result from unilateral adrenal adenoma (**Conn's syndrome**).

HISTORY/PE

- Presents with hypertension, headache, polyuria, and muscle weakness.
- Tetany, paresthesias, and peripheral edema are seen in severe cases.
- Consider hyperaldosteronism in younger adults who are diagnosed with hypertension without risk factors or a family history of hypertension.

DIAGNOSIS

- Patients have diastolic hypertension without edema.
- Labs show **hypokalemia, mild hypernatremia,** metabolic alkalosis, hypomagnesemia, hyperaldosteronism, and an ↑ **aldosterone/plasma renin activity ratio** (usually > 30).
- CT or MRI may reveal an adrenal mass. Adrenal venous sampling may be needed to localize the adenoma or to confirm bilateral adrenal hyperplasia.

TREATMENT

- Surgical resection for adrenal tumors (after correction of BP and potassium).
- Treat bilateral hyperplasia with spironolactone, an aldosterone receptor antagonist.

CONGENITAL ADRENAL HYPERPLASIA (CAH)

A condition of adrenal insufficiency due to a variety of inherited enzyme deficiencies that impair cortisol synthesis and result in the accumulation of cortisol precursors. Without the ⊖ feedback of cortisol on the hypothalamus and pituitary, ACTH secretion ↑, leading to the overproduction of adrenal androgens. Most cases are due to **21-hydroxylase deficiency** (95%, autosomal recessive), but other causes include 11- and 17-hydroxylase deficiencies. CAH can manifest either in a salt-losing form or in a non-salt-losing form.

HISTORY/PE

Presentation varies with gender:

- **Females:** In both forms, presents at birth with ambiguous genitalia.
- **Males:** Presents at birth with adrenal crisis in the salt-losing form, but presents with precocious puberty in the non-salt-losing form.

DIAGNOSIS

- Electrolyte abnormalities include hyponatremia, hyperkalemia, and metabolic acidosis. In severe cases, mineralocorticoid deficiency may lead to life-threatening salt wasting.
- An **elevated serum 17-hydroxyprogesterone level** is diagnostic.

TREATMENT

- **Medical: Immediate fluid resuscitation and salt repletion.** Administer cortisol to ↓ ACTH and adrenal androgens. Fludrocortisone is appropriate for severe 21-hydroxylase deficiency.
- **Surgical:** Correct ambiguous genitalia in female infants.
- Refer to the Gynecology chapter for information on the diagnosis and treatment of late-onset CAH.

Multiple Endocrine Neoplasias (MEN)

A family of tumor syndromes with autosomal dominant inheritance.

- **MEN type 1 (Wermer's syndrome):** Pancreatic islet cell tumors (eg, gastrinomas [Zollinger-Ellison syndrome], insulinomas, VIPomas), parathyroid hyperplasia, and pituitary adenomas.
- **MEN type 2A (Sipple's syndrome):** Medullary carcinoma of the thyroid, pheochromocytoma or adrenal hyperplasia, parathyroid gland hyperplasia. Due to mutations in the RET proto-oncogene.
- **MEN type 2B:** Medullary carcinoma of the thyroid, pheochromocytoma, oral and intestinal ganglioneuromatosis (mucosal neuromas), marfanoid habitus. Due to mutations in the RET proto-oncogene.

MNEMONIC

MEN 1 affects "P" organs:

Pancreas
Pituitary
Parathyroid

NOTES

EPIDEMIOLOGY

KEY FACT

Incidence can be measured in a cohort study; prevalence can be measured in a cross-sectional study.

KEY FACT

As the mortality of a disease ↓, the prevalence of that disease ↑ (eg, HIV infection) because the duration of disease has lengthened. Remember: P = I × D.

KEY FACT

Another name for a prevalence study is a cross-sectional study.

Assessment of Disease Frequency

- The **prevalence** of a disease is the number of existing cases in the population at a specific moment in time.

$$\text{Prevalence} = \frac{\text{total number of cases in the population at 1 point in time}}{\text{total population}}$$

- Prevalence depends on incidence and duration:

$$\text{Prevalence (P)} = \text{incidence (I)} \times \text{average duration of disease (D)}$$

- The **incidence** of a disease is the number of new cases in the disease-free population that develop over a period of time.

$$\text{Incidence} = \frac{\text{number of \textbf{new} cases in the population over a given time period}}{\text{total population at risk during the specified time period}}$$

- Remember to subtract the number of new cases of disease (numerator) from the total population at risk (denominator) because these individuals are no longer at risk.

CROSS-SECTIONAL STUDIES

A **cross-sectional study** that is undertaken to estimate prevalence is called a **prevalence study**. In a prevalence study, people in a population are examined for the presence of a disease of interest at a given point in time.

- The **advantages** of prevalence studies are as follows:
  - They provide an efficient means of examining a population, allowing cases and noncases to be assessed all at once.
  - They can be used as a basis for diagnostic testing.
  - They can be used to plan which health services to offer and where.
- Their **disadvantages** include the following:
  - One cannot determine causal relationships because information is obtained only at a **single point in time.**
  - The risk or incidence of disease cannot be directly measured.

Assessment of Diagnostic Studies

SENSITIVITY AND SPECIFICITY

Physicians often use tests to try to ascertain a diagnosis, but because no test is perfect, a given result may be falsely ⊕ or ⊖ (see Figure 2.4-1). When deciding whether to administer a test, one should thus consider both its sensitivity and its specificity.

	Disease Present	No Disease	
Positive test	a	b	PPV = a / (a + b)
Negative test	c	d	NPV = d / (c + d)

Sensitivity = a / (a + c)   Specificity = d / (b + d)

FIGURE 2.4-1. **Sensitivity, specificity, PPV, and NPV.**

- **Sensitivity:** The probability that a patient with a disease will have a ⊕ test result. A sensitive test will **rarely miss people** with the disease and is therefore good at **RULING OUT** those who do not have the disease.

$$\text{False-}\ominus \text{ ratio} = 1 - \text{sensitivity}$$

- **Specificity:** The probability that a patient without a disease will have a ⊖ test result. A specific test will rarely determine that someone has the disease when in fact they do not and is therefore good at **RULING IN those who have the disease.**

$$\text{False-}\oplus \text{ ratio} = 1 - \text{specificity}$$

- The ideal test is both sensitive and specific, but a trade-off must often be made between sensitivity and specificity. When sensitivity ↑, specificity ↓ (and vice versa).
  - **High sensitivity** is particularly desirable when there is a significant penalty for missing a disease. It is also desirable early in a **diagnostic workup or screening test,** when it is necessary to reduce a broad differential. **Example:** An initial ELISA test for HIV infection.
  - **High specificity** is useful for **confirming a likely diagnosis** or for situations in which false-⊕ results may prove harmful. **Example:** A Western blot confirmatory HIV test.

POSITIVE AND NEGATIVE PREDICTIVE VALUES

Once a test has been administered and a patient's result has been made available, that result must be interpreted through use of predictive values (**or post-test probabilities**):

- **Positive predictive value (PPV):** The probability that a patient with a ⊕ test result truly **has** the disease. The more specific a test, the higher its PPV. **The higher the disease prevalence, the higher the PPV of the test for that disease.**
- **Negative predictive value (NPV):** The probability that a patient with a ⊖ test result truly **does not have** the disease. **The more sensitive a test, the higher its NPV. The lower the disease prevalence, the higher the NPV of the test for that disease.**

LIKELIHOOD RATIO (LR)

Another way to describe the performance of a diagnostic test involves the use of **likelihood ratios (LRs),** which express how much more or less likely a given test result is in diseased as opposed to nondiseased people:

$$\oplus \text{ LR} = \frac{\text{diseased people with a } \oplus \text{ test result}}{\text{nondiseased people with a } \oplus \text{ test result}} = \frac{\text{sensitivity}}{1 - \text{specificity}}$$

$$\ominus \text{ LR} = \frac{\text{diseased people with a } \ominus \text{ test result}}{\text{nondiseased people with a } \ominus \text{ test result}} = \frac{1 - \text{sensitivity}}{\text{specificity}}$$

- The **⊕ LR** represents the fraction of patients with a disease who have a ⊕ test divided by the fraction of patients without a disease who have a ⊕ test. In other words, the ⊕ LR answers the following question: What is the proportion of patients with a target disorder who have a ⊕ test compared with the proportion of healthy patients who have a ⊕ test?
- The **⊖ LR** represents the fraction of patients with a disease who have a ⊖ test divided by the fraction of patients without a disease who have a ⊖ test.

In other words, the ⊖ LR answers the following question: What is the proportion of patients with a target disorder who have a ⊖ test compared with the proportion of healthy patients who have a ⊖ test?

- The ⊕ **LR** shows how much the odds (or probability) of disease are ↑ if the test result is ⊕.
- The ⊖ **LR** shows how much the odds (or probability) of disease are ↓ if the test result is ⊖.

$$\text{Posttest odds} = \text{pretest odds} \times \text{LR}$$

COHORT STUDIES

In a **cohort study,** a group of people is assembled, **none of whom has the outcome of interest** (ie, the disease), but **all of whom could potentially experience that outcome.** For each possible risk factor, the members of the cohort are classified as either exposed or unexposed. All the cohort members are then followed over time, and the **incidence of outcome events is compared in the 2 exposure groups.**

- **Advantages** of cohort studies are as follows:
  - They follow the same logic as the clinical question (if people are exposed, will they get the disease?).
  - They are the only way to **directly determine incidence** (because they follow a cohort over time to assess disease development).
  - They can be used to assess the relationship of a given exposure to many diseases.
  - In prospective studies, exposure is elicited without bias from a known outcome.
- **Disadvantages** of cohort studies include the following:
  - They can be time consuming and expensive.
  - Studies assess only the relationship of the disease to the few exposure factors recorded at the start of the study.
  - They require many subjects, which makes it difficult to study rare diseases.

Cohort studies may be either **prospective,** in which a cohort is assembled in the present and followed into the future, or **retrospective,** in which a cohort is identified from past records and is followed to the present.

CASE-CONTROL STUDIES

Case-control studies can be thought of as an efficient way to study a population. A series of **cases** are identified and a set of **controls** are sampled from the underlying population to estimate the frequency of exposure in the population at risk of the outcome. In such studies, a researcher **compares the frequency of exposure to a possible risk factor** in the 2 groups.

- The validity of a case-control study depends on appropriate selection of cases and controls, the manner in which exposure is measured, and the manner in which extraneous variables (confounders) are dealt with.
- Cases and controls should be comparable in terms of opportunity for exposure (ie, they should be members of the same base population with an equal opportunity of risk factor exposure).
- "**Matching**" in case-control studies occurs when the researcher chooses controls that match cases on a particular characteristic. For example, if matching on gender, female cases would be matched to female controls and male cases would be matched to male controls. The purpose of matching, followed by the appropriate analysis, is to ↓ confounding.

1 **A**

A test with high sensitivity such as a fingerstick lead test (capillary blood) is preferred for initial screening because it can ensure that no children who might have the disease—and who might therefore benefit from further testing and treatment—will be missed. The children with a ⊕ fingerstick test should subsequently have a serum blood level drawn (higher specificity).

2 **A**

PPV ↓ and NPV ↑. Remember that if prevalence is low, even a test with high sensitivity or specificity will have a low PPV.

- **Advantages** of case-control studies are as follows:
    - They use smaller groups than cohorts, thereby reducing cost.
    - They can be used to study rare diseases and can easily examine multiple risk factors.
- **Disadvantages** include the following:
    - Studies cannot calculate disease prevalence or incidence or directly estimate the relative risk because the numbers of subjects with and without a disease are determined artificially by the investigator rather than by nature; **however, an odds ratio can be used to estimate a measure of relative risk (rate ratio).**
    - Retrospective data may be inaccurate owing to recall or survivorship biases.

Measures of Effect

There are several ways to express and compare risk. These include the following:

- **Absolute risk:** Defined as the incidence of disease.
- **Attributable risk (or risk difference):** The difference in risk between the exposed and unexposed groups.

Attributable risk = incidence of disease in exposed − incidence in unexposed

- **Relative risk (or risk ratio):** Expresses how much more likely an exposed person is to get the disease in comparison to an unexposed person. This indicates the **relative strength of the association between exposure and disease,** making it useful when one is considering disease etiology.

$$\text{Relative risk} = \frac{\text{incidence in exposed}}{\text{incidence in unexposed}}$$

- **Odds ratio:** An **estimate of relative risk that is used in case-control studies.** The odds ratio tells how much more likely it is that a person with a disease has been exposed to a risk factor than someone without the disease. The lower the disease incidence, the more closely it approximates relative risk. In case-control studies, the odds ratio also describes how many times more likely an exposed individual is to have disease compared to an unexposed individual (see Figure 2.4-2).

$$\text{Odds ratio} = \frac{\text{odds that a diseased person is exposed}}{\text{odds that a nondiseased person is exposed}}$$

Survival Curves

Once a diagnosis has been established, it is important to be able to describe the associated prognosis. **Survival analysis is used to summarize the aver-**

Disease Develops   No Disease

	Disease Develops	No Disease
Exposure	a	b
No exposure	c	d

$$RR = \frac{a/(a+b)}{c/(c+d)}$$

$$OR = ad/bc$$

FIGURE 2.4-2.   Relative risk (RR) vs. odds ratio (OR).

KEY FACT

If alcohol intake among individuals with breast cancer is compared with that of individuals without breast cancer, think case-control study.

KEY FACT

In **case-control studies,** the researcher determines whether the participants have the disease or not and determines if they were exposed or unexposed. The odds ratio is calculated as an estimate of relative risk because it can't be calculated directly.

KEY FACT

$$\text{Odds} = \frac{\text{probability of event}}{1 - \text{probability of event}}$$

$$\text{Probability} = \frac{\text{odds}}{1 + \text{odds}}$$

Q

Assume that the data below are from a hypothetical case-control study. Calculate and interpret the odds ratio (OR).

	Exposed	Not Exposed
Cases	734	433
Controls	563	538

age time from 1 event (eg, presentation, diagnosis, or start of treatment) **to any outcome that can occur only once during follow-up** (eg, death or recurrence of cancer). The usual method is with a **Kaplan-Meier curve** (see Figure 2.4-3) describing the survival (or time-to-event if the measured outcome is not death) in a cohort of patients, with the probability of survival decreasing over time as patients die or drop out (are censored) from the study.

Treatment

Studies are typically used to compare treatments for a disease. Although **the gold standard for such evaluation is a randomized, double-blinded controlled trial,** other types of studies may be used as well (eg, an observational study, in which the exposure in question is a therapeutic intervention). In descending order of quality, published studies regarding treatment options include randomized controlled trials, observational studies, and case series/case reports. Meta-analyses are often used to systematically synthesize information across studies to help summarize the totality of the evidence.

RANDOMIZED CONTROLLED TRIALS (RCTs)

An RCT is defined as **an experimental, prospective study in which subjects are randomly assigned to a treatment or control group.** Random assignment helps ensure that the 2 groups are truly comparable. The control group may be treated with a placebo or with the accepted standard of care. The study may be masked in 1 of 2 ways: single blinded, in which patients do not know which treatment group they are in, or **double blinded,** in which neither the patients nor their physicians know who is in which group. **Double-blinded studies are the gold standard** for studying treatment effects.

- **Advantages** of RCTs are as follows (see also Table 2.4-1):
  - They minimize bias.
  - They have the potential to demonstrate **causal relationships** because exposure is assigned randomly, which minimizes confounding.
- **Disadvantages** include the following:
  - They are costly and time intensive.
  - Some interventions (eg, surgery) are not amenable to masking.

KEY FACT

Randomization minimizes bias and confounding; double-blinded studies prevent observation bias.

OR = ad / bc = (734 × 538) / (433 × 563) = 1.62. Interpretation: The exposed group had 1.62 times the odds of having disease compared to the unexposed group.

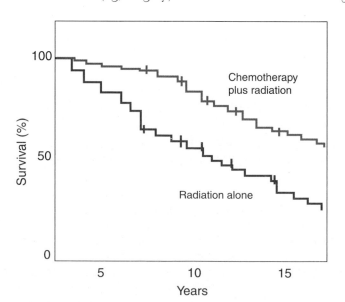

FIGURE 2.4-3. Example of a Kaplan-Meier curve.

TABLE 2.4-1.   Comparison of Study Designs

VARIABLE	RCT	COHORT	CROSS-SECTIONAL	CASE CONTROL
Purpose	Tests causality through random assignment of exposure; randomization removes confounding.	Tests association over a specified period of time to capture the development of disease.	Determines prevalence in a snapshot of time.	Tests association (usually retrospectively).
Outcomes	Any outcomes that are reported represent causal relationships.	Relative risk, odds ratio, incidence, prevalence.	Prevalence (not incidence).	Odds ratio.
Design	Subjects are randomly assigned to be in exposed (treatment A) or nonexposed (treatment B) groups.	Subjects are not assigned to groups. Determines if subjects are in exposed or nonexposed groups and follows them until they develop the disease (or do not).	Determines disease prevalence at 1 point in time; cannot determine the directionality of association between exposure and outcome.	Identifies cases (disease) and controls (no disease) groups first and then goes backward to determine if they are exposed or not (the opposite of RCT and cohort studies).
Advantages	Can determine causality; minimizes bias and confounding.	Temporality can be determined; incidence can be determined.	Less time consuming and costly.	Predetermined number of cases; less time consuming and costly.
Disadvantages	RCT is not possible when: ■ The treatment has an adverse outcome. ■ The outcome is very rare. ■ The treatment is in widespread use or represents the best option (because it is unethical to withhold treatment).	Follows large groups over long time periods. Selection bias in retrospective cohort studies.	Directionality of association cannot be determined. Incidence cannot be determined.	Recall bias, selection bias.

BIAS

Defined as **any process that causes results to systematically differ from the truth.** Common types of bias include the following:

■ **Selection bias:** Occurs when samples or participants are selected that differ from other groups in additional determinants of outcome. **Example:** Individuals concerned about a family history of breast cancer may be more likely to self-select in entering a mammography program, giving the impression of a prevalence that is higher than it is in reality.
■ **Measurement bias:** Occurs when measurement or data-gathering methods differ between groups. **Example:** One group is assessed by CT while another group is assessed by MRI.
■ **Confounding bias:** Occurs when a third variable is either positively or negatively associated with both the exposure and outcome variables, inducing an incorrect association. **Example:** Fishermen in an area may

KEY FACT

Studies that are masked and randomized are better protected from the effects of bias, whereas observational studies are particularly susceptible to bias.

experience a higher incidence of lung cancer than that found in the general population. However, if smokers are more likely to become fishermen and are also more likely to develop lung cancer than nonsmokers, becoming a fisherman will not in itself lead to lung cancer. Rather, it is the smoking to which those fishermen are exposed that causes the association.

- **Recall bias:** Results from a difference between 2 groups in the retrospective recall of past factors or outcomes. **Example:** A patient with cancer may be more motivated than would a healthy individual to recall past episodes of chemical exposure.
- **Lead-time bias:** Results from earlier detection of disease, giving an appearance of prolonged survival when in fact the natural course is not altered. **Example:** A new and widely used screening test that detects cancer 5 years earlier may yield the impression that patients are living longer with the disease.
- **Length bias:** Occurs when screening tests detect a disproportionate number of slowly progressive diseases but miss rapidly progressive ones, leading to overestimation of the benefit of the screen. **Example:** A better prognosis for patients with cancer is celebrated following the implementation of a new screening program. However, this test disproportionately detects slow-growing tumors, which generally tend to be less aggressive.

CHANCE

Even with bias reduction, unsystematic random error is unavoidable owing to chance variation in studied data. Types of errors are as follows:

- **Type I (α) error:**
  - Defined as the probability of **concluding that there is a difference** in treatment effects between groups **when in fact there is not** (ie, a false-$\oplus$ conclusion)—in other words, rejecting the null hypothesis (of no effect) when it should not be rejected.
  - The **p-value** is an estimate of the probability that differences in treatment effects in a study **could have happened by chance alone if no true association exists.** Often, differences associated with a $p < 0.05$ are statistically significant. A p-value alone **does not give any information about the direction or size of the effect.**
- **Type II (β) error:**
  - Defined as the probability of **concluding that there is no difference** in treatment effects **when in fact a difference exists** (ie, a false-$\ominus$ conclusion)—in other words, **not** rejecting the null hypothesis (of no effect) when it should be rejected.
  - **Power** is the probability that a study will find a statistically significant difference when one is truly there. Increasing the number of subjects in a study $\uparrow$ the power.

$$\text{Power} = 1 - \beta$$

- The **confidence interval (CI)** is a way of expressing statistical significance (p-value) that shows the **size of the effect and the statistical power (the narrower the CI, the greater the statistical power).** CIs are interpreted as follows:
  - If one is using a 95% CI, there is a **95% chance that the interval contains the true value.** By definition, the 95% CI contains the point estimate 100% of the time (in other words, if the calculated OR is 2.4, then the CI will always contain that value by definition).
  - **Example:** You would like to estimate the percentage of women with a specific disease. A 10% result from a sample of 3000 women would provide a 95% CI of 9–11%, whereas a 10% finding from a sample of

30 women would yield a CI of −1% of 21%. The first case has **more power because the sample size is larger, producing a narrow interval.** In the latter case, you cannot state with 95% certainty that women in general even have the disease because the interval contains 0%, which is the null value.

- If the CI includes the null value (relative risk or odds ratio of 1.0 or 0%), the results are not statistically significant.

Prevention

- There are 3 levels of prevention:
  - **1° prevention:** Includes preventive measures to ↓ the incidence of disease.
  - **2° prevention:** Focuses on identifying the disease early, when it is asymptomatic or mild, and implementing measures that can halt or slow disease progression. Includes screening tests that are designed to identify subclinical disease.
  - **3° prevention:** Includes measures that ↓ morbidity or mortality resulting from the presence of disease.
- Prevention may be accomplished by a **combination of immunization, chemoprevention, behavioral counseling, and screening. A good screening test** has the following characteristics:
  - It has **high sensitivity and specificity** (usually more important to have high sensitivity to **rule out** those that don't have the disease).
  - It has a **high PPV.**
  - It is inexpensive, easy to administer, and safe.
  - Treatment after screening is more effective than subsequent treatment without screening.

VACCINATION

- Vaccines work by mimicking infections and triggering an immune response in which memory cells are formed to recognize and fight any future infection. There are several different vaccine formulations, as indicated in Table 2.4-2.
- Recommended vaccination schedules for children and adults are outlined in Figures 2.4-4 through 2.4-6.

TABLE 2.4-2.   Types of Vaccinations

VACCINE TYPE	TARGETED DISEASES
Live attenuated	Measles, mumps, rubella, polio (Sabin), yellow fever, influenza (nasal spray).
Inactivated (killed)	Cholera, HAV, polio (Salk), rabies, influenza (injection).
Toxoid	Diphtheria, tetanus.
Subunit	HBV, pertussis, *Streptococcus pneumoniae*, HPV, meningococcus.
Conjugate	Hib, *S pneumoniae*.

KEY FACT

- **1° prevention:** A woman reduces dietary intake of fat or alcohol to reduce her risk of developing breast cancer.
- **2° prevention:** A woman obtains a mammogram to screen for breast cancer.
- **3° prevention:** A woman undergoes adjuvant therapy with tamoxifen for breast cancer.

Vaccine ▼ Age ▶	Birth	1 month	2 months	4 months	6 months	12 months	15 months	18 months	19–23 months	2–3 years	4–6 years
Hepatitis B	HepB	HepB			HepB						
Rotavirus			RV	RV	RV						
Diphtheria, Tetanus, Pertussis			DTaP	DTaP	DTaP		DTaP				DTaP
Haemophilus influenzae type b			Hib	Hib	Hib	Hib					
Pneumococcal			PCV	PCV	PCV	PCV				PPSV	
Inactivated Poliovirus			IPV	IPV		IPV					IPV
Influenza						Influenza (Yearly)					
Measles, Mumps, Rubella						MMR					MMR
Varicella						Varicella					Varicella
Hepatitis A						HepA (2 doses)				HepA Series	
Meningococcal										MCV4	

■ Range of recommended ages for all children
■ Range of recommended ages for certain high-risk groups

FIGURE 2.4-4. Recommended vaccinations for children 0–6 years of age. (Reproduced with permission from the Centers for Disease Control and Prevention, Atlanta, GA, www.cdc.gov/vaccines/recs/schedules/child-schedule.htm. Data from 2011.)

■ Live vaccines should not be administered to immunosuppressed patients. They are also contraindicated in pregnant women owing to a theoretical risk of maternal-fetal transmission. A possible exception to this rule can be some asymptomatic HIV/AIDS patients who may be candidates for the MMR vaccine.

BEHAVIORAL COUNSELING

In offering counsel, physicians should tailor their education and suggestions to the individual patient as well as to his or her **stage of change** (see Table 2.4-3).

Vaccine ▼ Age ▶	7–10 years	11–12 years	13–18 years
Tetanus, Diphtheria, Pertussis		Tdap	Tdap
Human Papillomavirus		HPV (3 doses)(females)	HPV Series
Meningococcal	MCV4	MCV4	MCV4
Influenza	Influenza (Yearly)		
Pneumococcal	Pneumococcal		
Hepatitis A	HepA Series		
Hepatitis B	Hep B Series		
Inactivated Poliovirus	IPV Series		
Measles, Mumps, Rubella	MMR Series		
Varicella	Varicella Series		

■ Range of recommended ages for all children
■ Range of recommended ages for catch-up immunization
■ Range of recommended ages for certain high-risk groups

FIGURE 2.4-5. Recommended vaccinations for children 7–18 years of age. (Reproduced with permission from the Centers for Disease Control and Prevention, Atlanta, GA, www.cdc.gov/vaccines/recs/schedules/child-schedule.htm. Data from 2011.)

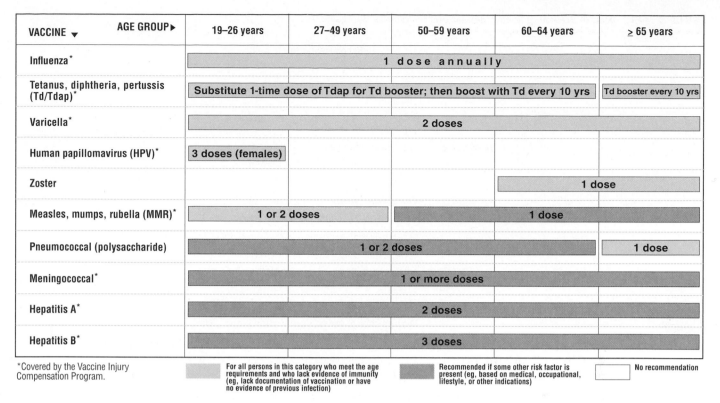

VACCINE ▼ AGE GROUP ▶	19–26 years	27–49 years	50–59 years	60–64 years	≥ 65 years
Influenza*	1 dose annually				
Tetanus, diphtheria, pertussis (Td/Tdap)*	Substitute 1-time dose of Tdap for Td booster; then boost with Td every 10 yrs				Td booster every 10 yrs
Varicella*	2 doses				
Human papillomavirus (HPV)*	3 doses (females)				
Zoster				1 dose	
Measles, mumps, rubella (MMR)*	1 or 2 doses		1 dose		
Pneumococcal (polysaccharide)	1 or 2 doses				1 dose
Meningococcal*	1 or more doses				
Hepatitis A*	2 doses				
Hepatitis B*	3 doses				

*Covered by the Vaccine Injury Compensation Program.

For all persons in this category who meet the age requirements and who lack evidence of immunity (eg, lack documentation of vaccination or have no evidence of previous infection)

Recommended if some other risk factor is present (eg, based on medical, occupational, lifestyle, or other indications)

No recommendation

FIGURE 2.4-6. Recommended vaccinations for adults. (Reproduced with permission from the Centers for Disease Control and Prevention, Atlanta, GA, www.cdc.gov/vaccines/recs/schedules/adult-schedule.htm. Data from 2011.)

Screening Recommendations

Tables 2.4-4 and 2.4-5 outline recommended health care screening measures by gender and age.

TABLE 2.4-3. Stages of Change in Behavioral Counseling

STAGE OF CHANGE	CHARACTERIZATION	EXAMPLE
Precontemplation	Denial or ignorance of the problem.	A 51-year-old smoker has not even thought about cessation.
Contemplation	Ambivalence or conflicted emotions; assessing benefits and barriers to change.	A 43-year-old crack cocaine addict considers treatment for her addiction.
Preparation	Experimenting with small changes; collecting information about change.	A 28-year-old heroin addict visits his doctor to ask questions about quitting.
Action	Taking direct action toward achieving a goal.	A 33-year-old enters a rehabilitation facility for treatment of addiction to prescription narcotics.
Maintenance	Maintaining a new behavior; avoiding temptation.	A 41-year-old continues to visit Alcoholics Anonymous meetings to gain support and reinforcement against relapse.

TABLE 2.4-4. Health Screening Recommendations for Women by Age

	RECOMMENDATION		
AGE	CARDIOVASCULAR	BREAST/REPRODUCTIVE	OTHER
19–39	BP screening at least once every 2 years. Cholesterol screening starting at age 20.	Discuss clinical breast examination with physician or nurse. Pap test every 2 years starting at age 21; then every 3 years for women ≥ 30. Pelvic exam yearly starting at age 21; chlamydia test yearly until age 24 if sexually active. Women ≥ 25 should be tested only if there is an ↑ risk. HIV test at least once to ascertain status.	N/A
40–49	BP screening at least once every 2 years. Discuss cholesterol screening with physician or nurse.	Discuss clinical breast examination with physician or nurse. Pap test every 3 years. Pelvic examination yearly; chlamydia test if the patient has new or multiple partners. HIV test at least once to ascertain status.	**Diabetes:** Blood glucose or HbA$_{1c}$ screening starting at age 45 and then every 3 years.
50–64	BP screening at least once every 2 years. Discuss cholesterol screening with physician or nurse.	Mammogram every 2 years. Discuss clinical breast examination with physician or nurse. Pap test every 3 years. Pelvic exam yearly; chlamydia test if the patient has new or multiple partners. HIV test at least once to ascertain status.	**Diabetes:** Blood glucose or HbA$_{1c}$ screening every 3 years. **Bone:** Discuss bone mineral density (BMD) test with physician or nurse. **Colorectal:** Discuss which test is best with physician or nurse.
≥ 65	BP screening at least once every 2 years. Discuss cholesterol screening with physician or nurse.	Mammogram every 2 years. Discuss clinical breast examination with physician or nurse. Discuss Pap test with physician or nurse. Pelvic examination yearly; chlamydia test if the patient has new or multiple partners. Discuss HIV test with physician or nurse.	**Diabetes:** Blood glucose or HbA$_{1c}$ screening every 3 years. **Bone:** BMD test at least once. **Colorectal:** Discuss which test is best with physician or nurse.

(Adapted with permission from the U.S. Department of Health and Human Services, Washington, DC, www.womenshealth.gov/pub/women.cfm.)

TABLE 2.4-5. Health Screening Recommendations for Men by Age

	RECOMMENDATION		
AGE	CARDIOVASCULAR	REPRODUCTIVE	OTHER
19–39	BP screening at least once every 2 years. Cholesterol screening starting at age 20.	Discuss testicular examination with physician or nurse. Both partners should be tested for STDs, including HIV, before initiating sexual intercourse.	N/A
40–49	BP screening at least once every 2 years. Discuss cholesterol screening with physician or nurse.	Discuss DRE and PSA with physician or nurse. Discuss testicular examination with physician or nurse. HIV test at least once to ascertain status.	**Diabetes:** Blood glucose or HbA$_{1c}$ screening starting at age 45 and then every 3 years.
50–64	BP screening at least once every 2 years. Discuss cholesterol screening with physician or nurse.	Discuss DRE and PSA with physician or nurse. Discuss testicular examination with physician or nurse. HIV test at least once to ascertain status.	**Diabetes:** Blood glucose or HbA$_{1c}$ screening every 3 years. **Colorectal:** Fecal occult blood test (FOBT) yearly; flexible sigmoidoscopy every 5 years or colonoscopy every 10 years.
≥ 65	BP screening at least once every 2 years. Discuss cholesterol screening with physician or nurse.	Discuss DRE and PSA with physician or nurse. Discuss testicular examination with physician or nurse. Discuss HIV test with physician.	**Diabetes:** Blood glucose or HbA$_{1c}$ screening every 3 years. **Colorectal:** FOBT yearly (patients > 75 should discuss with physician); flexible sigmoidoscopy every 5 years or colonoscopy every 10 years (patients > 75 should discuss with physician).

(Adapted with permission from the U.S. Department of Health and Human Services, Washington, DC, www.womenshealth.gov/pub/women.cfm.)

Causes of Death

The leading cause of cancer mortality in the United States is lung cancer. Prostate and breast cancers are the most prevalent cancers in men and women, respectively, with lung and colorectal cancers ranking second and third most common in both sexes. Table 2.4-6 lists the principal causes of death in the United States by age group.

Reportable Diseases

By law, disease reporting is mandated at the state level, and the list of diseases that must be reported to public health authorities varies slightly by state. The CDC has a list of nationally notifiable diseases that states voluntarily report to the CDC. These diseases include but are not limited to those listed in Table 2.4-7.

Q

A hypothetical study finds a ⊕ association between poor sleep habits and the risk of Parkinson's disease. The relative risk is 10 and the *p*-value is 0.4. How do you interpret these results?

TABLE 2.4-6.   Leading Causes of Death by Gender

Rank	Men	Women
1	Heart disease (26.3%)	Heart disease (25.8%)
2	Cancer (24.1%)	Cancer (22%)
3	Unintentional injuries (6.6%)	Stroke (6.7%)
4	Chronic lower respiratory diseases (4.9%)	Chronic lower respiratory diseases (5.3%)
5	Stroke (4.5%)	Alzheimer's disease (4.2%)
6	Diabetes (3%)	Unintentional injuries (3.5%)
7	Suicide (2.2%)	Diabetes (3%)
8	Influenza and pneumonia (2.1%)	Influenza and pneumonia (2.5%)
9	Kidney disease (1.8%)	Kidney disease (1.9%)
10	Alzheimer's disease (1.8%)	Septicemia (1.5%)

(Adapted with permission from the Centers for Disease Control and Prevention, Atlanta, GA, www.cdc.gov/men/lcod/ and www.cdc.gov/women/lcod/. Data from 2006.)

TABLE 2.4-7.   Common Reportable Diseases

Disease Category	Examples
STDs	HIV, AIDS, syphilis, gonorrhea, chlamydia, chancroid, HCV.
Tick-borne disease	Lyme disease, ehrlichiosis, Rocky Mountain spotted fever.
Potential bioweapons	Anthrax, smallpox, plague.
Vaccine-preventable disease	Diphtheria, tetanus, pertussis, measles, mumps, rubella, polio, varicella, HAV, HBV, *H influenzae* (invasive), meningococcal disease.
Water-/food-borne disease	Cholera, giardiasis, *Legionella*, listeriosis, botulism, shigellosis, shiga toxin–producing *E coli*, salmonellosis, trichinellosis, typhoid.
Zoonoses	Tularemia, psittacosis, brucellosis, rabies.
Miscellaneous	TB, leprosy, toxic shock syndrome, SARS, West Nile virus, vancomycin-resistant *S aureus* (VRSA), coccidioidomycosis, cryptosporidiosis. Methicillin-resistant *S aureus* (MRSA) is reportable in several states.

A

There is **not** sufficient evidence to reject the null hypothesis, and therefore there is insufficient evidence to support an association between poor sleep habits and the risk of Parkinson's disease. Remember that the null hypothesis always assumes that there is no association between the exposure and outcome variables. If the *p*-value is > 0.05, then you cannot reject the null hypothesis.

ETHICS AND LEGAL ISSUES

General Principles

- **Respect for autonomy:** Clinicians are obligated to respect patients as individuals and to honor their preferences. **Example:** A surgeon presents the risks and benefits of tumor resection to her patient before consent is given to proceed with the procedure.
- **Beneficence:** Physicians have a responsibility to act in the patient's best interest. As a fiduciary, the physician stands in a special relationship of trust and responsibility to patients. Respect for patient autonomy may conflict with beneficence. **Example:** An elderly woman is adamant that she does not want to go to a rehabilitation facility and thus refuses amputation of a potentially gangrenous foot. The procedure is necessary to prevent life-threatening complications. The physician has a responsibility to recommend what is in the patient's best interest.
- **Nonmaleficence:** "Do no harm." All medical interventions involve benefits and risks, and the physician should avoid recommending treatments where the risks are high and the benefits are negligible, remote, or improbable. Sometimes harm cannot be averted, but the benefits of an intervention outweigh the harms and risks. **Example:** A surgeon declines to perform a procedure because she thinks the patient will die intraoperatively.
- **Justice:** With regard to individual patients, fairness is expressed as the notion that similar persons should be treated similarly. Health care is an important resource, and access to quality health care gives individuals a greater chance for a healthy and productive life. Fair distribution of this resource is an ongoing challenge for health policy and in the clinical arena.

Informed Consent

- Defined as willing and voluntary acceptance of a medical intervention by a patient after adequate discussion with a physician about the **nature** of the intervention along with its **indications, risks, benefits,** and potential **alternatives** (including no treatment).
- **Patients may change their minds at any time.**
- Informed consent is required for significant procedures unless:
    - Emergency treatment is required. **Examples:** An unconscious patient presents with cerebral edema after a motor vehicle collision, or a patient without previously indicated DNR/DNI status undergoes cardiac arrest.
    - Patients lack decision-making capacity (consent is still required but must be obtained from a surrogate decision maker). When possible, assent should be obtained from the patient lacking capacity. **Examples:** Patients may present with dementia or significant psychiatric disturbances. Minors generally require surrogate decision makers until they demonstrate adequate decision-making capacity or are of legal age.

BRAIN of informed consent:

Benefits
Risks
Alternatives
Indications
Nature

KEY FACT

In general, it is ethically acceptable for a physician to honor a pregnant woman's refusal of treatment directed toward the fetus if the treatment poses a significant risk of harm to the woman. Physicians should not harm one patient in order to benefit another.

Minors

In general, minors (persons < 18 years of age) cannot consent for their own medical treatment and require parents or guardians to consent on their behalf, except in the following situations:

- **Life-threatening emergencies** when parents cannot be contacted.
- **Legal emancipation:** Emancipated minors do not require parental consent for medical care. Minors are emancipated if they are married, are in

the armed services, or are financially independent of their parents and have sought legal emancipation.

■ **Sexually transmitted infections and substance abuse treatment:** Rules concerning contraception, pregnancy, and abortion services and treatment for drug and alcohol dependency vary across the United States. Some states leave the decision of informing parents about adolescent use of confidential services to the physician based on the best interest of the patient; other states limit disclosure.

■ **Refusal of treatment:** A parent has the right to refuse treatment for his/her child as long as those decisions do not pose a serious threat to the child's well-being (eg, refusing immunizations is not considered a serious threat). If a parental decision is not in the best interest of the child, a physician may provide treatment against parental wishes. In emergent situations, if withholding treatment jeopardizes the child's safety, treatment can be initiated on the basis of legal precedent. **Example:** A physician provides blood transfusion to save the life of a 6-year-old child seriously injured in a motor vehicle collision despite parental requests to withhold such a measure.

Competence and Decision-Making Capacity

■ **Competence:** Refers to a person's **global and legal capacity to make decisions** and be held accountable in a court of law. Competence is assessed by the courts and is distinct from the term *decision-making capacity*.

■ **Decision-making capacity:** A medical term that refers to the ability of a patient to understand relevant information, appreciate the severity of the medical situation and its consequences, communicate a choice, and deliberate rationally about one's values in relation to the decision being made. This can be **assessed by the physician.**

■ Decision-making capacity is best understood as varying with the complexity of the decision involved. **Example:** The level of capacity needed for a decision about liver transplantation is different from that needed to choose between 2 types of pain medication for fracture-related pain.

■ Incompetent patients, as assessed by the courts, or temporarily incapacitated patients may still be able to provide assent or dissent for treatment. However, the need to treat supersedes the dissent of an incapacitated patient in emergency situations. **Example:** An extremely hypertensive patient with altered mental status who refuses treatment must receive antihypertensive therapy, as this constitutes a medical emergency.

■ In general, patients who have decision-making capacity have the right to refuse or discontinue treatment. **Example:** Jehovah's Witnesses can refuse blood products.

■ A patient's decision to refuse treatment can be overruled if the choice endangers the health and welfare of others. **Example:** A patient with active TB must undergo antibiotic treatment because not treating would pose a public health threat.

End-of-Life Issues

WRITTEN ADVANCE DIRECTIVES

■ **Living will:** Addresses a patient's wishes to maintain, withhold, or withdraw life-sustaining treatment in the event of terminal disease or a persistent vegetative state. **DNR** (do not resuscitate) and **DNI** (do not intubate) orders are based on patient preferences regarding CPR and intubation only.

KEY FACT

Patients with psychiatric illness can still give consent if their decision-making capacity is intact.

KEY FACT

In the absence of a living will or DPOAHC, the **Spouse CHIPS** in **F**or the patient: **Spouse, CHI**ldren, **P**arent, **S**ibling, **F**riend.

Q **1**

A 47-year-old male is diagnosed with pancreatic cancer. His diagnosis and treatment options are discussed, but the patient refuses any intervention. He states that he would like to go home to his wife and children to die peacefully. What is the most appropriate next step in management?

Q **2**

A 5-year-old girl with hydrocephalus needs another revision of her ventriculoperitoneal shunt. There are no satisfactory alternative options available to relieve her symptoms. Her father consents but her mother refuses, arguing that she has been through enough procedures in her young life. What is the most appropriate next step in management?

Q **3**

A 51-year-old male is brought to the ER after he was struck by a motor vehicle. He is unresponsive and in need of emergent surgery. His wife and children cannot be reached. What is the most appropriate next step in treatment?

- **Durable power of attorney for health care (DPOAHC):** Legally designates a surrogate health care decision maker if a patient lacks decision-making capacity. **More flexible than a living will.** Surrogates should make decisions consistent with the person's stated wishes.
- If no living will or DPOAHC exists, decisions should be made by close family members (spouse, adult children, parents, and adult siblings) or friends, in that order.

WITHDRAWAL OF CARE

- Patients and their decision makers have the right to forego or withdraw life-sustaining treatment. Nevertheless, physicians should seek to understand patients and their reasons for refusing beneficial treatments.
- **No ethical distinction is made between *withholding* a treatment and *withdrawing* a treatment because a patient may choose to refuse an intervention either *before* or *after* it is initiated.** This may include ventilation, fluids, nutrition, and medications such as antibiotics.
- If the intent is to relieve suffering and medications administered are titrated for that purpose, it is considered ethical to provide palliative treatment to relieve pain and suffering even if it may hasten a patient's death. **Example:** A physician may prescribe an ↑ dose of an opioid analgesic to a patient who is expected to die within a day, even though it may suppress respiration and hasten death.

EUTHANASIA AND PHYSICIAN-ASSISTED SUICIDE

- **Euthanasia** is the administration of a lethal agent with the intent to end life.
  - It is opposed by the AMA Code of Medical Ethics and is **illegal in all states.**
  - Patients who request euthanasia should be evaluated for inadequate pain control and comorbid depression.
- **Physician-assisted suicide** (also known as physician aid-in-dying) is prescribing a lethal agent to a patient who will self-administer it to end his/her own life. This is currently illegal except in the states of Oregon, Washington, and Montana.

FUTILE TREATMENT

Physicians are not ethically obligated to provide treatment and may refuse a patient's or family member's request for further intervention on the grounds of futility under any of the following circumstances:

- There is no evidence or pathophysiologic rationale for the treatment.
- The intervention has already failed.
- Maximal intervention is currently failing.
- Treatment will not achieve the goals of care.

Disclosure

FULL DISCLOSURE

- Patients have a right to know about their medical status, prognosis, and treatment options (full disclosure). They have the legal right to obtain copies of their medical records.

- A patient's family cannot require that a physician withhold information from the patient without the knowledge and consent of the patient.
- A physician may withhold information only if the patient requests not to be told, or perhaps in the rare and controversial case in which a physician determines that disclosure would cause severe and immediate harm to the patient (**therapeutic privilege**).

MEDICAL ERRORS

- **Physicians are obligated to inform patients of mistakes made in their medical treatment.**
- If the cause of a specific error or series of errors is not known, the physician should communicate this with the family promptly and maintain contact with the patient as investigations reveal more facts.

CLINICAL RESEARCH

- Physicians are obligated to inform patients considering involvement in a clinical research protocol about the purpose of the research study and the entire study design as it will affect the patient's treatment. This includes the possible risks, benefits, and alternatives to the research protocol.
- An informed consent form approved by the overseeing research institutional review board (IRB) must be completed for participation in any clinical research protocol, describing the possible risks and benefits of involvement in the research study.

Confidentiality

- Information disclosed by a patient to his/her physician and information about a patient's medical condition are confidential and cannot be divulged to anyone not directly involved in the patient's care without expressed patient consent, with few exceptions (described below).
- A patient may waive the obligation of the physician to protect confidentiality (eg, with insurance companies), preferably by way of written consent.
- It is ethically and legally necessary to override confidentiality in the following situations:
  - **Patient intent to commit a violent crime (Tarasoff decision):** Physicians have a **duty to protect** the intended victim through reasonable means (eg, warn the victim, notify police).
  - Suicidal patients.
  - Child abuse/neglect and elder mistreatment.
  - Reportable infectious diseases (duty to warn public officials and identifiable people at risk). It is normally best to encourage patients themselves to inform loved ones who are at risk for contracting the illness.
  - Gunshot and knife wounds (duty to notify the police).
  - Impaired automobile drivers. Currently, only 6 states have mandatory physician reporting laws. **Example:** A patient begins to drive 1 week after hospitalization for seizures, although the department of motor vehicles in his state requires that licensed drivers be without seizures for at least 3 months.

KEY FACT

Mandatory reporting of intimate-partner violence is controversial and varies by state; regardless of location, physicians should document the encounter, offer support, and have resources available for assistance.

KEY FACT

Potential signs of elder mistreatment:
- Cuts, bruises, pressure ulcers, burns
- Uncommon fractures
- Malnutrition or dehydration
- Anogenital injury or infection
- Evidence of poor caretaking

KEY FACT

Signs of suspected child abuse:
- History given is not consistent with injury
- Subdural hematomas
- Retinal hemorrhages
- Spiral, bucket-handle, or rib fractures
- Injuries in different stages of healing
- Unusual child or parental behavior

MNEMONIC

Overriding confidentiality—

WAIT a SEC before letting a dangerous patient go!

Wounds
Automobile-driving impairment
Infectious disease
Tarasoff—violent crimes
Suicide
Elder mistreatment
Child abuse

A 35-year-old female visits a primary care physician after hurting her wrist. Physical examination reveals circumferential bruises of her wrist, neck, and arms. The patient admits that the injuries were inflicted by her husband. What is the most appropriate next step in management?

Conflict of Interest

- Occurs when physicians find themselves having a personal interest in a given situation that influences their professional obligations. **Example:** A physician may own stock in a pharmaceutical company (financial interest) that produces a drug he is prescribing to his patient (patient care interest).
- Physicians should disclose existing conflicts of interest to affected parties (eg, patients, institutions, audiences of journal articles or scientific meetings).

Malpractice

- The essential elements of a civil suit under negligence include the **4 D's:**
  - The physician has a **Duty** to the patient.
  - **Dereliction** of duty occurs.
  - There is **Damage** to the patient.
  - Dereliction is the **Direct** cause of damage.
- Unlike a criminal suit, in which the burden of proof is "beyond a reasonable doubt," the burden of proof in a malpractice suit is "a preponderance of the evidence."

A

Offer support and acknowledge the courage it takes to discuss abuse. Assess the safety of the woman and of any children involved, introduce the concept of an emergency plan, and encourage the use of community resources.

GASTROINTESTINAL

Esophageal Disease

DYSPHAGIA/ODYNOPHAGIA

Difficulty swallowing (dysphagia) or pain with swallowing (odynophagia) due to abnormalities of the oropharynx or esophagus.

HISTORY/PE

- The presentation of dysphagia varies according to location:
  - **Oropharyngeal dysphagia:** Usually involves aspiration of food into the lungs **(liquids more than solids)**, leading to coughing or choking. Causes can be neurologic or muscular and include stroke, Parkinson's disease, myasthenia gravis, prolonged intubation, and Zenker's diverticula.
  - **Esophageal dysphagia:** If due to obstruction, usually involves **solids more than liquids** (strictures, Schatzki rings, webs, carcinoma) and is progressive. If due to a motility disorder (achalasia, scleroderma, esophageal spasm), usually presents with **both liquid and solid dysphagia.**
- Examine for masses (eg, goiter, tumor) and anatomic defects.

DIAGNOSIS

- **Oropharyngeal dysphagia:** Video fluoroscopy.
- **Esophageal dysphagia:** Barium swallow (aka esophagram) followed by endoscopy, manometry, and/or pH monitoring. If an obstructive lesion is suspected, proceed directly to endoscopy with biopsy.
- **Odynophagia:** Upper endoscopy.

TREATMENT

Etiology dependent.

INFECTIOUS ESOPHAGITIS

Table 2.6-1 outlines the etiology, diagnosis, and treatment of infectious esophagitis.

DIFFUSE ESOPHAGEAL SPASM

- A motility disorder in which normal peristalsis is periodically interrupted by high-amplitude **nonperistaltic** contractions. Also known as **nutcracker esophagus** (see Figure 2.6-2A).
- **Hx/PE:** Presents with chest pain, dysphagia, and odynophagia. **Often precipitated by ingestion of hot or cold liquids; relieved by nitroglycerin.**
- **Dx:** Barium swallow may show a **corkscrew-shaped esophagus.** Esophageal manometry reveals high-amplitude, simultaneous contractions.
- **Tx:** Nitrates and calcium channel blockers (CCBs) for symptomatic relief; surgery (esophageal myotomy) for severe, incapacitating symptoms.

ACHALASIA

- A motility disorder of the esophagus characterized by **impaired relaxation of the lower esophageal sphincter (LES)** and **loss of peristalsis** in the distal two-thirds of the esophagus. Results from degeneration of the inhibitory neurons in the myenteric (Auerbach's) plexus.

KEY FACT

Esophageal webs are associated with iron deficiency anemia and glossitis (Plummer-Vinson syndrome).

KEY FACT

Candidal esophagitis is an AIDS-defining illness.

KEY FACT

The musculature of the upper third of the esophagus is skeletal, whereas that of the lower two-thirds is smooth muscle.

TABLE 2.6-1. Causes of Infectious Esophagitis

Etiologic Agent	Exam Findings	Upper Endoscopy	Treatment
Candida albicans	Oral thrush (see Figure 2.6-1).	Yellow-white plaques adherent to the mucosa.	Nystatin oral suspension or fluconazole PO.
HSV	Oral ulcers.	Small, deep ulcerations; multinucleated giant cells with intranuclear inclusions on biopsy + Tzanck smear.	Acyclovir IV.
CMV	Retinitis, colitis.	Large, superficial ulcerations; intranuclear and intracytoplasmic inclusions on biopsy.	Ganciclovir IV.

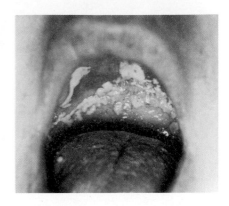

FIGURE 2.6-1. Oropharyngeal candidiasis. Multiple thick, yellowish-white plaques are seen on the palate and buccal mucosa. (Reproduced with permission from Kantarjian HM et al. *MD Anderson Manual of Medical Oncology,* 1st ed. New York: McGraw-Hill, 2006, Fig. 37-1.)

- **Hx/PE:** Common symptoms include progressive dysphagia, chest pain, regurgitation of undigested food, weight loss, and nocturnal cough.
- **Dx:**
  - Barium swallow reveals esophageal **dilation with a "bird's beak" tapering** of the distal esophagus (see Figure 2.6-2B).
  - Manometry shows ↑ **resting LES pressure, incomplete LES relaxation** upon swallowing, and ↓ **peristalsis** in the body of the esophagus.
  - Endoscopy is indicated to rule out mechanical causes of obstruction.
- **Tx:** Nitrates, CCBs, or endoscopic injection of botulinum toxin into the LES may provide short-term relief of symptoms. Pneumatic balloon dilation and surgical (Heller) myotomy are definitive treatment options.

 KEY FACT

Beware: malignancy may mimic achalasia (pseudoachalasia).

ESOPHAGEAL DIVERTICULA

- Diverticula can be present in any location. **Zenker's diverticulum** is defined as cervical outpouching through the cricopharyngeus muscle.
- **Hx/PE:** Presents with chest pain, dysphagia, halitosis, and regurgitation of undigested food.
- **Dx:** Barium swallow will demonstrate outpouchings.
- **Tx:** If symptomatic, treat with surgical excision of the diverticulum. For Zenker's diverticulum, **myotomy** of the cricopharyngeus is required to relieve the high-pressure zone.

ESOPHAGEAL CANCER

- **Squamous cell carcinoma (SCC)** is the **most common type of esophageal cancer worldwide,** whereas **adenocarcinoma is most prevalent in the United States, Europe, and Australia.**
- Risk factors include the following:
  - **SCC:** Alcohol and tobacco use.
  - **Adenocarcinoma:** Barrett's esophagus (columnar metaplasia of the distal esophagus 2° to chronic GERD).

KEY FACT

Squamous cell esophageal cancer is associated with tobacco and alcohol use.

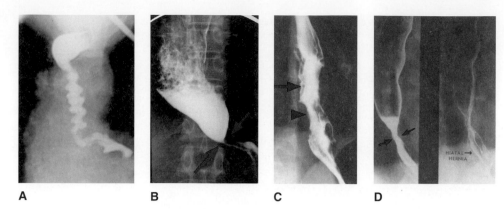

FIGURE 2.6-2. Esophageal disease on barium esophagram. (A) Esophageal spasm.
(B) Achalasia. Note the dilated esophagus tapering to a "bird's beak" narrowing (arrows) at the
LES. **(C)** Barrett's esophagus with adenocarcinoma. Note the nodular mucosa of Barrett's esophagus (arrow) and the raised filling defect (arrowhead) representing adenocarcinoma in this patient.
(D) Peptic stricture (arrows) 2° to GERD above a hiatal hernia (right). (Image A reproduced with permission from USMLERx.com. Image B reproduced with permission from Doherty GM. *Current Diagnosis & Treatment: Surgery*, 13th ed.
New York: McGraw-Hill, 2010, Fig. 20-5. Images C and D reproduced with permission from Chen MY et al. *Basic Radiology*, 1st ed.
New York: McGraw-Hill, 2004, Figs. 10-19 and 10-14.)

KEY FACT

Esophageal cancer metastasizes early because the esophagus lacks a serosa.

KEY FACT

SCC of the esophagus tends to occur in the upper and middle thirds of the esophagus, whereas adenocarcinoma occurs in the lower third.

KEY FACT

GERD can mimic cough-variant asthma.

KEY FACT

Patients with GERD should avoid caffeine, alcohol, chocolate, garlic, onions, mints, and nicotine.

- **Hx/PE:** Progressive dysphagia, initially to solids and later to liquids, is common. Weight loss, odynophagia, GERD, GI bleeding, and vomiting are also seen.
- **Dx:** Barium study shows narrowing of the esophagus with an irregular border protruding into the lumen (see Figure 2.6-2C). EGD with biopsy confirms the diagnosis. CT and endoscopic ultrasound are used for staging.
- **Tx:** Chemoradiation and surgical resection are first-line treatment. Resection is also indicated in cases of high-grade Barrett's dysplasia. Has a poor prognosis.

GASTROESOPHAGEAL REFLUX DISEASE (GERD)

Symptomatic reflux of gastric contents into the esophagus, most commonly from **transient LES relaxation.** Can also result from an incompetent LES, gastroparesis, or hiatal hernia.

HISTORY/PE

- Patients present with **heartburn** that commonly occurs 30–90 minutes **after a meal, worsens with reclining,** and often improves with antacids, sitting, or standing.
- Sour taste ("water brash"), a globus sensation (a sensation of a lump in the throat), unexplained cough, and morning hoarseness are also common.
- **Examination is usually normal** unless a systemic disease (eg, scleroderma) is present.

DIAGNOSIS

- Primarily a clinical diagnosis.
- An empiric trial of lifestyle modification and medical treatment is often attempted first. Studies may include barium swallow (to look for hiatal hernia and demonstrate reflux; see Figure 2.6-2D), esophageal manometry, and 24-hour pH monitoring.
- EGD with biopsies should be performed in patients whose symptoms are unresponsive to initial empiric therapy, long standing (to rule out Barrett's

esophagus and adenocarcinoma; see Figure 2.6-3), or associated with alarm symptoms (eg, blood in the stool, weight loss, dysphagia/odynophagia).

TREATMENT

- **Lifestyle:** Weight loss, head-of-bed elevation, small but frequent meals, and avoidance of nocturnal meals and substances that ↓ LES tone.
- **Pharmacologic:** Start with **antacids** in patients with mild, intermittent symptoms; use **H_2 receptor antagonists** (cimetidine, ranitidine) or **PPIs** (omeprazole, lansoprazole) in patients with chronic and frequent symptoms. PPIs are preferred for severe or erosive disease.
- **Surgical: Nissen fundoplication** may offer significant relief for refractory or severe disease.

COMPLICATIONS

Erosive esophagitis, esophageal peptic stricture, aspiration pneumonia, upper GI bleeding, **Barrett's esophagus.**

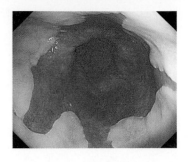

FIGURE 2.6-3. Barrett's esophagus on upper endoscopy. Shown is an irregular Z line (squamocolumnar junction between the esophagus and stomach) due to columnar metaplasia of the lower esophagus. (Reproduced with permission from Fauci AS et al. *Harrison's Principles of Internal Medicine,* 17th ed. New York: McGraw-Hill, 2008, Fig. 285-3A.)

HIATAL HERNIA

- Herniation of the stomach upward into the chest through the diaphragm. There are 3 common types:
  - **Sliding hiatal hernia (95%):** The gastroesophageal junction and a portion of the stomach are displaced above the diaphragm (see Figure 2.6-4A).
  - **Paraesophageal hiatal hernia (5%):** The gastroesophageal junction remains below the diaphragm, while the fundus herniates into the thorax (see Figure 2.6-4B).
  - **Mixed hiatal hernias** (rare).
- **Hx/PE:** May be asymptomatic. Patients with sliding hernias may present with GERD.
- **Dx:** Commonly an incidental finding on CXR; also frequently diagnosed by barium swallow or EGD.
- **Tx:**
  - **Sliding hernias:** Medical therapy and lifestyle modifications to ↓ GERD symptoms.

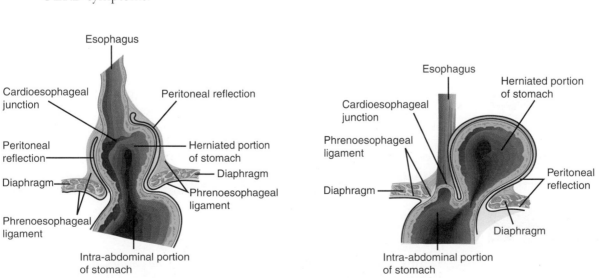

A **B**

FIGURE 2.6-4. Hiatal hernia. (A) Sliding hiatal hernia. (B) Paraesophageal hiatal hernia. (Reproduced with permission from Doherty GM. *Current Diagnosis & Treatment: Surgery,* 13th ed. New York: McGraw-Hill, 2010, Figs. 20-9 and 20-11.)

■ **Paraesophageal hernias:** Surgical gastropexy (attachment of the stomach to the rectus sheath and closure of the hiatus) is recommended to prevent gastric volvulus.

Disorders of the Stomach and Duodenum

GASTRITIS

Inflammation of the gastric mucosa. Subtypes are as follows:

■ **Acute gastritis:** Rapidly developing, superficial lesions that are often due to **NSAID** use, alcohol, *H pylori* infection, and stress from severe illness (eg, burns, CNS injury).
■ **Chronic gastritis:**
  ■ **Type A (10%):** Occurs in the fundus and is due to **autoantibodies to parietal cells.** Causes **pernicious anemia** and is associated with other autoimmune disorders. Associated with an ↑ risk of gastric adenocarcinoma and carcinoid tumors.
  ■ **Type B (90%):** Occurs in the antrum and may be caused by NSAID use or *H pylori* infection. Often asymptomatic, but associated with an ↑ risk of PUD and gastric cancer.

HISTORY/PE

Patients may be asymptomatic or may complain of epigastric pain, nausea, vomiting, hematemesis, or melena.

DIAGNOSIS

■ Upper endoscopy to visualize the gastric mucosa. A double-contrast upper GI series can also be used but is less sensitive than EGD.
■ *H pylori* infection can be detected by the **urease breath test,** serum IgG antibodies (which point to a history of exposure, not current infection), *H pylori* stool antigen (indicates current infection), or endoscopic biopsy.

TREATMENT

■ ↓ intake of exacerbating agents. Antacids, sucralfate, H_2 blockers, and/or PPIs may help.
■ Administer triple therapy (amoxicillin, clarithromycin, omeprazole) to treat *H pylori* infection unless the patient is penicillin allergic, in which case metronidazole should be substituted for amoxicillin.
■ Give prophylactic PPIs to patients at risk for stress ulcers (eg, ICU patients).

GASTRIC CANCER

■ A malignant tumor with a poor prognosis that is particularly common in Korea and Japan. Most are adenocarcinomas, which exhibit 2 morphologic types:
  ■ **Intestinal type:** Differentiated cancer that originates from the intestinal metaplasia of **gastric mucosal cells.** Risk factors include a diet high in nitrites and salt and low in fresh vegetables (antioxidants), *H pylori* colonization, and chronic gastritis.
  ■ **Diffuse type:** Undifferentiated cancer not associated with *H pylori* infection or chronic gastritis. Risk factors are unknown; signet ring cells on biopsy are characteristic.

KEY FACT

Type A gastritis is associated with pernicious anemia due to lack of intrinsic factor necessary for the absorption of vitamin B_{12}.

KEY FACT

Stress ulcers include Curling ulcers, which are associated with burn injuries, and Cushing ulcers, which are associated with traumatic brain injury.

KEY FACT

H pylori antibodies stay ⊕ even when the infection is cleared. Use the urease breath test or a repeat stool antigen as a test of cure.

KEY FACT

A gastric adenocarcinoma that metastasizes to the ovary is called a Krukenberg tumor.

KEY FACT

MALT (mucosa-associated lymphoid tissue) lymphoma is a rare gastric tumor that presents in patients with chronic *H pylori* infection. It is the only malignancy that can be cured with antibiotics. Treat with triple therapy.

- **Hx/PE:** Early-stage disease is usually asymptomatic but may be associated with indigestion and loss of appetite. Late-stage disease presents with abdominal pain, weight loss, and upper GI bleeding.
- **Dx:** Upper endoscopy with biopsy is necessary to rule out other etiologies and confirm the diagnosis.
- **Tx:** If detected early, treatment is surgical resection. Most patients present with late-stage, incurable disease. Five-year survival is < 10% for advanced disease.

PEPTIC ULCER DISEASE (PUD)

Although commonly thought to result from stress, PUD is now known to result from damage to the gastric or duodenal mucosa caused by impaired mucosal defense and/or ↑ acidic gastric contents. *H pylori* is the causative factor in > 90% of duodenal ulcers and 70% of gastric ulcers. Other risk factors include **corticosteroid, NSAID, alcohol,** and **tobacco use.** Males are affected more often than females.

HISTORY/PE

- Presents with chronic or periodic **dull, burning epigastric pain** that is often related to meals and can radiate to the back.
- Patients may also complain of nausea, hematemesis ("coffee-ground" emesis), or blood in the stool.
- Examination is usually normal but may reveal **epigastric tenderness** and ⊕ stool guaiac.
- Acute perforation presents with a rigid abdomen, rebound tenderness, and/or guarding.

DIAGNOSIS

- **Rule out perforation:**
  - **Gastric ulcers:** AXR reveals free air under the diaphragm (see Figure 2.6-5).
  - **Duodenal ulcers:** CT scan with contrast shows air in the retroperitoneal space. Order a CBC to detect GI bleeding.
- **Upper endoscopy** with biopsy to confirm and to rule out active bleeding or gastric adenocarcinoma (10% of gastric ulcers).
- *H pylori* testing.
- In recurrent or refractory cases, check serum gastrin levels to screen for Zollinger-Ellison syndrome.

TREATMENT

- **Acute management:**
  - If perforation is suspected, CT with IV contrast is indicated. If the diagnosis is confirmed, surgical laparotomy will likely be required. Carefully monitor BP.
  - Rule out active bleeding with rectal vault examination, NG lavage, and serial hematocrits. Monitor BP and treat with IV hydration, blood transfusion, and IV PPIs. Urgent EGD should be performed to control suspected bleeding.
- **Long-term management:**
  - Medical therapy is indicated to protect the mucosa, ↓ acid production, and eradicate *H pylori* infection.
    - For mild disease, treat with antacids, PPIs, or H₂ blockers.
    - Patients with *H pylori* infection should receive triple therapy.
    - Discontinue use of exacerbating agents.

KEY FACT

Gastric cancer may present with Virchow's node (an enlarged left supraclavicular lymph node).

KEY FACT

Stress is not a risk factor for PUD.

KEY FACT

After a meal, pain from a **G**astric ulcer is **G**reater, whereas **D**uodenal pain **D**ecreases.

KEY FACT

All gastric ulcers must be biopsied to rule out malignancy.

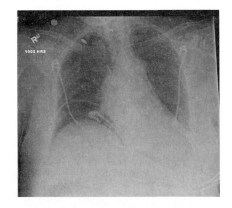

FIGURE 2.6-5. Pneumoperitoneum. Upright CXR reveals free air under the diaphragm. (Reproduced with permission from USMLERx.com.)

- Endoscopy with targeted biopsy is indicated in patients with symptoms refractory to medical therapy to rule out gastric cancer.
- Surgical therapy (eg, partial cell vagotomy) is indicated in severe cases.

COMPLICATIONS

Hemorrhage (posterior ulcers that erode into the gastroduodenal artery), gastric outlet obstruction, perforation, intractable pain.

ZOLLINGER-ELLISON SYNDROME

- A rare condition characterized by **gastrin-producing tumors** in the duodenum and/or pancreas that lead to oversecretion of gastrin.
- Oversecretion of gastrin ↑ gastric acid production, leading to recurrent or intractable **ulcers** in the stomach and duodenum (may occur more distally).
- In 20% of cases, gastrinomas are associated with multiple endocrine neoplasia (MEN) type 1.
- **Hx/PE:** Patients may present with unresponsive, recurrent **gnawing, burning abdominal pain** as well as with **diarrhea,** nausea, vomiting, fatigue, weakness, weight loss, and **GI bleeding.**
- **Dx:** ↑ fasting serum gastrin levels and ↑ gastrin with the administration of secretin are diagnostic; CT is indicated to characterize and stage disease.
- **Tx:**
  - Moderate- to high-dose PPIs often control symptoms.
  - Surgical resection of the gastrinoma after localization by CT or octreotide scan to identify suspected carcinoid tumors.

Disorders of the Small Bowel

DIARRHEA

Defined as the production of > **200 g of feces per day along with ↑ frequency or ↓ consistency of stool.** The most common mechanisms are malabsorption/maldigestive/osmotic, secretory, inflammatory/infectious, and ↑ motility (see also Table 2.6-2).

HISTORY/PE

- **Acute diarrhea:** Acute onset with a duration of < 2 weeks; usually infectious and self-limited.
  - Multiple pathogens may be responsible (see Table 2.6-2).
  - One of the most common causes of **pediatric diarrhea** is **rotavirus infection.**
- **Chronic diarrhea:** Insidious onset with a duration of > 4 weeks.
  - **Secretory:** Carcinoid tumors, VIPomas.
  - **Malabsorption/maldigestive/osmotic:** Bacterial overgrowth, pancreatic insufficiency, mucosal damage, lactose intolerance, celiac disease, laxative abuse, postsurgical short bowel syndrome.
  - **Inflammatory/infectious:** IBD.
  - **Increased motility:** IBS.

DIAGNOSIS

- For acute diarrhea, no further studies are indicated unless the patient has a high fever, bloody diarrhea, or diarrhea lasting > 4–5 days.

TABLE 2.6-2.   Causes of Infectious Diarrhea

INFECTIOUS AGENT	HISTORY	EXAM	COMMENTS	TREATMENT
Campylobacter	**The most common etiology of bacterial diarrhea.** Caused by ingestion of contaminated food or water. Affects young children and young adults; generally lasts 7–10 days.	Fecal RBCs and WBCs. Frequently presents with bloody diarrhea.	Rule out appendicitis and IBD.	Erythromycin.
Clostridium difficile	Associated with recent treatment with antibiotics (penicillins, quinolones, **clindamycin**). Affects hospitalized adult patients. **Watch for toxic megacolon.**	Presents with fever, abdominal pain, and possible systemic toxicity. Fecal RBCs and WBCs.	Most commonly causes colitis, but can involve the small bowel. Identify *C difficile* toxin in the stool. Sigmoidoscopy shows pseudomembranes.	**Cessation of the inciting antibiotic.** Treat with PO metronidazole or vancomycin; give IV metronidazole if the patient cannot tolerate PO.
Entamoeba histolytica	Caused by ingestion of contaminated food or water; look for a history of travel in developing countries. The incubation period can last up to 3 months.	Presents with severe abdominal pain and fever. Fecal RBCs and WBCs. Endoscopy shows "flask-shaped" ulcers.	Chronic amebic colitis mimics IBD.	Steroids can lead to fatal perforation. Treat with metronidazole.
E coli O157:H7	Caused by ingestion of contaminated food (raw meat). Affects children and the elderly; generally lasts 5–10 days.	Presents with severe abdominal pain, low-grade fever, and vomiting. Fecal RBCs and WBCs.	It is important to rule out GI bleed and ischemic colitis. Hemolytic-uremic syndrome (HUS) is a potential complication, primarily in children.	Avoid antibiotic or antidiarrheal therapy, which ↑ HUS risk.
Salmonella	Caused by ingestion of contaminated poultry or eggs. Affects young children and the elderly; generally lasts 2–5 days.	Presents with a prodromal headache, fever, myalgia, and abdominal pain. Fecal WBCs.	Sepsis is a concern, as 5–10% of patients become bacteremic. Sickle cell patients are susceptible to invasive disease leading to osteomyelitis.	Treat bacteremia or at-risk patients (eg, sickle cell patients) with oral quinolone or TMP-SMX.
Shigella	Extremely contagious; transmitted between people by the fecal-oral route. Affects young children and institutionalized patients.	Fecal RBCs and WBCs.	May lead to severe dehydration. Can also cause febrile seizures in the very young.	Treat with TMP-SMX to ↓ person-to-person spread.

KEY FACT

Organisms that cause watery diarrhea include *Vibrio cholerae*, rotavirus, *E coli* (ETEC), *Cryptosporidium,* and *Giardia.*

KEY FACT

Diarrhea after ingestion of raw eggs or dairy: think *Salmonella.*

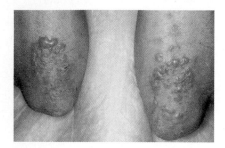

FIGURE 2.6-6. **Dermatitis herpetiformis.** Grouped, papulovesicular, pruritic skin lesions are shown. Lesions tend to be symmetrically located on the extensor surfaces of the elbows, knees, buttocks, and posterior scalp and are associated with celiac disease. (Reproduced with permission from Fauci AS et al. *Harrison's Principles of Internal Medicine,* 17th ed. New York: McGraw-Hill, 2008, Fig. 52-8.)

KEY FACT

The classic presentation of pellagra is the 4 D's: diarrhea, dementia, dermatitis, and death.

KEY FACT

Carcinoid tumors must metastasize to the liver in order to manifest with carcinoid syndrome.

- For chronic diarrhea, the history and physical examination are critical to narrowing the differential diagnosis. Additional studies include the following:
    - **Stool analysis:** Leukocytes, culture, *C difficile* toxin, and O&P.
    - **Sigmoidoscopy:** In patients with bloody diarrhea.

TREATMENT

- **Acute diarrhea:**
    - The most important treatment is oral rehydration.
    - Antibiotics do not shorten the course of illness and thus are not indicated (except in *C difficile* infection).
    - Symptomatic treatment includes antidiarrheal agents (eg, loperamide, bismuth salicylate). Avoid if the patient has high fever or bloody stools.
- **Chronic diarrhea:** Treatment is etiology specific.

MALABSORPTION/MALDIGESTION

- Inability to absorb macro- and/or micronutrients. Common etiologies include the following:
    - **Mucosal abnormalities:** Celiac disease (associated with dermatitis herpetiformis; see Figure 2.6-6), Whipple's disease, tropical sprue.
    - **Bile salt deficiency:** Bacterial overgrowth, ileal disease.
    - **Other:** Pancreatic insufficiency, short bowel syndrome.
- **Hx/PE:** Presents with **frequent, loose, watery stools** (carbohydrate malabsorption) and/or **pale, foul-smelling, bulky stools** (steatorrhea of fat maldigestion) associated with abdominal pain, **flatus, bloating,** weight loss, **nutritional deficiencies,** and fatigue.
- **Tx:** Etiology dependent. In severe cases, patients may require TPN, immunosuppressants, and anti-inflammatory medications.

LACTOSE INTOLERANCE

- Results from a **deficiency of lactase,** a brush-border enzyme that hydrolyzes lactose into glucose and galactose.
- Common among populations of African, Asian, and Native American descent.
- Transient lactose intolerance can occur after an acute episode of gastroenteritis.
- **Hx/PE:** Presents with **abdominal bloating, flatulence, cramping,** and **watery diarrhea following milk ingestion.**
- **Dx:** An empiric lactose-free diet that improves symptoms is highly suggestive of the diagnosis. **Hydrogen breath test** reveals ↑ hydrogen following the ingestion of lactose.
- **Tx:** Avoidance of dairy products; oral lactase enzyme replacement.

CARCINOID SYNDROME

- Due to the metastasis of **carcinoid tumors,** which most commonly arise from the ileum and appendix and produce serotonin. Prior to metastasis, most secreted hormones undergo first-pass metabolism by the liver and do not reach systemic circulation.
- **Hx/PE:** Cutaneous **flushing, diarrhea, abdominal cramps, wheezing,** and right-sided **cardiac valvular lesions** are the most common manifestations.
- **Dx:** High urine levels of the serotonin metabolite 5-HIAA are diagnostic. CT and In-111 octreotide scans are used to localize the tumor.
- **Tx:** Treatment includes **octreotide** and surgical resection.

IRRITABLE BOWEL SYNDROME (IBS)

An idiopathic functional disorder characterized by chronic, intermittent abdominal pain and changes in bowel habits. It is commonly diagnosed in women in their 20s to 30s but affects men and women of all ages. Half of all IBS patients who seek medical care have comorbid psychiatric disorders (eg, depression, anxiety, fibromyalgia).

HISTORY/PE

- Patients present with abdominal pain that is relieved by bowel movements, diarrhea and/or constipation, abdominal distention, and mucous stools. Symptoms often worsen with stress.
- IBS rarely awakens patients from sleep; vomiting, significant weight loss, and constitutional symptoms are uncommon.
- Examination is usually unremarkable.

DIAGNOSIS

- Exclude organic disorders such as IBD. The Rome III diagnostic criteria for IBS involve at least 3 months of episodic abdominal discomfort that is (1) relieved by defecation and (2) associated with a change in stool frequency or consistency.
- Tests to exclude other etiologies include CBC, TSH, electrolytes, stool cultures, abdominal films, barium contrast studies, and, rarely, colonoscopy with biopsy.

TREATMENT

- **Psychosocial:** Patients benefit from a strong patient-physician relationship. Physicians should offer reassurance and should not dismiss the symptoms.
- **Diet:** Fiber supplements (psyllium); exclude gas-producing foods.
- **Pharmacologic:** Symptomatic treatment with antispasmodics. Long-term medical therapy is usually not indicated.

SMALL BOWEL OBSTRUCTION (SBO)

Defined as blocked passage of bowel contents through the small bowel. Common etiologies include **adhesions** from prior abdominal surgery (60% of cases), **hernias** (10–20%), neoplasms (10–20%), intussusception, gallstone ileus, stricture due to IBD, and volvulus. The obstruction can be complete or partial:

- **Partial SBO:** Continued passage of flatus, but no stool.
- **Complete SBO:** No passage of flatus or stool (obstipation).

HISTORY/PE

- Patients experience crampy abdominal pain at 4- to 5-minute intervals.
- **Vomiting** typically follows the pain. In proximal obstruction, emesis is early, bilious, and nonfeculent; in distal obstruction, it is late and feculent.
- Abdominal examination often reveals distention, tenderness, prior surgical scars, or hernias.
- Hyperactive bowel sounds are characterized by **high-pitched tinkles** and **peristaltic rushes.**
- In prolonged obstruction, ischemic necrosis and bowel rupture are concerns. Patients present with peritonitis manifested by fever, hypotension, rebound tenderness, and tachycardia.

KEY FACT

The leading cause of SBO in children is hernia. The leading cause of SBO in adults is adhesions.

Q

A 53-year-old woman with a history of carcinoid tumor of the appendix (status post resection) presents to a local clinic with symmetric, dry, hyperpigmented skin lesions and persistent diarrhea. Her husband expresses concern that the patient does not seem to be herself anymore; he reports that she has been irritable, confused, and forgetful. What is the most likely diagnosis?

DIAGNOSIS

- Abdominal films demonstrate a **stepladder pattern of dilated small-bowel loops, air-fluid levels** (see Figure 2.6-7), and a paucity of gas in the colon.
- CBC may demonstrate **leukocytosis** if there is ischemia or necrosis of bowel.
- Labs often reveal **dehydration** and **metabolic alkalosis.** Lactic acidosis is a prognostic sign, as it suggests necrotic bowel.

TREATMENT

- Initial management involves fluid resuscitation.
- For partial obstruction, supportive care alone may be sufficient and should include NPO status, NG suction, IV hydration, correction of electrolyte abnormalities, and Foley catheterization to monitor fluid status.
- Exploratory laparotomy is indicated in cases of complete SBO, ischemic necrosis, or partial SBO symptoms lasting > 3 days without resolution.

ILEUS

Loss of peristalsis without structural obstruction. Risk factors include recent surgery/GI procedures, severe medical illness, immobility, hypokalemia or other electrolyte imbalances, hypothyroidism, diabetes mellitus (DM), and medications that slow GI motility (eg, anticholinergics, opioids).

HISTORY/PE

- Patients present with diffuse, constant abdominal discomfort, **nausea and vomiting,** and an **absence of flatus or bowel movements.**
- Examination may reveal diffuse tenderness, **abdominal distention,** and ↓ **or absent bowel sounds.**
- A **rectal examination is required** to rule out fecal impaction in elderly patients.

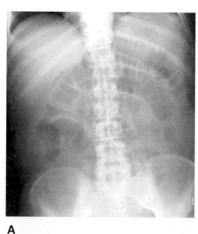
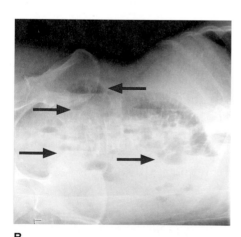

A **B**

FIGURE 2.6-7. **Small bowel obstruction.** (A) Supine abdominal radiograph shows dilated air-filled small bowel loops with relatively little gas in the colon. (B) Left lateral decubitus radiograph on the same patient demonstrates multiple air-fluid levels (arrows) at different levels. These are typical plain film findings of complete SBO. (Reproduced with permission from Doherty GM. *Current Diagnosis & Treatment: Surgery,* 13th ed. New York: McGraw-Hill, 2010, Fig. 29-5.)

DIAGNOSIS

- The clinical history must be considered in diagnosis.
- Abdominal films show **distended loops of small and large bowel,** with air seen throughout the colon and rectum (SBO has no air distal to the obstruction).

TREATMENT

- ↓ or discontinue the use of narcotics and any other drugs that reduce **bowel motility.**
- Temporarily ↓ or discontinue oral feeds.
- Initiate **NG suction/parenteral feeds** as necessary.
- Replete electrolytes as needed; hydrate with IV fluids.

> **KEY FACT**
>
> In ileus, there is air present throughout the small and large bowel on AXR.

MESENTERIC ISCHEMIA

Insufficient blood supply to the small intestine, resulting in ischemia and, potentially, necrosis. The 2 most common causes are as follows:

- **Acute arterial occlusion from thrombosis:** Most commonly occurs in the proximal SMA. The 1° risk factor is atherosclerosis.
- **Embolism:** Emboli most commonly originate in the heart. Risk factors include atrial fibrillation and stasis from a ↓ ejection fraction.

Other causes include nonocclusive arterial disease (low cardiac output, arteriolar vasospasm, atherosclerosis of mesenteric vessels) and venous thrombosis (due to hypercoagulable states).

HISTORY/PE

- Patients present with **severe abdominal pain out of proportion to the examination.**
- Patients may have a history of prior episodes of abdominal pain after eating ("intestinal angina"). If severe, this can lead to fear of eating and weight loss.
- Other symptoms may include nausea, vomiting, diarrhea, and bloody stools.
- Abdominal examination is often unremarkable until late in the disease course.

DIAGNOSIS

- Lab tests may show **leukocytosis, metabolic acidosis** with ↑ lactate, ↑ amylase, ↑ LDH, and ↑ CK.
- AXR and CT may reveal bowel wall edema ("thumbprinting") and air within the bowel wall (pneumatosis intestinalis).
- Mesenteric **angiography** is the gold standard for the diagnosis of arterial occlusive disease.

TREATMENT

- Volume resuscitation; broad-spectrum antibiotics.
- For acute arterial thrombosis or embolism, treat with anticoagulation and either laparotomy or angioplasty.
- For venous thrombosis, treat with anticoagulation.
- For all other etiologies, address the underlying cause.
- Surgical resection of infarcted bowel.

COMPLICATIONS

Sepsis/septic shock, multisystem organ failure, death.

APPENDICITIS

See the Emergency Medicine chapter.

Disorders of the Large Bowel

DIVERTICULAR DISEASE

Outpouchings of mucosa and submucosa (false diverticula) that herniate through the colonic muscle layers in areas of high intraluminal pressure; most commonly found in the sigmoid colon. Diverticulosis is the **most common cause of acute lower GI bleeding** in patients > 40 years of age. Risk factors include a **low-fiber and high-fat diet,** advanced age (65% occur in those > 80 years of age), and connective tissue disorders. **Diverticulitis** is inflammation and, potentially, perforation of a diverticulum 2° to fecalith impaction.

HISTORY/PE

- Diverticulosis is often **asymptomatic.**
- When symptomatic, patients present with sudden, intermittent, painless bleeding. If severe, patients may present with symptoms of anemia (fatigue, lightheadedness, dyspnea on exertion).
- **Diverticulitis** presents with **LLQ abdominal pain, fever,** nausea, and vomiting. Perforation is a serious complication that presents with peritonitis and shock.

DIAGNOSIS

- Clinical history is important to diagnosis.
- CBC may show **leukocytosis** or anemia.
- In diverticulitis, CT scan may reveal inflammation or abscess (see Figure 2.6-8).
- Colonoscopy provides the definitive diagnosis in diverticular disease. Avoid sigmoidoscopy/colonoscopy in patients with early diverticulitis in view of the risk of perforation.

TREATMENT

- **Uncomplicated diverticulosis:** Routine follow-up. Encourage a high-fiber diet or fiber supplements.
- **Diverticular bleeding:** Bleeding usually stops spontaneously; transfuse and hydrate as needed. If bleeding does not stop, hemostasis by colonoscopy, angiography with embolization, or **surgery** is indicated.
- **Diverticulitis:** Treat with **bowel rest (NPO),** NG tube placement, and **broad-spectrum antibiotics** (metronidazole and a fluoroquinolone or a second- or third-generation cephalosporin).
- For perforation, perform immediate surgical resection of diseased bowel via a Hartmann's procedure with a temporary colostomy.

LARGE BOWEL OBSTRUCTION (LBO)

Table 2.6-3 describes features that distinguish SBO from LBO. Figure 2.6-9 demonstrates the classic radiographic findings of LBO.

KEY FACT

Diverticulosis is the most common cause of acute lower GI bleeding in patients > 40 years of age.

KEY FACT

Following resolution of an acute episode of lower GI bleeding, all patients must have a colonoscopy to rule out colon cancer if they have not been screened within the last 5–10 years.

KEY FACT

Sigmoidoscopy should be avoided in the initial stages of diverticulitis in light of the risk of perforation.

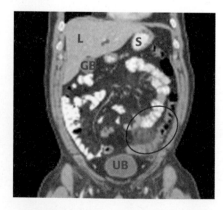

FIGURE 2.6-8. Acute diverticulitis. Coronal reconstruction from a contrast-enhanced CT demonstrates sigmoid diverticula with perisigmoid inflammatory "fat stranding." The area of abnormality is circled in red. L = liver; S = stomach; GB = gallbladder; UB = urinary bladder. (Reproduced with permission from USMLERx.com.)

TABLE 2.6-3. Characteristics of Small and Large Bowel Obstruction

VARIABLE	SBO	LBO
History	Moderate to severe acute abdominal pain; **copious emesis.** Cramping pain with distal SBO. Fever, signs of dehydration, and hypotension may be seen.	Constipation/obstipation, deep and cramping abdominal pain (less intense than SBO), nausea/vomiting (less than that of SBO, but more commonly **feculent**).
Exam	**Abdominal distention** (distal SBO), abdominal tenderness, visible peristaltic waves, fever, hypovolemia. Look for **surgical scars/hernias;** perform a rectal exam. **High-pitched "tinkly" bowel sounds;** later, absence of bowel sounds.	Significant **distention,** tympany, and tenderness; examine for peritoneal irritation or mass. Fever or signs of shock suggest perforation/peritonitis or ischemia/necrosis. **High-pitched "tinkly" bowel sounds;** later, absence of bowel sounds.
Etiologies	**Adhesions** (postsurgery), **hernias,** neoplasm, volvulus, intussusception, gallstone ileus, foreign body, Crohn's disease, cystic fibrosis (CF), stricture, hematoma.	**Colon cancer,** diverticulitis, volvulus, fecal impaction, benign tumors. **Assume colon cancer until proven otherwise.**
Differential	LBO, paralytic ileus, gastroenteritis.	SBO, paralytic ileus, appendicitis, IBD, Ogilvie's syndrome (pseudo-obstruction).
Diagnosis	CBC, electrolytes, lactic acid, AXR (see Figure 2.6-7); contrast studies (determine if it is partial or complete), CT scan.	CBC, electrolytes, lactic acid, AXR (see Figure 2.6-9), CT scan; water contrast enema (if perforation is suspected); sigmoidoscopy/colonoscopy if stable.
Treatment	Hospitalize. Partial SBO can be treated conservatively with **NG decompression** and NPO status. Patients with complete SBO should be managed aggressively with NPO status, NG decompression, IV fluids, electrolyte replacement, and **surgical correction.**	Hospitalize. Obstruction can be relieved with a Gastrografin enema, colonoscopy, or a **rectal tube;** however, **surgery** is usually required. Ischemic colon usually requires partial colectomy with a diverting colostomy. Treat the underlying cause (eg, neoplasm).

COLORECTAL CANCER

The second leading cause of cancer mortality in the United States. There is an ↑ incidence with age, with a peak incidence at 70–80 years. Risk factors and screening recommendations are summarized in Tables 2.6-4 and 2.6-5.

HISTORY/PE

Most patients are asymptomatic. When they are symptomatic, symptoms depend on the location of the lesion:

- **Right-sided lesions:** Often bulky, ulcerating masses that lead to **anemia from chronic occult blood loss.** Patients may complain of weight loss, anorexia, diarrhea, weakness, or vague abdominal pain. Obstruction is rare.
- **Left-sided lesions:** Typically **"apple-core" obstructing** masses (see Figure 2.6-10). Patients complain of a **change in bowel habits** (eg, ↓ stool caliber, constipation, obstipation) and/or blood-streaked stools. Obstruction is common.
- **Rectal lesions:** Usually present with bright red blood per rectum, often with tenesmus and/or rectal pain. Rectal cancer must be ruled out in all patients with rectal bleeding.

KEY FACT

Iron deficiency anemia in an elderly patient is colorectal cancer until proven otherwise.

Q

A 60-year-old male with no past medical history presents with fever, dyspnea, and orthopnea of 2 weeks' duration. Physical examination reveals splinter hemorrhages and a new IV/VI diastolic decrescendo murmur. Echocardiogram confirms aortic valve endocarditis, and IV antibiotics are started. Blood cultures are ⊕ for *Streptococcus bovis.* What is the next diagnostic step?

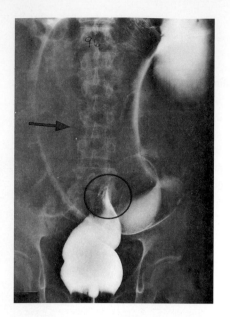

FIGURE 2.6-9. Large bowel obstruction. AP radiograph from a barium enema in a patient with an LBO reveals a massively dilated sigmoid colon (arrow) and a "bird's beak" appearance of the barium column at the site of volvulus (circle). (Reproduced with permission from Doherty GM. *Current Diagnosis & Treatment: Surgery,* 13th ed. New York: McGraw-Hill, 2010, Fig. 30-16.)

Colonoscopy. Although the mechanism of association has yet to be determined, there is a well-established association between *S bovis* and colon cancer.

TABLE 2.6-4. Risk Factors for Colorectal Cancer

RISK FACTOR	COMMENTS
Age	Risk ↑ with age; peak incidence is at 70–80 years.
Hereditary polyposis syndromes	Familial adenomatous polyposis (FAP; 100% risk by age 40); hereditary nonpolyposis colorectal cancer (HNPCC).
⊕ family history	–
IBD	Ulcerative colitis > Crohn's disease.
Adenomatous polyps	Villous > tubular; sessile > pedunculated.
High-fat, low-fiber diet	–

DIAGNOSIS

- Colonoscopy with biopsy can yield a definitive diagnosis.
- Order a CXR, LFTs, and an abdominal/pelvic CT to evaluate for metastases.
- Staging is based on the depth of tumor penetration into the bowel wall and the presence of lymph node involvement and distant metastases.

TREATMENT

- Surgical resection of the tumor is first-line treatment.
- **Adjuvant chemotherapy** is appropriate in cases with ⊕ lymph nodes.
- Follow with serial CEA levels to detect recurrence, colonoscopy, LFTs, CXR, and abdominal CT to screen for metastases.

TABLE 2.6-5. Screening Recommendations for Colorectal Cancer

RISK CATEGORY	RECOMMENDATIONS
No past medical or family history	Starting at age 50: ■ DRE and stool guaiac annually **and** ■ Colonoscopy every 10 years **or** ■ Sigmoidoscopy every 5 years.
First-degree relative with colon cancer	Colonoscopy every 10 years starting at age 40 **or** Colonoscopy every 10 years starting 10 years prior to the age of the affected family member at the time of diagnosis (whichever comes first).
Ulcerative colitis	Colonoscopy every 1–2 years starting 8–10 years after diagnosis.

ISCHEMIC COLITIS

- Insufficient blood supply to the colon that results in ischemia and, potentially, necrosis.
- Most commonly affects the left colon, particularly the "watershed area" at the splenic flexure.
- **Hx/PE:** Presents with crampy **lower abdominal pain** and **bloody diarrhea.** Fever and peritoneal signs suggest bowel necrosis.
- **Dx:**
    - CT scan with contrast may show thickened bowel wall.
    - **Colonoscopy** reveals pale mucosa with petechial bleeding.
- **Tx:**
    - Supportive therapy with bowel rest, IV fluids, and broad-spectrum antibiotics.
    - Surgical bowel resection is indicated for infarction, fulminant colitis, or obstruction.

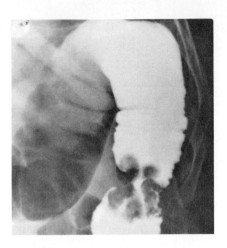

FIGURE 2.6-10. **Colon carcinoma.** The encircling carcinoma appears as an "apple-core" filling defect in the descending colon on barium enema x-ray. (Reproduced with permission from Way LW. *Current Surgical Diagnosis & Treatment*, 10th ed. Stamford, CT: Appleton & Lange, 1994: 658.)

Gastrointestinal Bleeding

Bleeding from the GI tract may present as hematemesis, hematochezia, and/or melena. Upper GI tract bleeding is defined as bleeding from lesions proximal to the ligament of Treitz (the anatomic boundary between the duodenum and jejunum). Table 2.6-6 presents the features of upper and lower GI bleeding.

> **KEY FACT**
>
> One unit of packed RBCs should ↑ hemoglobin by 1 g/dL and hematocrit by 3–4 units.

TABLE 2.6-6. **Features of Upper and Lower GI Bleeding**

VARIABLE	UPPER GI BLEEDING	LOWER GI BLEEDING
History/exam	Hematemesis ("coffee-ground" emesis), melena > hematochezia, hypovolemia (eg, tachycardia, lightheadedness, hypotension).	Hematochezia > melena, but can be either.
Diagnosis	NG tube and lavage; if stable, endoscopy.	Rule out upper GI bleed with NG lavage if brisk. Anoscopy/sigmoidoscopy for patients < 45 years of age with small-volume bleeding. Colonoscopy if stable; arteriography or exploratory laparotomy if unstable.
Etiologies	**PUD,** esophagitis/gastritis, Mallory-Weiss tear, esophageal varices.	**Diverticulosis** (60%), angiodysplasia, IBD, hemorrhoids/fissures, neoplasm, AVM.
Initial management	Protect the airway (intubation may be needed). Stabilize the patient with IV fluids and packed RBCs (hematocrit may be normal early in acute blood loss).	Similar to that of upper GI bleed.
Long-term management	Endoscopy followed by therapy directed at the underlying cause.	Depends on the underlying etiology. Endoscopic therapy (eg, epinephrine injection), intra-arterial vasopressin infusion or embolization, or surgery for diverticular disease or angiodysplasia.

Inflammatory Bowel Disease (IBD)

Includes **Crohn's disease** (see Figure 2.6-11) **and ulcerative colitis** (see Figure 2.6-12). Most common in Caucasians and **Ashkenazi Jews,** with onset most frequently occurring in the teens to early 30s or in the 50s. Table 2.6-7 summarizes the features of IBD.

Inguinal Hernias

Protrusions of abdominal contents (usually the small intestine) into the inguinal region through a weakness or defect in the abdominal wall. Classified as either direct or indirect:

- **Indirect:** Herniation of abdominal contents through the internal and external inguinal rings (see Figure 2.6-13A).
    - The **most common hernia in both genders.**
    - Due to a **congenital patent processus vaginalis.**
    - Protrudes **lateral** to the inferior epigastric vessels.
- **Direct:** Herniation of abdominal contents through the floor of **Hesselbach's triangle** (see Figure 2.6-13B).
    - Protrudes **medial** to the epigastric vessels.
    - Due to an **acquired** defect in the transversalis fascia from mechanical breakdown that occurs with age.

TREATMENT

Because of the risk of **incarceration** and **strangulation,** surgical correction is indicated.

Biliary Disease

CHOLELITHIASIS AND BILIARY COLIC

Colic results from transient cystic duct blockage from impacted stones. Although risk factors include the **4 F's**—Female, Fat, Fertile, and Forty—the disorder is common and can occur in any patient. Additional risk factors

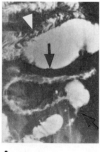

A

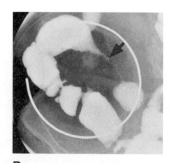

B

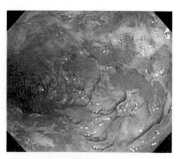

C

FIGURE 2.6-11. **Crohn's disease.** (**A**) Small bowel follow-through (SBFT) barium study shows skip areas of narrowed small bowel with nodular mucosa (arrows) and ulceration. Compare with normal small bowel (arrowhead). (**B**) Spot compression image from SBFT shows "string sign" narrowing (arrow) due to stricture. (**C**) Deep ulcers in the colon of a patient with Crohn's disease, seen at colonoscopy. (Image A reproduced with permission from Chen MY et al. *Basic Radiology,* 1st ed. New York: McGraw-Hill, 2004, Fig. 10-30. Image B reproduced with permission from USMLERx.com. Image C reproduced with permission from Fauci AS et al. *Harrison's Principles of Internal Medicine,* 17th ed. New York: McGraw-Hill, 2008, Fig. 285-48).

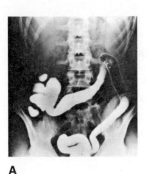
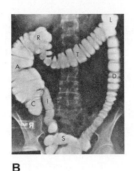
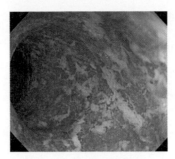

A **B** **C**

FIGURE 2.6-12. **Ulcerative colitis.** (A) Radiograph from a barium enema showing a featureless ("lead pipe") colon with small mucosal ulcerations (arrow). Compare with normal haustral markings in (B). (C) Diffuse mucosal ulcerations and exudates at colonoscopy in chronic ulcerative colitis. (Image A reproduced with permission from Doherty GM. *Current Diagnosis & Treatment: Surgery,* 13th ed. New York: McGraw-Hill, 2010, Fig. 30-17. Image B reproduced with permission from Chen MY et al. *Basic Radiology,* 1st ed. New York: McGraw-Hill, 2004, Fig. 10-10A. Image C reproduced with permission from Fauci AS et al. *Harrison's Principles of Internal Medicine,* 17th ed. New York: McGraw-Hill, 2008, Fig 285-4A.)

include OCP use, rapid weight loss, chronic hemolysis (pigment stones in sickle cell disease), small bowel resection (loss of enterohepatically circulated bile), and TPN.

HISTORY/PE

- Patients present with **postprandial abdominal pain** (usually in the **RUQ**) that radiates to the right subscapular area or the epigastrium.
- Pain is often associated with **nausea and vomiting,** dyspepsia, and flatulence.
- Gallstones may be asymptomatic in up to 80% of patients. Examination may reveal RUQ tenderness and a palpable gallbladder.

DIAGNOSIS

- Plain x-rays are rarely diagnostic; only 10–15% of stones are radiopaque.
- **RUQ ultrasound** is the imaging modality of choice (see Figure 2.6-14).
- Table 2.6-8 contrasts lab findings with those of other forms of biliary disease.

TREATMENT

Cholecystectomy is curative and recommended for patients with symptomatic gallstones. Asymptomatic gallstones do not require treatment.

ACUTE CHOLECYSTITIS

Prolonged blockage of the cystic duct by a gallstone that leads to progressive distention, inflammation, and superinfection. **Acalculous cholecystitis** occurs in the absence of cholelithiasis in patients who are chronically debilitated or critically ill.

HISTORY/PE

- Patients present with **RUQ pain, nausea, vomiting, and fever.**
- Look for a history notable for RUQ pain and nausea. Examination may reveal RUQ tenderness, inspiratory arrest with deep palpation of the RUQ (**Murphy's sign**), and low-grade fever.

KEY FACT

Pigmented gallstones result from hemolysis (black) or infection (brown).

KEY FACT

Most gallstones are precipitations of cholesterol and are not radiopaque.

Q

A 35-year-old male with a 12-year history of ulcerative colitis presents to a clinic for annual follow-up. He has no current complaints. What is the most important screening test he should undergo?

TABLE 2.6-7. Features of Ulcerative Colitis and Crohn's Disease

VARIABLE	ULCERATIVE COLITIS	CROHN'S DISEASE
Site of involvement	The **rectum** is always involved. May extend proximally in a **continuous fashion.** Inflammation and ulceration are **limited to the mucosa and submucosa.**	May involve **any portion** of the GI tract, particularly the **ileocecal region**, in a **discontinuous pattern** ("skip lesions"). The rectum is often spared. **Transmural inflammation** is seen, sometimes leading to fistulas to other organs.
History/exam	**Bloody diarrhea,** lower abdominal cramps, tenesmus, urgency. Examination may reveal orthostatic hypotension, tachycardia, abdominal tenderness, frank blood on rectal examination, and extraintestinal manifestations.	Abdominal pain, abdominal mass, low-grade fever, weight loss, watery diarrhea. Examination may reveal fever, abdominal tenderness or mass, **perianal fissures or tags, fistulas,** and extraintestinal manifestations.
Extraintestinal manifestations	Aphthous stomatitis, episcleritis/uveitis, arthritis, **primary sclerosing cholangitis,** erythema nodosum, and pyoderma gangrenosum.	The same as ulcerative colitis in addition to fistulas to the skin, to the bladder, or between bowel loops.
Diagnosis	CBC, AXR, stool cultures, O&P, stool assay for *C difficile.* Colonoscopy can show diffuse and continuous rectal involvement, friability, edema, and **pseudopolyps.** Definitive diagnosis can be made with biopsy.	The same lab workup as that of ulcerative colitis. Upper GI series with small bowel follow-through. Colonoscopy may show aphthoid, linear, or stellate ulcers, strictures, **"cobblestoning,"** and **"skip lesions."** "Creeping fat" may also be present during laparotomy. Definitive diagnosis can be made with biopsy.
Treatment	**5-ASA agents** (eg, sulfasalazine, mesalamine), topical or oral; corticosteroids and immunomodulating agents (eg, azathioprine) for refractory disease. **Total proctocolectomy can be curative** for long-standing or fulminant colitis or **toxic megacolon;** also ↓ cancer risk.	**5-ASA agents;** corticosteroids and immunomodulating agents (eg, azathioprine, infliximab) are indicated if no improvement is seen. Surgical resection may be necessary for suspected perforation, stricture, fistula, or abscess; **may recur** anywhere in the GI tract.
Incidence of cancer	There is a **markedly ↑ risk of colorectal cancer** in long-standing cases (monitor with frequent fecal occult blood screening and yearly colonoscopy with multiple biopsies after 8 years of disease).	The incidence of 2° malignancy is lower than that of ulcerative colitis but is greater than that of the general population.

Colonoscopy. Patients with ulcerative colitis are at significantly ↑ risk of colon cancer. Thus, colonoscopies are recommended for such patients every 1–2 years beginning 8–10 years after diagnosis. If dysplasia is present on random biopsy, total colectomy is recommended.

DIAGNOSIS

- Fever is sometimes present, and CBC shows leukocytosis (see Table 2.6-8).
- Ultrasound may demonstrate stones, bile sludge, pericholecystic fluid, a thickened gallbladder wall, gas in the gallbladder, and/or an ultrasonic Murphy's sign (see Figure 2.6-14).
- When ultrasound is equivocal, obtain a HIDA scan. In this nuclear medicine scan, which uses a radiotracer excreted through the biliary system, nonvisualization of the gallbladder suggests acute cholecystitis.

TREATMENT

- Give broad-spectrum **IV antibiotics** and **IV fluids;** replete electrolytes.
- Nonemergent **cholecystectomy** is indicated.

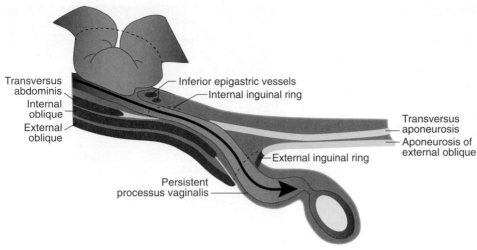

A

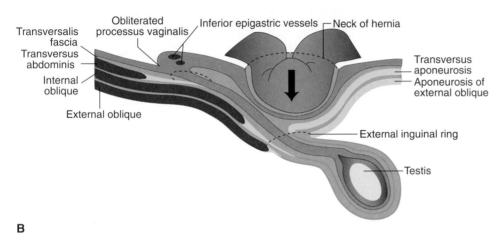

B

FIGURE 2.6-13. **Indirect (A) and direct (B) inguinal hernias.** (Reproduced with permission from Tintinalli JE et al. *Tintinalli's Emergency Medicine: A Comprehensive Study Guide,* 7th ed. New York: McGraw-Hill, 2010, Figs. 87-4 and 87-3.)

CHOLEDOCHOLITHIASIS

- Gallstones in the common bile duct. Symptoms vary according to the degree of obstruction, the duration of the obstruction, and the extent of bacterial infection.
- **Hx/PE:** Presents with biliary colic, jaundice, fever, and/or pancreatitis.
- **Dx:** The hallmark is ↑ **alkaline phosphatase** and **total and direct bilirubin** (see Table 2.6-8).
- **Tx:** Management consists of ERCP with sphincterotomy followed by cholecystectomy.

ASCENDING CHOLANGITIS

An acute bacterial infection of the biliary tree that commonly occurs 2° to **obstruction,** usually from **gallstones (choledocholithiasis).** Other etiologies include bile duct stricture, primary sclerosing cholangitis, and malignancy. Gram-⊖ enterics are commonly identified pathogens.

Q

A 43-year-old female presents to the ER with nausea, vomiting, and epigastric pain. She has complained of intermittent RUQ pain for the past several months. Physical examination reveals marked epigastric tenderness. Labs show leukocytosis, ↑ AST and ALT, and ↑ lipase. AXR is unremarkable. What is the most likely diagnosis?

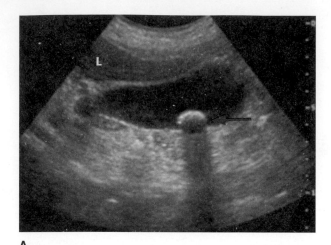
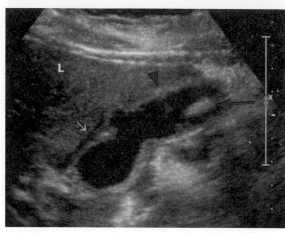

A   **B**

FIGURE 2.6-14. **Gallstone disease.** **(A) Cholelithiasis.** Ultrasound image of the gallbladder shows a gallstone (arrow) with posterior shadowing. **(B) Acute cholecystitis.** Ultrasound image shows a gallstone (red arrow), a thickened gallbladder wall (arrowheads), and pericholecystic fluid (white arrow). L = liver. (Reproduced with permission from USMLERx.com.)

KEY FACT

Charcot's triad consists of RUQ pain, jaundice, and fever/chills. Reynolds' pentad consists of RUQ pain, jaundice, fever/chills, shock, and altered mental status.

History/PE

- Charcot's triad—RUQ pain, jaundice, and fever/chills—is classic.
- Reynolds' pentad—Charcot's triad plus septic **shock** and **altered mental status**—may be present in acute suppurative cholangitis and suggests sepsis.

Diagnosis

- Labs reveal **leukocytosis**, ↑ **bilirubin**, and ↑ **alkaline phosphatase** (see Table 2.6-8).
- Obtain blood cultures to rule out sepsis.
- **ERCP** is both diagnostic and therapeutic.

Treatment

- Patients often require **ICU admission** for monitoring, hydration, BP support, and broad-spectrum **IV antibiotic treatment.**
- Patients with acute suppurative cholangitis require **emergent bile duct decompression** via ERCP/sphincterotomy, percutaneous transhepatic drainage, or open decompression.

A

Gallstone pancreatitis results from a gallstone that travels through the common bile duct and lodges at the ampulla of Vater, which obstructs the flow of both pancreatic exocrine enzymes and bile. It most commonly occurs in women, who often report a history of biliary colic. Treatment involves management of the pancreatitis with supportive care and elective cholecystectomy.

TABLE 2.6-8. **Differential Diagnosis of Biliary Disease**

	Fever/Elevated WBC Count	Elevated Total Bilirubin/ Alkaline Phosphatase	Elevated Serum Amylase
Cholelithiasis (colic)	−	−	−
Acute cholecystitis	+	−	−
Choledocholithiasis/ ascending cholangitis	+	+	−
Gallstone pancreatitis	+	+	+

GALLSTONE ILEUS

- A mechanical obstruction resulting from the passage of a large (> 2.5-cm) stone into the bowel through a cholecystoduodenal fistula. Obstruction is often at the ileocecal valve.
- **Hx/PE:** The classic presentation is a subacute SBO in an elderly woman. Patients may have no history of biliary colic.
- **Dx:** AXR with characteristics of SBO and pneumobilia (gas in the biliary tree) confirms the diagnosis. Upper GI barium contrast images will demonstrate no contrast in the colon.
- **Tx:** Laparotomy with stone extraction; closure of the fistula and cholecystectomy.

PRIMARY SCLEROSING CHOLANGITIS

- An idiopathic disorder characterized by progressive inflammation and fibrosis accompanied by strictures of extra- and intrahepatic bile ducts. The disease usually presents in **young males with ulcerative colitis.** Patients are at ↑ **risk for cholangiocarcinoma.**
- **Hx/PE:** Presents with progressive **jaundice, pruritus,** and **fatigue.**
- **Dx:**
  - Laboratory findings include ↑ **alkaline phosphatase** and ↑ **bilirubin.**
  - MRCP/ERCP show **multiple bile duct strictures** and dilatations ("beading").
  - Liver biopsy reveals periductal sclerosis ("onion skinning").
- **Tx:** High-dose ursodiol; ERCP with dilation and stenting of strictures. Liver transplantation is the definitive treatment.

KEY FACT

Primary sclerosing cholangitis is strongly associated with ulcerative colitis.

Liver Disease

ABNORMAL LIVER FUNCTION TESTS

Liver diseases can be divided into several patterns based on LFT results:

- **Hepatocellular injury:** ↑ AST and ALT.
- **Cholestasis:** ↑ alkaline phosphatase and bilirubin.
- **Isolated hyperbilirubinemia:** ↑ bilirubin.

Jaundice is a clinical sign that occurs when bilirubin levels exceed 2.5 mg/dL. Figures 2.6-15 and 2.6-16 summarize the clinical approaches toward cholestasis and isolated hyperbilirubinemia.

KEY FACT

H**C**V is **C**hronic; 60–70% of patients with HCV infection will develop chronic hepatitis.

HEPATITIS

Inflammation of the liver leading to cell injury and necrosis. Hepatitis can be either acute or chronic.

- **Acute:** The most common causes are viruses (HAV, HBV, HCV, HDV, HEV) and drugs (alcohol, acetaminophen, INH, methyldopa).
- **Chronic:** The most common causes are chronic viral infection, alcohol, autoimmune hepatitis, and metabolic syndromes (Wilson's disease, hemochromatosis, α_1-antitrypsin deficiency).
- HAV and HEV are transmitted by the fecal-oral route.
- HBV and HCV are transmitted by body fluids, although the risk of acquiring HCV sexually is very low.

A 21-year-old male college student in the midst of final exams presents to a local clinic with "yellow eyes." His physical examination is unremarkable except for scleral icterus, and a CBC and blood smear show no abnormalities. A comprehensive metabolic profile reveals a normal AST and ALT but elevated unconjugated bilirubin. What is the most likely diagnosis?

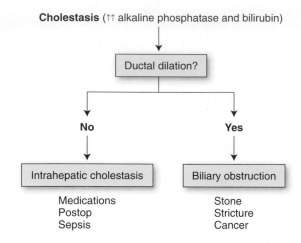

FIGURE 2.6-15.   **Approach to cholestasis.**

HISTORY/PE

- **Acute hepatitis:**
    - Often begins with a nonspecific viral prodrome (**malaise,** fever, joint pain, fatigue, URI symptoms, **nausea, vomiting,** changes in bowel habits) followed by **jaundice** and RUQ tenderness. Examination often reveals jaundice, scleral icterus, and tender hepatomegaly.
    - HAV and HEV have only a self-limited acute phase; HBV and HCV may feature a mild acute phase or none at all. Acetaminophen toxicity can cause a life-threatening hepatitis.
- **Chronic hepatitis:** Usually presents with symptoms only when the liver scars to the point of cirrhosis (jaundice, fatigue, ascites). At least 80% of those infected with HCV and 10% of those with HBV will develop persistent infection with chronic active hepatitis.

DIAGNOSIS

- **Acute hepatitis:** Labs reveal markedly ↑ **ALT and AST** and ↑ bilirubin/alkaline phosphatase.
- **Chronic hepatitis:** ALT and AST are persistently elevated for > 3–6 months.
- The diagnosis of viral hepatitis is made by **hepatitis serology** (see Table 2.6-9 and Figure 2.6-17 for a description and timing of serologic markers) and by liver biopsy in chronic or severe cases.

Gilbert's syndrome is an autosomal recessive disorder of bilirubin glucuronidation due to ↓ activity of the enzyme glucuronyl transferase. Patients present with unconjugated hyperbilirubinemia but have a normal CBC, blood smear, and LFTs. The condition is benign, and no treatment is indicated.

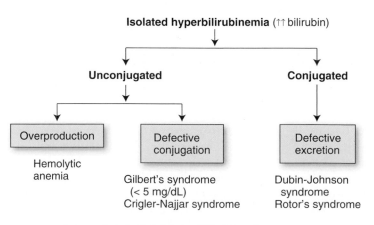

FIGURE 2.6-16.   **Approach to isolated hyperbilirubinemia.**

TABLE 2.6-9.   Key Hepatitis Serologic Markers

Serologic Marker	Description
IgM HAVAb	IgM antibody to HAV; the best test to detect acute HAV.
HBsAg	Antigen found on the surface of HBV; continued presence indicates carrier state.
HBsAb	Antibody to HBsAg; **indicates immunity** to HBV.
HBcAg	Antigen associated with core of HBV. Not measured in clinical practice.
HBcAb	Antibody to HBcAg; IgM ⊕ during the **window period.** IgG HBcAb is an indicator of prior or current infection.
HBeAg	A different antigenic determinant in the HBV core. An important indicator of transmissibility (**BE**ware!).
HBeAb	Antibody to e antigen; indicates low transmissibility.

- Other diagnostic studies include the following:
  - **Autoimmune hepatitis:** ⊕ anti–smooth muscle antibodies.
  - **Hemochromatosis:** High ferritin and transferrin saturation > 50%.
  - **Wilson's disease:** Low ceruloplasmin, high urine copper.

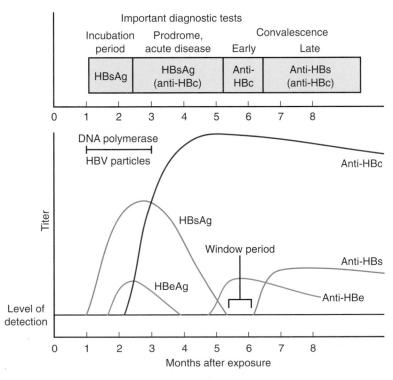

FIGURE 2.6-17.   Time course of hepatitis B with serologic markers.

KEY FACT

The sequelae of chronic hepatitis include cirrhosis, liver failure, and hepatocellular carcinoma.

TREATMENT

- **Acute hepatitis:** Supportive care.
- **Chronic hepatitis:** Treatment is etiology specific.
  - **Chronic HBV infection: Interferon** and **lamivudine (3TC)** or **adefovir.**
  - **Chronic HCV infection: Interferon** and **ribavirin.**
- **Liver transplantation** is the definitive treatment for patients with end-stage liver failure. Emergent transplantation is indicated in cases of fulminant hepatic failure.

COMPLICATIONS

Cirrhosis, liver failure, hepatocellular carcinoma (3–5%).

CIRRHOSIS

Defined as **fibrosis and nodular regeneration** resulting from chronic hepatic injury. Etiologies can be intra- or extrahepatic:

- **Intrahepatic:** All causes of chronic hepatitis.
- **Extrahepatic:**
  - Biliary tract disease (primary biliary cirrhosis, primary sclerosing cholangitis).
  - Posthepatic causes include right-sided heart failure, constrictive pericarditis, and Budd-Chiari syndrome (hepatic vein thrombosis 2° to hypercoagulability).

HISTORY/PE

KEY FACT

Spontaneous bacterial peritonitis is diagnosed by > 250 PMNs/mL in the ascitic fluid.

- Presents with **jaundice, ascites, spontaneous bacterial peritonitis, hepatic encephalopathy** (asterixis, altered mental status), **gastroesophageal varices,** coagulopathy, and renal dysfunction. Ascites can be complicated by **spontaneous bacterial peritonitis.**
- Examination may reveal an enlarged, palpable, or firm liver and other signs of portal hypertension and liver failure (see Figures 2.6-18 and 2.6-19).

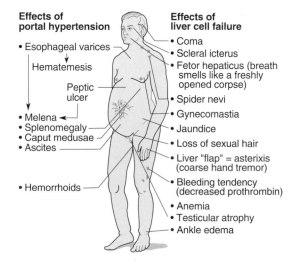

FIGURE 2.6-18. Presentation of cirrhosis/portal hypertension. (Adapted with permission from Chandrasoma P, Taylor CE. *Concise Pathology,* 3rd ed. Stamford, CT: Appleton & Lange, 1998: 654.)

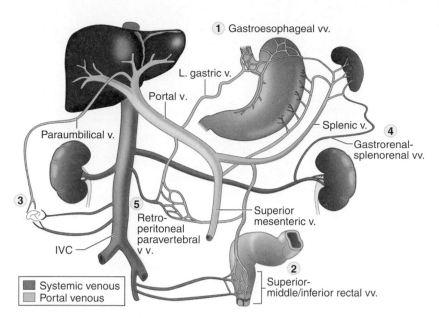

FIGURE 2.6-19. Portosystemic anastomoses. 1. Left gastric–azygos → esophageal varices. 2. Superior–middle/inferior rectal → hemorrhoids. 3. Paraumbilical–inferior epigastric → caput medusae (navel). 4. Gastrorenal-splenorenal. 5. Retroperitoneal paravertebral.

DIAGNOSIS

- Lab studies show ↓ **albumin**, ↑ **PT/INR**, and ↑ **bilirubin.** Anemia or thrombocytopenia (2° to hypersplenism and bone marrow suppression) may also be seen.
- Other studies, including hepatitis serologies, serum ferritin, ceruloplasmin, and α_1-antitrypsin, will identify other causes, such as infection, hemochromatosis, Wilson's disease, and α_1-antitrypsin deficiency, respectively.
- If ascites is present, the etiology of ascites can be determined by the **serum-ascites albumin gradient** (**SAAG** = serum albumin – ascites albumin); see Table 2.6-10.
- Liver biopsy will show bridging fibrosis and nodular regeneration.

TREATMENT

The goal is to slow the progression of cirrhosis and prevent associated complications (see Table 2.6-11).

TABLE 2.6-10. Etiologies of Cirrhosis by SAAG

SAAG > 1.1	SAAG < 1.1
Related to portal hypertension:	Not related to portal hypertension:
▪ **Presinusoidal:** Splenic or portal vein thrombosis, schistosomiasis	▪ Nephrotic syndrome
▪ **Sinusoidal:** Cirrhosis	▪ TB
▪ **Postsinusoidal:** Right heart failure, constrictive pericarditis, Budd-Chiari syndrome	▪ Malignancy with peritoneal carcinomatosis (eg, ovarian cancer)

Q

A 36-year-old woman with a past medical history of hypercholesterolemia and type 2 DM presents with intermittent dull RUQ discomfort. The patient does not drink alcohol. Her physical examination is unremarkable. Lab studies show elevated AST and ALT but are otherwise normal. Hepatitis serologies are ⊖. What is the most likely diagnosis?

TABLE 2.6-11. Complications of Cirrhosis

COMPLICATION	MECHANISM/HISTORY	MANAGEMENT
Ascites	↑ portal hypertension results in transudative effusion. Physical examination reveals abdominal distention, fluid wave, and shifting dullness to percussion.	Sodium restriction and diuretics (furosemide, spironolactone); large-volume paracentesis. Treat underlying liver disease if possible.
Spontaneous bacterial peritonitis	Presents with fever, abdominal pain, chills, nausea, and vomiting. Diagnostic paracentesis reveals > 250 PMNs/mL and a ⊕ Gram stain.	IV antibiotics acutely (third-generation cephalosporin), IV albumin; prophylaxis with a fluoroquinolone to prevent recurrence.
Hepatorenal syndrome	Acute prerenal failure in the setting of advanced cirrhosis. A diagnosis of exclusion. Urinary sodium is < 10 mEq/L.	Difficult to treat; often requires dialysis. The only cure is liver transplantation.
Hepatic encephalopathy	↓ clearance of ammonia; often precipitated by dehydration, infection, electrolyte abnormalities, and GI bleeding.	Protein restriction, lactulose, and/or rifaximin. Correct underlying triggers (eg, replete potassium).
Esophageal varices	Portal hypertension leads to ↑ flow through portosystemic anastomoses.	Endoscopic surveillance in all patients with cirrhosis; medical prophylaxis with β-blockers to prevent bleeding. For acute bleeding, endoscopy with band ligation or sclerotherapy is indicated.
Coagulopathy	Impaired synthesis of all clotting factors (except VIII).	For acute bleeding, administer fresh frozen plasma. **Vitamin K will not correct coagulopathy.**

KEY FACT

Primary biliary cirrhosis is an autoimmune disease that presents with jaundice and pruritus in middle-aged women.

Nonalcoholic fatty liver disease, a condition that is associated with insulin resistance and metabolic syndrome. In its earliest stage, the condition can be reversed with weight loss and a fat-restricted diet. Later, however, it can progress to irreversible nonalcoholic steatohepatitis and cirrhosis.

PRIMARY BILIARY CIRRHOSIS

- An **autoimmune** disorder characterized by **destruction of intrahepatic bile ducts.** Most commonly presents in **middle-aged women** with other autoimmune conditions.
- **Hx/PE:** Presents with progressive **jaundice, pruritus,** and fat-soluble vitamin deficiencies (A, D, E, K).
- **Dx:** Laboratory findings include ↑ **alkaline phosphatase,** ↑ bilirubin, ⊕ **antimitochondrial antibody,** and ↑ cholesterol.
- **Tx:** Ursodeoxycholic acid (slows progression of disease); cholestyramine for pruritus; liver transplantation.

HEPATOCELLULAR CARCINOMA

One of the most common cancers worldwide despite its relatively low incidence in the United States. 1° risk factors for the development of hepatocellular carcinoma in the United States are **cirrhosis** from alcohol and **chronic hepatitis** (HCV). In developing countries, **aflatoxins** (in various food sources) and **HBV infection** are major risk factors.

HISTORY/PE

- Patients commonly present with **RUQ tenderness, abdominal distention,** and signs of chronic liver disease such as **jaundice, easy bruisability,** and **coagulopathy.**
- Examination may reveal tender **enlargement** of the liver.

DIAGNOSIS

Often suggested by the presence of a mass on **ultrasound** or **CT** as well as by abnormal LFTs and significantly elevated α-fetoprotein (AFP) levels.

TREATMENT

- **Surgical:** Partial hepatectomy for single lesions < 5 cm with no cirrhosis; orthotopic liver transplantation in patients with cirrhosis.
- **Nonsurgical:** Transarterial chemoembolization (TACE) and/or sorafenib for advanced disease.
- Monitor AFP levels to screen for recurrence.

HEMOCHROMATOSIS

A state of iron overload in which hemosiderin accumulates in the liver, pancreas (islet cells), heart, adrenals, testes, and pituitary.

- **1° hemochromatosis:** An autosomal recessive disease characterized by mutations in the HFE gene that result in excessive absorption of dietary iron.
- **2° hemochromatosis:** Occurs in patients receiving chronic transfusion therapy (eg, α-thalassemia).

HISTORY/PE

- Patients may present with abdominal pain, **DM, hypogonadism, arthropathy of the MCP joints, heart failure,** or cirrhosis.
- Examination may reveal **bronze skin pigmentation, cardiac dysfunction** (CHF), hepatomegaly, and testicular atrophy. Labs may reveal evidence of DM.
- Hemochromatosis does not affect the lung, kidney, or eye.

DIAGNOSIS

- ↑ **serum iron,** percent saturation of iron, and ferritin with ↓ serum transferrin.
- A transferrin saturation (serum iron divided by TIBC) > 45% is highly suggestive of iron overload.
- In severe cases, patients may be report being repeatedly interrogated at airport security because they can accumulate so much iron that it activates metal detectors.
- Perform a **liver biopsy** (to determine hepatic iron index), MRI, or HFE gene mutation screen.

TREATMENT

- **Weekly phlebotomy** to normalize serum iron levels, and then maintenance phlebotomy every 2–4 months.
- **Deferoxamine** can be used for maintenance therapy.

COMPLICATIONS

Cirrhosis, hepatocellular carcinoma, restrictive cardiomyopathy, arrhythmias, DM, impotence, arthropathy, hypopituitarism.

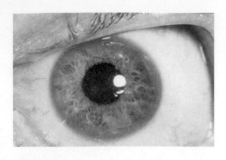

FIGURE 2.6-20. Kayser-Fleischer ring. Note the brown ring encircling the iris. This is a result of copper deposition in Descemet's membrane and is a classic finding in Wilson's disease. (Reproduced with permission from USMLERx.com.)

WILSON'S DISEASE (HEPATOLENTICULAR DEGENERATION)

- An autosomal recessive disorder that results in defective copper transport and subsequent accumulation and deposition of copper in the liver and brain. Usually occurs in patients < 30 years of age; 50% are symptomatic by age 15.
- **Hx:** Patients present with hepatitis/cirrhosis, neurologic dysfunction (ataxia, **tremor**), and **psychiatric abnormalities** (psychosis, anxiety, mania, depression).
- **PE:** May reveal **Kayser-Fleischer rings** (green-to-brown deposits of copper in Descemet's membrane; see Figure 2.6-20) as well as jaundice, hepatomegaly, asterixis, choreiform movements, and rigidity.
- **Dx:** ↓ **serum ceruloplasmin;** ↑ urinary copper excretion.
- **Tx: Dietary copper restriction** (avoid shellfish, liver, legumes), **penicillamine** (a copper chelator that ↑ urinary copper excretion), and zinc (↑ fecal excretion).

Pancreatic Disease

PANCREATITIS

Table 2.6-12 outlines the features of acute and chronic pancreatitis. Table 2.6-13 lists Ranson's criteria for predicting mortality in acute pancreatitis.

PANCREATIC CANCER

Most (75%) are adenocarcinomas in the head of the pancreas. Risk factors include smoking, chronic pancreatitis, and a first-degree relative with pancreatic cancer. Incidence ↑ after age 45; slightly more common in males.

HISTORY/PE

- Presents with **abdominal pain** radiating toward the back as well as with **obstructive jaundice,** loss of appetite, nausea, vomiting, **weight loss,** weakness, fatigue, and indigestion.
- Often asymptomatic, and thus presents late in the disease course.
- Examination may reveal a palpable, nontender gallbladder (**Courvoisier's sign**) or migratory thrombophlebitis (**Trousseau's sign**).

DIAGNOSIS

- CT scan with contrast to localize the tumor and assess the extent of local invasion and distant metastases.
- If a mass is not visualized on CT, use endoscopic ultrasound +/– ERCP.
- CA-19-9 is often elevated but is neither sensitive nor specific.

TREATMENT

- Most patients present with locally advanced or metastatic disease, so treatment is palliative.
- Patients with small tumors in the pancreatic head with no metastasis or major vessel involvement are eligible for surgical resection using the Whipple procedure (pancreaticoduodenectomy).
- Chemotherapy with 5-FU and gemcitabine may improve short-term survival, but long-term prognosis is poor (5–10% 5-year survival).

 KEY FACT

The hallmark finding in pancreatic cancer is a nontender, palpable gallbladder.

TABLE 2.6-12. **Features of Acute and Chronic Pancreatitis**

Variable	Acute Pancreatitis	Chronic Pancreatitis
Pathophysiology	Leakage of pancreatic enzymes into pancreatic and peripancreatic tissue.	Irreversible parenchymal destruction leading to pancreatic dysfunction and insufficiency.
Time course	Abrupt onset of severe pain.	Persistent, recurrent episodes of severe pain.
Risk factors	**Gallstones, alcohol abuse,** hypercalcemia, hypertriglyceridemia, trauma, drug side effects (thiazide diuretics), viral infections, post-ERCP, scorpion bites.	**Alcohol abuse** (90%), gallstones, CF, smoking, pancreatic divisum, family history.
History/exam	**Severe epigastric pain (radiating to the back);** nausea, vomiting, weakness, fever, shock. Flank discoloration **(Grey Turner's sign)** and periumbilical discoloration **(Cullen's sign)** may be evident on examination.	Recurrent episodes of **persistent epigastric pain;** anorexia, nausea, constipation, flatulence, **steatorrhea,** weight loss, DM.
Diagnosis	↑ **amylase,** ↑ **lipase,** ↓ **calcium** if severe; **"sentinel loop"** or **"colon cutoff sign"** on AXR. Abdominal ultrasound or CT may show an enlarged pancreas with stranding, abscess, hemorrhage, necrosis, or pseudocyst (see Figure 2.6-21A).	↑ to normal amylase and lipase, ↓ stool elastase, **pancreatic calcifications** (see Figure 2.6-21B), and mild ileus on AXR and CT **("chain of lakes").**
Treatment	Removal of the offending agent if possible. Supportive care, including IV fluids/electrolyte replacement, analgesia, bowel rest, NG suction, nutritional support, and O_2. Treat severe necrotizing pancreatitis with IV antibiotics, respiratory support, and surgical debridement.	Analgesia, pancreatic enzyme replacement, avoidance of causative agents (EtOH), celiac nerve block; surgery for intractable pain or structural causes.
Prognosis	Roughly 85–90% are mild and self-limited; 10–15% are severe, requiring ICU admission. Mortality may approach 50% in severe cases.	Patients can have chronic pain and pancreatic dysfunction.
Complications	**Pancreatic pseudocyst, fistula formation,** hypocalcemia, renal failure, pleural effusion, chronic pancreatitis, sepsis. Mortality 2° to acute pancreatitis can be predicted with Ranson's criteria (see Table 2.6-13).	**Chronic pain,** opiate addiction, malnutrition/weight loss, pancreatic cancer.

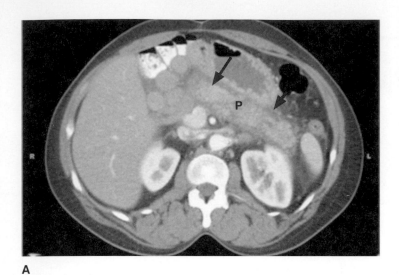
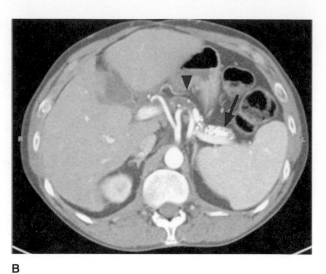

FIGURE 2.6-21. **Pancreatitis. (A) Uncomplicated acute pancreatitis.** Peripancreatic fluid and fat stranding can be seen (arrows). P = pancreas. **(B) Chronic pancreatitis.** Note the dilated pancreatic duct (arrowhead) and pancreatic calcifications (arrow). (Reproduced with permission from USMLERx.com.)

TABLE 2.6-13. **Ranson's Criteria for Acute Pancreatitis[a]**

On Admission	Within 48 Hours
"GA LAW":	**"C HOBBS":**
Glucose > 200 mg/dL	**C**a^{2+} < 8.0 mg/dL
Age > 55 years	**H**ematocrit ↓ by > 10%
LDH > 350 IU/L	Pa**O**$_2$ < 60 mm Hg
AST > 250 IU/dL	**B**ase deficit > 4 mEq/L
WBC > 16,000/mL	**B**UN ↑ by > 5 mg/dL
	Sequestered fluid > 6 L

[a] The risk of mortality is 20% with 3–4 signs, 40% with 5–6 signs, and 100% with ≥ 7 signs.

HEMATOLOGY/ONCOLOGY

Coagulation Disorders

COAGULATION CASCADE

Hemostasis requires the interaction of blood vessels, platelets, monocytes, and coagulation factors. This activates the clotting cascade, as shown in Figure 2.7-1.

- **Heparin:** ↑ PTT, activates antithrombin III and affects the **intrinsic pathway,** and ↓ fibrinogen levels. **Protamine sulfate** is the antidote.
- **Warfarin:** ↑ **PT,** inhibits vitamin K and affects the **extrinsic pathway** (factors II, VII, IX, and X and protein C and S), and is teratogenic, as its small size allows it to cross the placenta. **Vitamin K** is the antidote. The **goal INR is 2.0–3.0** (2.5–3.5 in patients with mechanical valves).
- **Enoxaparin** (low-molecular-weight heparin, or LMWH): Inhibits factor Xa and does not have to be monitored in most situations; dosing is once or twice daily.

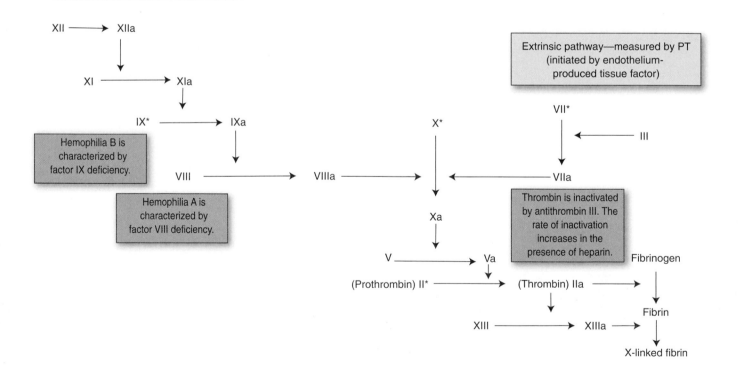

* Vitamin K–dependent clotting factors (II, VII, IX, X). Their synthesis is inhibited by warfarin.

FIGURE 2.7-1. Coagulation cascade.

Heparin-to-warfarin conversion is necessary because warfarin inhibits proteins C and S before other vitamin K–dependent factors (II, VII, IX, and X), leading to a transient period of **paradoxical hypercoagulability** before proper anticoagulation.

HEMOPHILIA

A deficiency of a clotting factor that leads to a bleeding diathesis. Subtypes are distinguished on the basis of which factor is lacking (see Table 2.7-1). The condition is usually hereditary but may be **acquired** through the development of an antibody to a clotting factor. This may occur with autoimmune or lymphoproliferative disease, postpartum, or following a blood transfusion. Patients are nearly always male and may have a ⊕ family history.

HISTORY/PE

- Presents with spontaneous hemorrhage into the tissues and joints that, if left untreated, can lead to **arthropathy and joint destruction.**
- Spontaneous intracerebral hemorrhages as well as renal, retroperitoneal, and GI bleeding may also be seen.
- Mild cases may have major hemorrhage after surgery or trauma but are otherwise asymptomatic.

DIAGNOSIS

- **Order labs:**
  - **PT:** Usually normal, but isolated elevations are seen in congenital factor VII deficiency.
  - **aPTT: Prolonged** (the more prolonged, the more severe the hemophilia).
  - **Thrombin time, fibrinogen, bleeding time:** Usually normal.
- **Conduct a mixing study:** Mix the patient's plasma with normal plasma; if this corrects the aPTT, a factor deficiency is likely. If the aPTT does not correct, the patient may have a clotting factor inhibitor.
- **Obtain factor assays:** Specific factor assays should then be performed for factors VII, VIII, IX, XI, and XII. Hemophilia is characterized according to factor level as follows:
- **Mild:** > 5% of normal.
- **Moderate:** 1–3% of normal.
- **Severe:** ≤ 1% of normal.

TABLE 2.7-1. **Types of Hemophilia**

SUBTYPE/INCIDENCE	PATHOGENESIS
Hemophilia A (factor VIII deficiency) (90%)	X-linked inheritance; the most common severe congenital clotting deficiency.
Hemophilia B (factor IX deficiency) (9%)	X-linked inheritance.
Hemophilia C (factor XI deficiency) (< 1%)	Most common in Ashkenazi Jews.
Factor VII deficiency (< 1%)	Presents in a milder, likely heterozygous form.

KEY FACT

Cryoprecipitate consists mainly of factor VIII and fibrinogen, with smaller concentrations of factor XIII, vWF, and fibronectin. It is a more concentrated source of factor VIII and fibrinogen than fresh frozen plasma (FFP).

KEY FACT

DDAVP helps the body release extra factor VIII.

KEY FACT

Ristocetin cofactor assay measures the ability of vWF to agglutinate platelets in vitro in the presence of ristocetin.

TREATMENT

- Treat bleeding episodes with immediate **transfusion of clotting factors (or cryoprecipitate) to at least 40% of normal concentration.**
- The length of treatment varies with the lesion, extending up to several weeks after orthopedic surgery.
- Mild hemophilia may be treated with desmopressin (**DDAVP**); if so, patients should be **fluid restricted** to prevent the side effect of **hyponatremia.**
- Depending on the degree of blood loss, it may be necessary to transfuse RBCs.

VON WILLEBRAND'S DISEASE (vWD)

An **autosomal dominant** condition in which patients have deficient or defective von Willebrand's factor (vWF) with low levels of factor VIII, which is carried by vWF (see Figure 2.7-2). Symptoms are due to platelet dysfunction and to deficient factor VIII. The disease is milder than hemophilia. vWD is the **most common inherited bleeding disorder** (1% of the population is affected).

HISTORY/PE

Presents with easy bruising, mucosal bleeding (eg, epistaxis, oral bleeding), menorrhagia, and postincisional bleeding. Platelet dysfunction is not severe enough to produce petechiae. Symptoms worsen with ASA use.

DIAGNOSIS

- Look for a family history of bleeding disorders.
- Platelet count and **PT** are **normal,** but a **prolonged aPTT and prolonged bleeding time** may be seen as a result of factor VIII deficiency.
- A **ristocetin cofactor assay** of patient plasma can measure the capacity of vWF to agglutinate platelets.

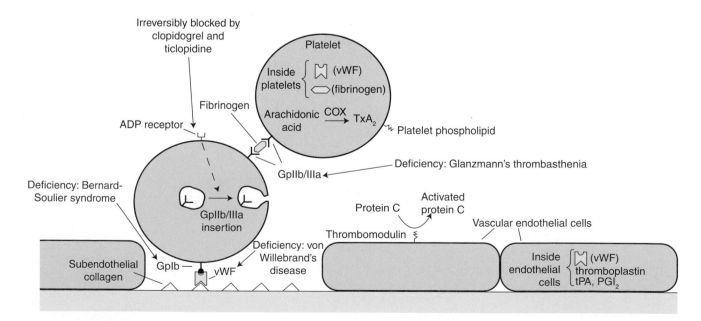

FIGURE 2.7-2. Thrombogenesis deficiencies.

TREATMENT

- Bleeding episodes can be treated with **DDAVP**; menorrhagia can be controlled with **OCPs.**
- Avoid ASA and other inhibitors of platelet function.

HYPERCOAGULABLE STATES

Also called **thrombophilias** or **prothrombotic states,** *hypercoagulable states* is an all-inclusive term describing conditions that ↑ a patient's risk of developing thromboembolic disease. Causes are multiple and may be **genetic, acquired, or physiologic** (see Table 2.7-2). Inherited causes are collectively called *hereditary thrombotic disease,* of which **factor V Leiden** (a polymorphism in factor V, rendering it resistant to inactivity by activated protein C, or APC) is the most common.

HISTORY/PE

- Presents with **recurrent** thrombotic complications, including **DVT, pulmonary embolism (PE), arterial thrombosis, MI, and stroke.** Women may have recurrent miscarriages.
- Although patients may have no recognizable predisposing factors, they usually have 1 or more of the causative factors outlined in Table 2.7-2. They may also have a ⊕ family history.

DIAGNOSIS

- Under ideal circumstances, patients should be diagnosed before they are symptomatic, but this rarely occurs.
- Before a workup is conducted for hereditary causes (see Table 2.7-2), acquired causes of abnormal coagulation values should be ruled out. **Confirmation of a hereditary abnormality requires 2 abnormal values that are obtained while the patient is asymptomatic and untreated, with similar values obtained in 2 other family members.**

TREATMENT

- Treatment should address the type of thrombotic event as well as the area of thrombosis.
- Treat DVT and PE with heparin (unfractionated or LMWH) followed by 3–6 months of oral warfarin anticoagulation for the first event, 6–12 months for the second, and lifelong anticoagulation for subsequent events.

TABLE 2.7-2. Causes of Hypercoagulable States

GENETIC	ACQUIRED	PHYSIOLOGIC
Antithrombin III deficiency	Surgery	Age
Protein C deficiency	Trauma	Pregnancy
Protein S deficiency	Malignancy	
Factor V Leiden	Immobilization	
Hyperhomocysteinemia	Smoking	
Dysfibrinogenemia	Obesity	
Plasminogen deficiency	Antiphospholipid syndrome	
Prothrombin G20210A mutation	Nephrotic syndrome	
	OCPs/hormone replacement	
MTHFR gene mutation	therapy	

KEY FACT

ASA ↑ the risk of bleeding in patients with vWD.

KEY FACT

Suspect PE in a patient with rapid onset of dyspnea, pleuritic chest pain, hypoxia, tachycardia, and an ↑ alveolar-arterial oxygen gradient without another obvious explanation.

Q

A 33-year-old female was admitted to the hospital for anticoagulation after a PE. On day 4 of her stay, her platelet level ↓ from 100,000 to 60,000/mm³ and her INR remains < 2. What is the next best step, and what complications can result from this condition?

- An IVC filter is the best means of preventing PE in DVT patients who have contraindications to anticoagulation (eg, recent trauma, hemorrhage, severe hypertension) and is also recommended for patients who have recurrent DVTs on anticoagulation.

DISSEMINATED INTRAVASCULAR COAGULATION (DIC)

A common disorder among hospitalized patients, second only to liver disease as a cause of acquired coagulopathy. It is caused by **deposition of fibrin in small blood vessels,** leading to thrombosis and end-organ damage. **Depletion of clotting factors and platelets** leads to a bleeding diathesis. It may be associated with almost any severe illness.

HISTORY/PE

- Disorders commonly associated with DIC include obstetric complications, infections with septicemia, neoplasms, acute promyelocytic leukemia, pancreatitis, intravascular hemolysis, vascular disorders (eg, aortic aneurysm), massive tissue injury and trauma, drug reactions, acidosis, and ARDS.
- Clinical presentation is as follows:
  - **Acute:** Presents with generalized bleeding from venipuncture sites and into organs, with ecchymoses and petechiae.
  - **Chronic:** Presents with bruising and mucosal bleeding, thrombophlebitis, renal dysfunction, and transient neurologic syndromes.

DIAGNOSIS

- Diagnosed as outlined in Table 2.7-3.
- DIC may be confused with severe liver disease, but **unlike liver disease, factor VIII is depressed.**

TREATMENT

Reverse the underlying cause; RBC transfusion, platelet transfusion, and shock management.

THROMBOTIC THROMBOCYTOPENIC PURPURA (TTP)

A bleeding disorder due to **platelet microthrombi** that block off small blood vessels, leading to end-organ ischemia and dysfunction. **RBCs are frag-**

KEY FACT

DIC is characterized by both thrombosis and hemorrhage.

This patient is experiencing heparin-induced thrombocytopenia (HIT), which occurs 2° to the formation of antibodies that activate platelets. Because HIT can lead to a hypercoagulable state, heparin must be stopped immediately, and the patient must be switched to lepirudin, danaparoid, or argatroban.

TABLE 2.7-3. **DIC and TTP Features**

VARIABLE	DIC	TTP
Clotting factors	↓	Normal
PT and aPTT	↑	Normal
Platelets	↓	↓
D-dimer and fibrin degradation products	↑	Normal
Fibrinogen level	↓	Normal
Microangiopathic hemolytic anemia	Present	Present

mented by contact with the microthrombi, leading to hemolysis (microangiopathic hemolytic anemia). The cause of initial microthrombus formation is unknown but may be infectious (bacterial toxins), drug related, autoimmune, or idiopathic.

HISTORY/PE

- A **clinical syndrome** characterized by **5 signs/symptoms:**
  - **Low platelet count**
  - **Microangiopathic hemolytic anemia**
  - **Neurologic changes (delirium, seizure, stroke)**
  - **Impaired renal function**
  - **Fever**
- Maintain high clinical suspicion for TTP if 3 of 5 of these symptoms are present.

DIAGNOSIS

- Diagnosis is largely clinical (see Table 2.7-3).
- It is rare for all signs to be present, but the presence of schistocytes (broken RBCs) on peripheral smear (see Figure 2.7-3) with low platelets and rising creatinine is highly suggestive. Nucleated RBCs are also often seen in the peripheral smear.
- Part of a spectrum of diseases that includes hemolytic-uremic syndrome (HUS) and HELLP syndrome (see the Obstetrics chapter).
  - **HUS:** Characterized by renal failure, hemolytic anemia, and low platelets. **Severe elevations in creatinine levels are more typical of HUS than of TTP.**
  - **HELLP syndrome:** Affects pregnant women, often occurring in conjunction with preeclampsia.

TREATMENT

Plasma replacement and plasmapheresis; steroids to ↓ microthrombus formation. **Platelet transfusion is contraindicated,** as it often worsens the patient's condition 2° to added platelet aggregation and microvascular thrombosis.

IDIOPATHIC THROMBOCYTOPENIC PURPURA (ITP)

A relatively common cause of thrombocytopenia. **IgG antibodies** are formed against the patient's platelets. Bone marrow production of platelets is ↑, with ↑ megakaryocytes in the marrow. The **most common immunologic disorder in women of childbearing age.** May be acute or chronic.

HISTORY/PE

- Patients often feel well and present with no systemic symptoms. They may have minor bleeding, easy bruising, petechiae, hematuria, hematemesis, or melena. Bleeding is mucocutaneous. Generally there is no splenomegaly.
- ITP is associated with a range of conditions, including lymphoma, leukemia, SLE, HIV, and HCV. Presentation is as follows:
  - **Acute:** Abrupt onset of hemorrhagic complications following a viral illness. Commonly affects children 2–6 years of age, with males and females affected equally.
  - **Chronic:** Insidious onset that is unrelated to infection. Most often affects adults 20–40 years of age; females are 3 times more likely to be affected than males.

An 8-year-old girl presents to the ER with 2 days of fever, vomiting, bloody diarrhea, and irritability. She began feeling unwell after attending a classmate's birthday party. Her labs reveal thrombocytopenia and an ↑ creatinine level. What is the best antibiotic therapy?

 KEY FACT

The 3 causes of microangiopathic hemolytic anemia are HUS, TTP, and DIC.

 KEY FACT

Remember: **DIC**k's **HoUS**e got **TP**ed because he caused microangiopathic hemolytic anemia.

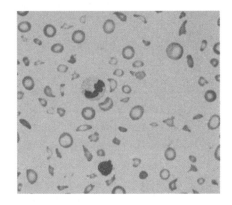

FIGURE 2.7-3. Schistocytes. These fragmented RBCs may be seen in microangiopathic hemolytic anemia and in mechanical hemolysis. (Courtesy of Peter McPhedran, MD, Yale Department of Hematology.)

HUS is the most common cause of acute renal failure in children. Supportive therapy includes IV fluids, BP control, blood transfusion, and, if necessary, dialysis. Antibiotics are not indicated, as they are thought to ↓ expulsion of the toxin and may ↑ toxin from the destruction of bacteria.

MNEMONIC

Differential diagnosis of thrombocytopenia—

HIT SHOC

HIT or **H**US
ITP
TTP or **T**reatment (meds)
Splenomegaly
Hereditary (eg, Wiskott-Aldrich syndrome)
Other causes (eg, malignancy)
Chemotherapy

KEY FACT

Anti-D (Rh) immunoglobulin and rituximab are second-line therapies for ITP.

KEY FACT

Anti-D (Rh) immunoglobulin and IVIG act as "decoys" so that WBCs will recognize them instead of IgG on platelets.

DIAGNOSIS

- A **diagnosis of exclusion,** as the test for platelet-associated antibodies is a poor one.
- Once other causes of thrombocytopenia have been ruled out, a diagnosis can be made on the basis of the history and physical, a CBC, and a peripheral blood smear showing normal RBC morphology.
- Most patients do not require bone marrow biopsy, which would show ↑ megakaryocytes as the only abnormality.

TREATMENT

- Most patients with acute childhood ITP spontaneously remit, but this is rarely the case with chronic ITP.
- Treatment is reserved for patients with symptomatic bleeding. Those with platelet counts > 20,000/mm³ are generally asymptomatic.
- Platelet transfusions are of no benefit, as patients' IgG levels will lead to destruction of platelets.
- The main therapies are **corticosteroids, high-dose gamma globulin (IVIG), and splenectomy.** Most patients respond to corticosteroids, but if they cannot be tapered after 3–6 months, splenectomy should be considered.
- In **pregnant patients, severe thrombocytopenia may occur in the fetus.**

Blood Cell Differentiation

Figure 2.7-4 illustrates the various blood cell categories and lineages.

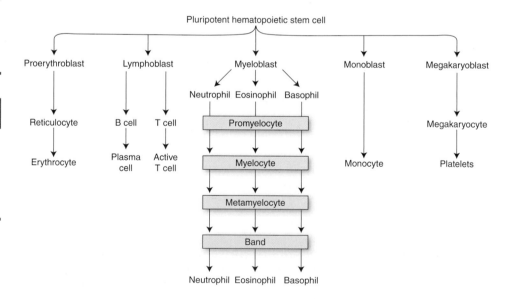

FIGURE 2.7-4. Blood cell differentiation.

Red Blood Cell (RBC) Disorders

ANEMIAS

Anemia is a disorder of **low hematocrit and hemoglobin.** There are several subtypes, which are classified according to RBC morphology and reticulocyte count (see Figure 2.7-5). Once anemia has been diagnosed by a low hemoglobin/hematocrit, the approach starts with the mean corpuscular volume (MCV):

- < 80 fL: **Microcytic anemia.**
- 80–100 fL: **Normocytic anemia.**
- > 100 fL: **Macrocytic anemia.**

Iron Deficiency Anemia (a Microcytic Anemia)

A condition in which iron loss exceeds intake. May occur when **dietary intake is insufficient** for the patient's needs (eg, when needs are ↑ by growth or pregnancy) or in the setting of **chronic blood loss,** usually 2° to menstruation or GI bleeding. **Toddlers, adolescent girls,** and **women of childbearing age** are most commonly affected.

KEY FACT

Iron deficiency anemia in an elderly patient may be due to colorectal cancer and must therefore be evaluated to rule out malignancy.

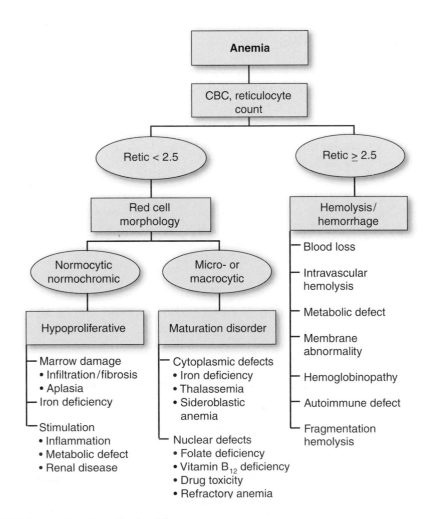

FIGURE 2.7-5.   Anemia algorithm.

MNEMONIC

Causes of microcytic anemia—

TICS

Thalassemia
Iron deficiency
Chronic disease
Sideroblastic anemia

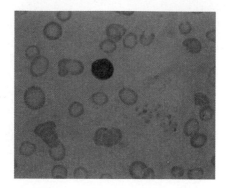

FIGURE 2.7-6. Iron deficiency anemia. Note the microcytic, hypochromic RBCs ("doughnut cells") with enlarged areas of central pallor. (Courtesy of Peter McPhedran, MD, Yale Department of Hematology.)

KEY FACT

Most macrocytic anemias are caused by processes that interfere with normal DNA synthesis and replication.

HISTORY/PE

- Symptoms include **fatigue, weakness, brittle nails,** and **pica.** If the anemia develops slowly, patients are generally asymptomatic.
- Physical findings include **glossitis, angular cheilitis,** and **koilonychia** ("spoon nails").

DIAGNOSIS

- Bone marrow biopsy looking for evidence of iron stores is the gold standard but is seldom performed.
- Iron deficiency is often confused with **anemia of chronic disease,** in which iron use by the body is impaired. Labs can help differentiate these conditions (see Table 2.7-4).
- Peripheral blood smear shows **hypochromic and microcytic RBCs** (see Figure 2.7-6) with a **low reticulocyte count.**
- Low serum ferritin reflects low body stores of iron and confirms the diagnosis. However, ferritin is also an acute-phase reactant and may thus obscure evidence of iron deficiency.
- Red cell distribution width (RDW) elevation is a highly specific test for iron deficiency anemia.

TREATMENT

- Treat with **replacement iron for 4–6 months.** Oral iron sulfate may lead to nausea, constipation, diarrhea, and abdominal pain. Antacids may interfere with iron absorption.
- If necessary, IV iron dextran can be administered but is associated with a 10% risk of serious side effects, including anaphylaxis. Other parenteral preparations are available with less allergic risk, such as iron sucrose.

Megaloblastic Anemia (a Macrocytic Anemia)

Vitamin B$_{12}$ (cobalamin) and **folate deficiency** interfere with DNA synthesis, leading to a delay in blood cell maturation. Cobalamin deficiency is due to intestinal malabsorption, traditionally from **pernicious anemia** (destruction of parietal cells, which produce the intrinsic factor needed for cobalamin absorption), although this is a rare disorder. Folate deficiency results from insufficient dietary folate, malabsorption, alcoholism, or use of certain drugs. **Drugs that interfere with DNA synthesis,** including many chemotherapeutic agents, may lead to megaloblastic anemia.

HISTORY/PE

- Presents with **fatigue, pallor, diarrhea, loss of appetite,** and **headaches.**
- Cobalamin deficiency affects the nervous system, so patients lacking that vitamin may develop a **demyelinating disorder** and may present with

TABLE 2.7-4. Iron Deficiency Anemia vs. Anemia of Chronic Disease

	IRON DEFICIENCY	CHRONIC DISEASE	BOTH
Serum iron	↓	↓	↓
TIBC or transferrin	↑	↓	Normal/↑
Ferritin	↓	↑	Normal/↓
Serum transferrin receptor	↑	Normal	Normal/↑

symptoms of motor, sensory, autonomic, and/or neuropsychiatric dysfunction, known as **subacute combined degeneration of the cord.**

DIAGNOSIS

- Peripheral smear shows RBCs with an **elevated MCV.** Hypersegmented (> 5) granulocytes can also be seen (see Figure 2.7-7).
- Bone marrow sample reveals **giant neutrophils** and **hypersegmented mature granulocytes.**
- The **Schilling test** (ingestion of radiolabeled cobalamin both with and without added intrinsic factor) is classic for measuring the absorption of cobalamin. Although this test is rarely performed, its interpretation is frequently tested. The patient is first given unlabeled B_{12} IM to saturate B_{12} receptors in the liver, followed by an oral challenge of radiolabeled B_{12}. The radiolabeled B_{12} will pass into the urine if it is properly absorbed, as the liver's B_{12} receptors will be saturated from the IM dose.
  - **Radiolabeled B_{12} in urine:** Dietary B_{12} deficiency.
  - **No radiolabeled B_{12} in urine:** Consider pernicious anemia, bacterial overgrowth, or pancreatic enzyme deficiency; test the hypothesis with the addition of intrinsic factor, antibiotics, or pancreatic enzymes to radiolabeled B_{12}.
- Serum vitamin levels are poorly diagnostic of deficiencies and are thus used with adjunctive tests, including red cell folate levels and methylmalonic acid (MMA) and homocysteine levels:
  - **B_{12} deficiency:** Elevated MMA and homocysteine.
  - **Folate deficiency:** Normal MMA; elevated homocysteine.

TREATMENT

Address the cause of the anemia, and correct the underlying cause.

Hemolytic Anemia (a Normocytic Anemia)

Occurs when bone marrow production is unable to compensate for ↑ destruction of circulating blood cells. Etiologies include the following:

- **G6PD deficiency:** An X-linked recessive disease that ↑ RBC sensitivity to oxidative stress.
- **Paroxysmal nocturnal hemoglobinuria:** A disorder in which blood cell sensitivity to complement activation is ↑. Patients are prone to thrombotic events.
- **Hereditary spherocytosis:** An abnormality of the RBC membrane. **Diagnose with a peripheral smear** (see Figure 2.7-8) **and an osmotic fragility test.**
- **Autoimmune RBC destruction:** Occurs 2° to EBV infection, mycoplasmal infection, CLL, rheumatoid disease, or medications.
- **Sickle cell disease:** A recessive β-globin mutation (see the following section).
- **Microangiopathic hemolytic anemia:** TTP, HUS, DIC.
- **Mechanical hemolysis:** Associated with mechanical heart valves.
- **Other:** Malaria, hypersplenism.

HISTORY/PE

- Presents with **pallor, fatigue, tachycardia,** and **tachypnea.**
- Patients are typically **jaundiced,** with low haptoglobin and elevated indirect bilirubin and LDH. Urine is dark with **hemoglobinuria,** and there is ↑ excretion of urinary and fecal urobilinogen. **Reticulocyte count is elevated.**

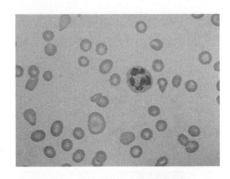

FIGURE 2.7-7. Hypersegmentation. The nucleus of this hypersegmented neutrophil has 6 lobes (6 or more nuclear lobes are required). This is a characteristic finding of megaloblastic anemia. (Courtesy of Peter McPhedran, MD, Yale Department of Hematology.)

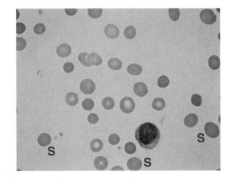

FIGURE 2.7-8. Spherocytes. These RBCs (S) lack areas of central pallor. Spherocytes are seen in autoimmune hemolysis and in hereditary spherocytosis. (Courtesy of Peter McPhedran, MD, Yale Department of Hematology.)

KEY FACT

Causes of oxidative stress in G6PD deficiency include infection, metabolic acidosis, fava beans, antimalarials, dapsone, sulfonamides, and nitrofurantoin.

KEY FACT

Patients with Fanconi's anemia may be identified on physical examination by café au lait spots, short stature, and radial/thumb hypoplasia/aplasia.

KEY FACT

The indirect Coombs' test detects antibodies to RBCs in the patient's serum. The direct Coombs' test detects sensitized erythrocytes.

DIAGNOSIS

Diagnosed by the history and clinical presentation. High LDH, elevated indirect bilirubin, and ↓ haptoglobin levels are consistent with a diagnosis of hemolytic anemia. Also obtain a reticulocyte count. A **Coombs' test** (see Figure 2.7-9) is used to detect autoimmune hemolysis.

TREATMENT

Treatment varies with the cause of hemolysis but typically includes **corticosteroids** to address immunologic causes and **iron supplementation** to replace urinary losses. Splenectomy may be helpful, and transfusion may be necessary to treat severe anemia.

Aplastic Anemia

A rare condition caused by failure of blood cell production due to **destruction of bone marrow cells**. It may be hereditary, as in **Fanconi's anemia;** may have an **autoimmune** or a **viral** etiology (eg, HIV, parvovirus B19); or may result from exposure to **toxins** (eg, drugs, cleaning solvents) or **radiation.**

HISTORY/PE

Patients are typically **pancytopenic,** with symptoms resulting from a lack of RBCs, WBCs, and platelets—eg, **pallor, weakness, a tendency to infection, petechiae, bruising, and bleeding.**

DIAGNOSIS

Diagnosed by clinical presentation and CBC; **verified by a bone marrow biopsy** revealing hypocellularity and space occupied by fat.

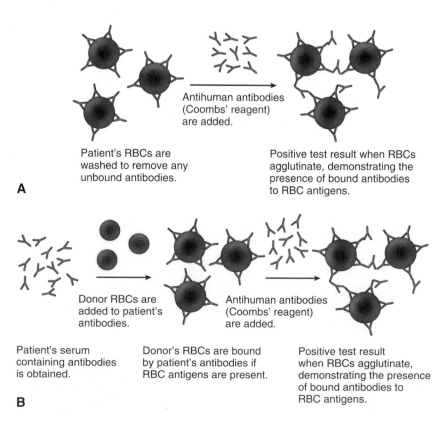

Antihuman antibodies
(Coombs' reagent)
are added.

Patient's RBCs are
washed to remove any
unbound antibodies.

Positive test result when RBCs
agglutinate, demonstrating the
presence of bound antibodies
to RBC antigens.

A

Donor RBCs are
added to patient's
antibodies.

Antihuman antibodies
(Coombs' reagent)
are added.

Patient's serum
containing antibodies
is obtained.

Donor's RBCs are bound
by patient's antibodies if
RBC antigens are present.

Positive test result
when RBCs agglutinate,
demonstrating the presence
of bound antibodies to
RBC antigens.

B

FIGURE 2.7-9.   **Direct (A) and indirect (B) Coombs' tests.**

TREATMENT

Blood transfusion and stem cell transplantation to replace absent cells; immunosuppression with cyclosporin A and antithymocyte globulin to prevent autoimmune destruction of marrow. **Infections** are a major cause of mortality and should be treated aggressively.

Sickle Cell Disease (SCD)

An **autosomal recessive** disorder most commonly caused by a mutation of adult hemoglobin (the β chain has glu replaced by val). Signs and symptoms are due to ↓ **RBC survival** and a tendency of sickled cells to lead to **vaso-occlusion.**

HISTORY/PE

- Asymptomatic during the first 1–2 years of life; may first present with dactylitis in childhood. Later, hemolysis results in **anemia, jaundice, cholelithiasis, ↑ cardiac output (murmur and cardiomegaly),** and **delayed growth.**
- Vaso-occlusion leads to ischemic organ damage, especially **splenic infarction,** which predisposes to pneumococcal sepsis and acute chest syndrome (pneumonia and/or pulmonary infarction; see Figure 2.7-10). Patients also experience painful crises of unknown etiology. Common triggers for a vaso-occlusive crisis (VOC) include cold temperatures, dehydration, and infection.
- Other potential complications include splenic sequestration, which occurs in patients who have not infarcted their spleens, and aplastic crisis, which is usually 2° to infection with parvovirus B19. These complications both present with ↓ hematocrit but are distinguished clinically by ↓ platelets in aplastic crisis (2° to bone marrow involvement) and normal to ↑ platelets in splenic sequestration.

DIAGNOSIS

The sickle cell screen is based on a blood smear with sickle cells and target cells (see Figure 2.7-11). The gold standard is quantitative hemoglobin electrophoresis.

> **KEY FACT**

SCD represents a qualitative defect in the β-globin chain.

> **KEY FACT**

The most common cause of osteomyelitis in SCD patients is *S aureus*. However, SCD patients are especially prone to *Salmonella* infections causing osteomyelitis. They are also at ↑ risk for AVN of the hip.

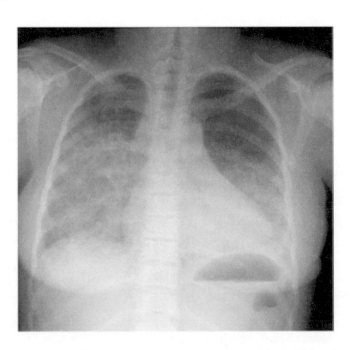

FIGURE 2.7-10.   Acute chest syndrome. Frontal CXR of a 19-year-old female with sickle cell disease and acute chest pain. Note the bilateral lower and midlung opacities and mild cardiomegaly. (Reproduced with permission from USMLERx.com.)

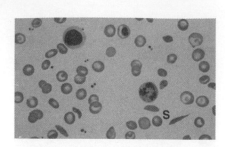

FIGURE 2.7-11. Sickle cell disease. Sickle-shaped RBCs (S) are almost always seen on blood smear, regardless of whether the patient is having a sickle cell crisis. Anisocytosis, poikilocytosis, target cells, and nucleated RBCs can also be seen. (Courtesy of Peter McPhedran, MD, Yale Department of Hematology.)

TREATMENT

- Treat with **hydroxyurea,** which stimulates the **production of fetal hemoglobin** (hydroxyurea is teratogenic, so it is contraindicated in pregnancy).
- If hydroxyurea does not prove effective, chronic transfusion therapy, which carries the risk of iron overload, can be tried.
- Health maintenance includes treating cholelithiasis with cholecystectomy, chronic folate supplementation, pneumococcal vaccination, and, when the patient is < 5 years of age, penicillin BID.
- VOCs must be treated with adequate pain management, O_2 therapy, IV fluid rehydration, and antibiotics (if infection is suspected to be the trigger).
- To prevent VOCs from progressing to acute chest syndrome, initiate aggressive hydration and incentive spirometry, and keep the sickle variant < 40%. This can be done with simple transfusions or, if necessary, exchange transfusion in an ICU setting.

THALASSEMIAS

Hereditary disorders involving ↓ or absent production of normal globin chains of hemoglobin. α-thalassemia is caused by a mutation of 1 or more of the 4 genes for α-hemoglobin; β-thalassemia results from a mutation of 1 or both of the 2 genes for β-hemoglobin.

HISTORY/PE

Thalassemia is most common among people of **African, Middle Eastern,** and **Asian descent.** Disease presentation and prognosis vary with the number of genes missing (see Table 2.7-5).

DIAGNOSIS

Diagnosed by hemoglobin electrophoresis evaluation (but note that this is normal in α-thalassemia) and DNA studies.

TABLE 2.7-5. Differential Diagnosis of Thalassemias

SUBTYPE	NUMBER OF GENES PRESENT	CLINICAL FEATURES
β-thalassemia major	0/2 β	Patients develop severe microcytic anemia in the first year of life and need chronic transfusions or marrow transplant to survive.
β-thalassemia minor	1/2 β	Patients are asymptomatic, but their cells are microcytic and hypochromic on peripheral smear.
Hydrops fetalis	0/4 α	Patients die in utero.
Hemoglobin H disease	1/4 α	Patients have severe hypochromic, microcytic anemia with chronic hemolysis, splenomegaly, jaundice, and cholelithiasis. **The reticulocyte count elevates to compensate,** and one-third of patients have skeletal changes due to expanded erythropoiesis.
α-thalassemia trait	2/4 α	Patients have low MCV but are usually asymptomatic.
Silent carrier	3/4 α	Patients have no signs or symptoms of disease.

TREATMENT

Most patients do not require treatment, but those with β-thalassemia major and hemoglobin H disease are commonly transfusion dependent and should be given iron chelators (deferoxamine) to prevent overload.

POLYCYTHEMIAS

Erythrocytosis (an abnormal elevation of hematocrit) may be either 1° (due to ↑ RBC production) or 2° (due to ↓ plasma volume and hemoconcentration).

HISTORY/PE

- Characterized by ↑ hematocrit, ↓ tissue blood flow and oxygenation, and ↑ cardiac work.
- Patients present with **"hyperviscosity syndrome,"** which consists of easy bleeding/bruising, blurred vision, neurologic abnormalities, plethora, pruritus (especially after a warm bath), hepatomegaly, splenomegaly, and CHF.
- 1° erythrocytosis is associated with hypoxia (from lung disease, smoking, high altitudes, or a poor intrauterine environment), neoplasia (erythropoietin-producing tumors), or polycythemia vera (PCV).
  - PCV results from clonal proliferation of a pluripotent marrow stem cell due to a JAK2 mutation. Although all marrow cell lines ↑, RBCs are most significantly affected.
  - This blood disorder primarily affects the elderly.
- 2° erythrocytosis is associated with excessive diuresis, severe gastroenteritis, and burns.

DIAGNOSIS

- Erythrocytosis is diagnosed clinically and by cell counts, with ABGs used to assess hypoxia or imaging to demonstrate neoplasia.
- Patients with PCV have excess RBCs, WBCs, and platelets. **Levels of erythropoietin** may be useful in distinguishing PCV, in which levels are low, from other causes of polycythemia. JAK2 mutation tests often confirm the diagnosis.

TREATMENT

- **Phlebotomy** relieves symptoms of erythrocytosis, but treatment should also address the underlying cause.
- PCV can be treated with **cytoreductive drugs** such as hydroxyurea or interferon. Because PCV is prothrombotic, **ASA** should also be used. With treatment, survival is 7–10 years.

TRANSFUSION REACTIONS

Blood transfusion is generally safe but may result in a variety of adverse reactions (see Table 2.7-6). Nonhemolytic febrile reactions and minor allergic reactions are the most common, each occurring in 3–4% of all transfusions.

PORPHYRIA

The porphyrias are a group of inherited disorders that include acute intermittent porphyria, porphyria cutanea tarda, and erythropoietic porphyria. Some porphyrias are **autosomal dominant** (eg, acute intermittent porphyria) and

KEY FACT

Premedication with acetaminophen and diphenhydramine is sometimes used to prevent transfusion reactions.

KEY FACT

Hemoglobinuria in hemolytic transfusion reaction may lead to acute tubular necrosis and subsequent renal failure.

KEY FACT

Heme is necessary for the production of hemoglobin, myoglobin, and cytochrome molecules.

A 15-year-old female sees her pediatrician after being diagnosed with mononucleosis. Her WBC count returns at 56,000/mm³. The physician orders a leukocyte alkaline phosphatase (LAP) to distinguish between a leukemoid reaction and a hematologic malignancy. What is the expected result in a leukemoid reaction?

TABLE 2.7-6. Transfusion Reactions

VARIABLE	NONHEMOLYTIC FEBRILE REACTION	MINOR ALLERGIC REACTION	HEMOLYTIC TRANSFUSION REACTION
Mechanism	Cytokine formation during storage of blood.	Antibody formation against donor proteins, usually after receiving plasma-containing product.	Antibody formation against donor erythrocytes, resulting either from ABO incompatibility or from minor antigen mismatch.
Presentation	Fever, chills, rigors, and malaise 1–6 hours after transfusion.	Prominent urticaria.	Fevers, chills, nausea, flushing, burning at the IV site, tachycardia, hypotension during or shortly after the transfusion.
Treatment	Stop the transfusion and give acetaminophen.	Give antihistamines. If the reaction is severe, it may be necessary to stop the transfusion and give epinephrine.	Stop the transfusion immediately! Give vigorous IV fluids and maintain good urine output.

KEY FACT

The telltale sign of porphyria is pink urine. The classic case involves a college student who consumes alcohol and barbiturates at a party and then has an acute episode of abdominal pain and brown urine the next day.

others **autosomal recessive** (eg, erythropoietic porphyria). All involve **abnormalities of heme production** that lead to an accumulation of porphyrins.

HISTORY/PE

- Signs and symptoms vary with the type of porphyria. In general, however, porphyrias are characterized by a combination of **photodermatitis, neuropsychiatric complaints,** and **visceral complaints** that typically take the form of **colicky abdominal pain and seizures.**
- Physical examination reveals **tachycardia, skin erythema and blisters, areflexia, and a nonspecific abdominal examination.**
- Patients with the erythropoietic form present with **hemolytic anemia.** Acute attacks are associated with stimulants of ↑ heme synthesis such as fasting or chemical exposures; well-known triggers are alcohol, barbiturates, and OCPs. Urine may appear red, pink, or brown after an acute attack. Patients may have a ⊕ family history.

DIAGNOSIS

Diagnosed by a combination of the history and physical along with labs showing elevated blood, urine, and stool porphyrins. Enzyme assays may also be helpful.

TREATMENT

- Avoidance of triggers and symptomatic treatment during acute attacks.
- High doses of **glucose** may be administered to ↓ heme synthesis during attacks (provides ⊖ feedback to the heme synthetic pathway).

LAP would be elevated. Hematologic malignancies, in contrast, have low LAP values.

White Blood Cell (WBC) Disorders

LEUKEMIAS

Malignant proliferations of hematopoietic cells, categorized by the type of cell involved and their level of differentiation.

Acute Leukemias

Acute myelogenous and lymphocytic leukemias are clonal disorders of early hematopoietic stem cells. They are characterized by rapid growth of immature blood cells (blasts) that overwhelms the ability of bone marrow to produce normal cells.

HISTORY/PE

- Acute myelogenous leukemia (AML) and acute lymphocytic leukemia (ALL) affect children as well as adults. **ALL is the most common childhood malignancy.**
- Disease onset and progression are rapid; patients present with signs and symptoms of anemia (pallor, fatigue) and thrombocytopenia (**petechiae, purpura, bleeding**). Medullary expansion and periosteal involvement may lead to **bone pain** (common in ALL).
- On examination, patients may have **hepatosplenomegaly** and **swollen/ bleeding gums** from leukemic infiltration and ↓ platelets. Leukemic cells also infiltrate the skin and CNS.

DIAGNOSIS

- Based on examination of the patient's bone marrow, obtained by biopsy and aspiration, or peripheral blood if circulating blasts are present. Marrow that is infiltrated with blast cells (> 20–30%) is consistent with a leukemic process. **In AML, the leukemic cells are myeloblasts; in ALL they are lymphoblasts.** These cells may be distinguished by examination of morphology (see Figure 2.7-12), cytogenetics, cytochemistry, and immunophenotyping (see Table 2.7-7).
- The WBC count is usually elevated, but the cells are dysfunctional, and patients may be neutropenic with a **history of frequent infection.** If the WBC count is very high (> 100,000/mm³), there is a risk of **leukostasis** (blasts occluding the microcirculation, leading to pulmonary edema, CNS symptoms, ischemic injury, and DIC).
- The type of acute leukemia is further classified according to the **FAB system** (ALL: L1–L3; AML: M0–M7) and karyotype analysis. Prognosis varies with leukemic cytogenetics.

A 41-year-old male is diagnosed with acute myelogenous leukemia (AML). Fluorescence in situ hybridization (FISH) analysis reveals that he has acute promyelocytic leukemia (APL), FAB subtype M3. What is the preferred therapy for this subtype of AML?

KEY FACT

A characteristic sign for AML type M3 (APL) is the **Auer rod** (see Figure 2.7-13), although Auer rods can be seen in other AML subtypes as well.

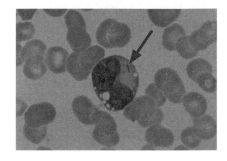

FIGURE 2.7-13.   Auer rod in AML. The red rod-shaped structure (arrow) in the cytoplasm of the myeloblast is pathognomonic. (Courtesy of Peter McPhedran, MD, Yale Department of Hematology.)

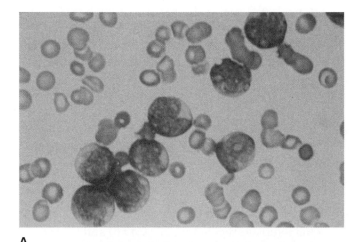

A

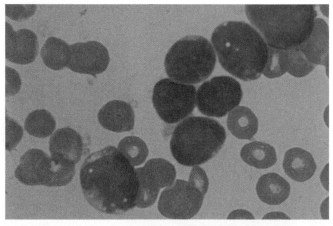

B

FIGURE 2.7-12.   AML vs. ALL on peripheral smear. (A) AML. Large, uniform myeloblasts with round or kidney-shaped nuclei and prominent nucleoli are characteristic. **(B) ALL.** Peripheral blood smear reveals numerous large, uniform lymphoblasts, which are large cells with a high nuclear-to-cytoplasmic ratio. Some lymphoblasts have visible clefts in their nuclei. (Courtesy of Peter McPhedran, MD, Yale Department of Hematology.)

APL has a good prognosis because it is responsive to all-*trans*-retinoic acid (ATRA) therapy. This AML subtype is also associated with an ↑ incidence of DIC and a chromosomal translocation involving chromosomes 15 and 17.

TABLE 2.7-7. Myeloblasts vs. Lymphoblasts

VARIABLE	MYELOBLAST	LYMPHOBLAST
Size	Larger (2–4 times RBC)	Smaller (1.5–3.0 times RBC)
Amount of cytoplasm	More	Less
Nucleoli	Conspicuous	Inconspicuous
Granules	Common, fine	Uncommon, coarse
Auer rods	Present in 50% of cases (see Figure 2.7-13)	Absent
Myeloperoxidase	⊕	⊖

KEY FACT

Eighty-five percent of children with ALL achieve complete remission with chemotherapy.

TREATMENT

- ALL and AML are treated primarily with chemotherapeutic agents, although transfusions, antibiotics, and colony-stimulating factors are also used. Patients with unfavorable genetics or those who do not achieve remission may be candidates for bone marrow transplantation.
- Prior to therapy, patients should be well hydrated; if their WBC counts are high, they may be started on **allopurinol** to prevent hyperuricemia and renal insufficiency resulting from blast lysis (**tumor lysis syndrome**).
- Leukostasis syndrome may be treated with hydroxyurea +/– leukapheresis to rapidly ↓ WBC count.
- Indicators of a poor prognosis are as follows:
    - **ALL:** Age < 1 year or > 10 years; an ↑ in WBC count to > 50,000/mm³; the presence of the Philadelphia chromosome t(9,22) (associated with B-cell cancer); CNS involvement at diagnosis.
    - **AML:** Age > 60 years; elevated LDH; poor-risk or complex karyotype.

Chronic Lymphocytic Leukemia (CLL)

A malignant, clonal proliferation of functionally incompetent lymphocytes that accumulate in the bone marrow, peripheral blood, lymph nodes, spleen, and liver. The most common type of leukemia. Almost all cases involve **well-differentiated B lymphocytes.** Primarily affects **older adults** (median age 65); the male-to-female ratio is 2:1.

HISTORY/PE

Often asymptomatic, but many patients present with **fatigue, malaise, and infection.** Common physical findings are **lymphadenopathy and splenomegaly.**

DIAGNOSIS

- Diagnosed by the clinical picture; may be confirmed by flow cytometry demonstrating the presence of CD5—normally found only on T cells—on leukemic cells with the characteristic B-cell antigens CD20 and CD21.
- CBC shows lymphocytosis (lymphocyte count > 5000/mm³) with an abundance of small, normal-appearing lymphocytes and ruptured **smudge cells** on peripheral smear (see Figure 2.7-14). **Granulocytopenia, anemia, and thrombocytopenia** are common owing to marrow infiltration with leukemic cells. Abnormal function by the leukemic cells leads to **hypogammaglobulinemia.**

KEY FACT

Look for smudge cells to point you toward CLL. Smudge cells result from the coverslip crushing the fragile leukemia cells.

- Bone marrow biopsy is rarely required for diagnosis or staging but may provide prognostic information and may help assess response to therapy.

TREATMENT

- The clinical stage correlates with expected survival.
- Treatment is palliative. The degree of peripheral lymphocytosis does not correlate with prognosis, nor does it dictate when treatment should be initiated. **Treatment is often withheld until patients are symptomatic**—eg, when they present with recurrent infection, severe lymphadenopathy or splenomegaly, anemia, and thrombocytopenia.
- Treatment consists primarily of chemotherapy, although radiation may be useful for localized lymphadenopathy.
- Although CLL is not curable, long disease-free intervals may be achieved with adequate treatment of symptoms.

Chronic Myelogenous Leukemia (CML)

Involves clonal expansion of myeloid progenitor cells, leading to leukocytosis with excess granulocytes and basophils and sometimes ↑ erythrocytes and platelets as well. To truly be CML, the BCR-ABL translocation must be present. In > 90% of patients, this is reflected by the **Philadelphia chromosome t(9,22)**. CML primarily affects **middle-aged** patients.

HISTORY/PE

- With routine blood testing, many patients are diagnosed while asymptomatic. However, typical signs and symptoms are those of **anemia.**
- Patients frequently have **splenomegaly** with LUQ pain and early satiety. Hepatomegaly may be present as well. The **constitutional symptoms** of weight loss, anorexia, fever, and chills may also be seen.
- Patients with CML go through 3 disease phases:
    - **Chronic:** Without treatment, typically lasts 3.5–5.0 years. Signs and symptoms are as described above. Infection and bleeding complications are rare.
    - **Accelerated:** A transition toward blast crisis, with an ↑ in peripheral and bone marrow blood counts. Should be suspected when the differential shows an abrupt ↑ in basophils and thrombocytopenia (platelet count < 100,000/mm³).
    - **Blast crisis:** Resembles acute leukemia; survival is 3–6 months.

DIAGNOSIS

- Diagnosed by the clinical picture, including labs; cytogenetic analysis usually reveals the Philadelphia chromosome.
- CBC shows a **very high WBC count**—often > 100,000/mm³ at diagnosis, and sometimes reaching > 500,000/mm³. The differential shows granulocytes in all stages of maturation. Rarely, the WBC count will be so elevated as to cause a **hyperviscosity syndrome.**
- LAP is low; LDH, uric acid, and B₁₂ levels are elevated.

TREATMENT

Varies with disease phase and is undergoing rapid change, particularly since the introduction of targeted therapies.

- **Chronic:** Treated with imatinib. Younger patients can be treated with allogeneic stem cell transplantation if a suitable matched sibling donor is available.

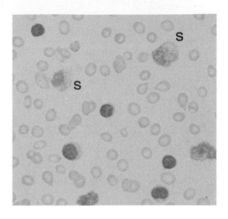

FIGURE 2.7-14. CLL with characteristic smudge cells. The numerous small, mature lymphocytes and smudge cells (S; fragile malignant lymphocytes are disrupted during blood smear preparation) are characteristic. (Courtesy of Peter McPhedran, Yale Department of Hematology.)

> **KEY FACT**

Likely diagnosis based on age at presentation:
- **ALL:** < 13 years (but can present in any age group)
- **AML:** 13–40 years (but can present in any age group)
- **CML:** 40–60 years
- **CLL:** > 60 years

A 71-year-old male seeks care for marked lethargy and constipation that are worsening. He also notes a dull back pain that is present at most times, even at night. His lab studies have been normal with the exception of an ↑ creatinine level. What is most likely responsible for the patient's worsening renal function?

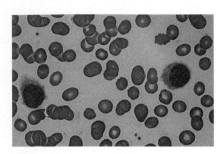

FIGURE 2.7-15. Hairy cell leukemia. Note the hairlike cytoplasmic projections from neoplastic lymphocytes. Villous lymphoma can also have this appearance. (Courtesy of Peter McPhedran, MD, Yale Department of Hematology.)

■ **Blast:** Treatment is the same as that for acute leukemia, or it may involve dasatinib plus hematopoietic stem cell transplantation or a clinical trial.

Hairy Cell Leukemia (HCL)

A malignant disorder of well-differentiated B lymphocytes with an unclear cause. HCL is a **rare** disease that accounts for 2% of adult leukemia cases and most commonly affects **older males.**

HISTORY/PE

■ Typically presents with pancytopenia, bone marrow infiltration, and splenomegaly.
■ Patients complain of weakness, fatigue, petechiae and bruising, infection (especially with atypical mycobacteria such as *Mycobacterium avium–intracellulare*), abdominal pain, early satiety, and weight loss. Symptoms are similar to those of CLL except that patients rarely have lymphadenopathy.

DIAGNOSIS

■ Diagnosed by the history, physical examination, and labs; confirmed through the identification of hairy cells in the blood, marrow, or spleen (see Figure 2.7-15).
■ **Tartrate-resistant acid phosphatase (TRAP) staining of hairy cells,** electron microscopy, and flow cytometry are helpful in distinguishing the pathognomonic hairy cells.
■ CBC usually demonstrates **leukopenia** (making the name *leukemia* a misnomer); roughly 85% of the time a peripheral smear shows **hairy cells, or mononuclear cells with abundant pale cytoplasm and cytoplasmic projections.**

TREATMENT

■ Ten percent of patients have a benign course and never require therapy, but the remainder develop progressive pancytopenia and splenomegaly, requiring therapy. **Nucleoside analogs** (the first-line therapy is cladribine) are currently the initial treatment of choice and effectively induce remission.
■ Other treatment options include splenectomy and IFN-α. The median survival without treatment is 5 years.

LYMPHOMAS

Malignant transformations of lymphoid cells residing primarily in lymphoid tissues, especially the lymph nodes. Classically organized into Hodgkin's and non-Hodgkin's varieties.

Non-Hodgkin's Lymphoma (NHL)

NHL represents a diverse group of diseases characterized by a progressive clonal expansion of B cells, T cells, and/or natural killer (NK) cells stimulated by chromosomal translocations, most commonly t(14,18); by the inactivation of tumor suppressor genes; or by the introduction of exogenous genes by oncogenic viruses (eg, EBV, HTLV-1, HCV). There is a strong association between *H pylori* infection and MALT gastric lymphoma. **Most NHLs (almost 85%) are of B-cell origin.** NHL is the **most common hematopoietic neoplasm** and is 5 times more common than Hodgkin's lymphoma.

HISTORY/PE

The median patient age is > **50 years,** but NHL may also be found in children, who tend to have more aggressive, higher-grade disease. Patient presentation varies with disease grade (see Table 2.7-8).

DIAGNOSIS

- **Excisional lymph node biopsy** is necessary for diagnosis; the disease may first present at an extranodal site, which should be biopsied for diagnosis as well.
- A CSF examination should be done in patients with HIV, neurologic signs or symptoms, or 1° CNS lymphoma. **Disease staging (Ann Arbor classification) is based on the number of nodes and on whether the disease involves sites on both sides of the diaphragm.**

TREATMENT

- Treatment is based on histopathologic classification rather than on stage. Symptomatic patients are treated with radiation and chemotherapy.
- The rule of thumb is for low-grade, indolent NHL to be treated with palliative intent in symptomatic patients and for high-grade, aggressive NHL to be treated aggressively with a curative approach.

Hodgkin's Disease (HD)

A **predominantly B-cell malignancy** with an unclear etiology. There is a possible association with EBV. HD has a **bimodal age distribution,** peaking first in the third decade (primarily the nodular sclerosing type) and then in the elderly at around age 60 (mainly the lymphocyte-depleted type). It has a male predominance in childhood.

HISTORY/PE

- HD commonly presents **above the diaphragm (classically as cervical adenopathy;** see Figure 2.7-16), with infradiaphragmatic involvement suggesting more widely disseminated disease.

KEY FACT

The treatment of high-grade NHL may be complicated by tumor lysis syndrome, in which rapid cell death releases intracellular contents and leads to hyperkalemia, hyperphosphatemia, hyperuricemia, and hypocalcemia.

TABLE 2.7-8. Presentation of Non-Hodgkin's Lymphoma

GRADE	HISTORY	PHYSICAL
Low	Painless peripheral adenopathy. Cytopenia from bone marrow involvement; fatigue and weakness.	Peripheral adenopathy, splenomegaly, hepatomegaly.
Intermediate to high	Adenopathy. Extranodal disease (GI, GU, skin, thyroid, CNS). B symptoms (temperature > 38.5°C [101.3°F], night sweats, weight loss). Mass formation (eg, abdominal mass with bowel obstruction in Burkitt's lymphoma; mediastinal mass and SVC syndrome in lymphoblastic lymphoma).	Bulky adenopathy, splenomegaly, hepatomegaly. Masses (abdominal, testicular, mediastinal). Skin findings.

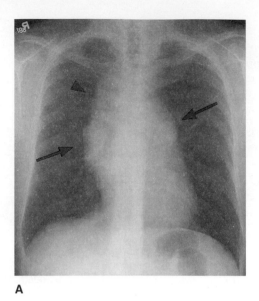

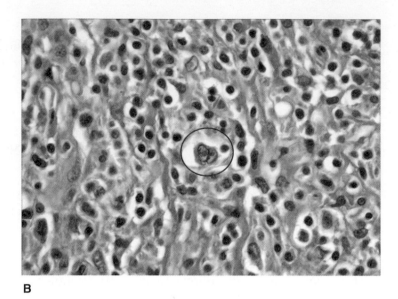

FIGURE 2.7-16. **Hodgkin's lymphoma.** (A) CXR of a 27-year-old male presenting with several weeks of fevers and night sweats shows bulky bilateral hilar (arrows) and right paratracheal (arrowhead) lymphadenopathy. (B) Lymph node sampling shows a mixed inflammatory infiltrate and a classic binucleate Reed-Sternberg cell (circle) consistent with Hodgkin's lymphoma. (Reproduced with permission from USMLERx.com.)

- Patients also have **systemic B symptoms** (see Table 2.7-8), **pruritus, and hepatosplenomegaly. Pel-Ebstein fevers** (1–2 weeks of high fever alternating with 1–2 afebrile weeks) and **alcohol-induced pain** at nodal sites are rare signs that are specific for HD.

DIAGNOSIS

- Fine-needle biopsy is usually nondiagnostic, so diagnosis is typically made by **excisional lymph node biopsy,** which is examined for the classic **Reed-Sternberg cells** (giant abnormal B cells with bilobar nuclei and huge, eosinophilic nucleoli, which create an "owl's-eye" appearance; see Figure 2.7-16) and for abnormal nodal morphology.
- Staging is based on the **number of nodes, the presence of B symptoms, and whether the disease involves sites on both sides of the diaphragm;** staging laparotomy is not recommended.

TREATMENT

- Treatment is stage dependent, involving chemotherapy and/or radiation.
- Five-year survival rates are very good and are 90% for stage I and II disease (nodal disease limited to 1 side of the diaphragm), 84% for stage III, and 65% for stage IV. **Lymphocyte-predominant HD has the best prognosis.**

> **KEY FACT**
>
> Chemotherapy and radiation can lead to 2° neoplasms such as AML, NHL, breast cancer, and thyroid cancer. Preventive measures such as mammography are warranted.

Plasma Cell Disorders

MULTIPLE MYELOMA

Clonal proliferation of malignant plasma cells at varying stages of differentiation, with **excessive production of monoclonal immunoglobulins (typically IgA or IgG) or immunoglobulin fragments** (kappa/lambda light chains). It is commonly believed to be a disease of the elderly, with a peak incidence in the seventh decade. Risk factors for disease development include radiation; monoclonal gammopathy of undetermined significance (MGUS); and, possibly, petroleum, pesticides, and other chemicals.

> **KEY FACT**
>
> The triad of anemia, renal failure, and bone pain must always raise suspicion for multiple myeloma.

HISTORY/PE

Patients present with **anemia, plasmacytosis of the bone marrow, lytic bone lesions, hypercalcemia,** and **renal abnormalities.** They are prone to **infection** and have **elevated monoclonal (M) proteins** in the serum and/or urine.

DIAGNOSIS

- The classic triad of diagnostic criteria are > 10% plasma cells in the bone marrow and/or histologically proven plasma cell infiltration, M protein in serum or urine, and evidence of lytic bone lesions.
- The **presence of M proteins alone is insufficient for the diagnosis of multiple myeloma;** MGUS is relatively common. Other lymphoproliferative diseases may also result in M proteins, including CLL, lymphoma, Waldenström's macroglobulinemia, and amyloidosis.
- Patients should be evaluated with a skeletal survey (see Figure 2.7-17), a bone marrow biopsy, serum and urine protein electrophoresis, and CBC.

TREATMENT

- Treat with chemotherapy.
- Common initial treatment involves a combination of **melphalan** (an oral alkylating agent), prednisone, and other agents.

KEY FACT

Bone pain at rest should raise concern for malignancy.

KEY FACT

Hypercalcemia manifests in symptoms of polyuria, constipation, confusion, nausea, vomiting, and lethargy.

KEY FACT

Because multiple myeloma is an osteoclastic process, a bone scan, which detects osteoblastic activity, may be ⊖.

WALDENSTRÖM'S MACROGLOBULINEMIA

A clonal disorder of B cells that leads to a malignant monoclonal gammopathy. **Elevated levels of IgM** result in hyperviscosity syndrome, coagulation abnormalities, cryoglobulinemia, cold agglutinin disease (leading to autoimmune hemolytic anemia), and amyloidosis. Tissue is infiltrated by IgM and neoplastic plasma cells. A **chronic, indolent disease of the elderly.**

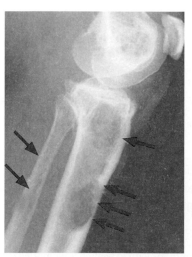

A

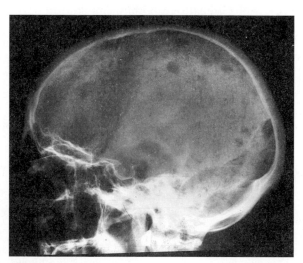

B

FIGURE 2.7-17. **Multiple myeloma skeletal survey.** Characteristic lytic bony lesions of multiple myeloma involving the tibia and fibula (**A**) and the skull (**B**) are seen. (Image A reproduced with permission from Lichtman MA et al. *Williams Hematology,* 8th ed. New York: McGraw-Hill, 2010, Fig. 109-13A. Image B reproduced with permission from Kantarjian HM. *MD Anderson Manual of Medical Oncology,* 1st ed. New York: McGraw-Hill, 2006, Fig. 8-1.)

HISTORY/PE

- Presents with nonspecific symptoms of lethargy and weight loss along with **Raynaud's phenomenon** from cryoglobulinemia. Patients complain of **neurologic problems** ranging from mental status changes to sensorimotor peripheral neuropathy and blurry vision. Organomegaly and organ dysfunction affecting the skin, GI tract, kidneys, and lungs are also seen.
- As with multiple myeloma, **MGUS is a precursor** to disease.

DIAGNOSIS

- Labs show elevated ESR, uric acid, LDH, and alkaline phosphatase.
- Bone marrow biopsy and aspirate are required to establish the diagnosis. Marrow shows abnormal plasma cells, classically with **Dutcher bodies** (PAS-⊕ IgM deposits around the nucleus). Serum and urine protein electrophoresis and immunofixation are also used.

TREATMENT

Excess immunoglobulin is removed with plasmapheresis; underlying lymphoma is treated with chemotherapy.

AMYLOIDOSIS

A generic term referring to extracellular deposition of protein fibrils. There are many different kinds of amyloidosis (see Table 2.7-9). Classically a disease of the **elderly.**

HISTORY/PE

- The clinical presentation depends on the type of precursor protein, tissue distribution, and the amount of amyloid deposition. In the 2 most common forms of systemic amyloidosis, 1° (AL) and 2° (AA), the major sites of clinically important amyloid deposition are in the kidneys, heart, and liver.
- In some disorders, clinically important amyloid deposition is limited to 1 organ (eg, the brain in **Alzheimer's disease**).

TABLE 2.7-9. Types of Amyloidosis

AMYLOID	CAUSE
AL	A plasma cell dyscrasia with deposition of monoclonal light-chain fragments. Associated with **multiple myeloma** and **Waldenström's macroglobulinemia.**
AA	Deposition of the acute-phase reactant serum amyloid A. Associated with **chronic inflammatory diseases** (eg, rheumatoid arthritis), infections, and neoplasms.
Dialysis related	Deposition of β_2 **microglobulin,** which accumulates in patients on long-term dialysis.
Heritable	Deposition of abnormal gene products (eg, transthyretin, aka prealbumin). A heterogeneous group of disorders.
Senile-systemic	Deposition of otherwise **normal transthyretin.**

DIAGNOSIS

Diagnosed by the clinical picture; confirmed by tissue biopsy with **Congo red staining** showing apple-green birefringence under polarized light.

TREATMENT

1° amyloidosis is treated with experimental chemotherapy to reduce protein burden; in 2° amyloidosis, the underlying condition should be addressed. Transplantation is also used.

Neutropenia

An **absolute neutrophil count (ANC) < 1500/mm³,** where ANC = (WBC count) × (% bands + % segmented neutrophils). Neutropenia may be due to a combination of ↓ production, sequestration to marginated or tissue pools, and ↑ destruction or utilization. It may be acquired or intrinsic.

HISTORY/PE

- Patients are at ↑ **risk of infection,** with the risk varying inversely with neutrophil count.
- **Acute neutropenia:** Associated with *S aureus, Pseudomonas, E coli, Proteus,* and *Klebsiella* **sepsis.**
- **Chronic and autoimmune neutropenia:** Presents with **recurrent sinusitis, stomatitis, gingivitis,** and **perirectal infections** rather than sepsis. Some chronic neutropenias are accompanied by splenomegaly (eg, Felty's syndrome, Gaucher's disease, sarcoidosis).

DIAGNOSIS

- The history (recent drug exposure or infection) and laboratory data are the cornerstones of diagnosis.
- A CBC with ANC may be used to follow neutropenia. If thrombocytopenia or anemia is present, bone marrow biopsy and aspirate should be performed.
- **Serum immunologic evaluation, ANA levels, and a workup for collagen vascular disease may be merited.**

TREATMENT

- Infection management is most important, as patients may not be able to mount an inflammatory response to infection owing to their lack of neutrophils.
- Fever in the context of neutropenia should be treated immediately with **broad-spectrum antibiotics such as cefepime.** Suspected fungal infections should be treated appropriately as well.
- Hematopoietic stem cell factors such as **G-CSF** can be used to shorten the duration of neutropenia. In some instances, **IVIG and allogeneic bone marrow transplantation** may be used.

KEY FACT

Hypothermia can be caused by fungemia.

Eosinophilia

An **absolute eosinophil count > 350/mm³.** Eosinophilia can be triggered by the overproduction of cytokines (IL-3, IL-5, and GM-CSF) or by chemokines that stimulate the migration of eosinophils into peripheral blood and tissues. Eosinophilia may be a 1° disorder but is usually 2° to another cause.

HISTORY/PE

- A **travel, medication, atopic, and diet history** should be elicited along with a history of symptoms relating to lymphoma/leukemia.
- Physical examination findings vary. Patients with hypereosinophilic syndrome (HES) may present with fever, anemia, and prominent cardiac findings (emboli from mural thrombi, abnormal ECGs, CHF, murmurs). Other affected organs include the lung, liver, spleen, skin, and nervous system (due to eosinophilic infiltration).

DIAGNOSIS

- In addition to a history and physical, a CBC and differential should be obtained, and **CSF should be analyzed for eosinophilia,** which is suggestive of a drug reaction or infection with coccidioidomycosis or a helminth.
- **Hematuria with eosinophilia may be a sign of schistosomiasis.**

TREATMENT

Medication should be tailored to the cause of the eosinophilia. HES is treated with corticosteroid and cytotoxic agents to ↓ the eosinophilia.

Transplant Medicine

- Tissue transplantation is increasingly used to treat a variety of diseases. Types of transplantation include the following:
  - **Autologous:** Transplantation from the patient to him/herself.
  - **Allogeneic:** Transplantation from a donor to a genetically different patient.
  - **Syngeneic:** Transplantation between identical twins (ie, from a donor to a genetically identical patient).
- With allogeneic donation, efforts are made to ABO and HLA match the donor and recipient. Even with antigenic matching and immunosuppression, however, transplants may be rejected. There are 3 types of rejection: hyperacute, acute, and chronic (see Table 2.7-10).
- Graft-versus-host disease (GVHD) is a complication specific to allogeneic bone marrow transplantation in which donated T cells attack host tissues, especially the skin, liver, and GI tract. It may be acute (occurring < 100 days posttransplant) or chronic (occurring > 100 days afterward).
  - **Minor histocompatibility antigens are thought to be responsible for GVHD,** which typically presents with **skin changes, cholestatic liver dysfunction, obstructive lung disease, or GI problems.**
  - Patients are treated with high-dose corticosteroids.

TABLE 2.7-10. Types of Transplant Rejection

VARIABLE	HYPERACUTE	ACUTE	CHRONIC
Timing after transplant	Within minutes.	Five days to 3 months.	Months to years.
Pathomechanism	Preformed antibodies.	T-cell mediated.	Chronic immune reaction causing fibrosis.
Tissue findings	Vascular thrombi; tissue ischemia.	Laboratory evidence of tissue destruction such as ↑ GGT, alkaline phosphatase, LDH, BUN, or creatinine.	Gradual loss of organ function.
Prevention	Check ABO compatibility.	N/A	N/A
Treatment	Cytotoxic agents.	Confirm with sampling of transplanted tissue; treat with corticosteroids, antilymphocyte antibodies (OKT3), tacrolimus, or MMF.	No treatment; biopsy to rule out treatable acute reaction.

- The typical regimen after transplant can include these commonly used drugs: prednisone, mycophenolate mofetil (MMF), FK506 (tacrolimus) to suppress immune-mediated rejection, TMP-SMX, ganciclovir, and keto-conazole to prevent subsequent infection in the immunosuppressed host.
- A variant of GVHD is the **graft-versus-leukemia effect,** in which leuke-mia patients who are treated with an allogeneic bone marrow transplant have significantly lower relapse rates than those treated with an autologous transplant. This difference is thought to be due to a reaction of donated T cells against leukemic cells.

Diseases Associated With Neoplasms

Table 2.7-11 outlines conditions that are commonly associated with neo-plasms.

TABLE 2.7-11. **Disorders Associated with Neoplasms**

CONDITION	NEOPLASM
Down syndrome	ALL ("We will **ALL** go **Down** together").
Xeroderma pigmentosum	Squamous cell and basal cell carcinomas of the skin.
Chronic atrophic gastritis, pernicious anemia, postsurgical gastric remnants	Gastric adenocarcinoma.
Tuberous sclerosis (facial angiofibroma, seizures, mental retardation)	Astrocytoma and cardiac rhabdomyoma.
Actinic keratosis	Squamous cell carcinoma of the skin.
Barrett's esophagus (chronic GI reflux)	Esophageal adenocarcinoma.
Plummer-Vinson syndrome (atrophic glossitis, esophageal webs, anemia; all due to iron deficiency)	Squamous cell carcinoma of the esophagus.
Cirrhosis (alcoholic, HBV or HCV)	Hepatocellular carcinoma.
Ulcerative colitis	Colonic adenocarcinoma.
Paget's disease of bone	2° osteosarcoma and fibrosarcoma.
Immunodeficiency states	Malignant lymphomas.
AIDS	Aggressive malignant NHLs and Kaposi's sarcoma.
Autoimmune diseases (eg, myasthenia gravis)	Benign and malignant thymomas.
Acanthosis nigricans (hyperpigmentation and epidermal thickening)	Visceral malignancy (stomach, lung, breast, uterus).
Multiple dysplastic nevi	Malignant melanoma.

INFECTIOUS DISEASE

Respiratory Infections

PNEUMONIA

Some common causes of pneumonia are outlined in Tables 2.8-1 and 2.8-2.

HISTORY/PE

- **May present classically or atypically.**
    - **Classic symptoms:** Sudden onset, fever, productive cough (purulent yellow-green sputum or hemoptysis), dyspnea, night sweats, pleuritic chest pain.
    - **Atypical symptoms:** Gradual onset, dry cough, headaches, myalgias, sore throat, GI symptoms.
- Lung examination may show ↓ or bronchial breath sounds, rales, wheezing, dullness to percussion, egophony, and/or tactile fremitus.
- Elderly patients as well as those with COPD, diabetes, or immune compromise may have minimal or atypical signs on physical examination.

KEY FACT

An adequate sputum Gram stain sample has many PMNs (> 25 cells/hpf) and few epithelial cells (< 10 cells/hpf).

DIAGNOSIS

- Diagnosis requires 2 or more symptoms of acute respiratory infection plus a new infiltrate on CXR or CT.
- Workup includes physical examination, **CXR** (see Figure 2.8-1), CBC, sputum Gram stain and culture (see Figure 2.8-2), nasopharyngeal aspirate, blood culture, and ABG.
- Tests for specific pathogens include the following:
    - *Legionella:* Urine *Legionella* antigen test (detects only serogroup 1), sputum staining with direct fluorescent antibody (DFA), culture.
    - *Chlamydia pneumoniae:* Serologic testing, culture, PCR.
    - *Mycoplasma:* Usually clinical. Serum cold agglutinins and serum *Mycoplasma* antigen may also be used.
    - *Streptococcus pneumoniae:* Urine pneumococcal antigen test, culture.
    - **Viral:** Nasopharyngeal aspirate, rapid tests for pathogens (eg, influenza, RSV), DFA, viral culture.

TREATMENT

- Table 2.8-3 summarizes the recommended initial treatment for pneumonia.
- Outpatient treatment with oral antibiotics is recommended in uncomplicated cases.

TABLE 2.8-1. Common Causes of Pneumonia by Age

CHILDREN (6 WEEKS–18 YEARS)	ADULTS (18–40 YEARS)	ADULTS (40–65 YEARS)	ELDERLY
Viruses (RSV)	Mycoplasma	S pneumoniae	S pneumoniae
Mycoplasma	C pneumoniae	H influenzae	Viruses
C pneumoniae	S pneumoniae	Anaerobes	Anaerobes
S pneumoniae		Viruses	H influenzae
		Mycoplasma	Gram-⊖ rods (GNRs)

TABLE 2.8-2.   Causes of Pneumonia by Category

CATEGORY	ETIOLOGY
Atypical	*Mycoplasma, Legionella, Chlamydia.*
Nosocomial (hospital acquired)	GNRs, *Staphylococcus,* anaerobes.
Immunocompromised	*Staphylococcus,* gram-⊕ rods, fungi, viruses, *Pneumocystis jiroveci* (with HIV), mycobacteria.
Aspiration	Anaerobes.
Alcoholics/IV drug users	*S pneumoniae, Klebsiella, Staphylococcus.*
Cystic fibrosis (CF)	*Pseudomonas, Burkholderia, S aureus,* mycobacteria.
COPD	*H influenzae, Moraxella catarrhalis, S pneumoniae.*
Postviral	*S pneumoniae, Staphylococcus, H influenzae.*
Neonates	Group B streptococci (GBS), *E coli.*
Recurrent	Obstruction, bronchogenic carcinoma, lymphoma, Wegener's granulomatosis, immunodeficiency, unusual organisms (eg, *Nocardia, Coxiella burnetii, Aspergillus, Pseudomonas*).

- **In-hospital treatment with IV antibiotics** is recommended for patients > 65 years of age and for those with comorbidities (alcoholism, COPD, diabetes, malnutrition), immunosuppression, malignancy, unstable vitals or signs of respiratory failure, altered mental status, and/or multilobar involvement.
- For patients with obstructive diseases (eg, CF or bronchiectasis), consider adding pseudomonal, staphylococcal, or anaerobic coverage.

COMPLICATIONS

Pleural effusion, empyema, lung abscess, necrotizing pneumonia, bacteremia.

TUBERCULOSIS (TB)

Infection due to *Mycobacterium tuberculosis.* Roughly 2 billion people worldwide are infected with TB. Initial infection usually leads to latent TB infection (LTBI) that is asymptomatic. Most symptomatic cases (ie, active disease) are due to reactivation of latent infection rather than to 1° exposure. Pulmonary TB is most common, but disseminated or extrapulmonary TB can occur as well. TB can infect almost any organ system, including the lungs, CNS, GU tract, bone, and GI tract. Risk factors include the following:

- **Risk factors for active disease** (ie, reactivation): Immunosuppression (HIV), alcoholism, preexisting lung disease, diabetes, advancing age.

Q

A 70-year-old male presents to the ER with 5 days of fever, productive cough, and altered mental status. He is also found to be hypotensive and tachypneic. Broad-spectrum antibiotics and fluid resuscitation are promptly administered, but the patient continues to be hypotensive. What is the next best step in treatment?

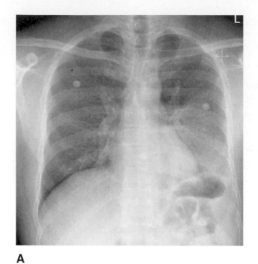
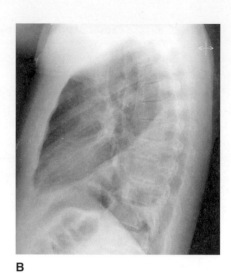

A   **B**

FIGURE 2.8-1. **Lobar pneumonia.** PA (**A**) and lateral (**B**) CXRs of a 41-year-old male with cough and shortness of breath show a left lower lobe opacity consistent with lobar pneumonia. *S pneumoniae* was confirmed by sputum Gram stain and culture. (Reproduced with permission from USMLERx.com.)

- **Risk factors for TB exposure in the United States: Homelessness** and crowded living conditions (eg, **prisons**), emigration/travel from developing nations, employment in a health profession, interaction with known TB contacts.

HISTORY/PE

- Presents with cough, **hemoptysis,** dyspnea, **weight loss, fatigue, night sweats, fever,** cachexia, hypoxia, tachycardia, lymphadenopathy, an abnormal lung examination, and a prolonged (> 3-week) symptom duration.
- TB is a common cause of fever of unknown origin.
- HIV patients can present with atypical signs and symptoms and have higher rates of extrapulmonary TB.

A

Administration of vasopressors and ICU admission. This patient is in septic shock, likely 2° to pneumonia. Patients with pneumonia who require vasopressors or mechanical ventilation warrant admission to an ICU.

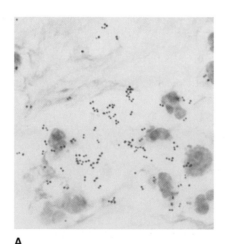
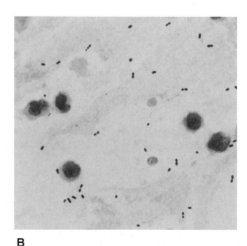

A   **B**

FIGURE 2.8-2. **Common pathogens causing pneumonia.** (**A**) *S aureus.* These clusters of gram-⊕ cocci were isolated from the sputum of a patient who developed pneumonia while hospitalized. (**B**) *S pneumoniae.* Sputum sample from a patient with pneumonia. Note the characteristic lancet-shaped gram-⊕ diplococci.

TABLE 2.8-3. Treatment of Pneumonia

PATIENT TYPE	SUSPECTED PATHOGENS	EMPIRIC COVERAGE
Outpatient community-acquired pneumonia, ≤ 65 years, otherwise healthy, no antimicrobials within 3 months	S pneumoniae, Mycoplasma pneumoniae, C pneumoniae, H influenzae, viral.	Macrolide or doxycycline.
> 65 years or comorbidity (COPD, heart failure, renal failure, diabetes, liver disease, EtOH abuse) or antimicrobial use within 3 months	S pneumoniae, H influenzae, aerobic GNRs (E coli, Enterobacter, Klebsiella), S aureus, Legionella, viruses.	Fluoroquinolone or β-lactam + macrolide.
Community-acquired pneumonia requiring hospitalization	S pneumoniae, H influenzae, anaerobes, aerobic GNRs, Legionella, Chlamydia.	Fluoroquinolone or antipneumococcal β-lactam + macrolide.
Community-acquired pneumonia requiring ICU care	S pneumoniae, Legionella, H influenzae, anaerobes, aerobic GNRs, Mycoplasma, Pseudomonas.	Antipneumococcal β-lactam + either azithromycin or fluoroquinolone.
Institution-/hospital-acquired pneumonia—hospitalized > 48 hours or in a long-term care facility > 14 days; ventilator-associated pneumonia	GNRs (including Pseudomonas and Acinetobacter), S aureus, Legionella, mixed flora.	Extended-spectrum cephalosporin or carbapenem with antipseudomonal activity. Add an aminoglycoside or a fluoroquinolone for coverage of resistant organisms (Pseudomonas) until lab sensitivities identify the best single agent.
Critically ill or worsening over 24–48 hours on initial antibiotic therapy	MRSA.	Add vancomycin or linezolid; broader gram-⊖ coverage.

DIAGNOSIS

- **Active disease:** Mycobacterial culture of sputum (or blood/tissue for extra-pulmonary disease) is the gold standard but can take weeks to obtain. A sputum **acid-fast stain** (see Figure 2.8-3) can yield rapid preliminary results but lacks sensitivity.
    - The most common finding among typical hosts is a cavitary infiltrate in the upper lobe on CXR (see Figure 2.8-4).
    - HIV patients or those with 1° TB may show lower lobe infiltrates with or without cavitation.
    - Multiple fine nodular densities distributed throughout both lungs are typical of miliary TB, which represents hematologic or lymphatic dissemination.
- **Latent disease (asymptomatic and previous exposure):** Diagnose with a ⊕ PPD test (see Figure 2.8-5).
    - Immunocompromised individuals with LTBI may have a ⊖ PPD (anergy).
    - All patients with a ⊕ PPD should be evaluated with a CXR to rule out active disease.

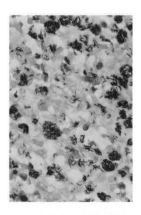

FIGURE 2.8-3. Tuberculosis. Note the red color ("red snappers") of tubercle bacilli on acid-fast staining. (Reproduced with permission from Milikowski C. *Color Atlas of Basic Histopathology*, 1st ed. Stamford, CT: Appleton & Lange, 1997: 193.)

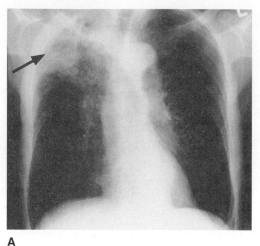
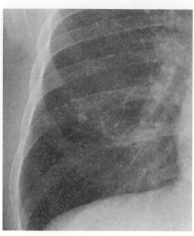

A   **B**

FIGURE 2.8-4. **Pulmonary TB.** (A) Right apical opacity with areas of cavitation (arrow) is seen in an elderly man with reactivation TB. (B) Coned-in view of a CXR in a young male with miliary TB shows innumerable 1- to 2-mm pulmonary nodules. (Image A reproduced with permission from Halter JB et al. *Hazzard's Geriatric Medicine and Gerontology,* 6th ed. New York: McGraw-Hill, 2009, Fig. 126-7. Image B reproduced with permission from USMLERx.com.)

KEY FACT

Rifampin turns body fluids orange (including tears); ethambutol can cause optic neuritis. INH causes peripheral neuropathy and hepatitis.

MNEMONIC

Patients with TB are RIPE for treatment:

Rifampin
INH
Pyrazinamide
Ethambutol

KEY FACT

Early antibiotic treatment of streptococcal pharyngitis can prevent rheumatic fever but not glomerulonephritis.

TREATMENT

All cases (both latent and active) must be reported to local and state health departments. Respiratory isolation should be instituted if active TB is suspected. Treatment measures are as follows:

- **Active disease:**
    - Directly observed multidrug therapy with a 4-drug regimen (**INH, pyrazinamide, rifampin, ethambutol**) × 2 months followed by INH and rifampin × 4 months.
    - Administer **vitamin B$_6$** (pyridoxine) with **INH** to prevent peripheral neuritis.
- **Latent disease:** For a ⊕ PPD without signs or symptoms of active disease, treat with **INH × 9 months.** Alternative regimens include INH × 6 months or rifampin × 4 months.

ACUTE PHARYNGITIS

Viral causes are more common (90% in adults), but it is important to identify streptococcal pharyngitis (**group A β-hemolytic *Streptococcus pyogenes***). Etiologies are as follows:

- **Bacterial:** Group A streptococci (GAS), *Neisseria gonorrhoeae, Corynebacterium diphtheriae,* M pneumoniae.
- **Viral:** Rhinovirus, coronavirus, adenovirus, HSV, EBV, CMV, influenza virus, coxsackievirus, acute HIV infection.

HISTORY/PE

- **Typical of streptococcal pharyngitis: Fever, sore throat, pharyngeal erythema, tonsillar exudate,** cervical lymphadenopathy, soft palate petechiae, headache, vomiting, scarlatiniform rash (indicates scarlet fever).
- **Atypical of streptococcal pharyngitis:** Coryza, hoarseness, rhinorrhea, **cough,** conjunctivitis, anterior stomatitis, ulcerative lesions, GI symptoms.

PPD is injected intradermally on the volar surface of the forearm. The diameter of induration is measured at 48–72 hours. BCG vaccination typically renders a patient PPD ⊕ but should not preclude prophylaxis as recommended for unvaccinated individuals. The size of induration that indicates a ⊕ test is interpreted as follows:

- **≥ 5 mm:** HIV or risk factors, close TB contacts, CXR evidence of TB.
- **≥ 10 mm:** Indigent/homeless, residents of developing nations, IV drug use, chronic illness, residents of health and correctional institutions, and health care workers.
- **≥ 15 mm:** Everyone else, including those with no known risk factors.

A ⊖ reaction with ⊖ controls implies anergy from immunosuppression, old age, or malnutrition and thus does not rule out TB.

FIGURE 2.8-5.   PPD interpretation.

DIAGNOSIS

Diagnosed by clinical evaluation, rapid GAS antigen detection, and throat culture. With 3 out of 4 of the Centor criteria, the sensitivity of rapid antigen testing is > 90%.

TREATMENT

If GAS is suspected, begin empiric antibiotic therapy with penicillin × 10 days. Cephalosporins, amoxicillin, and azithromycin are alternative options. Symptom relief can be attained with fluids, rest, antipyretics, and salt-water gargles.

COMPLICATIONS

- **Nonsuppurative:** Acute rheumatic fever (see the Cardiovascular chapter), poststreptococcal glomerulonephritis.
- **Suppurative:** Cervical lymphadenitis, mastoiditis, sinusitis, otitis media, retropharyngeal or peritonsillar abscess, and, rarely, thrombophlebitis of the jugular vein (**Lemierre's syndrome**) due to *Fusobacterium*, an oral anaerobe.
- **Peritonsillar abscess** may present with odynophagia, trismus ("lockjaw"), a muffled voice, unilateral tonsillar enlargement, and erythema, with the uvula and soft palate deviated away from the affected side. Culture abscess fluid and localize the abscess via intraoral ultrasound or CT. Treat with antibiotics and **surgical drainage.**

SINUSITIS

Refers to inflammation of the paranasal sinuses. The maxillary sinuses are most commonly affected. Subtypes include the following:

- **Acute sinusitis (symptoms lasting < 1 month):** Most commonly associated with viruses, *S pneumoniae*, *H influenzae*, and *M catarrhalis*. Bacterial causes are rare and characterized by purulent nasal discharge, facial or tooth tenderness, and symptoms lasting > 7 days.
- **Chronic sinusitis (symptoms persisting > 3 months):** A chronic inflammatory process often due to obstruction of sinus drainage and ongoing low-grade anaerobic infections. In patients with hematologic malignancy or poorly controlled diabetes mellitus (DM), mucormycosis should be considered.

KEY FACT

The Centor criteria for identifying streptococcal pharyngitis are fever, tonsillar exudate, tender anterior cervical lymphadenopathy, and lack of cough (3 of 4 are required).

KEY FACT

Always consider occult sinusitis in febrile ICU patients.

KEY FACT

Potential complications of sinusitis include meningitis, frontal bone osteomyelitis, cavernous sinus thrombosis, and abscess formation.

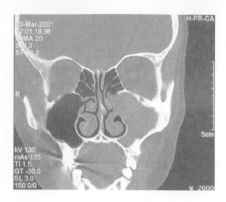

FIGURE 2.8-6. **Sinusitis.** Coronal CT image shows an opacified left maxillary sinus and marked associated bony thickening, consistent with chronic maxillary sinusitis. (Reproduced with permission from Lalwani AK. *Current Diagnosis & Treatment in Otolaryngology—Head and Neck Surgery*, 2nd ed. New York: McGraw-Hill, 2008, Fig. 14-2.)

HISTORY/PE

- Presents with **fever, facial pain/pressure, headache,** nasal congestion, and discharge. Examination may reveal tenderness, erythema, and swelling over the affected area.
- High fever, leukocytosis, and a purulent nasal discharge are suggestive of acute bacterial sinusitis.

DIAGNOSIS

- A clinical diagnosis. Culture and radiography are generally not required for acute sinusitis but may guide the management of chronic cases.
- Transillumination shows opacification of the sinuses (low sensitivity).
- CT is the test of choice for sinus imaging (see Figure 2.8-6) but is usually necessary only if symptoms persist after treatment.

TREATMENT

- Most cases of acute sinusitis are viral and/or self-limited and are treated with symptomatic therapy (decongestants, antihistamines, nasal saline lavage, pain relief).
- **Acute bacterial sinusitis:** Consider amoxicillin/clavulanate 500 mg PO TID × 10 days or clarithromycin, azithromycin, TMP-SMX, a fluoroquinolone, or a second-generation cephalosporin × 10 days.
- **Chronic sinusitis:**
  - Antibiotics are similar to those used for acute disease, although a **longer course** (3–6 weeks) may be necessary.
  - **Adjuvant** therapy with intranasal corticosteroids, decongestants, and antihistamines may be useful in combating the allergic/inflammatory component of the disease. **Surgical** intervention may be required.

COCCIDIOIDOMYCOSIS

A pulmonary fungal infection endemic to the **southwestern United States** (see Figure 2.8-7). Can present as an acute or subacute pneumonia or as a flulike illness, and may involve extrapulmonary sites, including bone, CNS, and skin. The incubation period is 1–4 weeks after exposure. Filipino, African American, pregnant, and HIV-⊕ patients are at ↑ risk for disseminated disease.

HISTORY/PE

Patients present with **fever,** anorexia, headache, chest pain, **cough,** dyspnea, arthralgias, and **night sweats.** Disseminated infection can present with meningitis, bone lesions, and soft tissue abscesses.

DIAGNOSIS

- Obtain bronchoalveolar lavage (BAL) as well as fungal cultures of sputum, wound exudate, or other affected tissue.
- Serum anti-coccidioidal antibodies are specific but not sensitive and lag behind clinical illness by weeks or months.
- Identify *Coccidioides immitis* spherules on H&E or other special sputum or tissue stains.
- CXR findings may be normal or may show infiltrates, nodules, cavities, mediastinal or hilar adenopathy, or pleural effusion.
- Consider bronchoscopy, fine-needle biopsy, open lung biopsy, or pleural biopsy if serology is indeterminate.

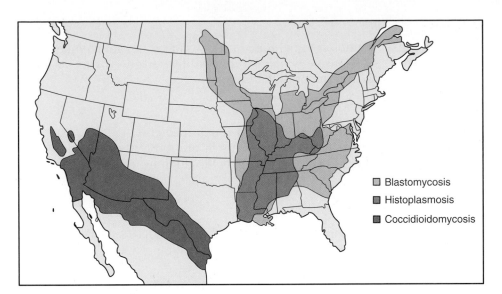

FIGURE 2.8-7. Geographic distribution of systemic fungal infection in the United States. (Reproduced with permission from Ryan KJ, Ray CG. *Sherris Medical Microbiology*, 5th ed. New York: McGraw-Hill, 2010, Fig. 46-4.)

TREATMENT

- **Acute:** PO fluconazole or itraconazole may be used for mild infection or continuation therapy once the patient is stable. IV therapy is rarely necessary; however, consider **IV amphotericin B** for severe or protracted 1° pulmonary infection and disseminated disease.
- **Chronic:** No treatment is needed for asymptomatic chronic pulmonary nodules or cavities. Progressive cavitary or symptomatic disease usually requires surgery plus long-term azole therapy for 8–12 months.

INFLUENZA

A highly contagious orthomyxovirus transmitted by droplet nuclei. There are 3 types of influenza: A, B, and C. Subtypes of influenza A (eg, H5N1, H1N1) are classified on the basis of glycoproteins (hemagglutinin and neuraminidase). Relevant terms are as follows:

- **Antigenic drift:** Refers to small, gradual changes in surface proteins through point mutations. These small changes are sufficient to allow the virus to escape immune recognition, accounting for the fact that individuals can be infected with influenza multiple times.
- **Antigenic shift:** Describes an acute, major change in the influenza A subtype (significant genetic reassortment) circulating among humans; leads to pandemics.

In the United States, the typical influenza season begins in November and lasts until March. **Vaccination with inactivated influenza virus is currently recommended for all patients ≥ 6 months of age.** Children 6 months to 9 years of age require 2 doses of the seasonal vaccine if they are receiving the vaccine for the first time. A high-dose flu vaccine is available for people ≥ 65 years of age.

HISTORY/PE

Patients typically present with abrupt onset of fevers, myalgias, chills, cough, coryza, and weakness. Elderly patients may have atypical presentations characterized only by confusion.

Q

A 70-year-old male presents to the ER in February with a high fever and a productive cough. One week ago he was treated for influenza, and his symptoms improved until 3 days ago, when they returned with greater severity. Examination now reveals cyanosis, tactile fremitus, and dullness to percussion over the left lower lobe. Against what organism should antibiotic therapy be directed?

DIAGNOSIS

Leukopenia is a common finding. Rapid influenza tests of viral antigens from nasopharyngeal swabs are available. More definitive diagnosis can be made with DFA tests, viral culture, or PCR assays.

TREATMENT

- Symptomatic care with analgesics and cough medicine.
- Antivirals such as oseltamivir or zanamivir are most effective when used within 2 days of onset and may shorten the duration of infection by 1–2 days.

COMPLICATIONS

- Severe 1° viral pneumonia, 2° bacterial pneumonia (see "Postviral" in Table 2.8-2), sinusitis, bronchitis, and exacerbation of COPD and asthma can occur.
- Reye's syndrome, or fatty liver encephalopathy, has been associated with ASA use in children with viral infections, including influenza.

CNS Infections

MENINGITIS

Acute bacterial meningitis is a **life-threatening** emergency. Viral (also called "aseptic") meningitis is more common and clinically less morbid. Risk factors for meningitis include recent ear infection, sinusitis, immunodeficiencies, recent neurosurgical procedures, and sick contacts. Causes by age group are listed in Table 2.8-4.

HISTORY/PE

Patients present with **fever,** malaise, **headache, neck stiffness, photophobia,** altered mental status, **nausea/vomiting,** seizures, or signs of meningeal irritation (⊕ Kernig's and Brudzinski's signs).

TABLE 2.8-4. Causes of Meningitis by Age Group[a,b]

NEWBORN (0–6 MONTHS)	CHILDREN (6 MONTHS–6 YEARS)	6–60 YEARS	60 YEARS +
GBS	S pneumoniae	N meningitidis	S pneumoniae
E coli/GNRs	Neisseria	Enteroviruses	GNRs
Listeria (see Figure 2.8-8)	meningitidis	S pneumoniae	Listeria
	H influenzae serotype b	HSV	N meningitidis
	Enteroviruses		

[a] Causes in HIV include *Cryptococcus,* CMV, HSV, VZV, TB, toxoplasmosis (brain abscess), and JC virus (PML).

[b] The incidence of *H influenzae* meningitis has greatly ↓ over the past 10–15 years as a result of the *H influenzae* vaccine.

DIAGNOSIS

- Order an **LP** for **CSF Gram stain and culture**; obtain glucose, protein, WBC count plus differential, RBC count, and opening pressure (in the absence of papilledema or focal neurologic deficits).
- **Viral PCRs** (eg, HSV); **cryptococcal antigen** (for HIV patients).
- **CT or MRI** to rule out other diagnoses. Obtain blood cultures. CBC may reveal leukocytosis; CSF findings vary (see Table 2.8-5).

TREATMENT

- Antibiotics should be administered rapidly (see Table 2.8-6) and may be given empirically up to 2 hours before an LP.
- Some cases of viral meningitis can be treated with supportive care and close follow-up.
- Close contacts of patients with meningococcal meningitis should receive **rifampin.** Second-line prophylactic regimens include ciprofloxacin, ceftriaxone, or azithromycin.
- **Dexamethasone** may be beneficial in bacterial meningitis, especially *S pneumoniae* or *H influenzae*, if given 15–20 minutes before antibiotics.

COMPLICATIONS

- **Cerebral edema:** Visible on CT/MRI. Presents with loss of oculocephalic reflex. Treat with IV mannitol.
- **Subdural effusions:** May be seen on CT scan. Occur in 50% of infants with *H influenzae* meningitis. No treatment is necessary.
- **Ventriculitis/hydrocephalus:** Presents as a worsening clinical picture with improved CSF findings. Requires ventriculostomy and possibly intraventricular antibiotics.
- **Seizures:** Treat with benzodiazepines and phenytoin.
- **Hyponatremia:** Assess intravascular volume status; if low, administer fluids to prevent ischemic stroke. Closely monitor sodium concentration and fluid intake/output.
- **Subdural empyema:** Presents with intractable seizures. Requires surgical evacuation.
- **Other:** Cranial nerve palsies, sensorineural hearing loss, coma, death.

ENCEPHALITIS

HSV and **arboviruses** are the most common causes of encephalitis. Rarer etiologies include CMV, toxoplasmosis, West Nile virus, VZV, *Borrelia, Rickettsia, Legionella,* enterovirus, *Mycoplasma,* and cerebral malaria. Children and the elderly are the most vulnerable.

HISTORY/PE

- Presents with **altered consciousness, headache, fever, and seizures.** Lethargy, confusion, coma, and focal neurologic deficits (cranial nerve deficits, accentuated DTRs) may also be present.
- The differential includes brain abscess, malignancy, toxic-metabolic encephalopathy, subdural hematoma, and SAH.

DIAGNOSIS

- CSF shows lymphocytic pleocytosis and moderately ↑ protein. RBCs without evidence of trauma suggest HSV encephalitis. The glucose level is low in tuberculous, fungal, bacterial, and amebic infections.
- Obtain a CSF Gram stain (bacteria), acid-fast stain (mycobacteria), India ink stain (*Cryptococcus*), a wet preparation (free-living amebae), and a

KEY FACT

Acute bacterial meningitis is a life-threatening emergency. Antibiotics should be started as soon as possible.

KEY FACT

Although other medications may be used, rifampin is the frequently tested prophylaxis of choice for close contacts of patients with meningococcal meningitis.

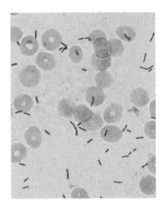

FIGURE 2.8-8.   *Listeria.* These numerous rod-shaped bacilli were isolated from the blood of a patient with *Listeria* meningitis.

KEY FACT

The presence of RBCs in CSF without a history of trauma is highly suggestive of HSV encephalitis.

A 19-year-old college student is brought to the ER from her dorm room, where she was found by her roommate in a confused state. She complains of fever, nausea, vomiting, and pain in her neck and head. She has a petechial rash on her legs. CSF examination reveals a glucose level of 22 mg/dL, a protein level of 140 mg/dL, and a WBC count of 1400/mm³. What is the most likely organism responsible for her condition?

TABLE 2.8-5. CSF Profiles

	RBCs (per mm³)	WBCs (per mm³)	GLUCOSE (mg/dL)	PROTEIN (mg/dL)	OPENING PRESSURE (cm H₂O)	APPEARANCE	GAMMA GLOBULIN (% PROTEIN)
Normal	< 10	< 5	~ 2/3 of serum	15–45	10–20	Clear	3–12
Bacterial meningitis	↔	↑ (> 1000 PMNs)	↓	↑	↑	Cloudy/purulent	↔ or ↑
Viral meningitis	↔	↑ (monos/ lymphs)	↔	↔ or ↑	↔ or ↑	Most often clear	↔ or ↑
Aseptic meningitis	↔	↑	↔	↔ or ↑	↔	Clear	↔
SAH	↑↑	↑	↔	↑	↔ or ↑	Yellow/red	↔ or ↑
Guillain-Barré syndrome	↔	↔	↔ or ↑	↑↑	↔	Clear or yellow (high protein)	↔
MS	↔	↔ or ↑	↔	↔	↔	Clear	↑↑
Pseudotumor cerebri	↔	↔	↔	↔	↑↑↑	Clear	↔

Giemsa stain (trypanosomes). Order a **PCR** for HSV, CMV, EBV, VZV, and enterovirus.

- **MRI** may demonstrate characteristic **temporal lobe signal abnormalities in HSV encephalitis** (see Figure 2.8-9).

TREATMENT

- **HSV encephalitis:** Requires immediate IV acyclovir.
- **CMV encephalitis:** Treat with IV ganciclovir +/− foscarnet.
- Give doxycycline for suspected Rocky Mountain spotted fever, Lyme disease, or ehrlichiosis.

BRAIN ABSCESS

A focal, suppurative infection of the brain parenchyma, usually with a "ring-enhancing" appearance due to fibrous capsule. The most common pathogens are **streptococci, staphylococci,** and **anaerobes; multiple** organisms are often implicated (80–90% are polymicrobial). Nonbacterial causes include *Toxoplasma, Aspergillus,* and *Candida;* zygomycosis should be considered in immunocompromised hosts, and neurocysticercosis should be considered in relevant epidemiologic settings. Modes of transmission include the following:

- **Direct spread:** Due to paranasal sinusitis (10% of cases; frequently affects young males, and often due to *Streptococcus milleri*), **otitis media** or **mastoiditis** (33%), or **dental infection** (2%).
- **Direct inoculation:** Affects patients with a history of head trauma or neurosurgical procedures.

TABLE 2.8-6.   Empiric Treatment of Bacterial Meningitis

AGE	CAUSATIVE ORGANISM	TREATMENT
< 1 month	GBS, *E coli*/GNRs, *Listeria*.	Ampicillin + cefotaxime or gentamicin.
1–3 months	Pneumococci, meningococci, *H influenzae*.	Vancomycin IV + ceftriaxone or cefotaxime.
3 months – adulthood	Pneumococci, meningococci.	Vancomycin IV + ceftriaxone or cefotaxime.
> 60 years/alcoholism/ chronic illness	Pneumococci, gram-⊖ bacilli, *Listeria,* meningococci.	Ampicillin + vancomycin + cefotaxime or ceftriaxone.

- **Hematogenous spread** (25% of cases): Often shows an **MCA distribution** with **multiple abscesses** that are poorly encapsulated and located at the **gray-white junction**.

HISTORY/PE

- **Headache,** drowsiness, inattention, confusion, and **seizures** are early symptoms, followed by signs of **increasing ICP** and then **a focal neurologic deficit.**
- **Headache** is the most common symptom and is often dull, constant, and refractory to treatment. ↑ ICP leads to CN III and CN VI deficits.

DIAGNOSIS

- **CT scan** will show a **ring-enhancing lesion** with a low-density core. MRI has higher sensitivity for early abscesses and posterior fossa lesions.
- **CSF analysis** is not necessary and **may precipitate brainstem herniation.**
- Lab values may show peripheral leukocytosis, ↑ ESR, and ↑ CRP.

KEY FACT

The classic clinical triad of headache, fever, and a focal neurologic deficit is present in 50% of cases of brain abscess.

KEY FACT

When fever is absent, 1° and metastatic brain tumors should be considered in the differential diagnoses.

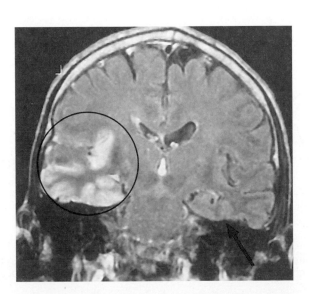

FIGURE 2.8-9.   HSV encephalitis. Coronal FLAIR image of a young male with HSV encephalitis shows the characteristic MRI pattern within the cortex of the right temporal lobe (circle). The left temporal lobe is also involved (arrow), but to a lesser extent. (Reproduced with permission from Fauci AS et al. *Harrison's Principles of Internal Medicine,* 17th ed. New York: McGraw-Hill, 2008, Fig. 376-3.)

TREATMENT

- **Initiate broad-spectrum IV antibiotics** and **surgical drainage** (aspiration or excision) if necessary for diagnostic and/or therapeutic purposes. Lesions < 2 cm can often be treated medically.
- Administer a third-generation cephalosporin + metronidazole +/– vancomycin; give IV therapy for 6–8 weeks. Obtain serial CT/MRIs to follow resolution.
- **Dexamethasone** with taper may be used in severe cases to ↓ cerebral edema; **IV mannitol** may be used to ↓ ICP. Give prophylactic anticonvulsants.

Human Immunodeficiency Virus (HIV)

A retrovirus that targets and destroys CD4+ T lymphocytes. Infection is characterized by a high rate of viral replication that leads to a progressive decline in CD4+ count (see Figure 2.8-10).

- **CD4+ count:** Indicates the **degree of immunosuppression;** guides therapy and prophylaxis and helps determine prognosis.
- **Viral load:** May predict the **rate** of disease progression; provides indications for treatment and gauges response to antiretroviral therapy.

HISTORY/PE

- In acute HIV (acute infection/seroconversion, acute retroviral syndrome), the initial infection is often **asymptomatic,** but patients may also present with **mononucleosis-like or flulike symptoms** (eg, fever, lymphadenopathy, maculopapular rash, pharyngitis, diarrhea, nausea/vomiting, weight loss, headache).
- HIV may later present as night sweats, weight loss, thrush, recurrent infections, or opportunistic infections. Complications are inversely correlated with CD4+ count (see Figure 2.8-11).

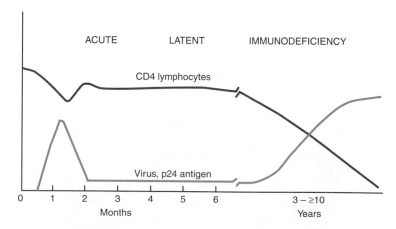

FIGURE 2.8-10. **Time course of HIV infection.** Note that the level of CD4 lymphocytes (red curve) remains normal for many years but then declines, resulting in the immunodeficiency stage, which is characterized by opportunistic infections and malignancies.

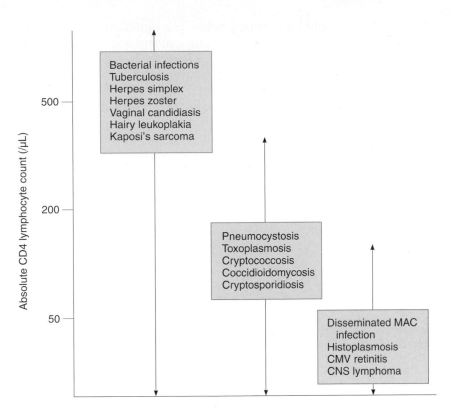

F I G U R E 2 . 8 - 1 1 .   Relationship of CD4+ count to development of opportunistic infections. (Reproduced with permission from McPhee SJ et al. *Current Medical Diagnosis & Treatment 2011.* New York: McGraw-Hill, 2011, Fig. 31-1.)

DIAGNOSIS

- **ELISA test** (high sensitivity, moderate specificity): Detects anti-HIV antibodies in the bloodstream (can take up to 6 months to appear after exposure).
- **Western blot** (low sensitivity, high specificity): Confirmatory.
- **Rapid HIV tests** are now available.
- Baseline evaluation should include HIV RNA PCR (viral load), CD4+ cell count, CXR, PPD skin test, Pap smear, mental status exam, VDRL/RPR, and serologies for CMV, viral hepatitis, toxoplasmosis, and VZV.
- Evaluation for acute retroviral syndrome (acute HIV) should include **HIV RNA PCR** (viral load); ELISA may be ⊖.

TREATMENT

- Initiate antiretroviral therapy for (1) **symptomatic patients** (those with AIDS-defining illness) regardless of CD4+ count or viral load; (2) patients with a **CD4+ count < 350/mm³**; (3) **pregnant patients;** and (4) those with specific HIV-related conditions (eg, HIV-associated nephropathy, neurocognitive deficits).
- The initial regimen should generally consist of a combination of 2 nucleoside/nucleotide reverse transcriptase inhibitors (NRTIs) plus either 1 non-nucleoside RTI (NNRTI) or 1 protease inhibitor. **The most important principle is to select multiple medications (usually at least 3)** in order to achieve a durable treatment response and limit the emergence of resistance.
- The goal of therapy is complete viral suppression (< 50 copies). After therapy is started, CD4+ count and viral load should be monitored monthly until suppression is achieved and every 3–6 months afterward.

KEY FACT

Common AIDS-defining illnesses:

- Esophageal candidiasis
- CMV retinitis
- Kaposi's sarcoma
- CNS lymphoma, toxoplasmosis, PML
- *P jiroveci* pneumonia or recurrent bacterial pneumonia
- HIV encephalopathy
- Disseminated mycobacterial or fungal infection
- Invasive cervical cancer

KEY FACT

If a pregnant HIV-⊕ patient is not on antiretroviral therapy at the time of delivery, she should be treated with zidovudine (AZT) intrapartum. Infants should receive AZT for 6 weeks after birth.

KEY FACT

MMR is the only live vaccine that should be given to HIV patients. Do not give oral polio vaccine to HIV-⊕ patients or their contacts.

MNEMONIC

AIDS pathogens—

The Major Pathogens Concerning Complete T-Cell Collapse

Toxoplasma gondii
Mycobacterium avium-intracellulare
Pneumocystis jiroveci
Candida albicans
Cryptococcus neoformans
Tuberculosis
CMV
Cryptosporidium parvum

- An HIV genotype should be obtained before the initiation of therapy and when resistance is suspected, as such testing can provide mutation information and identify resistance to specific antiretrovirals.
- The recommended prophylaxis for HIV exposure varies according to the severity of the source infection and the exposure. In the setting of a percutaneous injury, mucous membrane exposure, or nonintact skin exposure with an HIV-⊕ source, begin antiretroviral therapy as soon as possible with a basic 2-drug regimen or an expanded regimen of 3 or more drugs for 4 weeks, depending on the severity of the source infection.
- Table 2.8-7 outlines prophylactic measures against opportunistic infections.

Opportunistic Infections

Figure 2.8-12 illustrates the microscopic appearance of some common opportunistic organisms.

OROPHARYNGEAL CANDIDIASIS (THRUSH)

- Risk factors include xerostomia, antibiotic use, denture use, and immunosuppression (eg, HIV, leukemias, lymphomas, cancer, diabetes, corticosteroid inhaler use, immunosuppressive treatment).

TABLE 2.8-7. Prophylaxis for HIV-Related Opportunistic Infections

PATHOGEN	INDICATION FOR PROPHYLAXIS	TREATMENT	NOTES
P jiroveci pneumonia	CD4+ < 200/mm³, prior *P jiroveci* infection, unexplained fever × 2 weeks, or HIV-related oral candidiasis.	Single-strength TMP-SMX.	Discontinue prophylaxis when CD4+ is > 200/mm³ for ≥ 3 months.
Mycobacterium avium complex (MAC)	CD4+ < 50–100/mm³.	Weekly azithromycin.	Discontinue prophylaxis when CD4+ is > 100/mm³ for > 6 months.
Toxoplasma gondii	CD4+ < 100/mm³ + ⊕ IgG serologies.	Double-strength TMP-SMX.	—
M tuberculosis	PPD > 5 mm or "high risk" (see TB section).	INH × 9 months (+ pyridoxine) or rifampin × 4 months.	Include pyridoxine with INH-containing regimens.
Candida	Multiple recurrences.	**Esophagitis:** Fluconazole. **Oral:** Nystatin swish and swallow.	—
HSV	Multiple recurrences.	Daily suppressive acyclovir, famciclovir, or valacyclovir.	—
S pneumoniae	All patients.	Pneumovax.	Give every 5 years provided that CD4+ is > 200/mm³.
Influenza	All patients.	Influenza vaccine annually.	—

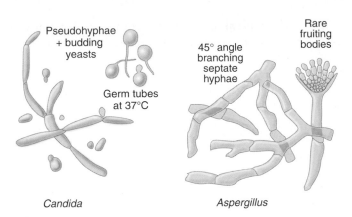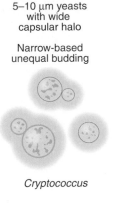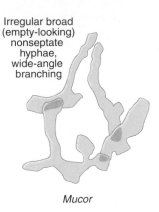

Pseudohyphae + budding yeasts

Germ tubes at 37°C

Candida

45° angle branching septate hyphae

Aspergillus

Rare fruiting bodies

5–10 μm yeasts with wide capsular halo

Narrow-based unequal budding

Cryptococcus

Irregular broad (empty-looking) nonseptate hyphae, wide-angle branching

Mucor

FIGURE 2.8-12. **Common opportunistic organisms.**

- **Hx/PE:** Presents with **soft white plaques that can be rubbed off,** with an erythematous base and possible mucosal burning. The differential includes oral hairy leukoplakia (affects the lateral borders of the tongue; not easily rubbed off). Odynophagia is characteristic of candidal esophagitis.
- **Dx:** Usually clinical. KOH or Gram stain shows **budding yeast and/or pseudohyphae.**
- **Tx:** Treat thrush with local therapy (eg, nystatin suspension, clotrimazole tablets, or a PO azole such as fluconazole). Treat candidal esophagitis with PO azole therapy.

CRYPTOCOCCAL MENINGITIS

- Risk factors include AIDS and exposure to **pigeon droppings.**
- **Hx/PE:** Presents with headache, fever, impaired mentation, and **absent meningeal signs.** The differential includes toxoplasmosis, lymphoma, TB meningitis, AIDS dementia complex, PML, HSV encephalitis, and other fungal disease.
- **Dx:** LP (↓ CSF glucose; ↑ protein; ↑ leukocyte count with monocytic predominance, ↑↑ opening pressure); ⊕ **cryptococcal antigen testing in CSF and/or blood, CSF India ink stain,** and fungal culture.
- **Tx:**
  - **IV amphotericin B** + flucytosine × 2 weeks; then fluconazole × 8 weeks. Lifelong **maintenance therapy** should be administered with fluconazole until symptoms resolve and CD4+ is > 100/mm³ for > 1 year.
  - ↑ opening pressure may require serial LPs or a ventriculoperitoneal shunt for management.

HISTOPLASMOSIS

Risk factors include HIV/AIDS, spelunking, and exposure to bird or bat excrement, especially in the **Ohio** and **Mississippi** river valleys (see Figure 2.8-7).

HISTORY/PE

- 1° exposure is often asymptomatic or causes a flulike illness.
- Presentation may range from no symptoms to fulminant disease with pulmonary and/or extrapulmonary manifestations.
- Fever, weight loss, hepatosplenomegaly, lymphadenopathy, a nonproductive cough, palatal ulcers, and pancytopenia indicate disseminated infection (most often within 14 days).

> **KEY FACT**
>
> The CSF antigen test for cryptococcal meningitis is highly sensitive and specific.

> **Q**
>
> A 35-year-old HIV-infected man from Ohio presents to his primary care provider with low-grade fever, dry cough, malaise, and a 5-lb weight loss over the past month. He is compliant with his HIV medications. Physical examination shows hepatosplenomegaly and palatal ulcers. His CBC reveals pancytopenia, and a CXR shows hilar lymphadenopathy. What is the next most appropriate step in management?

- The differential includes atypical bacterial pneumonia, blastomycosis, coccidioidomycosis, TB, sarcoidosis, pneumoconiosis, and lymphoma.

DIAGNOSIS

- **CXR** shows diffuse nodular densities, focal infiltrate, cavity, or hilar lymphadenopathy (chronic infection is usually cavitary).
- The **urine and serum polysaccharide antigen test** is the most sensitive test for making the initial diagnosis of disseminated disease, monitoring response to therapy, and diagnosing relapse. Culture is also diagnostic (blood, sputum, bone marrow, CSF).
- The yeast form is seen with special stains on biopsy (bone marrow, lymph node, liver) or BAL.

TREATMENT

Depends on the severity of disease and the host:

- **Mild pulmonary disease or stable nodules:** Treat supportively in the immunocompromised host. Consider itraconazole.
- **Chronic cavitary lesions:** Give itraconazole for > 1 year.
- **Severe acute pulmonary disease or disseminated disease:** Liposomal **amphotericin B** or amphotericin B × 14 days followed by itraconazole × 1 year or longer. Lifelong maintenance therapy with daily itraconazole may be necessary.

PNEUMOCYSTIS JIROVECI PNEUMONIA

Formerly known as *Pneumocystis carinii* pneumonia, or PCP. Risk factors include impaired cellular immunity and AIDS.

HISTORY/PE

- Presents with **dyspnea on exertion,** fever, a **nonproductive cough,** tachypnea, weight loss, fatigue, and **impaired oxygenation. Typically, symptoms have been present for weeks.**
- Can also present as disseminated disease or as local disease in other organ systems.
- The differential includes TB, histoplasmosis, and coccidioidomycosis.

DIAGNOSIS

- Diagnosed by cytology of induced sputum or bronchoscopy specimen with silver stain and immunofluorescence (see Figure 2.8-13A). Obtain an ABG to check Pa_{O_2}.
- CXR may show diffuse, bilateral interstitial infiltrates with a ground-glass appearance (see Figure 2.8-13B), but any presentation is possible.

A

Liposomal amphotericin B followed by itraconazole. The patient has clinical features of disseminated histoplasmosis (fever, malaise, weight loss, pancytopenia, hepatosplenomegaly, palatal ulcers).

TREATMENT

- Treat with **high-dose** TMP-SMX × 21 days.
- A prednisone taper should be used in patients with moderate to severe hypoxemia (Pa_{O_2} < 70 mm Hg or an arterial-alveolar oxygen gradient > 35).

CYTOMEGALOVIRUS (CMV)

Seventy percent of adults in the United States have been infected with CMV, and most are asymptomatic; reactivation generally occurs in immunocompromised patients.

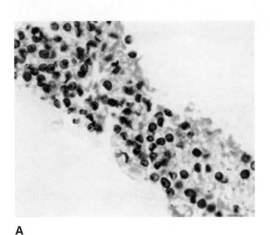
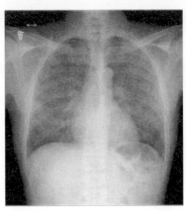

A   **B**

FIGURE 2.8-13. ***Pneumocystis* pneumonia.** (**A**) Lung tissue stained with silver uncovers folded cysts containing comma-shaped spores. (**B**) Frontal CXR shows diffuse "ground-glass" lung opacities characteristic of PCP in this patient with AIDS and a CD4+ count of 26. (Image A reproduced with permission from Ryan KJ, Ray CG. *Sherris Medical Microbiology,* 5th ed. New York: McGraw-Hill, 2010, Fig. 45-9. Image B reproduced with permission from USMLERx.com.)

- Transmission occurs via **sexual contact, breast milk, respiratory droplets** in nursery or day care facilities, and **blood transfusions.**
- Risk factors for reactivation include the first 100 days status post tissue or bone marrow transplant and HIV/AIDS (CD4+ < 100/mm³ or viral load > 10,000).

HISTORY/PE

- Systemic infection may resemble EBV mononucleosis (see the discussion of infectious mononucleosis).
- Specific manifestations include the following:
    - **CMV retinitis:** Associated with retinal detachment ("pizza pie" retinopathy); presents with floaters and visual field changes (CD4+ < 50/mm³).
    - **GI and hepatobiliary involvement:** Can present with multiple nonspecific GI symptoms, including bloody diarrhea. CMV, microsporidia, and cryptosporidia have been implicated in the development of **AIDS cholangiopathy.**
    - **CMV pneumonitis:** Presents with cough, fever, and sparse sputum production; associated with a high mortality rate. Much more common in patients with hematologic malignancies and transplant patients than in those with AIDS.
    - **CNS involvement:** Can include **polyradiculopathy, transverse myelitis,** and subacute **encephalitis** (CD4+ < 50/mm³; periventricular calcifications).

DIAGNOSIS

Virus isolation, culture, **tissue histopathology, serum PCR.**

TREATMENT

Treat with **ganciclovir** or foscarnet. Treat underlying disease if the patient is immunocompromised.

 KEY FACT

Treat CMV infection with ganciclovir.

MYCOBACTERIUM AVIUM COMPLEX (MAC)

Ubiquitous organisms causing **pulmonary** and **disseminated** infection in several demographic groups. The 1° pulmonary form occurs in **apparently healthy nonsmokers (Lady Windermere syndrome)**; a 2° pulmonary form affects patients with **preexisting pulmonary disease** such as COPD, TB, or CF. Disseminated infection occurs in AIDS patients with a **CD4+ < 50/mm³**.

HISTORY/PE

- Disseminated *M avium* infection in AIDS is associated with **fever, weakness,** and **weight loss in patients who are not on HAART or chemoprophylaxis for MAC.**
- Hepatosplenomegaly and lymphadenopathy are occasionally seen.
- Adrenal insufficiency is possible in the setting of adrenal infiltration.

DIAGNOSIS

- Obtain mycobacterial **blood cultures** (⊕ in 2–3 weeks).
- Labs show anemia, hypoalbuminemia, and ↑ **serum alkaline phosphatase and LDH.**
- Biopsy of bone marrow, intestine, or liver reveals **foamy macrophages** with **acid-fast bacilli.** Typical granulomas may be absent in immunocompromised patients.

TREATMENT

Treat with **clarithromycin** and consider **HAART if drug-naïve. Ethambutol +/– rifabutin is second line.** Continue for > 12 months and until CD4+ is > 100/mm³ for > 6 months.

PREVENTION

Weekly azithromycin for those with a CD4+ < 50/mm³ or AIDS-defining opportunistic infection.

TOXOPLASMOSIS

Risk factors include ingesting **raw or undercooked meat** and **changing cat litter.**

HISTORY/PE

- 1° infection is usually asymptomatic.
- Reactivated toxoplasmosis occurs in immunosuppressed patients and may present in specific organs (brain, lung, and eye > heart, skin, GI tract, and liver).
- Encephalitis is common in seropositive AIDS patients. Classically, CNS lesions present with fever, headache, altered mental status, seizures, and focal neurologic deficits.

DIAGNOSIS

- **Serology, PCR** (indicates exposure and risk for reactivation); tissue examination for histology, isolation of the organism in mice, or tissue culture.
- In the setting of CNS involvement, **obtain a CT scan (look for multiple isodense or hypodense ring-enhancing mass lesions)** or an **MRI** (has a predilection for the **basal ganglia;** more sensitive).

KEY FACT

Ring-enhancing lesions in patients with AIDS should always prompt consideration of toxoplasmosis and CNS lymphoma.

TREATMENT

- Induction with high-dose PO **pyrimethamine** + **sulfadiazine and leucovorin** (a folic acid analog to prevent hematologic toxicity) × 4–8 weeks; maintenance with a low-dose regimen until the disease has resolved clinically and radiographically.
- **TMP-SMX (Bactrim DS)** or pyrimethamine + dapsone can be used for prophylaxis in patients with a CD4+ count < $100/mm^3$ and a $\oplus$ toxoplasmosis IgG.

Sexually Transmitted Diseases (STDs)

CHLAMYDIA

The most common bacterial STD in the United States. Caused by *Chlamydia trachomatis*, which can infect the genital tract, urethra, anus, and eye. Risk factors include **unprotected sexual intercourse and new or multiple partners.** Often coexists with or mimics N *gonorrhoeae* infection (known as nongonococcal urethritis when gonorrhea is absent). LGV serovars of *Chlamydia* cause lymphogranuloma venereum, an emerging cause of proctocolitis.

HISTORY/PE

- Infection is often asymptomatic in men and may present with **urethritis, mucopurulent cervicitis,** or **PID** in women.
- Examination may reveal cervical/adnexal tenderness in women or penile discharge and testicular tenderness in men.
- The differential includes gonorrhea, endometriosis, PID, orchitis, vaginitis, and UTI.
- Lymphogranuloma venereum presents in its 1° form as a painless, transient papule or shallow ulcer. In its 2° form, it presents as painful swelling of the inguinal nodes, and in its 3° form it can present as an "anogenital syndrome" (anal pruritus with discharge, rectal strictures, rectovaginal fistula, and elephantiasis).

DIAGNOSIS

- Diagnosis is usually clinical; culture is the **gold standard.**
- Urine tests (nucleic acid amplification tests) are a rapid means of detection, whereas DNA probes and immunofluorescence (for gonorrhea/chlamydia) take 48–72 hours.
- **Gram stain** of urethral or genital discharge may show **PMNs but no bacteria (intracellular).**

TREATMENT

- **Doxycycline** × 7 days or azithromycin once. Use azithromycin or amoxicillin in pregnant patients.
- **Treat sexual partners,** and maintain a low threshold to treat for N *gonorrhoeae.* LGV serovars require prolonged therapy for 21 days.

COMPLICATIONS

- Chronic infection and pelvic pain, Reiter's syndrome (urethritis, conjunctivitis, arthritis), Fitz-Hugh–Curtis syndrome (perihepatic inflammation and fibrosis).

- Ectopic pregnancy/infertility can result from PID (in women) and epididymitis (in men).

GONORRHEA

A gram-⊖ intracellular diplococcus that can infect almost any site in the female reproductive tract. Infection in men tends to be limited to the urethra.

HISTORY/PE

- Presents with a **greenish-yellow discharge,** pelvic or **adnexal pain,** and swollen Bartholin's glands. Men experience a **purulent urethral discharge,** dysuria, and erythema of the urethral meatus.
- The differential includes chlamydia, endometriosis, pharyngitis, PID, vaginitis, UTI, salpingitis, and tubo-ovarian abscess.

DIAGNOSIS

- **Gram stain and culture** is the gold standard for any site (pharynx, cervix, urethra, or anus). **Nucleic acid amplification tests** can be sent on penile/vaginal tissue or from urine.
- Disseminated disease may present with **monoarticular septic arthritis,** rash, and/or **tenosynovitis.**

TREATMENT

- **Ceftriaxone IM or cefixime PO.** Also treat for presumptive chlamydia coinfection with doxycycline or a macrolide. Condoms are effective prophylaxis. Treat the sexual partner or partners if possible. Fluoroquinolones should not be used because of emerging resistance.
- Disseminated disease requires IV ceftriaxone for at least 24 hours.

COMPLICATIONS

Persistent infection with pain; infertility; tubo-ovarian abscess with rupture; disseminated gonococcal infection (see Figure 2.8-14).

SYPHILIS

Caused by *Treponema pallidum,* a spirochete. AIDS can accelerate the course of disease progression.

HISTORY/PE

- **1° (10–90 days after infection):** Presents with a **painless ulcer (chancre;** see Figure 2.8-15).
- **2° (4–8 weeks after chancre):** Presents with low-grade fever, headache, malaise, and generalized lymphadenopathy with a diffuse, symmetric, asymptomatic (nonpruritic) **maculopapular rash on the soles and palms.** Highly infective 2° eruptions include mucous patches or **condylomata lata** (see Figure 2.8-16). Meningitis, hepatitis, nephropathy, and eye involvement may also be seen.
  - **Early latent** (period from resolution of 1° or 2° syphilis to the end of the **first year** of infection): No symptoms; ⊕ serology.
  - **Late latent** (period of asymptomatic infection **beyond the first year**): No symptoms; ⊕ or ⊖ serology. One-third of cases progress to 3° syphilis.
- **3°** (late manifestations appearing 1–20 years after initial infection): Presents with destructive, granulomatous **gummas. Neurosyphilis** includes

Azithromycin. The patient has signs and symptoms of disseminated *Mycobacterium avium* complex. HIV-infected patients with CD4+ counts < 50 cells/mm³ should receive prophylaxis against MAC with azithromycin once a week.

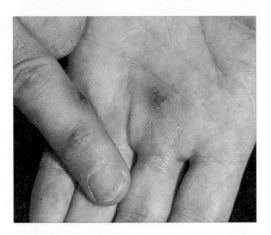

FIGURE 2.8-14. **Disseminated gonococcal infection.** Hemorrhagic, painful pustules are seen on erythematous bases. (Reproduced with permission from Wolff K et al. *Fitzpatrick's Dermatology in General Medicine,* 7th ed. New York: McGraw-Hill, 2008, Fig. 205-4.)

tabes dorsalis (posterior column degeneration), meningitis, and **Argyll Robertson pupil** (constricts with accommodation but not reactive to light). **Cardiovascular** findings include dilated aortic root, aortitis, **aortic root aneurysms,** and aortic regurgitation.

DIAGNOSIS

- Table 2.8-8 summarizes relevant diagnostic tests.
- **VDRL false ⊕s** are seen with **V**iruses (mononucleosis, HSV, HIV, hepatitis), **D**rugs/IV drug use, **R**heumatic fever/**R**heumatoid arthritis, and SLE/Leprosy.
- Neurosyphilis should be suspected and ruled out in patients with AIDS, neurologic symptoms, and a ⊕ RPR.

TREATMENT

- **1°/2°: Benzathine penicillin IM** × 1 day. Tetracycline or doxycycline × 14 days may be used for patients with penicillin allergies. Pregnant patients who are penicillin allergic and have ⊕ antibody titers must be desensitized and treated with penicillin.
- **Latent infection:** Treat with benzathine penicillin. Give 1 dose for early latent infection; give a weekly dose × 3 weeks for late latent infection or for asymptomatic infection of unknown duration.
- **Neurosyphilis:** Treat with penicillin IV × 10–14 days; penicillin-allergic patients should be desensitized prior to therapy.

TABLE 2.8-8. **Diagnostic Tests for Syphilis**

TEST	COMMENTS
Dark-field microscopy	Identifies motile spirochetes (only 1° and 2° lesions).
VDRL/RPR	Nontreponemal tests. Rapid and cheap, but sensitivity is only 75–85% in 1° disease. Many false ⊕s. Used for screening and quantitative measurement.
FTA-ABS, TP-PA, MHA-TP, TP-EIA	Treponemal tests. Sensitive and specific. Used as confirmatory tests.

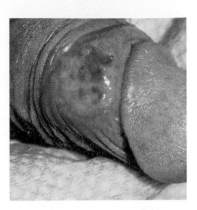

FIGURE 2.8-15. **1° syphilis.** The chancre is an ulcerated papule with a smooth, clean base; raised, indurated borders; and scant discharge. (Reproduced with permission from Bondi EE. *Dermatology: Diagnosis and Therapy,* 1st ed. Stamford, CT: Appleton & Lange, 1991: 394.)

 KEY FACT

Syphilis is the "great imitator" because its dermatologic findings resemble those of many other diseases.

 KEY FACT

Remember that treatment of syphilis can result in an acute flulike illness known as the Jarisch-Herxheimer reaction.

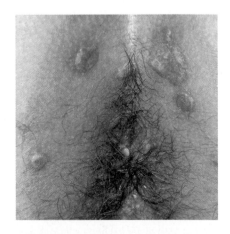

FIGURE 2.8-16. **Condylomata lata.** Typical appearance of the verrucous, heaped-up lesions of condylomata lata. (Reproduced with permission from Tintinalli JE et al. *Tintinalli's Emergency Medicine: A Comprehensive Study Guide,* 7th ed. New York: McGraw-Hill, 2011, Fig. 248-7.)

GENITAL LESIONS

See Table 2.8-9 for a description of common sexually transmitted genital lesions along with an outline of their diagnosis and treatment.

TABLE 2.8-9. Sexually Transmitted Genital Lesions

VARIABLE	*KLEBSIELLA GRANULOMATIS*[a] (GRANULOMA INGUINALE)	*HAEMOPHILUS DUCREYI* (CHANCROID)	HSV-1 OR HSV-2[b]	HPV[c]	*TREPONEMA PALLIDUM*
Lesion	Papule becomes a **beefy-red ulcer** with a characteristic rolled edge of granulation tissue.	Papule or pustule (chancroid; see Figure 2.8-17).	Vesicle (3–7 days postexposure).	Papule (condylomata acuminata; warts).	Papule (chancre).
Appearance	Raised red lesions with a white border.	Irregular, deep, well demarcated, necrotic.	Regular, red, shallow ulcer.	Irregular, pink or white, raised; cauliflower.	Regular, red, round, raised.
Number	1 or multiple	1–3	Multiple	Multiple	Single
Size	5–10 mm	10–20 mm	1–3 mm	1–5 mm	1 cm
Pain	No	**Yes**	**Yes**	No	No
Concurrent signs and symptoms	Granulomatous ulcers.	Inguinal lymphadenopathy.	Malaise, myalgias, and fever with vulvar burning and pruritus.	Pruritus.	Regional adenopathy.
Diagnosis	Clinical exam, biopsy (Donovan bodies).	Difficult to culture; diagnosis is made on clinical grounds.	Tzanck smear shows multinucleated giant cells; viral cultures; DFA or serology.	Clinical exam; biopsy for confirmation.	Spirochetes seen under dark-field microscopy; *T pallidum* identified by serum antibody test.
Treatment[d]	Doxycycline or azithromycin.	Azithromycin or ceftriaxone.	Acyclovir, famciclovir, or valacyclovir for 1° infection.	Cryotherapy, laser, or excision; topical agents such as podophyllotoxin, imiquimod, or trichloroacetic acid.	Penicillin IM.

[a] Previously known as *Calymmatobacterium granulomatis*.
[b] Some 85% of genital herpes lesions are caused by HSV-2.
[c] HPV serotypes 6 and 11 are associated with genital warts; types 16, 18, and 31 are associated with cervical cancer.
[d] For all, treat sexual partners.

Genitourinary Infections

URINARY TRACT INFECTIONS (UTIs)

Affect females more frequently than males, and ⊕ *E coli* cultures are obtained in 80% of cases. See the mnemonic **SEEKS PP** for other pathogens. Risk factors include the presence of catheters or other urologic instrumentation, anatomic abnormalities (eg, BPH, vesicoureteral reflux), previous UTIs or pyelonephritis, DM, recent antibiotic use, immunosuppression, and pregnancy.

HISTORY/PE

- Present with **dysuria, urgency, frequency,** suprapubic pain, and hematuria.
- Children may present with **bedwetting,** poor feeding, recurrent fevers, and foul-smelling urine.
- The differential includes vaginitis, STDs, urethritis or acute urethral syndrome, and prostatitis.

DIAGNOSIS

- Diagnosed by **clinical symptoms.** In the absence of symptoms, treatment is warranted only for children, patients with anatomical GU tract anomalies, pregnant women, those with instrumented urinary tracts, patients scheduled for GU surgery, and renal transplant patients.
- Urine dipstick/UA: ↑ **leukocyte esterase** (a marker of WBCs) is 75% sensitive and up to 95% specific. ↑ **nitrites** (a marker of bacteria), ↑ urine pH (*Proteus* infections), and hematuria (seen with cystitis) are also commonly seen.
- Microscopic analysis: **Pyuria** (> 5 WBCs/hpf) and **bacteriuria** (1 organism/hpf = 10^6 organisms/mL) are suggestive.
- Urine culture: The gold standard is > 10^5 **CFU/mL.**

TREATMENT

- **Uncomplicated UTI:** Treat on an outpatient basis with PO **TMP-SMX** or a **fluoroquinolone** × 3 days, or **nitrofurantoin** × 5 days. The use of fluoroquinolones should be reserved for severe symptoms in light of resistance and MRSA selection.
- **Complicated UTI** (urinary obstruction, men, renal transplant, catheters, instrumentation): Administer the same antibiotics as above, but for 7–14 days.
- **Pregnant patients:** Treat asymptomatic bacteruria or symptomatic UTI with **nitrofurantoin** or amoxicillin × 3–7 days. Avoid fluoroquinolones. Confirm clearance with a posttreatment urine culture.
- **Urosepsis:** Patients with urosepsis should be hospitalized and initially treated with **IV antibiotics.** Consider broader coverage to include resistant GNRs or enterococcus.
- Prophylactic antibiotics may be given to women with uncomplicated recurrent UTIs. Check for prostatitis in men.

PYELONEPHRITIS

Nearly 85% of community-acquired cases of pyelonephritis result from the same pathogens that cause cystitis. Cystitis and pyelonephritis have similar risk factors.

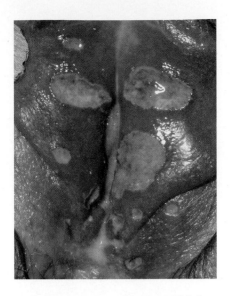

FIGURE 2.8-17. Chancroid. Multiple, painful ulcers are seen. (Reproduced with permission from Wolff K, Johnson RA. *Fitzpatrick's Color Atlas & Synopsis of Clinical Dermatology,* 6th ed. New York: McGraw-Hill, 2009, Fig. 30-28.)

MNEMONIC

Common UTI bugs—

SEEKS PP

Serratia
E coli
Enterobacter
Klebsiella pneumoniae
Staphylococcus saprophyticus
Pseudomonas
Proteus mirabilis

Q

A 45-year-old woman presents to the ER with fever, chills, nausea, vomiting, and severe flank pain. She has a history of multiple UTIs and was recently hospitalized for pyelonephritis. UA reveals pyuria and bacteriuria. Ultrasound performed in the ER shows what appears to be a perinephric abscess. What is the next most appropriate step in management?

HISTORY/PE

- Signs and symptoms are similar to those of cystitis but show evidence of **upper urinary tract disease.**
- Symptoms include **flank pain, fever/chills,** and nausea/vomiting. Dysuria, frequency, and urgency are also possible.

DIAGNOSIS

- **UA and culture:** Results are similar to those of cystitis, but with **WBC casts.** Send blood cultures to rule out urosepsis.
- **CBC:** Reveals leukocytosis.
- **Imaging:** In general, imaging is not necessary. Patients who relapse or do not respond to therapy within 48–72 hours should be evaluated by ultrasound or CT for obstruction, abscess, and other complications of pyelonephritis.

TREATMENT

- For mild cases, patients may be treated on an outpatient basis for 7–14 days. **Fluoroquinolones** are first-line therapy. Encourage ↑ PO fluids and monitor closely.
- Admit and administer IV antibiotics to patients who have serious medical complications or systemic symptoms, are **pregnant,** present with severe **nausea and vomiting,** or have suspected bacteremia. Fluoroquinolones, third- or fourth-generation cephalosporins, β-lactam/β-lactamase inhibitors, and carbapenem may be used depending on disease severity.

Hematologic Infections

SEPSIS

Defined as the presence of systemic inflammatory response syndrome (**SIRS**) with a **documented infection** induced by microbial invasion or toxins in the bloodstream. **Severe sepsis** refers to sepsis with end-organ dysfunction due to poor perfusion. **Septic shock** refers to sepsis with hypotension and organ dysfunction from vasodilation. Examples include the following:

- **Gram-⊕ shock** (eg, staphylococci and streptococci) 2° to fluid loss caused by exotoxins.
- **Gram-⊖ shock** (eg, *E coli, Klebsiella, Proteus,* and *Pseudomonas*) 2° to vasodilation caused by endotoxins (lipopolysaccharide).
- **Neonates:** GBS, *E coli, Listeria monocytogenes, H influenzae.*
- **Children:** *H influenzae,* pneumococcus, meningococcus.
- **Adults:** Gram-⊕ cocci, aerobic gram-⊖ bacilli, anaerobes (dependent on the presumed site of infection).
- **IV drug users/indwelling lines:** *S aureus,* coagulase-⊖ *Staphylococcus* species.
- **Asplenic patients:** Pneumococcus, *H influenzae,* meningococcus (encapsulated organisms).

HISTORY/PE

- Presents with abrupt onset of fever and chills, altered mental status, tachycardia, and tachypnea. Severe sepsis may lead to end-organ dysfunction such as renal or hepatic failure. **Hypotension** occurs in cases of septic shock.

- Septic shock is typically a warm shock with **warm skin and extremities.** This contrasts with cardiogenic shock, which typically presents with **cool skin and extremities.**
- Petechiae, ecchymoses, or abnormal coagulation tests suggest DIC (2–3% of cases).

DIAGNOSIS

- A clinical diagnosis.
- Labs show leukocytosis or leukopenia with ↑ bands, thrombocytopenia (50% of cases), evidence of ↓ tissue perfusion (↑ creatinine, ↑ LFTs, ↑ lactate), and abnormal coagulation studies (↑ INR).
- It is critical to obtain cultures of all appropriate sites (eg, blood, sputum, CSF, wound, urine).
- Imaging (CXR, CT) may aid in establishing the etiology or site of infection.

TREATMENT

- ICU admission may be required. Treat aggressively with IV fluids, empiric antibiotics (based on the likely source of infection), and vasopressors.
- Treat underlying factors (eg, remove Foley catheter or infected lines).
- The 1° goal is to **maintain BP** and **perfuse** end organs.

MALARIA

A protozoal disease caused by 4 strains of the genus ***Plasmodium*** (*P falciparum, vivax, ovale, malariae*) and transmitted by the bite of an infected female ***Anopheles*** mosquito. **P falciparum** has the highest morbidity and mortality, occasionally within 24 hours of symptom onset. Travelers to endemic areas should take chemoprophylaxis and use mosquito repellent and bed nets to minimize exposure.

HISTORY/PE

- Patients have a history of exposure in a malaria-endemic area, with **periodic** attacks of sequential **chills, fever** (> 41°C, or > 105.8°F), and **diaphoresis** occurring over 4–6 hours.
- **Splenomegaly** often appears 4 or more days after symptom onset. Patients are often asymptomatic between attacks, which recur every 2–3 days depending on the *Plasmodium* strain.
- Severely ill patients may present with hyperpyrexia, prostration, impaired consciousness, agitation, hyperventilation, and bleeding. The presence of rash, skin ulcer, eosinophilia, lymphadenopathy, neck stiffness, or photophobia suggests a different or additional diagnosis.

DIAGNOSIS

- Timely diagnosis of the correct strain is essential because *P falciparum* can be fatal and is often resistant to standard chloroquine treatment.
- **Giemsa- or Wright-stained thick and thin blood films** should be sent for expert microscopic evaluation to determine the species as well as the degree of parasitemia (see Figure 2.8-18).
- CBC usually demonstrates normochromic, normocytic anemia with reticulocytosis.
- If resources allow, more sensitive serologic tests are available, including rapid antigen detection methods, fluorescent antibody methods, and PCR.

KEY FACT

SIRS = 2 or more of the following:
1. **Temperature:** Either < 35°C or > 38.5°C (ie, hypothermia or fever).
2. **Tachypnea:** > 20 breaths per minute or $Paco_2$ < 32 mm Hg on ABG.
3. **Tachycardia:** Heart rate > 90 bpm.
4. **Leukocytosis/leukopenia:** WBC count < 4000 cells/mm³ or > 12,000 cells/mm³.

KEY FACT

Consider malaria in the differential for any patient who has emigrated from or recently traveled to tropical locations and presents with fever.

KEY FACT

P vivax, P ovale, and *P malariae* can all cause symptoms months to years after the initial infection.

KEY FACT

Obtain a fingerstick in a patient with malaria and mental status changes to rule out hypoglycemia.

KEY FACT

Nearly all malaria-endemic countries now have chloroquine-resistant malaria.

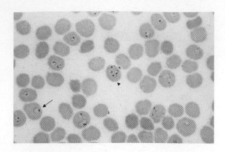

FIGURE 2.8-18. *Plasmodium falciparum* **hyperparasitemia in the thin smear of a patient with cerebral malaria.** (Courtesy of Dr. S. Glenn, Public Health Image Library, Centers for Disease Control and Prevention, Atlanta, GA, as published in Levinson W. *Review of Medical Microbiology and Immunology,* 11th ed. New York: McGraw-Hill, 2010, Fig. 52-2.)

KEY FACT

Cerebral malaria presents with headache, a change in mental status, neurologic signs, retinal hemorrhages, convulsions, and delirium. If left untreated, it may rapidly progress to coma and death.

KEY FACT

A young adult who presents with the triad of **fever, sore throat,** and **lymphadenopathy** may have infectious mononucleosis.

KEY FACT

The lymphocytosis in EBV infection is predominantly due to B-cell proliferation, but the atypical cells are T lymphocytes.

TREATMENT

- Uncomplicated malarial infection can be treated orally. **Chloroquine** has been the standard antimalarial medication, but increasing resistance often necessitates the use of other medications.
- In cases of *P vivax, P ovale,* or an unknown strain, **primaquine** is added to eradicate the hypnozoites in the liver.
- Severe infections can be treated with parenteral antimalarial medications (**IV quinidine**) with transition to oral regimens as tolerated. Symptoms can be treated with supportive care.
- **Mefloquine is the first-line chemoprophylaxis against chloroquine-resistant malaria.**

COMPLICATIONS

Cerebral malaria, severe hemolytic anemia, renal impairment, noncardiogenic pulmonary edema, hypoglycemia, lactic acidosis, acute hepatopathy, gram-$\ominus$ bacteremia.

INFECTIOUS MONONUCLEOSIS

Most commonly occurs in **young adult** patients; usually due to acute EBV infection. Transmission most often occurs through exchange of body fluids, most commonly saliva.

HISTORY/PE

- Presents with **fever** and **pharyngitis. Fatigue** invariably accompanies initial illness and may persist for 3–6 months. Examination may reveal low-grade fever, generalized lymphadenopathy (especially **posterior cervical**), tonsillar exudate and enlargement, palatal petechiae, a generalized maculopapular rash, splenomegaly, and **bilateral upper eyelid edema.**
- Patients who present with pharyngitis as their 1° symptom may be misdiagnosed with streptococcal pharyngitis (30% of patients with infectious mononucleosis are asymptomatic carriers of GAS in their oropharynx).
- The differential also includes CMV, toxoplasmosis, HIV, HHV-6, other causes of viral hepatitis, and lymphoma.
- Most patients with mononucleosis who are given ampicillin for suspected streptococcal pharyngitis develop a prolonged, pruritic maculopapular rash.

DIAGNOSIS

- Diagnosed by the **heterophil antibody (Monospot) test** (may be $\ominus$ in the first few weeks after symptoms begin).
- **EBV-specific antibodies** can be ordered in patients with suspected mononucleosis and a $\ominus$ Monospot test. Infectious mononucleosis syndromes that are Monospot $\ominus$ and EBV-antibody $\ominus$ are most often due to CMV infection. Acute HIV and other viral etiologies should be considered.
- CBC with differential often reveals mild **thrombocytopenia** with relative **lymphocytosis** and > 10% **atypical T lymphocytes.**
- CMP usually reveals mildly elevated transaminases, alkaline phosphatase, and total bilirubin.

TREATMENT

Treatment is mostly supportive, as there is no effective antiviral therapy. Corticosteroids are indicated for airway compromise due to tonsillar enlargement, severe thrombocytopenia, or severe autoimmune hemolytic anemia.

COMPLICATIONS

- **CNS infection:** Can present as aseptic meningitis, encephalitis, meningo-encephalitis, cranial nerve palsies (particularly CN VII), optic and peripheral neuritis, transverse myelitis, or Guillain-Barré syndrome.
- **Splenic rupture:** Occurs in < 0.5% of cases. More common in males, and presents with abdominal pain, referred shoulder pain, or hemodynamic compromise.
- **Upper airway obstruction:** Treat with steroids.
- **Bacterial superinfection:** Many patients develop a 2° streptococcal pharyngitis.
- **Fulminant hepatic necrosis:** More common in males; the most common cause of death in affected males.
- **Autoimmune hemolytic anemia:** Occurs in 2% of patients during the first 2 weeks. Coombs ⊕. Mild anemia lasts 1–2 months. Treat with corticosteroids if severe.

KEY FACT

Many patients with infectious mononucleosis have coexisting streptococcal pharyngitis that requires treatment.

 Fever

FEVER OF UNKNOWN ORIGIN (FUO)

A temperature of > 38.3°C (> 100.9°F) of at least 3 weeks' duration that remains undiagnosed following 3 outpatient visits or 3 days of hospitalization.

HISTORY/PE

Presents with fever, headache, myalgia, and malaise. The differential includes the following:

- **Infectious:** TB, endocarditis (eg, HACEK organisms; see the discussion of infective endocarditis), occult abscess, osteomyelitis, catheter infections. In HIV patients, consider MAC, histoplasmosis, CMV, or lymphoma.
- **Neoplastic:** Lymphomas, leukemias, hepatic and renal cell carcinomas.
- **Autoimmune:** Still's disease, SLE, cryoglobulinemia, polyarteritis nodosa, connective tissue disease, granulomatous disease (including sarcoidosis).
- **Miscellaneous:** Pulmonary emboli, alcoholic hepatitis, drug fever, familial Mediterranean fever, factitious fever.
- Undiagnosed (10–15%).

DIAGNOSIS

- Confirm the presence of fever and take a detailed history, including family, social, sexual, occupational, dietary, exposures (pets/animals), and travel.
- **Labs:** Obtain a CBC with differential, ESR, serum protein electrophoresis, multiple blood cultures, sputum Gram stain and culture, UA and culture, and PPD. Specific tests (ANA, RF, CK, viral cultures, viral serologies/antigen tests) can be obtained if an infectious or autoimmune etiology is suspected.
- **Imaging:** Obtain a CXR. CT of the chest, abdomen, and pelvis should be done early in the workup of a true FUO. Invasive testing (marrow/liver biopsy) is generally low yield. Laparoscopy and colonoscopy are higher yield as second-line tests (after CT).

TREATMENT

Stop unnecessary medications. Patients with FUO and a completely ⊖ workup have a good prognosis, with fevers resolving over months to years.

KEY FACT

Overall, infections and cancer account for the majority of cases of FUO (> 60%). Autoimmune diseases account for ~ 15%. In the elderly, rheumatic diseases account for one-third of cases.

KEY FACT

FUO patients without other symptoms do not require empiric antibiotic therapy.

Q

A 17-year-old male presents with 1 week of fever, sore throat, and progressive fatigue. Physical examination reveals palatal petechiae, large tonsils with whitish exudates, splenomegaly, and cervical and axillary lymphadenopathy. The patient says that he has been too tired to attend football practices and is concerned that he may lose his spot on the starting roster. What is the most appropriate advice to be given regarding his participation in athletics?

NEUTROPENIC FEVER

- Defined as a single oral temperature of ≥ 38.3°C (≥ 101°F) or a temperature of ≥ 38.0°C (≥ 100.4°F) for ≥ 1 hour in a neutropenic patient (ie, an absolute neutrophil count < 500 cells/mm³).
- **Hx/PE:** Common in cancer patients undergoing chemotherapy (neutropenic nadir 7–10 days postchemotherapy). Inflammation may be minimal or absent.
- **Dx:**
    - Conduct a thorough physical examination, but **avoid a rectal examination** in light of the bleeding risk if the patient is thrombocytopenic.
    - Obtain a CBC with differential, serum creatinine, BUN, and transaminases; send blood, urine, lesion, sputum, and stool cultures. Consider testing for viruses, fungi, and mycobacteria.
    - CXR for patients with respiratory symptoms; CT scan to evaluate for abscesses or other occult infection.
- **Tx:** Empiric antibiotic therapy. Admission and IV antibiotics are warranted for high-risk patients (eg, hematologic malignancy, chemotherapy, neutropenia > 14 days). Routine use of colony-stimulating factors is not indicated. If fevers persist after 72 hours despite antibiotic therapy, start antifungal treatment.

Tick-Borne Infections

LYME DISEASE

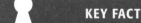

KEY FACT

Lyme disease is the most common vector-borne disease in North America.

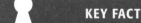

KEY FACT

Lyme arthritis can be very subtle and minimally inflammatory, and it can wax and wane.

Tell the patient to refrain from contact sports until his physical examination normalizes. Splenomegaly 2° to infectious mononucleosis puts him at ↑ risk for splenic rupture.

- A tick-borne disease caused by the spirochete *Borrelia burgdorferi.* Usually seen during the **summer months,** and carried by *Ixodes* ticks on white-tailed deer and white-footed mice. Endemic to the **Northeast,** northern Midwest, and Pacific coast.
- **Hx/PE:** Presents with the onset of rash with fever, malaise, fatigue, headache, myalgias, and/or arthralgias. Infection usually occurs after a tick feeds for > 18 hours.
    - **1° (early localized disease): Erythema migrans** begins as a small erythematous macule or papule that is found at the tick-feeding site and expands slowly over days to weeks. The border may be macular or raised, often with central clearing ("bull's eye"; see Figure 2.8-19).
    - **2° (early disseminated disease):** Presents with migratory polyarthropathies, neurologic phenomena (eg, Bell's palsy), meningitis and/or myocarditis, and conduction abnormalities (third-degree heart block).
    - **3° (late disease):** Arthritis and subacute encephalitis (memory loss and mood change).
- **Dx:**
    - **ELISA** and **Western blot:** Use the Western blot to confirm a ⊕ or indeterminate ELISA. A ⊕ ELISA denotes **exposure** but is not specific for active disease. Western blots sent without ELISA have high false-⊕ rates.
    - **Tissue culture/PCR:** Extremely difficult to obtain; not routinely done.
- **Tx:**
    - Treat early disease with **doxycycline** (or amoxicillin in children < 8 years of age and in pregnant patients); more advanced disease (eg, CNS or arthritic disease) should be treated with **ceftriaxone.**
    - Consider empiric therapy for patients with the characteristic rash, arthralgias, or a tick bite acquired in an endemic area. Prevent with tick bite avoidance.

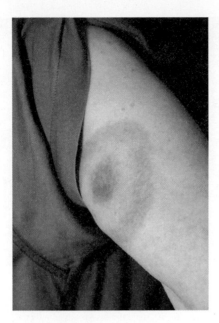

FIGURE 2.8-19. Erythema chronicum migrans seen in Lyme disease. Note the classic "bull's eye" lesion, which consists of an outer ring where the spirochetes are found, an inner ring of clearing, and central erythema due to an allergic response at the site of the tick bite. (Courtesy of James Gathany, Public Health Image Library, Centers for Disease Control and Prevention, Atlanta, GA, as published in McPhee SJ et al. *Current Medical Diagnosis & Treatment 2010.* New York: McGraw-Hill, 2010, Plate 32.)

ROCKY MOUNTAIN SPOTTED FEVER

- A disease caused by ***Rickettsia rickettsii*** and carried by the American dog tick (***Dermacentor variabilis***). The organism invades the endothelial lining of capillaries and causes **small vessel vasculitis.**
- **Hx/PE:** Presents with **headache, fever,** malaise, and **rash.** The characteristic rash is initially macular (beginning on the wrists and ankles) but becomes petechial/purpuric as it spreads centrally (see Figure 2.8-20). Altered mental status or DIC may develop in severe cases.
- **Dx:** Clinical diagnosis should be confirmed with biopsy and indirect immunofluorescence of the skin lesion.
- **Tx: Doxycycline** or chloramphenicol (for pregnant women). The condition can be rapidly fatal if left untreated. If clinical suspicion is high, begin treatment while awaiting testing. Prevent by avoiding tick bites.

Infections of the Eyes and Ears

INFECTIOUS CONJUNCTIVITIS

A common complaint in the ER setting, inflammation of the conjunctiva is most often bacterial or viral but can also be fungal, parasitic, allergic, or chemical. It is essential to differentiate potentially vision-threatening infectious etiologies from allergic or other causes of conjunctivitis, as well as to identify other vision-threatening conditions that may mimic conjunctivitis. Table 2.8-10 lists the common etiologies of infectious conjunctivitis.

MNEMONIC

With fever and rash, think—

Tiny GERMS

Typhoid fever
Gonococcemia
Endocarditis
Rocky Mountain spotted fever
Meningococcemia
Sepsis (bacterial)

KEY FACT

Rocky Mountain spotted fever starts on the wrists and ankles and then spreads centrally.

A 70-year-old female with a history of hypertension and lymphoma presents with nausea, vomiting, and fever for the past 2 days. She just underwent her second cycle of high-dose chemotherapy. She has a temperature of 38.5°C (101.3°F). Her CXR is unchanged, and her WBC count is 900 with 25% neutrophils. After urine and blood cultures have been sent, what is the next step in management?

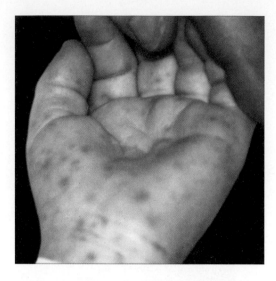

FIGURE 2.8-20. Rocky Mountain spotted fever. These erythematous macular lesions will evolve into a petechial rash that will spread centrally. (Reproduced with permission from Wolff K, Johnson RA. *Fitzpatrick's Color Atlas & Synopsis of Clinical Dermatology,* 6th ed. New York: McGraw-Hill, 2009, Fig. 26-1.)

ORBITAL CELLULITIS

- Commonly due to infection of the **paranasal sinuses;** can lead to endophthalmitis and blindness. Usually caused by **streptococci, staphylococci (including MRSA), and *H influenzae*** (in children). In diabetic and immunocompromised patients, the zygomycetes ***Mucor* and *Rhizopus*** must be included in the differential.
- **Hx/PE:** Presents with **acute-onset fever, proptosis, ↓ EOM,** ocular pain, and ↓ visual acuity. Look for a **history of ocular trauma/surgery or sinusitis.** Palatal or nasal mucosal ulceration with coexisting maxillary and/or ethmoid sinusitis suggests mucormycosis or *Rhizopus.*
- **Dx: Mostly clinical.** Blood and tissue fluid culture; CT scan (to rule out orbital abscess and intracranial involvement).
- **Tx:**
  - **Admit and give immediate IV antibiotics;** request an **ophthalmologic/ENT** consult.
  - Abscess formation or a worsening condition may necessitate surgery.
  - **Diabetic and immunocompromised patients** should be treated with **amphotericin B and surgical debridement** (often associated with **cavernous sinus thrombosis**) if *Mucor* or *Rhizopus* is diagnosed.

OTITIS EXTERNA

- An inflammation of the external auditory canal, also known as "swimmer's ear." ***Pseudomonas*** and Enterobacteriaceae are the most common etiologic agents. Both grow in the presence of excess moisture.
- **Hx/PE:** Presents with pain, pruritus, and possible purulent discharge. Examination reveals **pain with movement of the tragus/pinna** (unlike otitis media) and an edematous and erythematous ear canal. See the Pediatrics chapter for a discussion of otitis media.
- **Dx:** A clinical diagnosis. Obtain a culture for severe or refractory cases. Order a CT scan if the patient is toxic appearing.

TABLE 2.8-10. **Common Causes of Infectious Conjunctivitis**

PATHOGEN	CHARACTERISTICS	DIAGNOSIS	TREATMENT
BACTERIAL			
Staphylococci, streptococci, *Haemophilus*, *Pseudomonas*, *Moraxella*	Foreign body sensation, purulent discharge.	Gram stain and culture if severe.	Antibiotic drops/ointment.
N gonorrhoeae	**An emergency!** Corneal involvement can lead to perforation and blindness.	Gram stain shows gram-⊖ intracellular diplococci.	IM ceftriaxone, PO ciprofloxacin or ofloxacin. **Inpatient** treatment if complicated.
C trachomatis A–C	**Recurrent epithelial keratitis** in childhood; trichiasis, corneal scarring, and entropion. **The leading cause of preventable blindness worldwide.**	Giemsa stain, chlamydial cultures.	Azithromycin, tetracycline, or erythromycin × 3–4 weeks.
VIRAL			
Adenovirus (most common)	Copious **watery discharge,** severe ocular irritation, preauricular lymphadenopathy. Occurs in epidemics.		**Contagious;** self-limited. Topical corticosteroids with supervision by an ophthalmologist.

 Tx: **Clean the ear** and give **antibiotic** and steroid eardrops. Add systemic antibiotics in patients with severe disease, immunodeficiency, or diabetes. Elderly diabetics and immunocompromised individuals are at risk for necrotizing otitis externa and may require IV antibiotics.

Miscellaneous Infections

INFECTIVE ENDOCARDITIS

Infection of the endocardium. Most commonly affects the heart valves, especially the mitral valve. Risk factors include rheumatic, congenital, or valvular heart disease; prosthetic heart valves; IV drug abuse; and immunosuppression. Etiologies are as follows (see also Table 2.8-11):

- **S aureus:** The causative agent in > 80% of cases of acute bacterial endocarditis in patients with a history of IV drug abuse.
- **Viridans streptococci:** The most common pathogens for left-sided subacute bacterial endocarditis and following dental procedures in native valves.
- **Coagulase-⊖ *Staphylococcus*:** The most common infecting organism in prosthetic valve endocarditis.
- ***Streptococcus bovis:*** S bovis endocarditis is associated with coexisting GI malignancy.
- ***Candida*** and ***Aspergillus*** **species:** Account for most cases of fungal endocarditis. Predisposing factors include long-term indwelling IV catheters, malignancy, AIDS, organ transplantation, and IV drug use.

KEY FACT

Diabetics are at risk for malignant otitis externa.

KEY FACT

Otitis media should not cause pain with movement of the tragus/pinna.

TABLE 2.8-11. Causes of Endocarditis

Acute	Subacute	Marantic	Culture-⊖ (includes HACEK)	SLE
S aureus (IV drug abuse)	Viridans streptococci (native valve)	Cancer (poor prognosis) Mets seed valves; emboli can cause cerebral infarcts	*Haemophilus parainfluenzae*	Libman-Sacks endocarditis (autoantibody to valve)
S pneumoniae	*Enterococcus*		*Actinobacillus*	
N gonorrhoeae	*S epidermidis* (prosthetic valve)		*Cardiobacterium*	
	S bovis (GI insult)		*Eikenella*	
	Fungi		*Kingella*	
			Coxiella burnetii	
			Brucella	
			Bartonella	

MNEMONIC

Presentation of endocarditis—

JR = NO FAME

Janeway lesions
Roth's spots
Nail-bed (splinter) hemorrhage
Osler's nodes
Fever
Anemia
Murmur
Emboli

History/PE

- Constitutional symptoms are common (fever/FUO, weight loss, fatigue).
- Examination reveals a **heart murmur.** The mitral valve (mitral regurgitation) is more commonly affected than the aortic valve in non–IV drug users; more right-sided involvement is found in IV drug users (tricuspid valve > mitral valve > aortic valve).
- **Osler's nodes** (small, tender nodules on the finger and toe pads), **Janeway lesions** (small peripheral hemorrhages; see Figure 2.8-21A), **splinter hemorrhages** (subungual petechiae; see Figure 2.8-21B), **Roth's spots** (retinal hemorrhages), focal neurologic deficits from embolic stroke, and other embolic phenomena are also seen.

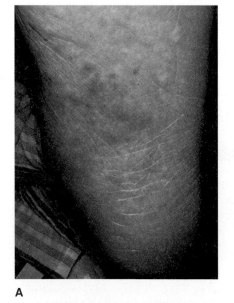

A

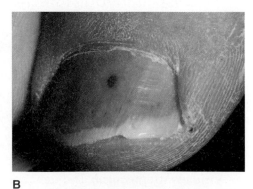

B

FIGURE 2.8-21. **Cutaneous manifestations of infective endocarditis. (A)** Janeway lesions. Peripheral embolization to the sole leads to a cluster of erythematous macules known as Janeway lesions. **(B) Splinter hemorrhages.** The splinter hemorrhages shown along the distal aspect of the nail plate are due to emboli from subacute bacterial endocarditis. (Image A courtesy of the Armed Forces Institute of Pathology, Bethesda, MD, as published in Knoop KJ et al. *Atlas of Emergency Medicine,* 2nd ed. New York: McGraw-Hill, 2002: 384. Image B Courtesy of the Department of Dermatology, Wilford Hall USAF Medical Center and Brooke Army Medical Center, San Antonio, TX, as published in Knoop KJ et al. *Atlas of Emergency Medicine,* 2nd ed. New York: McGraw-Hill, 2002: 384.)

DIAGNOSIS

- Diagnosis is guided by risk factors, clinical symptoms, and the **Duke criteria** (see Table 2.8-12). The presence of 2 major, 1 major + 3 minor, or 5 minor criteria all merit the diagnosis of endocarditis.
- **CBC** with leukocytosis and left shift; ↑ **ESR** and CRP.

TREATMENT

- **Early empiric IV antibiotic treatment** for acutely ill patients. Vancomycin is an appropriate choice for most patients. Tailor antibiotics once the causative agent is known. Acute valve replacement is sometimes necessary. The prognosis for prosthetic valve endocarditis is poor.
- Give antibiotic prophylaxis before dental work in patients with high-risk valvular disease (eg, those with previous endocarditis or a prosthetic valve).

ANTHRAX

Caused by the spore-forming gram-⊕ bacterium *Bacillus anthracis*. Infection is an occupational hazard for veterinarians, farmers, and individuals who handle **animal wool, hair, hides, or bone meal products.** Also a biological weapon. *B anthracis* can cause cutaneous (most common), inhalation (most deadly), or GI anthrax. **There is no person-to-person spread of anthrax.**

HISTORY/PE

- **Cutaneous:** Presents 1–7 days after skin exposure and penetration of spores. The lesion begins as a **pruritic papule** that enlarges to form an ulcer surrounded by a satellite bulbus/lesion with an edematous halo and a round, regular, raised edge. **Regional lymphadenopathy** is also characteristic. The lesion evolves into a **black eschar** within 7–10 days (see Figure 2.8-22).
- **Inhalational:** Presents with fever, dyspnea, hypoxia, hypotension, or symptoms of pneumonia (1–3 days after exposure), classically due to **hemorrhagic mediastinitis.** Patients typically do not have pulmonary infiltrates.

TABLE 2.8-12. Duke Criteria for the Diagnosis of Endocarditis

CRITERIA	COMPONENTS
Major	At least 2 separate ⊕ blood cultures for a typical organism, persistent bacteremia with any organism, or a single ⊕ culture of *Coxiella burnetii*.
	Evidence of endocardial involvement (via transesophageal echocardiography or new murmur).
Minor	Predisposing risk factors.
	Fever ≥ 38.3°C (≥ 100.9°F).
	Vascular phenomena: Septic emboli, septic infarcts, mycotic aneurysm, Janeway lesions.
	Immunologic phenomena: Glomerulonephritis, Osler's nodes. Roth's spots.
	Microbiological evidence that does not meet major criteria.

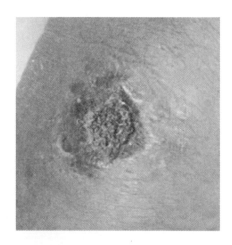

FIGURE 2.8-22. Cutaneous anthrax. Black eschar is seen on the forearm. (Courtesy of Dr. James H. Steele, Public Health Image Library, Centers for Disease Control and Prevention, Atlanta, GA, as published in Levinson W. *Review of Medical Microbiology and Immunology,* 11th ed. New York: McGraw-Hill, 2010, Fig. 5.)

1 **A**

Surgical debridement and amphotericin B. The patient has mucormycosis, a dangerous and aggressive infection found in diabetic and immunocompromised patients. Aggressive surgical debridement is warranted.

2 **A**

S aureus. Salmonella is the second most common organism that causes osteomyelitis in patients with sickle cell disease and should always be considered in these patients.

■ **GI:** Occurs after the ingestion of poorly cooked, contaminated meat; can present with dysphagia, nausea/vomiting, bloody diarrhea, and abdominal pain.

DIAGNOSIS

Criteria for diagnosis include culture isolation or 2 nonculture supportive tests (PCR, immunohistochemical staining, or ELISA). CXR is the most sensitive test for inhalational disease (shows a **widened mediastinum** and pleural effusions).

TREATMENT

■ **Ciprofloxacin** or doxycycline plus 1–2 additional antibiotics for at least 14 days are first-line therapy for inhalational disease or cutaneous disease of the face, head, or neck.
■ For other cutaneous disease, treat for 7–10 days. Postexposure prophylaxis (**ciprofloxacin**) to prevent inhalation anthrax should be continued for 60 days.

OSTEOMYELITIS

Bone or bone marrow infection 2° to **direct spread** from a soft tissue infection (80% of cases) is most common in adults, whereas infection due to **hematogenous seeding** (20% of cases) is more common in children (metaphyses of the long bones) and IV drug users (**vertebral bodies**). Common pathogens are outlined in Table 2.8-13.

HISTORY/PE

Presents with **localized bone pain and tenderness** along with warmth, swelling, erythema, and limited motion of the adjacent joint. Systemic symptoms (fevers, chills) and purulent drainage may be present.

TABLE 2.8-13. **Common Pathogens in Osteomyelitis**

IF	THINK
No risk factors	S aureus.
IV drug user	S aureus or Pseudomonas.
Sickle cell disease	Salmonella.
Hip replacement	S epidermidis.
Foot puncture wound	Pseudomonas.
Chronic	S aureus, Pseudomonas, Enterobacteriaceae.
Diabetic	Polymicrobial, Pseudomonas, S aureus, streptococci, anaerobes.

DIAGNOSIS

- **Labs:** ↑ WBC count; ↑ **ESR** and **CRP** levels in most cases. Blood cultures may be ⊕.
- **Imaging:**
    - X-rays are often ⊖ initially but may show **periosteal elevation** within 10–14 days. Bone scans are sensitive for osteomyelitis but lack specificity.
    - **MRI** (the test of choice) will show ↑ signal in the bone marrow and associated soft tissue infection (see Figure 2.8-23).
    - Definitive diagnosis is made by bone aspiration with Gram stain and culture. Clinical diagnosis made by probing through the soft tissue to bone is usually sufficient, as aspiration carries a risk of infection.

TREATMENT

- **Surgical debridement** of necrotic, infected bone followed by **IV antibiotics** × 4–6 weeks. Empiric antibiotic selection is based on the suspected organism and Gram stain.
- Consider clindamycin plus ciprofloxacin, ampicillin/sulbactam, or oxacillin/nafcillin (for methicillin-sensitive *S aureus*); vancomycin (for MRSA); or ceftriaxone or ciprofloxacin (for gram-⊖ bacteria).

COMPLICATIONS

Chronic osteomyelitis, sepsis, septic arthritis. Long-standing chronic osteomyelitis with a draining sinus tract may eventually lead to **squamous cell carcinoma** (Marjolin's ulcer).

KEY FACT

Osteomyelitis is associated with peripheral vascular disease, diabetes, penetrating soft tissue injuries, chronic decubitus ulcers, and IV drug abuse.

KEY FACT

Diabetic osteomyelitis should be treated with antibiotics targeting gram-⊕ organisms and anaerobes.

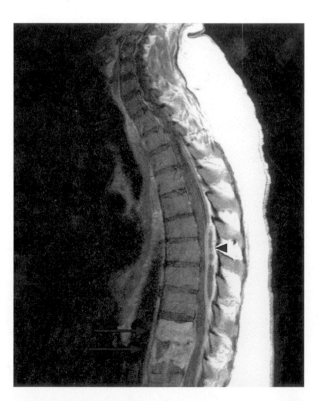

FIGURE 2.8-23. Diskitis/osteomyelitis. Sagittal contrast-enhanced MRI shows destruction of a lower thoracic intervertebral disk with abnormal enhancement throughout the adjacent vertebral bodies (arrows) and a posterior rim-enhancing epidural abscess (arrowhead) in the spinal canal. (Reproduced with permission from Tintinalli JE et al. *Tintinalli's Emergency Medicine: A Comprehensive Study Guide,* 6th ed. New York: McGraw-Hill, 2004, Fig. 305-5.)

NOTES

Common Adult Orthopedic Injuries

Table 2.9-1 outlines the presentation and treatment of orthopedic injuries that commonly affect adults.

TABLE 2.9-1.   Common Adult Orthopedic Injuries

INJURY	MECHANICS	TREATMENT
Shoulder dislocation	**Anterior dislocation:** Most common; the **axillary nerve is at risk.** Patients hold the arm in slight **abduction and external rotation** (see Figure 2.9-1). **Posterior dislocation:** Rare; associated with **seizure and electrocutions.** Patients hold the arm in adduction and internal rotation.	Reduction followed by a sling and swath. Recurrent dislocations may need surgical treatment.
Hip dislocation	**Anterior dislocation:** Can injure the obturator nerve. **Posterior dislocation: Most common** (> 90%); occurs via a posteriorly directed force on an internally rotated, flexed, adducted hip ("dashboard injury"). Associated with a risk of sciatic nerve injury and avascular necrosis (AVN) (see Figure 2.9-2).	Closed reduction followed by abduction pillow/bracing. Evaluate with CT scan after reduction.
Colles' fracture	Involves the distal radius. Often results from a **fall onto an outstretched hand,** leading to a dorsally displaced, dorsally angulated fracture. Commonly seen in the elderly (osteoporosis) and children.	Closed reduction followed by application of a long-arm cast; open reduction if the fracture is intra-articular.
Scaphoid fracture	The **most commonly fractured carpal bone.** May take 2 weeks for radiographs to show the fracture (see Figure 2.9-3). Assume a fracture if there is tenderness in the **anatomical snuff box.**	Thumb spica cast. If displacement or scaphoid nonunion is present, treat with open reduction. With proximal-third scaphoid fractures, AVN may result from disruption of blood flow.
Boxer's fracture	Fracture of the fifth metacarpal neck. Due to forward trauma of a closed fist (eg, punching a wall).	Closed reduction and ulnar gutter splint; percutaneous pinning if the fracture is excessively angulated. If skin is broken, assume infection by human oral pathogens and treat with surgical irrigation, debridement, and IV antibiotics (covering *Eikenella*).
Humerus fracture	Direct trauma. May have radial nerve palsy leading to wrist drop and loss of thumb extension.	Hanging-arm cast vs. coaptation splint and sling. Functional bracing.
"Nightstick fracture"	Ulnar shaft fracture resulting from self-defense with the arm against a blunt object.	Open reduction and internal fixation (ORIF) if significantly displaced.
Monteggia's fracture	Diaphyseal fracture of the proximal **ulna** with subluxation of the radial head.	ORIF of the shaft fracture and closed reduction of the radial head.
Galeazzi's fracture	Diaphyseal fracture of the **radius** with dislocation of the distal radioulnar joint. Results from a direct blow to the radius.	ORIF of the radius and casting of the fractured forearm in supination to reduce the distal radioulnar joint.

TABLE 2.9-1. **Common Adult Orthopedic Injuries** *(continued)*

INJURY	MECHANICS	TREATMENT
Hip fracture	↑ risk with osteoporosis. Presents with a shortened and externally rotated leg. Hip fractures can be radiographically occult, so a good clinical history with ⊖ radiographs warrants further evaluation with CT or MRI. **Displaced femoral neck fractures:** Associated with an ↑ **risk of AVN** and nonunion. Associated with DVTs.	ORIF. Displaced femoral neck fractures in elderly patients may require a hip hemiarthroplasty. Anticoagulate to ↓ the likelihood of DVTs.
Femoral fracture	Direct trauma. Beware of **fat emboli,** which present with fever, changes in mental status, dyspnea, hypoxia, petechiae, and ↓ platelets.	Intramedullary nailing of the femur. Irrigate and debride open fractures.
Tibial fracture	Direct trauma. Watch for compartment syndrome.	Casting vs. intramedullary nailing vs. ORIF.
Open fractures	**An orthopedic emergency;** patients must be taken to the OR within 8–24 hours in light of the ↑ risk of infection.	OR urgently for irrigation and debridement; repair fracture. Treat with antibiotics and tetanus prophylaxis.
Achilles tendon rupture	Presents with a sudden "pop" like a rifle shot. More likely with ↓ physical conditioning. Examination shows limited plantar flexion and a ⊕ Thompson's test (pressure on the gastrocnemius leading to absent foot plantar flexion).	Treat surgically followed by a long-leg cast for 6 weeks.
Knee injuries	Present with knee instability and hematoma. **ACL:** ▪ Result from a noncontact twisting mechanism, forced hyperextension, or impact to an extended knee. ▪ ⊕ anterior drawer and Lachman tests. ▪ Rule out a meniscal or MCL injury (MCL injury = ⊕ valgus stress test; LCL injury = ⊕ varus stress test). ▪ The "classic" **unhappy triad** of knee injury involves the ACL, the MCL, and the medial meniscus. However, **lateral** meniscal tears are more commonly seen in **acute** ACL injuries. **PCL:** ▪ Result from a posteriorly directed force on a flexed knee (eg, dashboard injury). ▪ ⊕ posterior drawer test. **Meniscal tears:** ▪ Result from an acute twisting injury or a degenerative tear in elderly patients. ▪ Clicking or locking may be present. ▪ Examination shows joint line tenderness and a ⊕ McMurray's test.	MRI is the diagnostic test of choice. Treatment of MCL/LCL and meniscal tears can be **conservative.** Treatment of ACL injuries in active patients is generally **surgical** with graft from the patellar or hamstring tendons. Operative PCL reconstruction is reserved for highly competitive athletes with high-grade injuries. Operative meniscal repair is for younger patients with reparable tears or older patients with mechanical symptoms who do not respond to conservative treatment.

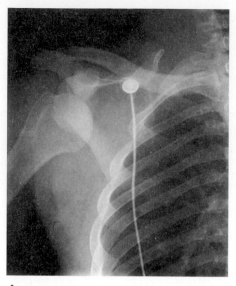
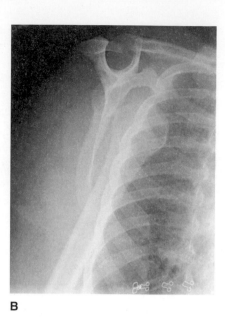

A   B

FIGURE 2.9-1. **Anterior shoulder dislocation.** AP (**A**) and scapular Y (**B**) radiographs of the right shoulder demonstrate anterior and inferior dislocation of the humeral head relative to the glenoid. (Reproduced with permission from USMLERx.com.)

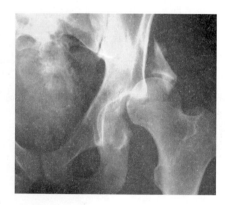

FIGURE 2.9-2. **Posterior hip dislocation.** Posterior hip dislocation with concomitant fracture of the posterior wall and dome of the acetabulum. (Reproduced with permission from Doherty GM. *Current Diagnosis & Treatment: Surgery,* 13th ed. New York: McGraw-Hill, 2010, Fig. 40-13.)

KEY FACT

Volkmann's contracture of the wrist and fingers is caused by compartment syndrome, which can be associated with supracondylar humerus fractures.

Common Peripheral Nerve Injuries

Table 2.9-2 outlines the clinical findings of the most common peripheral nerve injuries.

Compartment Syndrome

↑ **pressure** within a confined space that compromises nerve, muscle, and soft tissue perfusion. Occurs primarily in the anterior compartment of the lower leg and forearm 2° to trauma (fracture or muscle injury) to the affected limb.

HISTORY/PE

- Presents with pain out of proportion to physical findings; **pain with passive motion** of the fingers and toes; and paresthesias, pallor, poikilothermia, pulselessness, and paralysis (the **6 P's**).
- Pulselessness occurs late, so pulses are usually detectable!

DIAGNOSIS

Measure compartment pressures (positive if ≥ 30 mm Hg); measure delta pressures (diastolic pressure – compartment pressure; also ⊕ if ≤ 30 mm Hg).

TREATMENT

Immediate fasciotomy to ↓ pressures and ↑ tissue perfusion.

Carpal Tunnel Syndrome (CTS)

Entrapment of the median nerve at the wrist caused by ↓ size or space of the carpal tunnel, leading to paresthesias, pain, and occasionally paralysis. Can be precipitated by overuse of wrist flexors; associated with diabetes mellitus or thyroid dysfunction. Commonly occurs in pregnant and middle-aged women.

HISTORY/PE

- Presents with aching over the **thenar area of the hand** and proximal forearm.
- Paresthesias or numbness is seen in a median nerve distribution.
- Symptoms **worsen at night** or when the wrists are held in flexion.
- Examination shows thenar atrophy (if CTS is long-standing).
- **Phalen's maneuver** and **Tinel's sign** are ⊕.

DIAGNOSIS

A clinical diagnosis, although EMG testing can be used to confirm.

TREATMENT

- Splint the wrist in a neutral position at night and during the day if possible. Administer NSAIDs.
- Conservative treatment can include corticosteroid injection of the carpal canal.

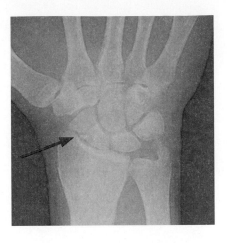

FIGURE 2.9-3. **Scaphoid fracture.** PA radiograph of the right wrist shows a fracture (arrow) through the waist of the scaphoid. (Reproduced with permission from USMLERx.com.)

TABLE 2.9-2. Common Peripheral Nerve Injuries

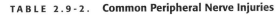

NERVE	MOTOR DEFICIT	SENSORY DEFICIT	COMMON CAUSES	CLINICAL FINDINGS
Radial	Wrist extension.	Dorsal forearm and hand (the first 3 fingers).	Humeral fracture.	**Wrist drop.**
Median	Pronation, thumb opposition.	Palmar surface (the first 3 fingers).	Carpal tunnel.	Weak wrist flexion and flat thenar eminence.
Ulnar	Finger abduction.	Palmar and dorsal surface (the last 2 fingers).	Elbow dislocation.	**Claw hand.**
Axillary	Abduction.	Lateral shoulder.	**Anterior** humeral dislocation.	—
Peroneal	Dorsiflexion, eversion.	Dorsal foot and lateral leg.	Knee dislocation.	**Foot drop.**

A 37-year-old male is seen after a motorcycle accident. He complains of intense leg pain, tingling in his foot, and inability to move his toes. Examination reveals pain with passive motion of his toes and palpable dorsalis pedis pulses. An x-ray confirms a tibial fracture. What is the best treatment?

■ Surgical release of the carpal tunnel is a widely accepted treatment, particularly for fixed sensory loss, thenar weakness, or intolerable symptoms.

COMPLICATIONS

Permanent loss of sensation, hand strength, and fine motor skills.

Bursitis

Inflammation of the bursae by **repetitive use, trauma, infection, or systemic inflammatory disease.** A bursa is a flattened sac filled with a small amount of synovial fluid that serves as a protective buffer between bones and overlapping muscles. Common sites of bursitis include subacromial, olecranon, trochanteric, prepatellar, and infrapatellar bursae.

HISTORY/PE

Presents with localized tenderness, ↓ range of motion (ROM), edema, and erythema; patients may have a history of trauma or inflammatory disease.

DIAGNOSIS

Needle aspiration is indicated if septic bursitis is suspected; no labs or imaging is needed.

TREATMENT

■ Conservative treatment includes rest, heat and ice, elevation, and NSAIDs.
■ Intrabursal corticosteroid injection can be considered but is **contraindicated if septic bursitis** is suspected.
■ Septic bursitis should be treated with 7–10 days of antibiotics.

Tendinitis

An **inflammatory condition** characterized by pain at tendinous insertions into bone associated with swelling or impaired function. It commonly occurs in the supraspinatus, **biceps,** wrist extensor, **patellar,** iliotibial band, posterior tibial, and **Achilles tendons.** Overuse is the most common cause.

HISTORY/PE

■ Presents with pain at a tendinous insertion that worsens with **repetitive stress** and **resisted strength testing** of the affected muscle group.
■ Wrist extensor tendinitis (lateral epicondylitis, or tennis elbow) worsens with resisted extension of the wrist.

DIAGNOSIS

A clinical diagnosis. Consider a radiograph if there is a history of trauma.

TREATMENT

■ Treat with rest and NSAIDs; apply ice for the first 24–48 hours.
■ Consider splinting, bracing, or immobilization.
■ Begin strengthening exercises once pain has subsided.
■ If conservative treatment fails, consider surgical debridement. **Never inject the Achilles tendon** in view of the ↑ risk of rupture. Avoid repetitive injection.

KEY FACT

Oral fluoroquinolones are associated with an ↑ risk of tendon rupture and tendinitis.

Immediate fasciotomy for compartment syndrome (within 6 hours to prevent muscle necrosis) followed by fracture stabilization. Remember that nonpalpable pulses are a late finding.

Low Back Pain (LBP)

Table 2.9-3 outlines the motor, reflex, and sensory deficits with which low back pain is associated.

HERNIATED DISK

Causes include degenerative changes, trauma, or neck/back strain or sprain. Most common (95%) in the lumbar region, especially at **L5–S1** (the most common site) and **L4–L5** (the second most common site).

HISTORY/PE

- Presents with sudden onset of severe, electricity-like LBP, usually preceded by several months of aching, "discogenic" pain.
- Common among middle-aged and older men.
- Exacerbated by ↑ intra-abdominal pressure or Valsalva (eg, coughing).
- Associated with **sciatica,** paresthesias, muscle weakness, atrophy, contractions, or spasms.
- A **passive straight-leg raise ↑ pain** (highly sensitive but not specific).
- A crossed straight-leg raise ↑ pain (highly specific but not sensitive). Large midline herniations can cause **cauda equina syndrome.**

DIAGNOSIS

- Obtain an ESR and a plain radiograph if other causes of back pain are suspected (eg, infection, trauma, compression fracture).
- Order a stat MRI for cauda equina syndrome or for a severe or rapidly progressing neurologic deficit.
- Order an MRI if symptoms are refractory to conservative management.
- X-ray may show disk herniation (see Figure 2.9-4).

TREATMENT

- **NSAIDs** in scheduled doses, physical therapy, and local heat lead to resolution within 4 weeks in 80% of cases. Do not prescribe bed rest; **continuation of regular activities** is preferred.

TABLE 2.9-3.   Motor and Sensory Deficits in Back Pain

| | ASSOCIATED DEFICIT | | |
NERVE ROOT	MOTOR	REFLEX	SENSORY
L4	Foot dorsiflexion (tibialis anterior).	Patellar.	Medial aspect of the lower leg.
L5	Big toe dorsiflexion (extensor hallucis longus), foot eversion (peroneus muscles).	None.	Dorsum of the foot and lateral aspect of the lower leg.
S1	Plantar flexion (gastrocnemius/ soleus), hip extension (gluteus maximus).	Achilles.	Plantar and lateral aspects of the foot.

KEY FACT

Most LBP is mechanical, so bed rest is contraindicated.

KEY FACT

Red flags for LBP include age > 50, > 6 weeks of pain, a previous cancer history, severe pain, constitutional symptoms, neurologic deficits, and loss of anal sphincter tone.

KEY FACT

Bowel or bladder dysfunction (urinary overflow incontinence), impotence, and saddle-area anesthesia are consistent with cauda equina syndrome, which is a surgical emergency.

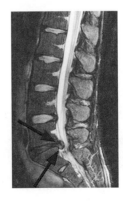

FIGURE 2.9-4.   Disk herniation.
Sagittal T2-weighted MRI of the lumbar spine shows posterior herniation of the L5–S1 disk. (Reproduced with permission from Fauci AS et al. *Harrison's Principles of Internal Medicine,* 17th ed. New York: McGraw-Hill, 2008, Fig. 16-4.)

A 55-year-old male with a history of prostate cancer presents with lower back pain and bilateral leg weakness. On examination, he is found to have point tenderness on the lumbar spine, hyperreflexia, and ↓ sensation in his legs. What is the best next step?

- Epidural injection or nerve block may be of benefit.
- Severe or rapidly evolving neurologic deficits and cauda equina syndrome are indications for surgical intervention.

SPINAL STENOSIS

Narrowing of the lumbar or cervical spinal canal, leading to compression of the nerve roots and spinal cord. Most commonly due to degenerative joint disease; typically occurs in middle-aged or elderly patients.

HISTORY/PE

- Presents with neck pain, back pain that **radiates to the arms or the buttocks and legs,** and leg numbness/weakness.
- In lumbar stenosis, leg cramping is worse with standing and with walking.
- In lumbar stenosis, symptoms **improve** with **flexion at the hips** and bending forward, which relieves pressure on the nerves.

DIAGNOSIS

- Radiographs show degenerative changes that include disk space narrowing, facet hypertrophy, and sometimes spondylolisthesis, leading to a narrowed spinal canal.
- MRI or CT shows spinal stenosis.

TREATMENT

- **Mild to moderate:** NSAIDs and abdominal muscle strengthening.
- **Advanced:** Epidural corticosteroid injections can provide relief.
- **Refractory:** Surgical laminectomy may achieve significant short-term success, but many patients will have a recurrence of symptoms.

Osteosarcoma

The second most common 1° malignant tumor of bone (after multiple myeloma). Tends to occur in the **metaphyseal** regions of the **distal femur, proximal tibia,** and proximal humerus; often metastasizes to the lungs. Risk factors include male gender and age 20–30.

HISTORY/PE

- Presents as progressive and eventually intractable **pain that worsens at night.**
- Constitutional symptoms such as fever, weight loss, and night sweats may be present.
- Erythema and enlargement over the site of the tumor may be seen.
- See the Endocrinology chapter for a discussion of osteosarcoma vs. Paget's disease.

DIAGNOSIS

- Radiographs can show **Codman's triangle** (periosteal new-bone formation at the diaphyseal end of the lesion) or a **"sunburst pattern"** of the osteosarcoma (see Figure 2.9-5)—in contrast to the multilayered **"onion skinning"** that is classic for Ewing's sarcoma and the **"soap bubble"** appearance of giant cell tumor of bone (see Figure 2.9-6).
- MRI and CT of the chest facilitate staging (soft tissue and bony invasion) and planning for surgery.

KEY FACT

The most common benign bone tumor is osteochondroma.

KEY FACT

Classic findings of **Ewing's sarcoma:** a child 10–20 years of age with a multilayered "onion-skinning" finding on x-ray in the diaphyseal regions of the femur.

KEY FACT

Classic findings of a **giant cell tumor of bone:** a female 20–40 years of age presenting with knee pain and a mass, along with a "soap bubble" appearance on x-ray in the epiphyseal/metaphyseal region of long bones.

Give steroids to relieve spinal cord compression resulting from likely bone metastasis. MRI is the best study, but preventing permanent neurologic disability is more important at this time. Remember to consider multiple myeloma, which presents almost identically.

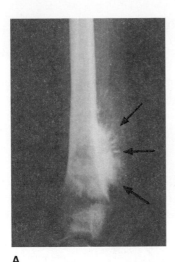
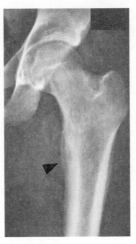

A   B

FIGURE 2.9-5.   Malignant bone tumors. (A) Osteosarcoma. Femoral radiograph shows the typical "sunburst" appearance of osteosarcoma (arrows). **(B) Ewing's sarcoma.** The characteristic "onion skinning" of Ewing's sarcoma (arrowhead) is evident in the proximal femur in this radiograph of the left hip. (Reproduced with permission from Kantarjian HM et al. *MD Anderson Manual of Medical Oncology,* 1st ed. New York: McGraw-Hill, 2006, Fig. 33-7A and B.)

TREATMENT

- Limb-sparing surgical procedures and pre- and postoperative chemotherapy (eg, methotrexate, doxorubicin, cisplatin, ifosfamide).
- Amputation may be necessary.

Septic Arthritis

An infection of the joint space that can occur after open injury or bacteremia. Prosthetic joints greatly ↑ the risk. Rheumatoid arthritis (RA) and osteoarthritis (OA) are also risk factors (see below). Bacteremia from endocarditis and IV drug use is also a major risk factor.

HISTORY/PE

Presents as a warm, red, immobile joint. Palpable effusions may also be present. Fevers and chills can be seen if the patient is bacteremic.

DIAGNOSIS

- The best test is **joint aspiration.**
- A **WBC count** > 80,000 mm³, a ⊕ Gram stain, or a ⊕ fluid culture all point to septic arthritis.
- The most common organisms are *Staphylococcus, Streptococcus,* and gram-⊖ rods.

TREATMENT

Empirically treat with **ceftriaxone and vancomycin** until cultures come back; then modify therapy for specific organisms. Septic joints are treated with surgical debridement or serial aspirations.

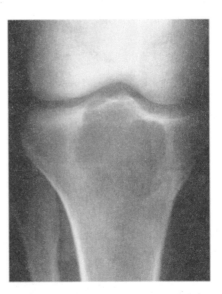

FIGURE 2.9-6.   Giant cell tumor of the bone. Note the "soap bubble" appearance at the proximal end of the tibia. The distal end of the femur (not shown) is another common location. (Reproduced with permission from Skinner HB. *Current Diagnosis & Treatment in Orthopedics,* 4th ed. New York: McGraw-Hill, 2006, Fig. 6-25.)

Osteoarthritis (OA)

A common, chronic, noninflammatory arthritis of the synovial joints. Characterized by deterioration of the articular cartilage and osteophyte bone formation at the joint surfaces. Risk factors include a ⊕ family history, **obesity**, and a **history of joint trauma.** Table 2.9-4 contrasts OA with RA.

HISTORY/PE

Presents with **crepitus**, ↓ ROM, and initially **pain that worsens with activity and weight bearing but improves with rest.** Morning stiffness generally lasts for < 30 minutes. Stiffness is also experienced after periods of rest ("gelling").

DIAGNOSIS

- Radiographs show **joint space narrowing**, osteophytes, subchondral sclerosis, and subchondral bone cysts (see Figure 2.9-7). Radiograph severity does not correlate with symptomatology.
- Synovial fluid shows straw-colored fluid, normal viscosity, and a WBC count < 2000 cells/μL.
- Laboratory tests, including inflammatory markers, are typically **normal.**

TREATMENT

- Physical therapy, **weight reduction**, and **NSAIDs.** Intra-articular corticosteroid injections may provide temporary relief.
- Consider **joint replacement** (eg, total hip/knee arthroplasty) in advanced cases.

KEY FACT

Heberden's nodes: DIP enlargement.
Bouchard's nodes: PIP enlargement.

KEY FACT

In a child with gout and inexplicable injuries, consider Lesch-Nyhan syndrome.

Gout

Recurrent attacks of **acute monoarticular arthritis** resulting from intra-articular deposition of **monosodium urate crystals** due to disorders of urate metabolism. Risk factors include male gender, obesity, postmenopausal status in females, and **binge drinking.**

TABLE 2.9-4. **Osteoarthritis vs. Rheumatoid Arthritis**

VARIABLE	OSTEOARTHRITIS	RHEUMATOID ARTHRITIS
History	Affects the elderly; has slow onset. Pain **worsens with use.**	Affects the young; presents with morning stiffness that **improves with use.**
Joint involvement	Affects the **DIP, PIP**, hips, and knees.	Affects the **wrists, MCP**, ankles, knees, shoulders, hips, and elbows. Has a **symmetrical** distribution.
Synovial fluid analysis and imaging	WBC count < 2000 cells/μL; osteophytes. Joint space narrowing is seen on x-ray.	Anti–cyclic citrullinated peptide (anti-CCP) antibodies.

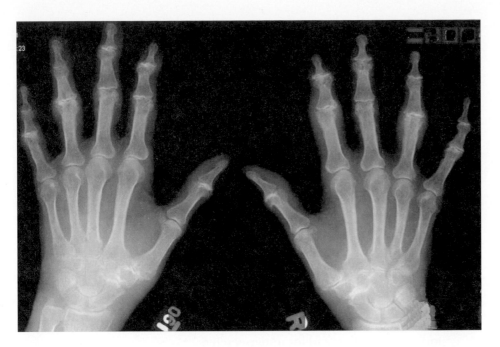

FIGURE 2.9-7.   Osteoarthritis. Plain radiographs show joint space narrowing, osteophytes, and subchondral degenerative cysts involving the DIP and PIP joints, with sparing of the MCP. (Reproduced with permission from USMLERx.com.)

HISTORY/PE

- Presents with excruciating joint pain of sudden onset.
- Most commonly affects the **first MTP joint** (podagra) and the midfoot, knees, ankles, and wrists; the hips and shoulders are generally spared.
- Joints are erythematous, swollen, and exquisitely tender.
- **Tophi** (urate crystal deposits in soft tissue) may be seen with chronic disease (see Figure 2.9-8).
- Uric acid kidney stones are seen with chronic disease.

KEY FACT

Gout crystals appear ye**LL**ow when para**LL**el to the condenser.

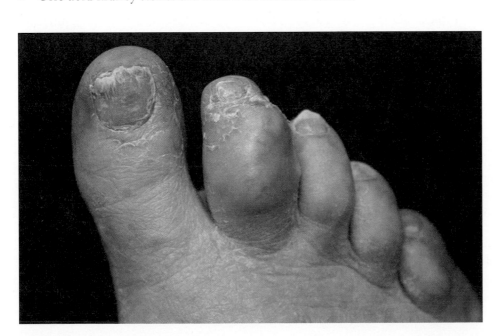

FIGURE 2.9-8.   Tophaceous gout. Note the slowly enlarging nodule of the right second toe in a 55-year-old alcoholic, hypertensive male on HCTZ. (Reproduced with permission from USMLERx. com.)

KEY FACT

Causes of hyperuricemia:

- ↑ cell turnover (hemolysis, blast crisis, tumor lysis, myelodysplasia, psoriasis)
- Cyclosporine
- Dehydration
- Diabetes insipidus
- Diet (eg, ↑ red meat, alcohol)
- Diuretics
- Lead poisoning
- Lesch-Nyhan syndrome
- Salicylates (low dose)
- Starvation

KEY FACT

Colchicine inhibits neutrophil chemotaxis and is most effective when used early during a gout flare. However, it can cause diarrhea and bone marrow suppression (neutropenia).

DIAGNOSIS

- Joint fluid aspirate shows **needle-shaped, negatively birefringent crystals** (vs. pseudogout; see Table 2.9-5).
- An elevated WBC count in the joint aspirate or peripheral blood may be seen during flares.
- Serum uric acid is usually ↑ (≥ 7.5 mg/dL), but patients may have normal levels.
- Punched-out erosions with overhanging cortical bone ("rat-bite" erosions) are seen in advanced gout.

TREATMENT

- **Acute attacks:**
  - High-dose **NSAIDs** (eg, indomethacin) are first line. Colchicine may also be used but is inferior to NSAIDs.
  - **Steroids** are used when NSAIDs are ineffective or contraindicated, as in renal disease.
- **Maintenance therapy:**
  - **Allopurinol** for overproducers, those with contraindications to probenecid treatment (tophi, renal stones, chronic kidney disease), and refractory cases; **probenecid** for undersecreters.
  - Allopurinol can ↓ the incidence of **acute urate nephropathy.**
- Weight loss and avoidance of triggers of hyperuricemia will prevent recurrent attacks in many patients. **Avoid alcohol consumption.**

Ankylosing Spondylitis

A chronic inflammatory disease of the spine and pelvis that leads to fusion of the affected joints. Strongly associated with **HLA-B27.** Risk factors include male gender and a ⊕ family history.

HISTORY/PE

- Typical onset is in the late teens and early 20s. Presents with fatigue, intermittent hip pain, and LBP that **worsens with inactivity and in the mornings.**
- ↓ spine flexion (⊕ Schober test), loss of lumbar lordosis, hip pain and stiffness, and ↓ chest expansion are seen as the disease progresses.
- Anterior **uveitis** and **heart block** may occur.

TABLE 2.9-5. Gout vs. Pseudogout

DISORDER	HISTORY	PHYSICAL FINDINGS	CRYSTAL SHAPE	CRYSTAL BIREFRINGENCE
Gout	Male, binge drinking, acute onset afterward.	The first big toe is affected.	Needle shaped.	⊖
Pseudogout (calcium pyrophosphate deposition disease [CPPD])	Hemochromatosis or hyperparathyroidism.	The wrists and knees are affected.	Rhomboid.	⊕

- Other forms of seronegative spondyloarthropathy must be ruled out, including the following:
    - **Reactive arthritis** (formerly known as **Reiter's syndrome**): A disease of young men. The characteristic arthritis, uveitis, conjunctivitis, and urethritis usually follow an infection with *Campylobacter*, *Shigella*, *Salmonella*, *Chlamydia*, or *Ureaplasma*.
    - **Psoriatic arthritis:** An oligoarthritis that can include the **DIP joints.** Associated with psoriatic skin changes and **sausage-shaped digits** (dactylitis). X-rays show a classic "pencil in cup" deformity.
    - **Enteropathic spondylitis:** An ankylosing spondylitis–like disease characterized by sacroiliitis that is usually asymmetric and is associated with IBD.

DIAGNOSIS

- $\oplus$ HLA-B27 is found in 85–95% of cases.
- Radiographs may show **fused sacroiliac joints,** squaring of the lumbar vertebrae, development of vertical syndesmophytes, and **bamboo spine** (see Figure 2.9-9).
- ESR or CRP is ↑ in 75% of cases.
- $\ominus$ **RF;** $\ominus$ ANA.

TREATMENT

- **NSAIDs** (eg, indomethacin) for pain; exercise to improve posture and breathing.
- **Tumor necrosis factor (TNF) inhibitors** or sulfasalazine can be used in refractory cases.

Polymyositis and Dermatomyositis

Polymyositis is a progressive, systemic connective tissue disease characterized by immune-mediated striated muscle inflammation. **Dermatomyositis** presents with symptoms of polymyositis plus cutaneous involvement, although the pathogenesis is different. Most often affect patients 50–70 years of age; the male-to-female ratio is 1:2. African Americans are affected more often than Caucasians.

HISTORY/PE

- Distinguished as follows:
    - **Polymyositis:** Presents with **symmetric,** progressive **proximal** muscle weakness, pain, and difficulty breathing or swallowing (advanced disease).
    - **Dermatomyositis:** Patients may have a **heliotrope rash** (a violaceous periorbital rash), **"shawl sign"** (a rash involving the shoulders, upper chest, and back), and/or **Gottron's papules** (a papular rash with scales located on the dorsa of the hands, over bony prominences).
- Patients may also develop myocarditis and cardiac conduction deficits.
- Can be associated with an underlying malignancy, especially lung and breast carcinoma.

DIAGNOSIS

- ↑ **serum CK and anti-Jo-1 antibodies** are seen (see Table 2.9-6).
- **Muscle biopsy** reveals inflammation and muscle fibers in varying stages of necrosis and regeneration.

KEY FACT

Reactive arthritis: "Can't see (uveitis), can't pee (urethritis), can't climb a tree (arthritis)."

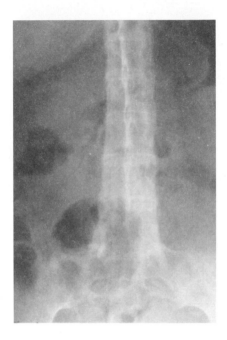

FIGURE 2.9-9. **Ankylosing spondylitis.** Frontal view of the thoracolumbar spine shows the classic "bamboo" appearance of the spine, which results from fusion of the vertebral bodies and posterior elements. (Reproduced with permission from Chen MY et al. *Basic Radiology,* 2nd ed. New York: McGraw-Hill, 2011, Fig. 7-45.)

Q

A 49-year-old male presents with a painful, swollen big toe after a night of heavy drinking. His home medications are lansoprazole, ASA, sildenafil, and psyllium. Which medication should he temporarily discontinue?

TABLE 2.9-6. **Common Antibodies and Their Disease Associations**

ANTIBODY	DISEASE ASSOCIATION
ANA	SLE
Anti-CCP	RA
Anticentromere	CREST syndrome
Anti-dsDNA	SLE
Antihistone	Drug-induced SLE
Anti-Jo-1	Polymyositis/dermatomyositis
Antimitochondrial	Primary biliary cirrhosis
Antinuclear	Scleroderma
Anti-Scl-70	Scleroderma
Anti-Sm	SLE
Anti–smooth muscle	Autoimmune hepatitis
Antitopoisomerase I	Scleroderma
Anti-TSHR	Graves' disease
c-ANCA	Vasculitis, especially Wegener's
p-ANCA	Vasculitis, microscopic polyangiitis
Rheumatoid factor	RA
U1RNP antibody	Mixed connective tissue disease

TREATMENT

- High-dose corticosteroids with taper after 4–6 weeks to ↓ the maintenance dose.
- Azathioprine and/or methotrexate can be used as steroid-sparing agents.

Rheumatoid Arthritis (RA)

A systemic autoimmune disorder characterized by chronic, destructive, inflammatory arthritis with **symmetric** joint involvement that results in synovial hypertrophy and pannus formation, ultimately leading to erosion of adjacent cartilage, bone, and tendons. Risk factors include female gender, age 35–50, and **HLA-DR4.**

ASA (aspirin). This patient is having an acute gout attack, and ASA can cause ↓ excretion of uric acid by the kidney.

HISTORY/PE

- Presents with insidious onset of **morning stiffness** for > 1 hour along with painful, warm swelling of multiple symmetric joints (**wrists, MCP joints,** ankles, knees, shoulders, hips, and elbows) for > 6 weeks.
- Fever, fatigue, malaise, anorexia, and weight loss may also be seen.
- In late cases, ulnar deviation of the fingers is seen with MCP joint hypertrophy (see Figure 2.9-10A).
- Also presents with ligament and tendon **deformations** (eg, swan-neck and boutonnière deformities), vasculitis, atlantoaxial subluxation (intubation risk), and keratoconjunctivitis sicca.

DIAGNOSIS

- **Labs:**
    - ↑ **RF** (IgM antibodies against Fc IgG) is seen in > 75% of cases.
    - The presence of **anti-CCP** antibodies is more specific than RF.
    - ↑ ESR may also be seen.
    - Anemia of chronic disease is common.
    - Synovial fluid aspirate shows turbid fluid, ↓ viscosity, and an ↑ WBC count (3000–50,000 cells/µL).
- **Radiographs:**
    - **Early:** Soft tissue swelling and juxta-articular demineralization.
    - **Late:** Symmetrical joint space narrowing and erosions (see Figure 2.9-10B).

TREATMENT

- **NSAIDs** (can be ↓ or discontinued following successful treatment with **disease-modifying antirheumatic drugs [DMARDs]**).
- DMARDs should be started early and include **methotrexate** (the best initial DMARD to start with), hydroxychloroquine, and sulfasalazine. Second-line agents include TNF inhibitors, rituximab (anti-CD20), and leflunomide.

 KEY FACT

Keratoconjunctivitis sicca 2° to Sjögren's syndrome is a common ocular manifestation of RA.

 KEY FACT

Felty's syndrome is characterized by RA, splenomegaly, and neutropenia.

 KEY FACT

The DIP joint is spared in RA but is involved in OA.

 KEY FACT

Hydroxychloroquine causes retinal toxicity.

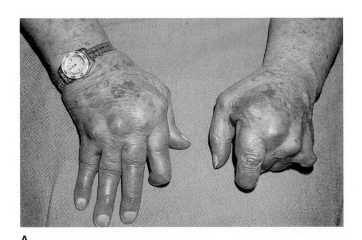

A

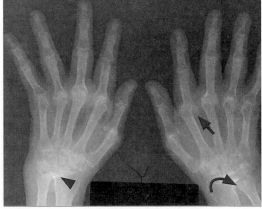

B

FIGURE 2.9-10. **Rheumatoid arthritis.** (A) Note the typical ulnar deviation of the MCP joints and swelling of the MCP and PIP joints. Multiple subcutaneous rheumatoid nodules are also seen. (B) Hand radiograph shows symmetric erosions and joint space narrowing involving the MCP (arrow), carpal (arrowhead), and radioulnar (curved arrow) joints. Ulnar deviation at the MCP joint is also noted. (Image A reproduced with permission from Wolff K et al. *Fitzpatrick's Dermatology in General Medicine,* 7th ed. New York: McGraw-Hill, 2008, Fig. 161-1A. Image B reproduced with permission from USMLERx.com.)

MNEMONIC

CREST syndrome:

Calcinosis
Raynaud's phenomenon
Esophageal dysmotility
Sclerodactyly
Telangiectasias

Scleroderma

Also called systemic sclerosis; characterized by inflammation that leads to progressive tissue fibrosis through excessive deposition of type I and type III collagen. Commonly manifests as **CREST syndrome** (limited form), but can also occur in a diffuse form involving the skin as well as the GI, GU, renal, pulmonary, and cardiovascular systems. Risk factors include female gender and age 35–50.

HISTORY/PE

- Examination may reveal symmetric thickening of the skin of face and/or distal extremities.
- **CREST syndrome** involves Calcinosis, Raynaud's phenomenon, Esophageal dysmotility, Sclerodactyly, and Telangiectasias.
- The diffuse form can lead to **pulmonary fibrosis,** cor pulmonale, acute renal failure, and malignant hypertension.

DIAGNOSIS

- RF and ANA may be ⊕.
- **Anticentromere antibodies** are specific for CREST syndrome (see Table 2.9-6).
- **Anti-Scl-70** (antitopoisomerase 1) **antibodies** are associated with diffuse disease and a poor prognosis (see Table 2.9-6).
- Eosinophilia may be seen.

TREATMENT

- Corticosteroids for acute flares; penicillamine can be used for skin changes.
- **Calcium channel blockers** for Raynaud's phenomenon.
- ACEIs for renal disease and for prevention of a scleroderma renal crisis.

COMPLICATIONS

Mortality is due to pulmonary hypertension and complications of pulmonary hypertension.

MNEMONIC

Criteria for SLE—

DOPAMINE RASH

Discoid rash
Oral ulcers
Photosensitivity
Arthritis
Malar rash
Immunologic criteria
Neurologic symptoms (lupus cerebritis, seizures)
Elevated ESR
Renal disease
ANA ⊕
Serositis (pleural or pericardial effusion)
Hematologic abnormalities

Systemic Lupus Erythematosus (SLE)

A multisystem autoimmune disorder related to antibody-mediated cellular attack and deposition of antigen-antibody complexes. African American women are at highest risk. Usually affects women of childbearing age.

HISTORY/PE

- Presents with nonspecific symptoms such as fever, anorexia, weight loss, and symmetric joint pain.
- The mnemonic **DOPAMINE RASH** summarizes the criteria for diagnosing SLE (see also Figure 2.9-11). Patients with 4 of the criteria are likely to have SLE (96% sensitive and specific).

DIAGNOSIS

- A ⊕ ANA is highly sensitive but not specific. **Anti-dsDNA** and **anti-Sm antibodies** are highly specific but not as sensitive (see Table 2.9-6).

- **Drug-induced SLE:** ⊕ antihistone antibodies are seen **in 100% of cases** but are nonspecific.
- **Neonatal SLE:** Associated with ⊕ anti-Ro antibodies transmitted from mother to neonate.
- The following may also be seen:
  - Antiphospholipid antibodies.
  - Anemia, leukopenia, and/or thrombocytopenia.
  - Proteinuria and/or casts.

TREATMENT

- **NSAIDs** for mild joint symptoms.
- **Corticosteroids** for **acute exacerbations.**
- Corticosteroids, hydroxychloroquine, cyclophosphamide, and azathioprine can be used for progressive or refractory cases. A few have specific uses:
  - **Hydroxychloroquine:** Can be used for isolated skin and joint involvement.
  - **Cyclophosphamide:** Used for severe cases of lupus nephritis. Be sure to get a renal biopsy for patients with nephritic symptoms!

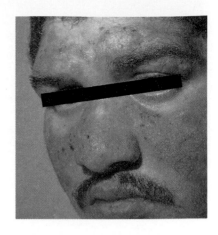

FIGURE 2.9-11. SLE. The malar rash of SLE is a red-to-purple, continuous plaque extending across the bridge of the nose and to both cheeks. (Reproduced with permission from Bondi EE. *Dermatology: Diagnosis and Therapy,* 1st ed. Stamford, CT: Appleton & Lange, 1991: 395.)

Temporal Arteritis

Also called giant cell arteritis; due to subacute granulomatous inflammation of the large vessels, including the aorta, external carotid (especially the **temporal** branch), and vertebral arteries. The most feared manifestation is **blindness** 2° to occlusion of the **central retinal artery** (a branch of the internal carotid artery). Risk factors include polymyalgia rheumatica (affects almost half of patients), age > 50, and female gender.

HISTORY/PE

- Presents with new headache (unilateral or bilateral); scalp pain and **temporal tenderness;** and **jaw claudication.**
- Fever, permanent **monocular blindness,** weight loss, and myalgias/arthralgias (especially of the shoulders and hips) are also seen.

DIAGNOSIS

- **ESR > 50** (usually > 100) mm/hr.
- Ophthalmologic evaluation.
- **Temporal artery biopsy:** Look for thrombosis; necrosis of the media; and lymphocytes, plasma cells, and giant cells.

TREATMENT

- Begin **high-dose prednisone** immediately to prevent ocular involvement (or involvement of the remaining eye after onset of monocular blindness).
- Obtain a biopsy, but do not delay treatment. Conduct a follow-up eye exam.

Complex Regional Pain Syndrome

A **pain syndrome** accompanied by **loss of function and autonomic dysfunction,** usually occurring after trauma. The disease has 3 phases: acute/traumatic → dystrophic phase → atrophic phase.

KEY FACT

Libman-Sacks endocarditis: Noninfectious vegetations often seen on the mitral valve in association with SLE and antiphospholipid syndrome.

KEY FACT

SLE can cause a ⊕ VDRL or RPR test!

KEY FACT

SLE and RA both affect the MCP and PIP joints; the difference is that SLE is nondeforming.

HISTORY/PE

- **Diffuse pain occurs** out of proportion to the initial injury, often in a **non-anatomic** distribution.
- Pain can occur at any time relative to the initial injury.
- **Loss of function** of the affected limb is seen.
- **Sympathetic dysfunction** occurs and may be documented by skin, soft tissue, or blood flow changes.
- Skin temperature, hair growth, and nail growth may ↑ or ↓. Edema may be present.

DIAGNOSIS

A clinical diagnosis, but objective evidence of changes in skin temperature, hair growth, or nail growth may be present.

TREATMENT

- Medications include NSAIDs, corticosteroids, low-dose TCAs, gabapentin, pregabalin, and calcitonin (no oral medications are consistently effective).
- Physical therapy modalities may be helpful.
- **Chemical sympathetic blockade** may relieve symptoms.
- Referral to a chronic pain specialist is appropriate for complicated cases.

Fibromyalgia

- A chronic pain disorder characterized by soft tissue and axial skeletal pain in the absence of joint pain. Inflammation is notably absent (see Table 2.9-7).
- **Hx/PE:** Most common in **women 30–50 years of age**; associated with depression, anxiety, sleep disorders, IBS, and cognitive disorders ("fibro fog").
- **Dx:** Multiple (≥ 11 of 18) tender points over all 4 body quadrants and the axial skeleton must be present for diagnosis. The presence of < 11 of 18 tender points or non-fibromyalgia-associated tender points is known as **myofascial pain syndrome.**

TABLE 2.9-7. Fibromyalgia vs. Polymyalgia Rheumatica

CHARACTERISTIC	FIBROMYALGIA	POLYMYALGIA RHEUMATICA
Age and sex	Middle-aged women (30–50 years of age).	Women > 50 years of age.
Location	Various.	Shoulder and pelvic girdle.
ESR	Normal.	Markedly ↑ (> 100 mm/hr).
Muscle biopsy	Normal.	Normal.
Classic findings	Anxiety, stress, point tenderness, ⊖ workup.	Temporal arteritis; response to steroids.
Treatment	Antidepressants, NSAIDs, rest.	Low-dose prednisone.

■ **Tx: Antidepressants** (an SSRI/TCA combination and 2 SNRIs have proven efficacy), gabapentin, pregabalin, muscle relaxants, and **physical therapy** (stretching, heat application, hydrotherapy). Avoid narcotics.

Polymyalgia Rheumatica

■ Risk factors include female gender and age > 50 (see Table 2.9-7).
■ **Hx/PE:**
  ■ Presents with pain and stiffness of **the shoulder and pelvic girdle** musculature with difficulty getting out of a chair or lifting the arms above the head.
  ■ Other symptoms include **fever,** malaise, and weight loss. Weakness is generally not appreciated on exam.
■ **Dx:** Labs reveal a markedly ↑ **ESR, often associated with anemia.**
■ **Tx: Low-dose prednisone** (10–20 mg/day).

Pediatric Musculoskeletal Disorders

COMMON PEDIATRIC ORTHOPEDIC INJURIES

Table 2.9-8 outlines the presentation and treatment of common pediatric orthopedic injuries.

DUCHENNE MUSCULAR DYSTROPHY (DMD)

An **X-linked recessive disorder** resulting from a deficiency of **dystrophin,** a cytoskeletal protein. Onset is usually at 3–5 years of age.

HISTORY/PE

■ Affects axial and proximal muscles more than distal muscles.
■ May present with progressive **clumsiness, fatigability,** difficulty standing or walking, difficulty walking on toes (gastrocnemius shortening), **Gowers' maneuver** (using the hands to push off the thighs when rising from the floor), and waddling gait.
■ **Pseudohypertrophy of the gastrocnemius muscles** is also seen.
■ Mental retardation is common.
■ Table 2.9-9 outlines the differential diagnosis of DMD and Becker muscular dystrophy.

DIAGNOSIS

■ ⊖ **dystrophin immunostain;** ↑ CK.
■ EMG shows polyphasic potentials and ↑ recruitment.
■ **Muscle biopsy** shows necrotic muscle fibers from degeneration and variation in fiber size with fibrosis from regeneration.

TREATMENT

Physical therapy is necessary to maintain ambulation and to prevent contractures. Liberal use of tendon release surgery may prolong ambulation.

TABLE 2.9-8. Orthopedic Injuries in Children

INJURY	MECHANICS	TREATMENT
Clavicular fracture	The most commonly fractured long bone in children. May be birth related (especially in large infants); can be associated with brachial nerve palsies. Usually involves the middle third of the clavicle, with the proximal fracture end displaced superiorly owing to the pull of the sternocleidomastoid.	Figure-of-eight sling vs. arm sling.
Greenstick fracture	Incomplete fracture involving the cortex of only 1 side (tension side) of the bone.	Reduction with casting. Order films at 10–14 days.
Nursemaid's elbow	Radial head subluxation that typically occurs as a result of being pulled or lifted by the hand. Presents with pain and refusal to bend the elbow.	Manual reduction by gentle supination of the elbow at 90 degrees of flexion. No immobilization.
Torus fracture	Buckling of the compression side of the cortex of a long bone 2° to trauma. Usually occurs in the distal radius or ulna.	Cast immobilization for 3–5 weeks.
Supracondylar humerus fracture	**The most common pediatric elbow fracture.** Tends to occur at 5–8 years of age. Proximity to the brachial artery ↑ the risk of Volkmann's contracture (results from compartment syndrome of the forearm). Beware of **brachial artery entrapment** (remember to do a radial artery pulse test). See Figure 2.9-12.	Cast immobilization; closed reduction with percutaneous pinning if significantly displaced.
Osgood-Schlatter disease	Overuse apophysitis of the tibial tubercle. Causes localized pain, especially with quadriceps contraction, in active young boys.	↓ activity for 2–3 months or until asymptomatic. A neoprene brace may provide symptomatic relief.
Salter-Harris fracture 	Fractures of the growth plate in children. Classified by fracture pattern: ■ **I:** Physis (growth plate). ■ **II:** Metaphysis and physis. ■ **III:** Epiphysis and physis. ■ **IV:** Epiphysis, metaphysis, and physis. ■ **V:** Crush injury of the physis.	Closed vs. open reduction to obtain appropriate alignment, followed by immobilization.

COMPLICATIONS

Mortality is due to pulmonary congestion caused by high-output cardiac failure (stemming from cardiac fibrosis).

DEVELOPMENTAL DYSPLASIA OF THE HIP

Also called congenital hip dislocation; can result in subluxed or dislocated femoral heads, leading to early degenerative joint disease of the hips. Dislocations result from poor development of the hip due to lax musculature and from **excessive uterine packing** in the flexed and adducted position (eg,

TABLE 2.9-9. **DMD vs. Becker Muscular Dystrophy**

VARIABLE	DMD	BECKER MUSCULAR DYSTROPHY
Onset	3–5 years.	5–15 years and beyond.
Life expectancy	Teens.	30s–40s.
Mental retardation	Common.	Uncommon.
Western blot	Dystrophin is markedly ↓ or absent.	Dystrophin levels are normal, but protein is abnormal.

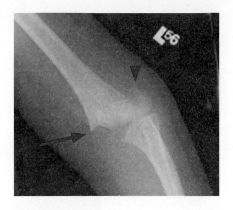

FIGURE 2.9-12. Supracondylar humerus fracture. Radiograph of the left elbow shows a medial supracondylar humerus fracture (arrow) with displacement of the distal fracture fragment (arrowhead) following trauma in a 9-year-old boy. (Reproduced with permission from USMLERx. com.)

breech presentation), leading to excessive stretching of the posterior hip capsule and contractures.

HISTORY/PE

- Most commonly found in **first-born females** born in the **breech position.**
- **Barlow's maneuver:** Posterior pressure is placed on the inner aspect of the abducted thigh, and the hip is then adducted, leading to an audible "clunk" as the femoral head dislocates posteriorly.
- **Ortolani's maneuver:** The thighs are gently abducted from the midline with anterior pressure on the greater trochanter. A **soft click** signifies reduction of the femoral head into the acetabulum.
- **Allis' (Galeazzi's) sign:** The knees are at unequal heights when the hips and knees are flexed (the dislocated side is lower).
- **Asymmetric skin folds** and limited abduction of the affected hip are also seen.

DIAGNOSIS

- **Early detection is critical** to allow for proper hip development.
- Ultrasound may be helpful, especially after 10 weeks of age.
- Radiographs are unreliable until patients are > 4 months of age because of the lack of ossification of the neonatal femoral head.

TREATMENT

- Begin treatment early.
- **< 6 months:** Splint with a **Pavlik harness** (maintains the hip flexed and abducted). To prevent AVN, do not flex the hips > 60 degrees.
- **6–15 months:** Spica cast.
- **15–24 months:** Open reduction followed by spica cast.

COMPLICATIONS

- Joint contractures and AVN of the femoral head.
- Without treatment, a significant defect is likely in patients < 2 years of age.

LEGG-CALVÉ-PERTHES DISEASE

Idiopathic AVN of the femoral head (see Figure 2.9-13). Most commonly found in boys 4–10 years of age. Usually a self-limited disease, with symptoms lasting < 18 months.

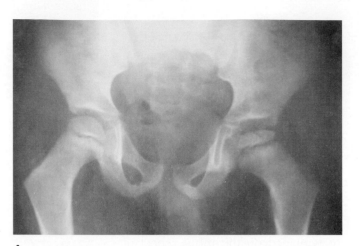

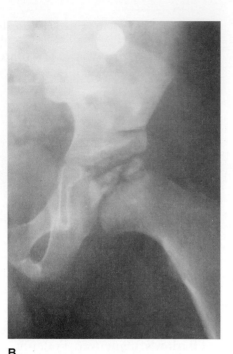

A   **B**

F I G U R E   2 . 9 - 1 3 .   **Legg-Calvé-Perthes disease.** AVN of the femoral head. (Reproduced with permission from Skinner HB. *Current Diagnosis & Treatment in Orthopedics,* 2nd ed. Stamford, CT: Appleton & Lange, 2000: 543.)

MNEMONIC

Differential diagnosis of pediatric limp—

STARTSS HOTT

Septic joint
Tumor
Avascular necrosis (Legg-Calvé-Perthes)
Rheumatoid arthritis/JIA
Tuberculosis
Sickle cell disease
SCFE
Henoch-Schönlein purpura
Osteomyelitis
Trauma
Toxic synovitis

HISTORY/PE

- Generally asymptomatic at first, but patients can develop a painless limp.
- If pain is present, it can be in the groin or anterior thigh, or it may be referred to the knee.
- **Limited abduction and internal rotation;** atrophy of the affected leg.
- Usually unilateral (85–90%).

TREATMENT

- **Observation** is sufficient if there is limited femoral head involvement or if full ROM is present.
- If extensive or if there is ↓ ROM, consider bracing, hip abduction with a Petrie cast, or an osteotomy.
- The prognosis is good if the patient is < 6 years of age and has full ROM, ↓ femoral head involvement, and a stable joint.

SLIPPED CAPITAL FEMORAL EPIPHYSIS (SCFE)

Separation of the proximal femoral epiphysis through the growth plate, leading to inferior and posterior displacement of the femoral head relative to the femoral neck. The name is misleading because the epiphysis remains within the acetabulum while the metaphysis moves anteriorly and superiorly. Risk factors include obesity, age 11–13, male gender, and African American ethnicity. Associated with hypothyroidism and other endocrinopathies.

HISTORY/PE

- Typically presents with acute or insidious **groin** or **knee pain** and a **painful limp.**
- Acute cases present with restricted ROM and, commonly, **inability to bear weight.**
- **Inability to bear weight differentiates unstable from stable SCFE.**

- Bilateral in 40–50% of cases.
- Characterized by limited internal rotation and abduction of the hip. Flexion of the hip results in an obligatory external rotation 2° to physical displacement that is observed as further loss of internal rotation with hip flexion.

DIAGNOSIS

- Radiographs of **both** hips in **AP and frog-leg lateral views** reveal **posterior and inferior displacement** of the femoral head (see Figure 2.9-14).
- In patients under the 10th percentile of height, rule out hypothyroidism with TSH.

TREATMENT

- The disease is progressive, so treatment should begin promptly.
- **No weight bearing** should be allowed until the defect is surgically stabilized.
- Percutaneous single-screw fixation is the most common treatment for stable SCFE.

COMPLICATIONS

Chondrolysis, AVN of the femoral head, and premature hip osteoarthritis leading to hip arthroplasty.

SCOLIOSIS

A **lateral curvature of the spine** > 10 degrees. It is sometimes associated with kyphosis or lordosis. **Most commonly idiopathic,** developing in early adolescence. Other etiologies are congenital or associated with neuromuscular, ver-

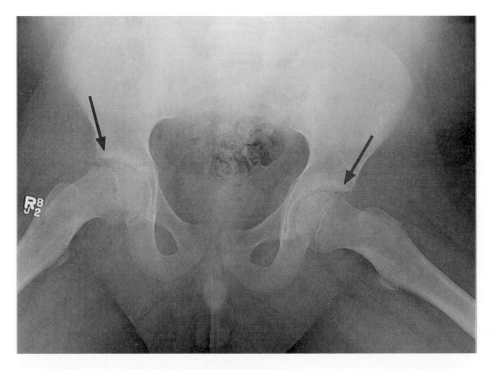

FIGURE 2.9-14. **Slipped capital femoral epiphysis.** Frog-leg AP radiograph demonstrates medial and inferior displacement of the right femoral epiphysis (red arrow) relative to the femoral neck. In comparison, the left side (blue arrow) is normal. (Reproduced with permission from USMLERx.com.)

tebral, or spinal cord disease. The male-to-female ratio is 1:7 for curves that progress and require treatment.

HISTORY/PE

- Idiopathic disease is usually identified during school physical screening.
- Vertebral and rib rotation deformities are accentuated by the Adams forward bending test.

DIAGNOSIS

Radiographs of the spine (posterior, anterior, and full-length views).

TREATMENT

- Close observation for < 20 degrees of curvature.
- Spinal bracing for 20–49 degrees of curvature in patients with remaining growth. **Curvature may progress even with bracing.**
- Surgical correction for > 50 degrees of curvature.

COMPLICATIONS

Severe scoliosis can create restrictive lung disease.

JUVENILE IDIOPATHIC ARTHRITIS (JIA)

A nonmigratory, nonsuppurative mono- and polyarthritis with bony destruction that occurs in patients ≤ 16 years of age and lasts > 6 weeks. Formerly known as juvenile rheumatoid arthritis. Approximately 95% of cases resolve by puberty. More common in girls than in boys.

HISTORY/PE

- Can be accompanied by **fever, nodules, erythematous rashes, pericarditis,** and **fatigue.**
- Subtypes are as follows:
  - **Pauciarticular:** An asymmetric arthritis that involves < 4 joints. Associated with an ↑ risk of **iridocyclitis** that leads to blindness if left untreated.
  - **Polyarticular:** Resembles RA with symmetric involvement of multiple (5 or more) small joints. Systemic features are less prominent; carries a ↓ risk of iridocyclitis.
  - **Acute febrile (systemic, Still's disease):** The least common subtype; manifests as arthritis with **daily high, spiking fevers** and a maculopapular, **evanescent, salmon-colored rash.** Hepatosplenomegaly and serositis may also be seen. No iridocyclitis is present; remission may occur within 1 year. Occurs equally in girls and boys.

DIAGNOSIS

- There is **no diagnostic test for JIA.**
- **Labs:**
  - A ⊕ RF is found in 15% of cases.
  - ANA may be ⊕, especially in the pauciarticular subtype.
  - ↑ ESR, WBC count, and platelets.
- **Imaging:** Soft tissue swelling and osteoporosis may be seen.

TREATMENT

NSAIDs or corticosteroids; methotrexate is second-line therapy.

NEUROLOGY

Clinical Neuroanatomy

Tables 2.10-1 through 2.10-4 and Figure 2.10-1 outline critical aspects of clinical neuroanatomy, including cranial nerve functions; the clinical presentation of common facial nerve lesions; spinal cord anatomy and functions; and pertinent clinical reflexes.

TABLE 2.10-1. **Cranial Nerve Functions**

NERVE	CN	FUNCTION	TYPE	MNEMONIC
Olfactory	I	Smell	Sensory	Some
Optic	II	Sight	Sensory	Say
Oculomotor	III	Eye movement, pupillary constriction, lens accommodation, eyelid opening	Motor	Marry
Trochlear	IV	Eye movement	Motor	Money
Trigeminal	V	Mastication, facial sensation (including orbits, sinuses, tongue, teeth, and buccal mucosa), intracranial sensation (including meninges and blood vessels)	Both	But
Abducens	VI	Eye movement	Motor	My
Facial	VII	Facial movement, taste from the anterior two-thirds of the tongue, lacrimation, salivation (submandibular and sublingual glands), eyelid closing	Both	Brother
Vestibulocochlear	VIII	Hearing, balance	Sensory	Says
Glossopharyngeal	IX	Taste from the posterior third of the tongue, oropharyngeal sensation, swallowing (stylopharyngeus), salivation (parotid gland), monitoring carotid body and sinus chemo- and baroreceptors, gag reflex	Both	Big
Vagus	X	Taste from the epiglottic region, swallowing, palatal elevation, talking, thoracoabdominal viscera, monitoring aortic arch chemo- and baroreceptors	Both	Brains
Accessory	XI	Head turning, shoulder shrugging	Motor	Matter
Hypoglossal	XII	Tongue movement	Motor	Most

(Adapted with permission from Le T et al. *First Aid for the USMLE Step 1 2011*. New York: McGraw-Hill, 2011: 416.)

TABLE 2.10-2. Facial Nerve Lesions

Type	Description	Comments
UMN lesion	Lesion of the motor cortex or the connection between the cortex and the facial nucleus. Contralateral paralysis of the lower face only.	**AL**exander **Bell** with **STD**: **A**IDS, **L**yme, **S**arcoid, **T**umors, **D**iabetes.
LMN lesion	Ipsilateral paralysis of the upper and lower face.	
Bell's palsy	Complete destruction of the facial nucleus itself or its branchial efferent fibers (facial nerve proper). Peripheral ipsilateral facial paralysis with inability to close the eye on the involved side. Can occur idiopathically; gradual recovery is seen in most cases. Seen as a complication in **A**IDS, **L**yme disease, **S**arcoidosis, **T**umors, and **D**iabetes.	

(Adapted with permission from Le T et al. *First Aid for the USMLE Step 1 2011.* New York: McGraw-Hill, 2011: 419.)

Vascular Disorders

STROKE

Acute onset of focal neurologic deficits resulting from disruption of cerebral circulation. Many classifications exist, but the most common comparison involves ischemic (80%) and hemorrhagic (20%). Table 2.10-5 contrasts modifiable and nonmodifiable risk factors associated with stroke. Etiologies are as follows:

 KEY FACT

Stroke is the third most common cause of death and the leading cause of major disability in the United States.

TABLE 2.10-3. Spinal Tract Functions

Tract	Function	Decussation	Origin
Lateral corticospinal	Movement of contralateral limbs.	Pyramidal, at the cervicomedullary junction.	1° motor cortex.
Dorsal column medial lemniscus	Fine touch, vibration, conscious proprioception.	Arcuate fibers at the medulla.	Pacini's and Meissner's tactile disks, muscle spindles, and Golgi tendon organs.
Spinothalamic	Pain, temperature.	Ventral white commissure at the spinal cord level.	Free nerve endings, pain fibers.

TABLE 2.10-4. **Clinical Reflexes**

DISTRIBUTION	LOCATION	COMMENTS
	Biceps = C5 nerve root.	Reflexes count up in order.
	Triceps = C7 nerve root.	S1, 2
C5, 6	Patella = L4 nerve root.	L3, 4
C7, 8	Achilles = S1 nerve root.	C5, 6
	Babinski—dorsiflexion of the big toe	C7, 8
L3, 4	and fanning of other toes; sign of	
S1, 2	UMN lesion, but normal reflex in	
	the first year of life.	

(Adapted with permission from Le T et al. *First Aid for the USMLE Step 1 2011.* New York: McGraw-Hill, 2011: 414.)

- **Atherosclerosis** of the extracranial vessels (internal/common carotid, basilar, and vertebral arteries).
- **Lacunar infarcts** in regions supplied by perforating vessels (result from chronic hypertension, hypercholesterolemia, or diabetes).
- **Cardiac or aortic emboli:**
  - **Thromboemboli:** Atrial fibrillation (AF), ventricular hypokinesis, prosthetic valves, marantic endocarditis.
  - **Atheroemboli:** Aortic arch atherosclerosis.

Poliomyelitis and Werdnig-Hoffmann disease: lower motor neuron lesions only, due to destruction of anterior horns; flaccid paralysis

Multiple sclerosis: mostly white matter of cervical region; random and asymmetric lesions, due to demyelination; scanning speech, intention tremor, nystagmus

ALS: combined upper and lower motor neuron deficits with no sensory deficit; both upper and lower motor neuron signs

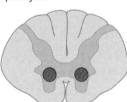 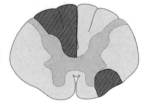 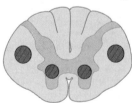

Complete occlusion of anterior spinal artery; spares dorsal columns and tract of Lissauer

Tabes dorsalis (3° syphilis): degeneration of dorsal roots and dorsal columns; impaired proprioception, locomotor ataxia

Syringomyelia: crossing fibers of spinothalamic tract damaged; bilateral loss of pain and temperature sensation

Vitamin B$_{12}$ neuropathy and Friedreich´s ataxia: demyelination of dorsal columns, lateral corticospinal tracts, and spinocerebellar tracts; ataxic gait, hyperreflexia, impaired position and vibration sense

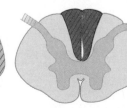 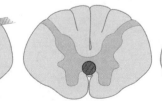 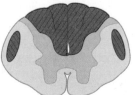

FIGURE 2.10-1. **Spinal cord lesions.** (Reproduced with permission from Le T et al. *First Aid for the USMLE Step 1 2009.* New York: McGraw-Hill, 2009: 389.)

TABLE 2.10-5.   Modifiable and Nonmodifiable Risk Factors for Stroke

MODIFIABLE RISK FACTORS	NONMODIFIABLE RISK FACTORS
"Live the way a **COACH SH**oul**DD**":	**FAME:**
CAD	**F**amily history of MI or stroke
Obesity	**A**ge > 60
Atrial fibrillation	**M**ale gender
Carotid stenosis	**E**thnicity (African American, Hispanic, Asian)
Hypercholesterolemia	
Smoking	
Hypertension	
Diabetes	
Drug use (cocaine, IV drugs)	

- **Infectious emboli:** Bacterial endocarditis.
- **Paradoxical emboli:** Via patent foramen ovale.
- **Hypercoagulable states:** Include those associated with antiphospholipid antibodies, activated protein C resistance, malignancy, and OCPs in the context of smoking.
- **Craniocervical dissection:** Trauma, fibromuscular dysplasia (young females), inflammatory/infectious diseases.
- **Other causes:** Venous sinus thrombosis, sickle cell anemia, vasculitis (eg, giant cell arteritis).

HISTORY/PE

Symptoms are dependent on the vascular territory affected:

- **Middle cerebral artery (MCA):** Aphasia (dominant hemisphere), neglect (nondominant hemisphere), contralateral paresis and sensory loss in the face and arm, gaze preference toward the side of the lesion, homonymous hemianopsia.
- **Anterior cerebral artery (ACA):** Contralateral paresis and sensory loss in the leg; cognitive or personality changes.
- **Posterior cerebral artery (PCA):** Homonymous hemianopsia, memory deficits, dyslexia/alexia.
- **Basilar artery:** Coma, "locked-in" syndrome, cranial nerve palsies (eg, diplopia), apnea, visual symptoms, drop attacks, dysphagia, dysarthria, vertigo, "crossed" weakness and sensory loss affecting the ipsilateral face and contralateral body.
- **Basal ganglia lacunar:** Pure motor or sensory stroke, dysarthria–clumsy hand syndrome, ataxic hemiparesis.
- **TIA:** A transient neurologic deficit that lasts < **24 hours** (most last < 1 hour) and is determined to be of ischemic etiology. Many TIAs have MRI-⊖ presentations, and some (~ 30–50%) are associated with small, asymptomatic strokes on diffusion-weighted MRI.

MNEMONIC

The 4 "deadly D's" of posterior circulation strokes—

Diplopia
Dizziness
Dysphagia
Dysarthria

DIAGNOSIS

- **Immediate labs** include CBC with platelets, cardiac enzymes and troponin, electrolytes, BUN, creatinine, serum glucose, PTT, PT, INR, lipid profile, and O_2 saturation.
- **Emergent head CT without contrast** (see Figure 2.10-2A) to differentiate ischemic from hemorrhagic stroke and to identify potential candidates for thrombolytic therapy. Strokes < 6 hours old are usually not visible on CT scan.

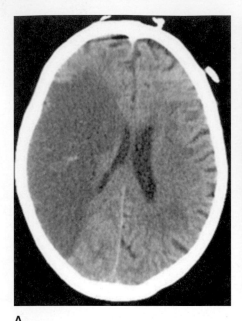
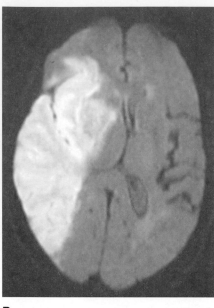
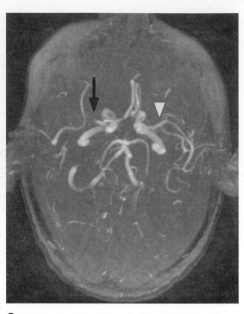

A   B   C

FIGURE 2.10-2. **Acute ischemic stroke.** Acute left hemiparesis in a 62-year-old woman. **(A)** Noncontrast head CT with loss of gray and white matter differentiation and asymmetrically decreased size of the right lateral ventricle in a right MCA distribution (indicating mass effect). **(B)** Diffusion-weighted MRI with reduced diffusion in the same distribution, consistent with an acute infarct; **diffusion-weighted sequences are the most sensitive modality for diagnosing an acute ischemic infarct.** **(C)** MRA shows the cause: an abrupt occlusion of the proximal right MCA (arrow). Compare with the normal left MCA (arrowhead). (Reproduced with permission from USMLERx.com.)

 MNEMONIC

***MCA stroke can cause* CHANGes:**

Contralateral paresis and sensory loss in the face and arm
Homonymous hemianopsia
Aphasia (dominant)
Neglect (nondominant)
Gaze preference toward the side of the lesion

- **MRI** (see Figure 2.10-2B) to identify early ischemic changes (eg, diffusion-weighted MRI is sensitive for acute stroke with changes as early as 20 minutes after an ischemic event).
- **ECG** and an **echocardiogram** if embolic stroke is suspected.
- **Vascular studies** of intracranial and extracranial disease include carotid ultrasound, transcranial Doppler, MRA, CT angiography, and conventional angiography (see Figure 2.10-2C).
- **Screen for hypercoagulable states** in patients with a history of thrombosis, in the setting of a first stroke, or in patients < 50 years of age.

TREATMENT

Acute treatment measures are as follows:

- **Hemorrhagic stroke:** See the discussion of parenchymal hemorrhage.
- **Ischemic stroke:**
  - **tPA** is indicated if administered within **3 hours** of symptom onset, but contraindications must first be ruled out. Be aware of potential bleeding or angioedema.
  - **Intra-arterial thrombolysis** can be used for select patients within **6 hours** of a major stroke from MCA occlusion if such patients are not suitable candidates for IV tPA.
  - **ASA** is associated with ↓ morbidity and mortality in acute ischemic stroke presenting ≤ 48 hours from onset.
  - **ICU admission** should be considered, especially for large strokes, comatose patients, or those who are unable to protect their airways for possible intubation.
  - Monitor for signs and symptoms of brain swelling, ↑ ICP, and herniation. Serial CTs are helpful in the evaluation of deteriorating patients. As a temporizing measure, treat with **mannitol** and **hyperventilation.**
  - **Allow permissive hypertension and hypoxemia** to maintain perfusion of ischemic cerebral tissue. However, in the setting of severe hyperten-

sion (systolic BP > 220 or diastolic BP > 120 mm Hg) or hemorrhagic stroke, treat with IV **labetalol** or **nicardipine** infusion. For the administration of tPA, the patient's systolic BP must be < 185 and diastolic BP < 110 mm Hg.

■ **Treat fever and hyperglycemia,** as both are associated with worse prognoses in the setting of acute stroke.

■ Prevent and treat poststroke complications such as aspiration pneumonia, UTI, and DVT.

Preventive and long-term treatment measures are as follows:

■ **ASA, clopidogrel:** If stroke is 2° to small vessel disease or thrombosis, or if anticoagulation is contraindicated.

■ **Carotid endarterectomy:** If stenosis is > 60% in symptomatic patients or > 70% in asymptomatic patients (contraindicated in 100% occlusion; see Figure 2.10-3).

■ **Anticoagulation:** In new AF or hypercoagulable states, the target INR is 2–3. In cases involving a prosthetic valve, the target INR is 3–4 or add an antiplatelet agent.

■ **Management of hypertension, hypercholesterolemia,** and **diabetes** (hypertension is the single greatest risk factor for stroke).

SUBARACHNOID HEMORRHAGE (SAH)

Etiologies of SAH include **trauma, berry aneurysms,** AVM, and trauma to the circle of Willis.

HISTORY/PE

■ Aneurysmal SAH presents with an **abrupt-onset, intensely painful "thunderclap" headache,** often followed by **neck stiffness.**

■ Other signs of meningeal irritation, including photophobia, nausea/vomiting, and meningeal stretch signs, may also be seen.

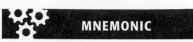

MNEMONIC

Contraindications to tPA therapy—

SAMPLE STAGES

Stroke or head trauma within the last 3 months
Anticoagulation with INR > 1.7 or prolonged PTT
MI (recent)
Prior intracranial hemorrhage
Low platelet count (< 100,000/mm³)
Elevated BP: Systolic > 185 or diastolic > 110 mm Hg
Surgery in the past 14 days
TIA (mild symptoms or rapid improvement of symptoms)
Age < 18
GI or urinary bleeding in the past 21 days
Elevated (> 400 mg/dL) or ↓ (< 50 mg/dL) blood glucose
Seizures present at the onset of stroke

KEY FACT

CN III palsy with pupillary involvement is associated with berry aneurysms.

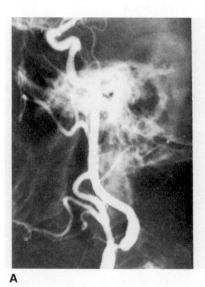
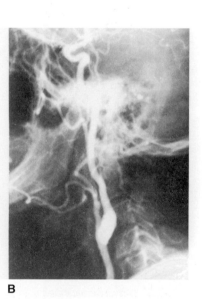

A   B

FIGURE 2.10-3. **Vascular studies pre- and postendarterectomy. (A)** Carotid arteriogram showing stenosis of the proximal internal carotid artery. **(B)** Postoperative arteriogram with restoration of the normal luminal size following endarterectomy. (Reproduced with permission from Way LW. *Current Surgical Diagnosis & Treatment,* 10th ed. Stamford, CT: Appleton & Lange, 1994: 763.)

SAH = "the worst headache of my life" with **sudden** onset. Migraine = a gradually worsening headache (peak intensity > 30 minutes).

- In the absence of neurosurgical intervention, rapid development of obstructive hydrocephalus or seizures often leads to ↓ arousal or frank coma and death.
- More than one-third of patients will give a history of a **"sentinel bleed"** days to weeks earlier marked by an abrupt-onset headache, often with nausea/vomiting, or transient diplopia that completely resolved in a matter of minutes to hours.

DIAGNOSIS

- Immediate head **CT without contrast** (see Figure 2.10-4, left panel) to look for blood in the subarachnoid space. Sensitivity is > 95% in patients with severe SAH but is much lower in those with normal mental status.
- Immediate **LP if CT is ⊖** to look for **RBCs, xanthochromia** (yellowish CSF due to breakdown of RBCs), ↑ protein (from the RBCs), and ↑ ICP. Note that LP results can be falsely ⊖ both in the first 6–12 hours (because xanthochromia has not yet developed) and after the first 24–28 hours (because xanthochromia has resolved).
- **Four-vessel angiography** (or equivalent noninvasive angiography such as CT angiography with 3D reconstructions) should be performed once SAH

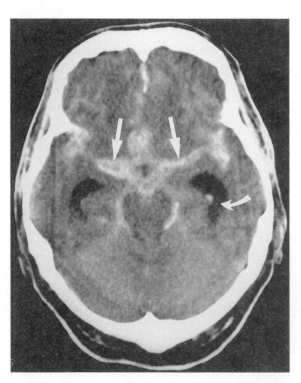

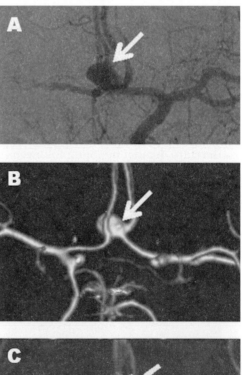

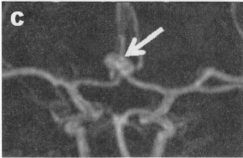

FIGURE 2.10-4.   Subarachnoid hemorrhage. Noncontrast CT (left) showing SAH filling the basilar cisterns and sylvian fissures (straight arrows). The curved arrow shows the dilated temporal horns of the lateral ventricles/hydrocephalus. Coned-down images (right) from a catheter angiogram (**A**), a CT angiogram (**B**), and an MRA (**C**) show a saccular aneurysm arising from the anterior communicating artery (arrow). (Left image reproduced with permission from Tintinalli JE et al. *Tintinalli's Emergency Medicine: A Comprehensive Study Guide,* 6th ed. New York: McGraw-Hill, 2004, Fig. 237-4. Right image reproduced with permission from Doherty GM. *Current Diagnosis & Treatment: Surgery,* 13th ed. New York: McGraw-Hill, 2010, Fig. 36-6.)

has been confirmed (see Figure 2.10-4A–C). Noninvasive angiography is warranted in high-risk cases and in those with high clinical suspicion even if CT and LP are unrevealing.

- Call neurosurgery.

TREATMENT

- **Prevent rebleeding** (most likely to occur in the first 48 hours) by maintaining systolic BP < 150 mm Hg until the aneurysm is clipped or coiled.
- **Prevent vasospasm and associated neurologic deterioration** (most likely to occur 5–7 days after SAH) by administering calcium channel blockers (CCBs), IV fluids, and pressors to maintain BP.
- ↓ **ICP** by raising the head of the bed and instituting hyperventilation in an acute setting (< 30 minutes after onset).
- **Treat hydrocephalus** through a lumbar drain or serial LPs.
- **Surgical clipping** is the **definitive treatment for aneurysms.** Endovascular coiling is also a safe option for many aneurysms.

MNEMONIC

Conditions associated with berry aneurysms that can MAKE an SAH more likely:

Marfan's syndrome
Aortic coarctation
Kidney disease (autosomal dominant, polycystic)
Ehlers-Danlos syndrome
Sickle cell anemia
Atherosclerosis
History (familial)

INTRACEREBRAL HEMORRHAGE

- Risk factors include hypertension, tumor, amyloid angiopathy (in the elderly), anticoagulation, and vascular malformations (AVMs, cavernous hemangiomas).
- **Hx/PE:** Presents with **focal motor and sensory deficits that often worsen as the hematoma expands.** A sudden-onset severe headache, nausea/vomiting, seizures, lethargy, or obtundation may also be seen.
- **Dx:** Immediate noncontrast head CT (see Figure 2.10-5). Look for mass effect or edema that may predict herniation.
- **Tx:** Similar to that of SAH. Elevate the head of the bed and institute antiseizure prophylaxis. Surgical evacuation may be necessary if mass effect is present. Several types of herniation may occur, including central, **uncal,** subfalcine, and tonsillar (see Figure 2.10-6 and Table 2.10-6).

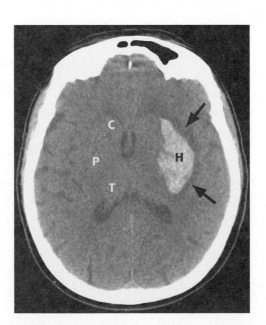

FIGURE 2.10-5.   Intracerebral hemorrhage. Noncontrast head CT shows an intraparenchymal hemorrhage (H) and surrounding edema (arrows) centered in the left putamen, a common location for hypertensive hemorrhage. C, P, and T denote the normal contralateral caudate, putamen, and thalamus. (Reproduced with permission from Fauci AS et al. *Harrison's Principles of Internal Medicine,* 17th ed. New York: McGraw-Hill, 2008, Fig. 364-17.)

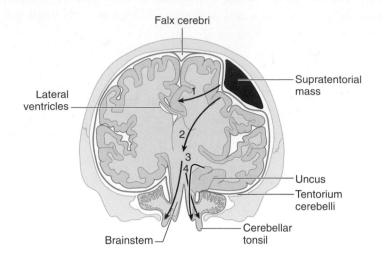

FIGURE 2.10-6. **Sites of herniation syndromes.** (1) Cingulate herniation under the falx cerebri. (2) Downward transtentorial (central) herniation. (3) Uncal herniation. (4) Cerebellar tonsillar herniation into the foramen magnum. Coma and death result when these herniations compress the brainstem. (Adapted with permission from Simon RP et al. *Clinical Neurology,* 4th ed. Stamford, CT: Appleton & Lange, 1999: 314.)

SUBDURAL HEMATOMA

- Typically occurs following head trauma (usually falls or assaults), leading to rupture of **bridging veins** and accumulation of blood between the dura and arachnoid membranes. Common in the **elderly** and **alcoholics.**
- Hx/PE: Presents with **headache, changes in mental status, contralateral hemiparesis,** and focal neurologic findings. Changes may be subacute or chronic. May present as pseudodementia in the elderly.

TABLE 2.10-6. **Clinical Presentation of Herniation Syndromes**

TYPE OF HERNIATION	PRESENTATION
Cingulate herniation	Occurs 2° to mass lesions of the frontal lobes. No specific signs or symptoms; frequently seen on head CT.
Downward transtentorial (central) herniation	Occurs when large supratentorial mass lesions push the midbrain inferiorly. Presents with a rapid change in mental status; bilaterally small and reactive pupils; Cheyne-Stokes respirations; and flexor or extensor posturing.
Uncal herniation	Occurs 2° to mass lesions of the middle fossa. CN III becomes entrapped, leading to a fixed and dilated ipsilateral pupil followed by an eye that is deviated "down and out." Ipsilesional hemiparesis ("false localizing") results from compression of the cerebral peduncle (opposite the mass lesion) against the tentorial edge.
Cerebellar tonsillar herniation into the foramen magnum	Occurs 2° to posterior fossa mass lesions. Tonsillar herniation → medullary compression → respiratory arrest. Usually rapidly fatal.

- **Dx:** CT demonstrates a **crescent-shaped, concave hyperdensity** acutely (isodense subacutely; hypodense chronically) that does **not cross the midline** (see Figure 2.10-7A).
- **Tx: Surgical evacuation if symptomatic.** Subdural hematomas may regress spontaneously.

EPIDURAL HEMATOMA

- Usually a result of a **lateral skull fracture** leading to a tear of the **middle meningeal artery.**
- **Hx/PE:** Obvious, severe **trauma** induces an **immediate loss of consciousness** followed by a **lucid interval (minutes to hours).** Uncal herniation leads to coma with a **"blown pupil"** (fixed and dilated ipsilateral pupil) and ultimately an **ipsilateral hemiparesis.**
- **Dx:** CT shows a **lens-shaped, convex hyperdensity limited by the sutures** (see Figure 2.10-7B).
- **Tx:** Emergent neurosurgical evacuation. May quickly evolve to brain herniation and death 2° to the arterial source of bleeding.

Headaches

Causes of headache include the following:

- **Acute** (onset seconds to minutes):
  - **Primary:** New migraine/cluster headache.
  - **Vascular/ischemic:** Aneurysmal SAH, cerebral venous thrombosis, cavernous sinus thrombosis, craniocervical dissection, acute severe hypertension (eg, pheochromocytoma), ischemic stroke/intraparenchymal hemorrhage (headache is usually not the presenting manifestation), pituitary apoplexy.
  - **↑ ICP:** Colloid cyst, obstructive hydrocephalus.
  - **Acute ocular disease:** Angle-closure glaucoma.

KEY FACT

Mental status changes associated with an expanding epidural hematoma occur within minutes to hours and classically include a lucid interval. With a subdural hematoma, such changes can occur within days to weeks.

KEY FACT

A "blown pupil" suggests impending brainstem compression.

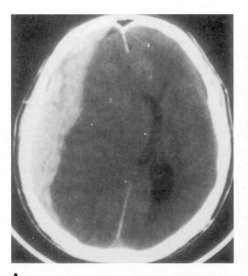
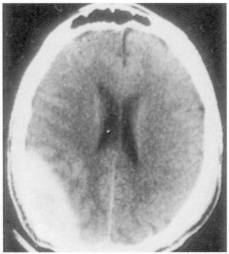

A   B

FIGURE 2.10-7. **Subdural vs. epidural hematoma.** (A) Subdural hematoma. Note the crescent shape and the mass effect with midline shift. (B) **Epidural hematoma** with a classic biconvex lens shape. (Reproduced with permission from Aminoff MJ. *Clinical Neurology*, 3rd ed. Stamford, CT: Appleton & Lange, 1996: 296.)

- Subacute (onset hours to days):
    - **Primary:** New migraine/tension-type headache.
    - **Infectious:** Viral syndrome, meningitis, cranial infections (acute sinusitis, dental infections, orbital infections, cavernous sinus infections, otitis media/mastoiditis), encephalitis.
    - **Vascular/ischemic:** Temporal arteritis, subacute severe hypertension (eg, hypertensive encephalopathy, eclampsia), intracranial hypotension (eg, spontaneous, post-LP), subdural hematoma, carbon monoxide, lead poisoning in children (rare).
    - **Subacutely ↑ ICP:** Large tumor, progressive hydrocephalus, altitude sickness, pseudotumor cerebri.
    - **Subacute ocular disease:** Keratitis, iritis, scleritis, orbital infection.
- Chronic/episodic:
    - **Primary:** Migraine, cluster headache, tension-type headache.
    - **Infectious:** Chronic sinusitis.
    - **Other:** Medication overuse (eg, caffeine withdrawal, "rebound" headaches from NSAID or analgesic overuse), trigeminal or other neuralgias (eg, glossopharyngeal, postherpetic), TMJ disorders, cervical arthritis.

History/PE

- Conduct full general and neurologic exams, including a **funduscopic** exam.
- Evaluate the following:
    - **Chronicity:** Recent or recently changed headaches warrant immediate workup if they are not clearly migraines or other 1° headache disorders.
    - **Intensity:** Severe headaches are more likely to be dangerous.
    - **Location:** Posterior headaches are less likely to be benign, especially in children.
    - **Duration:** Headaches lasting > 72 hours are atypical for migraines.
    - **Diurnal variation:** Cluster headaches and those from ↑ ICP usually occur or worsen at night.
    - **Triggers:** Examples include chocolate and red wine in migraines.
    - **Provocative factors:** Lying down may worsen high-ICP headaches; standing up may exacerbate low-ICP headaches.
    - **Palliative factors:** Examples include sleep alleviating migraine headaches.
    - **Associated symptoms/signs:**
        - Significant findings include **fever or rash** (consider meningitis or other infectious causes), **jaw claudication** (specific for temporal arteritis), or constitutional symptoms such as **weight loss** (associated with neoplastic, inflammatory, or infectious conditions).
        - **Photophobia, nausea, and vomiting** are associated with migraine, aneurysmal SAH, and meningitis; neck stiffness is more likely to accompany the last 2 conditions.
    - **Neurologic sequelae:** Look for **diplopia,** mental status changes or associated symptoms (numbness, weakness, dizziness, ataxia, visual disturbances), **papilledema,** or pupillary abnormalities (partial CN III palsy or Horner's syndrome).
    - **Patient risk factors:** High-risk patients are > 50 years of age, immunocompromised, or with preexisting malignancy.

Diagnosis

- If SAH is suspected, obtain a **head CT without contrast.**
- If CT is ⊖, LP is mandatory.
- Obtain a CBC to rule out systemic infections. If temporal arteritis is suspected, obtain an ESR.

- A CT/MRI is needed for suspected SAH, ↑ ICP, or focal neurologic findings. Use **CT without contrast** to evaluate acute hemorrhage.

MIGRAINE HEADACHE

- Affects **females** more often than males; may be familial. Associated with **vascular** and brain neurotransmitter (**serotonin**) changes. Pain is ultimately linked to trigeminal nucleus activation in the brainstem. Onset is usually by the **early 20s.**
- Auras may occur with or without the pain of migraine headache.
- **Triggers** include certain foods (eg, red wine), fasting, stress, menses, OCPs, bright light, and disruptions in normal sleep patterns.
- Hx/PE:
  - Presents with a throbbing headache (> 2 hours but usually < 24 hours, and almost always < 72 hours in duration) that is associated with **nausea, vomiting, photophobia,** and noise sensitivity. Headache is usually relieved by **sleep and darkness.**
  - **Classic migraines:** Often **unilateral** and preceded by a visual **aura** in the form of either scintillating scotomas (bright or flashing lights) or visual field cuts.
  - **Common migraines:** May be **bilateral** and periorbital **without preceding auras.**
- **Dx:** Based on the history and an otherwise ⊖ workup.
- **Tx:**
  - **Avoid known triggers.**
  - **Abortive therapy** includes **triptans** (first-line therapy after OTC NSAIDs have failed), **metoclopramide,** and various analgesics. Consider symptomatic treatment for nausea.
  - **Prophylaxis** for frequent or severe migraines includes **anticonvulsants** (eg, gabapentin, topiramate), **TCAs** (eg, amitriptyline), **β-blockers** (propranolol), and **CCBs.**

KEY FACT

If a 20-year-old female develops headaches after drinking red wine, think migraine.

CLUSTER HEADACHE

- **Males** are affected more often than females; average age of onset is 25.
- Hx/PE:
  - Presents as a brief, **excruciating, unilateral periorbital headache** that lasts 30 minutes to 3 hours, during which the patient tends to be extremely restless.
  - Attacks tend to occur in **clusters,** affecting the same part of the head at the same time of day (commonly during sleep) and in a certain season of the year.
  - Associated symptoms include **ipsilateral lacrimation** of the eye, conjunctival injection, Horner's syndrome, and nasal stuffiness.
- **Dx:** Classic presentations with a history of repeated attacks over an extended period of time require no evaluation. First episodes require a workup to exclude disorders associated with Horner's syndrome (eg, carotid artery dissection, cavernous sinus infection).
- **Tx:**
  - **Acute therapy:** High-flow O_2, dihydroergotamine, octreotide, sumatriptan or zolmitriptan.
  - **Prophylactic therapy:** Transitional (prednisone, ergotamine), maintenance (verapamil, methysergide, lithium, valproic acid, topiramate).

KEY FACT

If a 25-year-old male wakes up repeatedly during the night with unilateral periorbital pain associated with ipsilateral lacrimation, think cluster headache.

TENSION-TYPE HEADACHE

- Considered by some to be a milder form of migraine headache.
- Hx/PE: Presents with **tight, bandlike pain** that is not associated with sensory phobia, nausea/vomiting, or auras and is brought on by fatigue or stress. Nonspecific symptoms (eg, anxiety, poor concentration, difficulty sleeping) may also be seen. Usually occurs at the end of the day.
- Dx: A diagnosis of exclusion. Be particularly aware of giant cell arteritis in patients > 50 years of age with new headaches; always obtain an ESR even if headaches are mild and unassociated with constitutional or vascular symptoms.
- Tx: Relaxation, massage, hot baths, and **avoidance of exacerbating factors. NSAIDs** and **acetaminophen** are first-line abortive therapy, but triptans may also be considered.

CAVERNOUS SINUS THROMBOSIS

The usual etiology involves a **suppurative process** of the orbit, nasal sinuses, or central face that leads to **septic thrombosis** of the cavernous sinus. Nonseptic thrombosis is rare; *S aureus* is the most common causative agent. The syndrome can also be seen with nonbacterial agents, particularly fungi (*Mucor* or *Aspergillus* species). Current antimicrobials have greatly ↓ both incidence and mortality.

HISTORY/PE

- **Headache is the most common presenting symptom.**
- Patients may present with orbital pain, edema, diplopia (2° to oculomotor, abducens, or trochlear nerve involvement), or visual disturbances and may describe a recent history of sinusitis or facial infection. On examination, they typically appear ill and have a **fever.**
- Additional signs may include red eye, proptosis, ptosis, or ophthalmoplegia of the affected eye (partial or complete).
- Changes in mental status such as confusion, drowsiness, or coma suggest spread to the CNS or sepsis. Late findings include meningismus or systemic signs of sepsis.

DIAGNOSIS

- Lab studies show an ↑ WBC count.
- Blood cultures reveal the causative agent in up to 50% of cases.
- CSF exam may reveal ↑ protein consistent with a parameningeal reaction unless there is frank meningitis.
- **MRI** (with gadolinium and MR venography) is the principal means of confirming the anatomic diagnosis; CT angiography and CT venography are also often used for diagnosis.
- Biopsy of paranasal sinuses or other affected tissue is often necessary in fungal cases for organism identification by histology and culture.

TREATMENT

- Treat aggressively and empirically with a **penicillinase-resistant penicillin** (nafcillin or oxacillin) plus a **third- or fourth-generation cephalosporin** (eg, ceftriaxone or cefepime) to provide broad-spectrum coverage pending blood culture results. Potential anaerobic infection from sinus or dental sources should be covered with **metronidazole. Vancomycin** can be added to address potential MRSA involvement. Antifungal therapy is required for fungal cases.

- IV antibiotics are recommended for at least 3–4 weeks.
- Surgical drainage may be necessary if there is no response to antibiotics within 24 hours.

Seizure Disorders

Paroxysmal events associated with aberrant electrical activity in the brain detectable by EEG, leading to changes in neurologic perception or behavior. An aura is experienced by 50–60% of patients with epilepsy. See Table 2.10-7 for common etiologies by age. To further narrow down the etiology of a seizure, assess the following:

- Determine whether the patient has a history of epilepsy (ie, a history of unprovoked and recurrent seizures). Other seizures may be self-limited and may resolve once an underlying medical condition has been identified and treated.
- Elevated serum prolactin levels are consistent with an epileptic seizure in the immediate postictal period.
- Non-neurologic etiologies include **hypoglycemia, hyponatremia, hypocalcemia, hyperosmolar states, hepatic encephalopathy,** uremia, porphyria, **drug overdose** (cocaine, antidepressants, neuroleptics, methylxanthines, lidocaine), **drug withdrawal** (alcohol and other sedatives), eclampsia, hyperthermia, hypertensive encephalopathy, head trauma, and cerebral hypoperfusion.
- Seizures with a focal onset (or focal postictal deficit) suggest focal CNS pathology. They may be the presenting sign of a tumor, stroke, AVM, infection, hemorrhage, or developmental abnormality.
- First-time seizures that resolve after a single episode are usually not treated with antiseizure medications when the underlying cause is unknown.

PARTIAL SEIZURES

Arise from a **discrete region,** or an "epileptogenic focus," in 1 cerebral hemisphere and **do not** by themselves cause **loss of consciousness** unless they secondarily generalize.

TABLE 2.10-7. Causes of Seizure by Age Group

INFANTS	CHILDREN (2–10)	ADOLESCENTS	ADULTS (18–35)	ADULTS (35+)
Perinatal injury	Idiopathic	Idiopathic	Trauma	Trauma
Infection	Infection	Trauma	Alcoholism	Stroke
Metabolic	Trauma	Drug withdrawal	Brain tumor	Metabolic disorders
Congenital	Febrile	AVM		Alcoholism
				Brain tumor

Q

A 23-year-old female presents to the ER with a first-time seizure during the eighth month of her first pregnancy. Is this seizure more likely to be related to her pregnancy or to a preexisting condition?

KEY FACT

If a patient presents wth progressive jerking of successive body regions and hallucinations but without loss of consciousness, think simple partial seizures.

KEY FACT

If a patient presents with an episode of lip smacking associated with an impaired level of consciousness and followed by confusion, think complex partial seizures.

KEY FACT

Both simple partial and complex partial seizures may evolve into 2° generalized tonic-clonic (grand mal) seizures.

HISTORY/PE

- **Simple partial seizures:**
  - May include motor features (eg, jacksonian march, or the progressive jerking of successive body regions) as well as sensory, autonomic, or psychic features (eg, fear, déjà vu, hallucinations).
  - **Do not involve alteration of consciousness.**
  - A postictal focal neurologic deficit (eg, hemiplegia/hemiparesis, or Todd's paralysis) is possible and usually resolves within 24 hours. Often confused with acute stroke (ruled out by MRI).
- **Complex partial seizures:**
  - Typically involve the temporal lobe (70–80%) with bilateral spread of the aberrant electrical discharge.
  - **Involve an impaired level of consciousness.**
  - Characterized by auditory or visual hallucinations, déjà vu, and automatisms (eg, lip smacking, chewing, or even walking).
  - Postictal confusion/disorientation and amnesia are characteristic.

DIAGNOSIS

- Obtain an **EEG** to rule out pseudoseizures and to find an epileptogenic focus if present.
- Rule out systemic causes with a CBC, electrolytes, calcium, fasting glucose, LFTs, a renal panel, RPR, ESR, and a toxicology screen.
- A focal seizure implies a focal brain lesion. Evaluate by MRI or CT with contrast.

TREATMENT

- For acute seizures lasting longer than 2 minutes, use IV benzodiazepines and phenytoin.
- In cases of systemic 2° seizures, **treat the underlying cause.**
- **Recurrent partial seizures:** Phenytoin, oxcarbazepine, carbamazepine (Tegretol), phenobarbital, and valproic acid can be administered as monotherapy. In **children, phenobarbital** is the first-line anticonvulsant.
- **Intractable temporal lobe seizures:** Consider **anterior temporal lobectomy.**

KEY FACT

If a patient presents with clonic movements associated with loss of consciousness and incontinence, think tonic-clonic (grand mal) seizures.

A

This first-time seizure is most likely 2° to the patient's pregnancy as opposed to a preexisting seizure disorder. Her presentation is most consistent with eclampsia, which typically follows preeclampsia, a serious complication of high blood pressure during pregnancy.

TONIC-CLONIC (GRAND MAL) SEIZURES

Primarily idiopathic. Partial seizures can evolve into secondarily generalized tonic-clonic seizures.

HISTORY/PE

- Presents with sudden onset of loss of consciousness with tonic extension of the back and extremities, continuing with 1–2 minutes of repetitive, symmetric clonic movements.
- Marked by **incontinence** and **tongue biting.** Patients may appear **cyanotic** during the ictal period. Consciousness is slowly regained in the postictal period, but patients are confused and may prefer to sleep; muscle aches and headaches may be present.

DIAGNOSIS

Diagnosed by the **history and EEG** (typically shows 10-Hz activity during the tonic phase and slow waves during the clonic phase).

TREATMENT

- **Protect the airway.**
- Treat the underlying cause if known.
- **1° generalized tonic-clonic seizures: Phenytoin,** fosphenytoin, or valproate constitutes first-line therapy. Lamotrigine or topiramate may be used as adjunctive therapy.
- **Secondarily generalized tonic-clonic seizures:** Treatment is the same as that for partial seizures.

ABSENCE (PETIT MAL) SEIZURES

- Begin in **childhood;** subside before adulthood. Often **familial.**
- **Hx/PE:** Present with brief **(5- to 10-second),** often unnoticeable episodes of **impaired consciousness** occurring up to hundreds of times per day. Patients are **amnestic** during and immediately after seizures and may appear to be **daydreaming** or **staring.** Eye fluttering or lip smacking is common.
- **Dx: EEG** shows classic 3-per-second spike-and-wave discharges (remember classic EEG findings, but do **not** worry about learning how to read them!). Hyperventilation can trigger these seizures.
- **Tx: Ethosuximide** is the first-line agent. Valproic acid is second line.

STATUS EPILEPTICUS

A **medical emergency** consisting of prolonged (> **10-minute)** or repetitive seizures that occur without a return to baseline consciousness. May be either convulsive (the more medically urgent form) or nonconvulsive.

- Common causes include anticonvulsant withdrawal/noncompliance, anoxic brain injury, EtOH/sedative withdrawal or other drug intoxication, metabolic disturbances (eg, hyponatremia), head trauma, and infection.
- Death usually results from the underlying medical condition and may occur in 10% of cases of status epilepticus.

DIAGNOSIS

- Determine the underlying cause with pulse oximetry, CBC, electrolytes, calcium, glucose, ABGs, LFTs, BUN/creatinine, ESR, antiepileptic drug levels, and a toxicology screen.
- **Obtain an EEG and brain imaging, but defer testing until the patient is stabilized.**
- **Obtain a stat head CT** to evaluate for intracranial hemorrhage.
- Obtain an LP in the setting of fever or meningeal signs, but only after a CT scan has been obtained to assess the safety of the LP.

TREATMENT

- Maintain **ABCs;** consider rapid intubation for airway protection.
- Administer **thiamine, followed by glucose and naloxone** to presumptively treat potential etiologies.
- Give an **IV benzodiazepine** (lorazepam or diazepam) plus a loading dose of **fosphenytoin.**
- If seizures continue, intubate and load with **phenobarbital.** Consider an IV sedative (midazolam or pentobarbital) and initiate continuous EEG monitoring.
- Initiate a meticulous search for the underlying cause.

KEY FACT

If you see petit mal seizures, think about the classic EEG finding of 3-per-second spike-and-wave discharges.

KEY FACT

If a child is brought from school to her pediatrician after experiencing multiple intermittent 5-second episodes of staring into space, think absence (petit mal) seizures.

INFANTILE SPASMS (WEST SYNDROME)

- A form of **generalized epilepsy** that typically begins within 6 months of birth. May be idiopathic or 2° to a variety of conditions, including PKU, perinatal infections, hypoxic-ischemic injury, and tuberous sclerosis.
- Affects males more often than females; associated with a ⊕ family history.
- **Hx/PE:** Presents with tonic, bilateral, symmetric **jerks of the head, trunk, and extremities** that tend to occur in clusters of 5–10; **arrest of psychomotor development** occurs at the age of seizure onset. The majority of patients have mental retardation.
- **Dx:** Look for an **abnormal interictal EEG** characterized by **hypsarrhythmia**.
- **Tx:** Hormonal therapy with **ACTH**, prednisone, and clonazepam or valproic acid. Medications may treat the spasms but have little impact on patients' long-term prognosis.

LENNOX-GASTAUT SYNDROME

- A form of childhood onset seizures that is often refractory to treatment.
- **Hx/PE:** Presents with daily multiple seizures, often nocturnal tonic seizures. Classically appears between ages 2 and 6; more common in males than in females. Strongly associated with mental retardation, behavior disorders, and delayed psychomotor development.
- **Dx:** Look for an abnormal interictal EEG characterized by slow spike-and-wave complexes.
- **Tx:** Usually treatment resistant.

Vertigo and Dizziness

BENIGN PAROXYSMAL POSITIONAL VERTIGO (BPPV)

- A common cause of recurrent **peripheral vertigo** resulting from a **dislodged otolith** that leads to disturbances in the semicircular canals (95% posterior, 5% horizontal).
- **Hx/PE:** Patients present with **transient, episodic vertigo (lasting < 1 minute)** and mixed upbeat-**torsional nystagmus triggered by changes in head position** (eg, while turning in bed, getting in and out of bed, or reaching overhead). Patients may complain of nonvertiginous dizziness or lightheadedness. **Nausea and vomiting are uncommon** owing to the short-lived nature of the stimulus.
- **Dx:**
  - **Dix-Hallpike maneuver:** Have the patient turn his or her head 45 degrees right or left and go from a sitting to a supine position while quickly turning the head to the side. If vertigo and the typical nystagmus (upbeat and toward the affected shoulder) are reproduced, BPPV is the likely diagnosis.
  - Nystagmus that persists for > 1 minute, gait disturbance, or nausea/vomiting that is out of proportion to nystagmus should raise concern for a central lesion.
- **Tx:**
  - Eighty percent of cases can be resolved with a modified Epley maneuver (a 270-degree head rotation from the Dix-Hallpike testing position).

- The condition usually subsides spontaneously in weeks to months, but 30% recur within a year. Antivertigo medications (eg, meclizine) are generally contraindicated, as they inhibit central compensation, which may lead to chronic unsteadiness.

ACUTE PERIPHERAL VESTIBULOPATHY (LABYRINTHITIS AND VESTIBULAR NEURITIS)

- Hx/PE:
  - Presents with **acute onset of severe vertigo, head-motion intolerance, and gait unsteadiness** accompanied by **nausea, vomiting, and nystagmus.**
  - Auditory or aural symptoms (labyrinthitis) may include unilateral tinnitus, ear fullness, or hearing loss. Without auditory or aural symptoms, the condition is known as vestibular neuritis.
  - Labyrinthitis (with auditory symptoms) is mimicked by lateral pontine/cerebellar stroke (AICA territory). Vestibular neuritis (without auditory symptoms) is mimicked by lateral medullary/cerebellar stroke (PICA territory).
- Dx:
  - A **diagnosis of exclusion** once the more serious causes of vertigo (eg, cerebellar stroke) have been ruled out.
  - Acute peripheral vestibulopathy demonstrates the following:
    - An abnormal vestibulo-ocular reflex as determined by a bedside head impulse test (ie, rapid head rotation from lateral to center while staring at the examiner's nose).
    - A predominantly horizontal nystagmus that always beats in 1 direction, opposite the lesion.
    - No vertical eye misalignment by alternate cover testing.
  - If patients are "high risk"—ie, if they have atypical eye findings or neurologic symptoms or signs, cannot stand independently, have head or neck pain, are > 50 years of age, or have 1 or more stroke risk factors— MRI with diffusion-weighted imaging is indicated.
- Tx: Acute treatment consists of corticosteroids given < 72 hours after symptom onset and vestibular sedatives (eg, meclizine). The condition usually subsides spontaneously within weeks to months.

KEY FACT

If you see someone with vertigo and vomiting for 1 week after having been diagnosed with a viral infection, think acute vestibular neuritis.

MÉNIÈRE'S DISEASE

- A cause of recurrent **vertigo with auditory symptoms** that affects at least 1 in 500 in the United States. More common among females.
- Hx/PE: Presents with **recurrent episodes of severe vertigo, hearing loss, tinnitus, or ear fullness,** often lasting hours to days. **Nausea and vomiting are typical.** Patients progressively lose low-frequency hearing over years and may become deaf on the affected side.
- Dx: The **diagnosis is made clinically** and is based on a thorough history and physical. **Two episodes** lasting ≥ 20 minutes with remission of symptoms between episodes, hearing loss documented at least once with audiometry, and tinnitus or aural fullness are needed to make the diagnosis once other causes (eg, TIA, otosyphilis) have been ruled out.
- Tx:
  - Classically, a low-sodium diet and diuretic therapy were first-line treatments. As theories of pathogenesis have shifted, many clinicians have begun to treat patients with "migraine diets," lifestyle changes, prophy-

KEY FACT

Ménière's disease consists of recurrent episodes, but unlike BPPV, these usually last hours to days.

lactic antimigraine medications, and occasionally benzodiazepines or antiemetics.

- For severe unilateral cases, ablative therapies (eg, intratympanic gentamicin to ablate the labyrinth, vestibular nerve section) have been used with some success.

VESTIBULAR MIGRAINE

- A cause of recurrent **vertigo (usually without auditory symptoms)** that affects roughly 10% of migraine sufferers. More common among females.
- **Hx/PE:** Presents with **recurrent episodes of mild dizziness to severe vertigo** lasting minutes to days. Nausea, vomiting, and photophobia are common; headaches are variably present and may be mild or severe. Patients have no substantial deficits in between spells, but balance may deteriorate over decades.
- **Dx:**
  - **The diagnosis is usually made clinically** on the basis of a thorough history and physical to exclude other causes.
  - Patients who would otherwise qualify for a diagnosis of Ménière's save the absence of auditory symptoms and documented hearing loss are likely to have vestibular migraine. A history of photo- or phonophobia during the episode, particularly if dizziness is associated with headache, is highly suggestive.
  - The **diagnosis is one of exclusion,** and care should be taken to ensure that patients do not have intermittent dizziness due to TIA. In patients < 50 years of age, a history of recent trauma or of severe, abrupt-onset, or persistent pain (> 72 hours) should raise concern for vertebral artery dissection with TIAs.
  - A brain MRI with vascular imaging (eg, MRA) is sometimes indicated to assess potential intracranial pathology, particularly cerebrovascular disease.
- **Tx:** Can usually be prevented through migraine medication, diet, or lifestyle changes. Benzodiazepines or antiemetics may be tried. Surgical therapies are not indicated.

SYNCOPE

- One of the **most common causes** of loss of consciousness 2° to an abrupt drop in cerebral perfusion. Etiologies include cardiac arrhythmias and cardiac outflow obstruction, vasovagal syncope, orthostatic hypotension, micturition-related syncope, basilar TIAs, and idiopathic causes. Presyncope is described as a feeling of imminent loss of consciousness without actual fainting. Commonly **confused with seizures.**
- **Hx/PE:**
  - Patients may report a **trigger** (eg, standing for a long period of time, fear/sight of blood, Valsalva maneuver).
  - Typically follows a **prodrome of lightheadedness or dizziness,** muffled sounds, constricting vision, diffuse weakness, diaphoresis, or pallor. Leads to loss of consciousness and muscle tone for < 30 seconds and recovery within seconds.
- **Dx:**
  - Structural CNS causes (eg, basilar TIA, intermittent obstructive hydrocephalus) are rare among patients who return to normal mental status and have a normal neurologic examination after a brief loss of consciousness.

KEY FACT

Unlike Ménière's disease, vestibular migraine usually has no associated auditory or aural symptoms.

KEY FACT

Rule out vertebral artery dissection in those with persistent head or neck pain and intermittent isolated dizziness or vertigo.

- Seizures are more likely if limb jerking is unilateral or lasts > 30 seconds; if there is prolonged confusion after the episode; or if the patient bites the lateral aspect of his or her tongue.
- Unless there is a clear vasovagal faint in a young patient without cardiac disease or risk factors, place all patients on **telemetry** or **Holter monitoring** to evaluate for arrhythmia, and rule out myocardial ischemia with an **ECG** and **cardiac enzymes.** Obtain an **EEG** to rule out seizures. Consider an **echocardiogram,** a **tilt-table test,** or **neuroimaging,** especially vascular.
- **Tx:** Treat the underlying cause; avoid triggers.

Disorders of the Neuromuscular Junction

MYASTHENIA GRAVIS

An **autoimmune disorder** caused by antibodies that bind to **postsynaptic acetylcholine (ACh) receptors** located at the neuromuscular junction. Most often affects young adult females, and can be associated with **thyrotoxicosis, thymoma,** and other autoimmune disorders.

HISTORY/PE

- Presents with fluctuating **fatigable ptosis or double vision,** bulbar symptoms (eg, dysarthria, dysphagia), and **proximal muscle weakness. Symptoms typically worsen as the day progresses but fluctuate dramatically.**
- Patients may report difficulty climbing stairs, rising from a chair, brushing their hair, and swallowing.
- **Myasthenic crisis** is rare but includes the potentially lethal complications of respiratory compromise and aspiration.

DIAGNOSIS

- **Edrophonium (Tensilon test): Anticholinesterase** leads to **rapid** amelioration of symptoms. Rarely used today owing to the risk of bradycardia and discontinuation of production lines.
- **Ice test:** Place a pack of ice on 1 eye for 5 minutes; ptosis resolves transiently.
- An abnormal **single-fiber EMG** and/or a **decremental response to repetitive nerve stimulation** can yield additional confirmation.
- AChR antibodies are ⊕ in 80% of patients; anti–muscle-specific kinase (anti-MuSK) antibodies are ⊕ in 5%.
- Chest CT is used to evaluate for thymoma. Eighty-five percent of patients with myasthenia gravis and a thymoma have ⊕ antibodies against striated muscle.
- Follow serial FVCs to determine the need to intubate.

TREATMENT

- Anticholinesterases **(pyridostigmine)** are used for symptomatic treatment.
- **Prednisone** and other immunosuppressants (eg, azathioprine, cyclosporine, MMF) are the mainstays of treatment.
- In severe cases, plasmapheresis or IVIG may provide temporary relief (days to weeks).
- **Resection of thymoma** can be curative.
- **Avoid giving certain antibiotics** (eg, aminoglycosides) **and drugs** (eg, β-blockers) to patients with myasthenia gravis.

LAMBERT-EATON MYASTHENIC SYNDROME

- A paraneoplastic autoimmune disorder caused by antibodies directed toward presynaptic calcium channels in the neuromuscular junction. **Small cell lung carcinoma** is a significant risk factor (60% of cases).
- Hx/PE: Presents with weakness of proximal muscles along with depressed or absent DTRs. Extraocular, respiratory, and bulbar muscles are typically spared.
- **Dx: Repetitive nerve stimulation** reveals a characteristic incremental response. Also diagnosed by autoantibodies to presynaptic calcium channels and a chest CT indicative of a lung neoplasm.
- **Tx:**
  - Treat small cell lung carcinoma; tumor resection may reverse symptoms.
  - 3,4-diaminopyridine or guanidine can be given; acetylcholinesterase inhibitors (eg, pyridostigmine) can be added to either regimen.
  - Corticosteroids and azathioprine can be combined or used alone for immunosuppression in cases where a neoplasm cannot be identified and an autoimmune cause is suspected.

> **KEY FACT**
>
> Repetitive nerve stimulation reveals a characteristic incremental response in Lambert-Eaton myasthenic syndrome but shows a decremental response in myasthenia gravis.

MULTIPLE SCLEROSIS (MS)

Although the pathogenesis of MS is unclear, there is evidence of an autoimmune etiology in genetically susceptible individuals who are exposed to environmental triggers such as viral infections. Such potential etiologies are thought to be **T-cell mediated.** The female-to-male ratio is 3:2, and onset is typically between 20 and 40 years of age. MS becomes more common with increasing distance from the equator during childhood. Subtypes are **relapsing-remitting,** 1° progressive, 2° progressive, and progressive relapsing (see Table 2.10-8).

HISTORY/PE

- Presents with **multiple neurologic complaints that are separated in time and space and are not explained by a single lesion.** As the disease progresses, permanent deficits may accumulate.

TABLE 2.10-8. Subtypes of Multiple Sclerosis

	RELAPSING-REMITTING	1° PROGRESSIVE	2° PROGRESSIVE	PROGRESSIVE RELAPSING
Relapses	Yes.	No acute episodes.	Yes.	Yes.
Progression	None.	From onset.	Not at onset; begins to progress later.	From onset.
Course of symptoms	Full recovery, or deficits may remain after each episode.	Minor remissions and plateaus may take place during progression.	Relapses, minor remissions, and plateaus may take place during progression.	Full recovery, or progressive deficits may remain after each episode.
Percentage of cases at onset	66%	19%	Develops after relapsing-remitting type.	15%
Prognosis	Best.	Worse.	Worse.	Worse.

- Limb weakness, **optic neuritis,** paresthesias, diplopia, vertigo, nystagmus, gait unsteadiness, urinary retention, sexual and bowel dysfunction, depression, and cognitive impairment are also seen. Symptoms classically worsen transiently with hot showers.
- Attacks are unpredictable but on average occur every 1.5 years, lasting for 2–8 weeks.
- Neurologic symptoms can come and go or be progressive. Those with a **relapsing and remitting history** have the **best prognosis.**
- Lhermitte's sign, demonstrated by vibratory/electrical sensations traveling up or down the neck and back with flexion, generally suggests the presence of cervical myelitis.

Diagnosis

- MRI shows **multiple, asymmetric,** often **periventricular** white matter lesions (Dawson's fingers), especially in the **corpus callosum.** Active lesions enhance with gadolinium.
- CSF reveals mononuclear pleocytosis (> 5 cells/μL), an ↑ IgG index, or at least 2 oligoclonal bands not found in the serum (nonspecific).
- Abnormal somatosensory or visual evoked potentials may also be present.

Treatment

- **Corticosteroids** should be given during acute exacerbations.
- Immunomodulators alter relapse rates in relapsing-remitting MS and include interferon-β_{1a} (**A**vonex/**R**ebif), interferon-β_{1b} (**B**etaseron), and copolymer-1 (**C**opaxone).
- Natalizumab is an effective second-line therapy but carries a 1:500 risk for JC virus–mediated progressive multifocal leukoencephalopathy (PML).
- Mitoxantrone can be given for worsening relapsing-remitting or progressive MS.
- Alternative treatments include cyclophosphamide, IVIG, and plasmapheresis.
- **Symptomatic therapy** is crucial and includes baclofen for spasticity; cholinergics for urinary retention; anticholinergics for urinary incontinence; carbamazepine or amitriptyline for painful paresthesias; and antidepressants for clinical depression.

GUILLAIN-BARRÉ SYNDROME (GBS)

An **acute, rapidly progressive,** acquired demyelinating autoimmune disorder of the peripheral nerves that results in weakness. Also known as acute inflammatory demyelinating polyneuropathy. Associated with recent *Campylobacter jejuni* infection, viral infection, or influenza vaccination. Approximately 85% of patients make a complete or near-complete recovery (may take up to 1 year). The mortality rate is < 5%.

History/PE

- Classically presents with progressive (over days), symmetric, **ascending paralysis** (distal to proximal) involving the trunk, diaphragm, and cranial nerves. Atypical presentations are common, including variants that begin with cranial involvement or progress unpredictably to involve the respiratory muscles.
- Autonomic dysregulation, areflexia, and dysesthesias may be present.

Diagnosis

- Evidence of diffuse demyelination is seen on **nerve conduction studies,** which show ↓ nerve conduction velocity.

KEY FACT

The classic triad (Charcot's triad) in MS is scanning speech, intranuclear ophthalmoplegia, and nystagmus.

KEY FACT

Pregnancy may be associated with a ↓ in MS symptoms.

KEY FACT

For optic neuritis, give IV, not oral, corticosteroids.

MNEMONIC

The 5 A's of GBS:

Acute inflammatory demyelinating polyradiculopathy
Ascending paralysis
Autonomic neuropathy
Arrhythmias
Albuminocytologic dissociation

- Supported by a **CSF protein level > 55 mg/dL** with little or no pleocytosis (albuminocytologic dissociation).

TREATMENT

- Admit to the ICU for cases of impending **respiratory failure.**
- **Plasmapheresis** and **IVIG** are first-line treatments. Corticosteroids are **not indicated.**
- Aggressive physical rehabilitation is imperative.

AMYOTROPHIC LATERAL SCLEROSIS (ALS)

A **chronic, progressive degenerative disease** of unknown etiology characterized by loss of **upper and lower motor neurons.** Also known as **Lou Gehrig's disease.** ALS has an unrelenting course and almost always progresses to respiratory failure and death, usually within 5 years of diagnosis. Males are more commonly affected than females, and onset is generally between ages 40 and 80.

HISTORY/PE

- Presents with **asymmetric,** slowly progressive weakness (over months to years) affecting the arms, legs, diaphragm, and lower cranial nerves. Some patients initially present with **fasciculations.** Weight loss is common.
- Associated with **UMN** and/or **LMN signs** (see Table 2.10-9). Eye movements and sphincter tone are generally spared. Tongue atrophy and fasciculations may be apparent.
- Emotional lability is a common feature.

DIAGNOSIS

- The clinical presentation is usually diagnostic.
- Involvement of the tongue (CN XII) or oropharyngeal muscles (CN IX, X), known as "bulbar" involvement, suggests pathology above the foramen magnum and generally excludes the most common differential, cervical spondylosis with compressive myelopathy, as a cause.
- **EMG/nerve conduction studies** reveal widespread denervation and fibrillation potentials. Such studies are principally performed to exclude other demyelinating motor neuropathies.
- CT/MRI of the cervical spine is done to exclude structural lesions, particularly in those without bulbar involvement.

TREATMENT

Supportive measures and patient education; riluzole.

KEY FACT

A 55-year-old male presents with slowly progressive weakness in his left upper extremity and later his right, associated with fasciculations and atrophy, but without bladder disturbance and with a normal cervical MRI. Think ALS.

KEY FACT

Some 25% of people have "bulbar onset" ALS, which presents with difficulty swallowing, loss of tongue motility, and difficulty speaking (slurred or nasal quality).

TABLE 2.10-9. UMN vs. LMN Signs

CLINICAL FEATURES	UMN	LMN
Pattern of weakness	Pyramidal (arm extensors, leg flexors)	Variable
Tone	Spastic (↑); initially flaccid (↓)	Flaccid (↓)
DTRs	↑ (initially ↓ or normal)	↓
Miscellaneous signs	Babinski's, other CNS signs	Atrophy, fasciculations

Dementia

A chronic, progressive, global decline in multiple cognitive areas. Alzheimer's disease accounts for 60–80% of cases. The differential diagnosis is described in the mnemonic **DEMENTIAS.** Take care not to confuse delirium and dementia (see the Psychiatry chapter). Table 2.10-10 and the sections below contrast the time course, diagnostic criteria, and treatment of common types of dementia.

ALZHEIMER'S DISEASE (AD)

Risk factors include **age,** female gender, a **family history, Down syndrome,** and low educational status. Pathology involves **neurofibrillary tangles, neuritic plaques** with **amyloid** deposition, amyloid angiopathy, and neuronal loss.

HISTORY/PE

- **Amnesia** for newly acquired information is usually the first presenting sign, followed by language deficits, acalculia, depression, agitation, psychosis, and apraxia (inability to perform skilled movements).
- Mild cognitive impairment may precede AD by 10 years. **Survival is 5–10 years** from the onset of symptoms, with death usually occurring 2° to **aspiration pneumonia** or other infections. Except for the mental state, the physical examination is generally normal.

DIAGNOSIS

- **A diagnosis of exclusion** suggested by clinical features and by an insidiously progressive cognitive course without substantial motor impairment.

MNEMONIC

Differential diagnosis—

DEMENTIAS

Neuro**D**egenerative diseases
Endocrine
Metabolic
Exogenous
Neoplasm
Trauma
Infection
Affective disorders
Stroke/**S**tructural

TABLE 2.10-10. **Types of Dementia**

TYPE	TIME COURSE	PATHOLOGY	IMAGING/STUDIES
Alzheimer's disease (AD)	Gradual.	Diffuse atrophy with enlarged ventricles, senile plaques, and neurofibrillary tangles.	PET imaging shows nonspecific bilateral temporoparietal hypometabolism.
Vascular dementia	Abrupt.	–	Brain imaging reveals evidence of old infarctions or extensive deep white-matter changes 2° to chronic ischemia.
Pick's disease	Gradual.	**Pick bodies** (round intraneuronal inclusions).	MRI/CT show frontotemporal atrophy.
Normal pressure hydrocephalus (NPH)	Gradual/abrupt.	–	CT/MRI reveal ventricular enlargement.
Creutzfeldt-Jakob disease (CJD)	Abrupt.	Prion proteins on biopsy.	MRI with diffusion-weighted imaging may show ↑ T2 and FLAIR intensity in the putamen and the head of the caudate and is also used to exclude structural brain lesions. EEG shows **pyramidal signs and periodic sharp waves.**

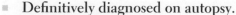

Pseudodementia. The key difference between pseudodementia and AD is that in pseudodementia, the patient is actively concerned about memory loss.

- **Definitively diagnosed on autopsy.**
- MRI or CT may show atrophy and can rule out other causes, particularly vascular dementia, NPH, and chronic subdural hematoma.
- CSF is normal.
- Neuropsychological testing can help distinguish dementia from depression. Hypothyroidism, vitamin B_{12} deficiency, and neurosyphilis should be ruled out in atypical cases.

TREATMENT

- **Prevention of associated symptoms:**
    - Provide supportive therapy for the patient and family.
    - Treat depression, agitation, sleep disorders, hallucinations, and delusions.
- **Prevention of disease progression: Cholinesterase inhibitors** (donepezil, rivastigmine, galantamine, tacrine) are first-line therapy for mild to moderate disease. Tacrine is associated with hepatotoxicity and is less often used. Memantine, an NMDA receptor antagonist, may slow decline in moderate to severe disease.

VASCULAR DEMENTIA

Dementia associated with a history of stroke and cerebrovascular disease is the second most common type of dementia. **Risk factors** include **age, hypertension, diabetes,** embolic sources, and a history of **stroke.**

DIAGNOSIS

Criteria for the diagnosis of vascular dementia include the presence of dementia and 2 or more of the following:

- Focal neurologic signs on examination.
- Symptom onset that was **abrupt,** stepwise, or related to stroke.

TREATMENT

Protocols for the prevention and treatment of vascular dementia are the same as those for stroke.

FRONTOTEMPORAL DEMENTIA (PICK'S DISEASE)

A **rare,** progressive form of dementia characterized by **atrophy of the frontal and temporal lobes.**

HISTORY/PE

- Patients present with **significant changes in behavior and personality early in the disease.** Other symptoms include speech disturbance, inattentiveness, compulsive behaviors, and occasionally extrapyramidal signs.
- Unlike Parkinson's disease, frontotemporal dementia rarely begins after age 75.

DIAGNOSIS

The diagnosis is suggested by clinical features and by evidence of circumscribed frontotemporal atrophy revealed by MRI or CT.

TREATMENT

Treatment is symptomatic.

KEY FACT

If a patient shows abrupt changes in symptoms over time rather than a steady decline, think vascular dementia.

NORMAL PRESSURE HYDROCEPHALUS (NPH)

A **potentially treatable** form of dementia that is thought to arise from impaired CSF outflow from the brain.

HISTORY/PE

Symptoms include the **classic triad of dementia, gait apraxia, and urinary incontinence.** Headaches and other signs of ↑ ICP (eg, papilledema) typically do not appear, although continuous ICP monitoring may reveal spikes of elevated pressure.

DIAGNOSIS

- The diagnosis is suggested by clinical features. The gait is classically described as "magnetic" or with "feet glued to the floor," as the forefoot is not completely dorsally extended.
- CT or MRI shows ventricular enlargement out of proportion to sulcal atrophy (see Figure 2.10-8).

TREATMENT

LP or continuous lumbar CSF drainage for several days may cause clinically significant improvement of the patient's symptoms. If so, surgical CSF shunting is the treatment of choice.

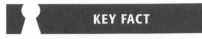

KEY FACT

NPH = "**W**et (incontinence), **W**obbly (apraxia), and **W**acky (dementia)."

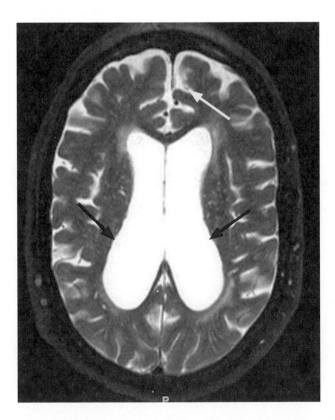

FIGURE 2.10-8.   Normal pressure hydrocephalus. T2-weighted MRI from a 60-year-old female with slowly developing urinary incontinence, gait instability, and early dementia shows marked dilation of the lateral ventricles (red arrows). This is out of proportion to the sulci (yellow arrow), which appear normal. (Reproduced with permission from USMLERx.com.)

CREUTZFELDT-JAKOB DISEASE (CJD)

Although it is the most common **prion disease,** CJD remains an extremely rare form of dementia. CJD is a member of the transmissible spongiform encephalopathies, all of which are characterized by spongy degeneration, neuronal loss, and astrocytic proliferation. In CJD, an abnormal protease-resistant prion protein accumulates in the brain.

HISTORY/PE

- CJD causes a **subacute dementia** with ataxia or startle-induced myoclonic jerks with rapid clinical decline that is noted weeks to months after symptom onset.
- New-variant CJD (mad cow disease) is a more slowly progressive prion disease seen in younger people with a history of eating contaminated beef or contaminated human brains (kuru).

DIAGNOSIS

- Suggested by clinical features.
- The differential diagnosis often includes limbic encephalitis, Hashimoto's (steroid-responsive) encephalopathy, and toxic encephalopathy (eg, lithium or bismuth).
- Elevated levels of CSF 14-3-3 and tau protein are seen.
- Definitive diagnosis can be made only by brain biopsy or autopsy. Specimens must be handled with special precautions to prevent transmission.

TREATMENT

Currently, there is no effective treatment. Most patients die within 1 year of symptom onset.

Movement Disorders

HUNTINGTON'S DISEASE (HD)

A rare, **hyperkinetic, autosomal dominant** disease involving multiple **abnormal CAG triplet repeats** (< 29 is normal) within the HD gene on chromosome 4. The number of repeats typically expands in subsequent generations, leading to earlier expression and more severe disease **(anticipation).** Life expectancy is 20 years from the time of diagnosis.

HISTORY/PE

- Presents at 30–50 years of age with gradual onset of **chorea** (sudden onset of purposeless, involuntary dancelike movements), **altered behavior,** and **dementia** (begins as irritability, clumsiness, fidgetiness, moodiness, and antisocial behavior).
- Weight loss and depression may also be seen.

DIAGNOSIS

- A clinical diagnosis confirmed by genetic testing.
- CT/MRI show cerebral atrophy (especially of the caudate and putamen; see Figure 2.10-9). Molecular genetic testing is conducted to determine the number of CAG repeats.

KEY FACT

If a patient presents with rapid cognitive decline over the course of weeks to months, think CJD.

KEY FACT

If a 43-year-old male patient presents with sudden onset of chorea, irritability, and antisocial behavior and his father experienced these symptoms at a slightly older age, think Huntington's disease.

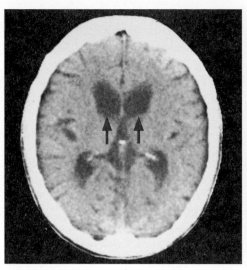
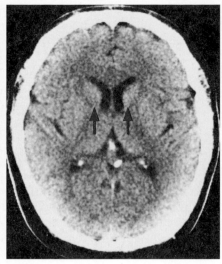

A   **B**

FIGURE 2.10-9. **Atrophy of the cerebral and caudate nuclei in Huntington's disease.**
(A) Noncontrast CT in a 54-year-old patient with Huntington's disease shows atrophy of the
caudate nuclei (arrows) and diffuse cerebral atrophy with ex vacuo dilation of the lateral ventricles. **(B)** A normal 54-year-old subject (arrows on caudate nuclei). (Reproduced with permission from
Ropper AH, Samuels MA. *Adams & Victor's Principles of Neurology,* 9th ed. New York: McGraw-Hill, 2009, Fig. 39-4.)

TREATMENT

- There is no cure, and disease progression cannot be halted. Treat symp-
  tomatically.
- Reserpine or tetrabenazine can be given to minimize unwanted movements. Psychosis should preferably be treated with atypical antipsychotics
  to ↓ the risk of extrapyramidal side effects or tardive dyskinesia. SSRIs are
  first-line therapy for depression.
- Genetic counseling should be offered to offspring.

PARKINSON'S DISEASE

An **idiopathic hypokinetic** disorder that usually begins after age 50–60 and
is attributable to **dopamine depletion** in the **substantia nigra.** It is characterized pathologically by **Lewy bodies,** which are intraneuronal eosinophilic
inclusions.

HISTORY/PE

- The **"Parkinson's tetrad"** consists of the following:
  - **Resting tremor** (eg, "pill rolling").
  - **Rigidity:** "Cogwheeling" due to the combined effects of rigidity and
    tremor.
  - **Bradykinesia:** Slowed movements as well as difficulty initiating move-
    ments. Festinating gait (a wide leg stance with short accelerating steps)
    without arm swing is also seen.
  - **Postural instability:** Stooped posture, impaired righting reflexes, freez-
    ing, falls.
- **Other manifestations:** Masked facies, memory loss, and micrographia.
- Parkinsonism is the broader clinical phenotype of bradykinesia and rigidity
  (with or without substantial tremor) and is often caused by disorders other
  than idiopathic Parkinson's disease, most commonly **multiple subcortical
  infarcts** ("vascular parkinsonism").

KEY FACT

A significant difference between the gait
abnormalities of Parkinson's and that
of NPH is preservation of arm swing in
NPH.

Q

A 65-year-old male presents to his
internist with 10 years of bilateral
hand tremors. His mother and older
brother have similar tremors. He
denies difficulty concentrating, trouble
with rising from seated positions, or
recent falls. What is the most likely
diagnosis?

- Nonidiopathic causes of parkinsonism include viral encephalitis (postencephalitic parkinsonism), trauma (dementia pugilistica), and toxins such as manganese, MPTP ("designer drugs"), and, iatrogenically, neuroleptics (tardive dyskinesia). These disorders are often diagnosed when levodopa/carbidopa fail to produce a clinical response.
- Other L-dopa-unresponsive mimics of Parkinson's disease include progressive supranuclear palsy and multiple-system atrophy.

TREATMENT

- **Levodopa/carbidopa** combination therapy is the mainstay of treatment. Levodopa is a dopamine precursor that can cross the blood-brain barrier. Carbidopa blocks the peripheral conversion of levodopa to prevent the side effects of levodopa (nausea and vomiting).
- Dopamine agonists (ropinirole, pramipexole, bromocriptine) can be used for treatment in early disease. Apomorphine is another dopamine agonist that can be used for rescue therapy if a sudden additional dose is needed.
- Selegiline (an MAO-B inhibitor) may be neuroprotective and may ↓ the need for levodopa.
- Catechol-O-methyltransferase (COMT) inhibitors (entacapone or tolcapone) are not given alone but ↑ the availability of levodopa to the brain and may ↓ motor fluctuations.
- Amantadine has mild antiparkinsonian activity and may improve akinesia, rigidity, and tremor. It can be used for temporary, short-term monotherapy early in the course of the disease.
- If medical therapy is insufficient, **surgical pallidotomy** or chronic **deep brain stimulators** may produce clinical benefit.

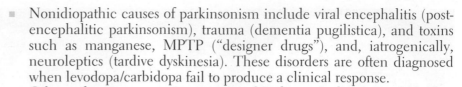

Neoplasms

Intracranial neoplasms may be 1° (30%) or **metastatic (70%)**.

- Of all 1° brain tumors, 40% are benign, and these rarely spread beyond the CNS.
- Metastatic tumors are most often from 1° **lung, breast, kidney, and GI tract neoplasms** and **melanoma.** They occur at the gray-white junction; may be multiple discrete nodules; and are characterized by rapid growth, invasiveness, necrosis, and neovascularization.
- More common in males than in females, except for meningiomas.

HISTORY/PE

- Symptoms depend on tumor type and location (see Tables 2.10-11 and 2.10-12), local growth and **resulting mass effect,** cerebral edema, or ↑ ICP 2° to ventricular obstruction. Although headaches are often thought of as the main presenting symptom, only 31% of patients present with headache at diagnosis, and only 8% have headache as the sole presenting feature.
- Seizures or slowly progressive focal motor deficits are the most common presenting features. When ↑ ICP is the presenting feature, symptoms include headache, nausea/vomiting, and diplopia (false localizing CN VI palsies). However, in the era of neuroimaging, it is relatively rare for patients to present with ↑ ICP.
- Hemispheric tumors often produce visual field abnormalities and neuropsychiatric symptoms, including personality changes, lethargy, syncope, cognitive decline, aphasia, apraxia, and depression. Parasellar lesions usually present with visual loss and/or diplopia. Posterior fossa lesions tend

TABLE 2.10-11. Common 1° Neoplasms in Adults

TUMOR	PATHOLOGY	PRESENTATION	TREATMENT
Astrocytoma	Arises in brain parenchyma. Low-grade astrocytomas are relatively uncommon.	Presents with seizures, focal deficits, or headache; has a **protracted course.** Has a better prognosis than glioblastoma multiforme.	Resection if possible; radiation.
Glioblastoma multiforme (grade IV astrocytoma)	High mitotic activity and either endothelial proliferation or necrosis in tumor, leading to ring-enhancing lesions on MRI.	The most common 1° brain tumor. Presents with headache, seizures, or focal deficits. Progresses rapidly and has a poor prognosis (< 1 year from the time of prognosis).	Surgical removal/resection. Radiation and chemotherapy have variable results.
Meningioma	Originates from the **dura mater or arachnoid.**	Presentation depends on location; often related to cranial neuropathy or is an incidental finding. Has a good prognosis; incidence ↑ with age. Imaging may reveal **dural tail.**	Surgical resection; radiation for unresectable tumors.
Acoustic neuroma (schwannoma)	Derived from **Schwann cells.**	Presents with ipsilateral tinnitus, hearing loss, vertigo, and late signs of CN V–VII or brainstem compression.	Observation; surgical removal.

- to present with gait ataxia or cranial nerve deficits and/or ↑ ICP from obstructive hydrocephalus.
- Metastases that tend to present with intracranial hemorrhage include renal cell carcinoma, thyroid papillary cancer, choriocarcinoma, and melanoma.

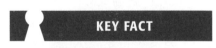
KEY FACT

Lung and **S**kin **G**o to the **BR**ain: **L**ung, **S**kin, **G**I, **B**reast, **R**enal.

TABLE 2.10-12. Common 1° Neoplasms in Children

TUMOR	PATHOLOGY	PRESENTATION	TREATMENT
Medulloblastoma	A primitive neuroectodermal tumor. Arises from the fourth ventricle and causes ↑ ICP.	**Highly malignant;** may seed the subarachnoid space. May cause obstructive hydrocephalus.	Surgical resection coupled with radiation and chemotherapy.
Ependymoma	May arise from the ependyma of a ventricle (commonly the fourth) or the spinal cord.	Low grade. May cause obstructive hydrocephalus.	Surgical resection; radiation.
Craniopharyngioma	The most common suprasellar tumor in children. Calcification is common.	Benign. May cause hypopituitarism.	Surgical resection.

KEY FACT

Two-thirds of 1° brain tumors in adults are supratentorial. One-third of those in children are supratentorial.

KEY FACT

Symptoms of ↑ ICP:
- Nausea
- Vomiting
- Diplopia
- Headache that is worse in the morning, with bending over, or with recumbency

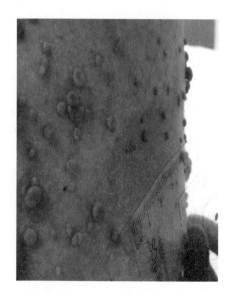

FIGURE 2.10-10. **Neurofibromas associated with neurofibromatosis.** (Reproduced with permission from USMLERx.com.)

KEY FACT

NF1 and NF2 are clinically evident by ages 15 and 20, respectively.

DIAGNOSIS

- Contrast CT and MRI with and without gadolinium to localize and determine the extent of the lesion. Gadolinium-enhanced MRI is generally better for visualizing soft tissue tumors and vascularity, but CT is preferred for evaluating skull base lesions and for emergencies (eg, obstructive hydrocephalus) when an MRI cannot be rapidly acquired.
- Histologic diagnosis via CT-guided biopsy or surgical tumor debulking/removal.

TREATMENT

- **Resection** (if possible), **radiation,** and **chemotherapy.**
- Therapy is highly dependent on tumor type, histology, progression, and site (see Tables 2.10-11 and 2.10-12).
- **Corticosteroids** can be used to ↓ vasogenic edema and ICP. Management is often palliative.
- Seizure prophylaxis can be used in patients who have had a seizure.

Neurocutaneous Disorders

NEUROFIBROMATOSIS (NF)

The most common neurocutaneous disorder. There are **2 major types:** neurofibromatosis 1 (NF1, or von Recklinghausen's syndrome) and neurofibromatosis 2 (NF2). Both obey **autosomal dominant inheritance.** The NF genes are located on **chromosome 17 and 22,** respectively, for NF1 and NF2.

HISTORY/PE

- Diagnostic criteria for **NF1** include 2 or more of the following:
  - Six **café au lait spots** (each ≥ 5 mm in children or ≥ 15 mm in adults).
  - Two neurofibromas of any type (see Figure 2.10-10).
  - **Freckling in the axillary or inguinal area.**
  - **Optic glioma.**
  - Two **Lisch nodules** (pigmented iris hamartomas).
  - Bone abnormality (eg, kyphoscoliosis).
  - A **first-degree relative** with NF1.
- Diagnostic criteria for **NF2** are as follows:
  - **Bilateral acoustic neuromas** or a first-degree relative with NF2 and **either** unilateral acoustic neuromas or 2 of any of the following: neurofibromas, meningiomas, gliomas, or schwannoma.
  - Other features include seizures, skin nodules, and café au lait spots.

DIAGNOSIS

- **MRI** of the brain, brainstem, and spine with gadolinium.
- Conduct a complete dermatologic exam, ophthalmologic exam, and family history. Auditory testing is recommended.

TREATMENT

- There is no cure; treatment is symptomatic (eg, surgery for kyphoscoliosis or debulking of tumors).
- Acoustic neuromas and optic gliomas can be treated with surgery or radiosurgery. Meningiomas may be resected.

TUBEROUS SCLEROSIS

Affects **many organ systems,** including the CNS, skin, heart, retina, and kidneys. Obeys **autosomal dominant** inheritance.

HISTORY/PE

- Presents with **convulsive seizures** (infantile spasms in infants), **"ash-leaf"** **hypopigmented lesions** on the trunk and extremities, and **mental retardation** (↑ likelihood with early age of onset).
- Other skin manifestations include **sebaceous adenomas** (small red nodules on the nose and cheeks in the shape of a butterfly) and a **shagreen patch** (a rough papule in the lumbosacral region with an orange-peel consistency).
- Two retinal lesions are recognized: (1) mulberry tumors, which arise from the nerve head; and (2) phakomas, which are round, flat, gray lesions located peripherally in the retina.
- Symptoms are 2° to small benign tumors that grow on the face, eyes, brain, kidney, and other organs.
- Mental retardation and CHF from cardiac rhabdomyoma may also be seen.
- Renal involvement may include hamartomas, angiomyolipomas, or, rarely, renal cell carcinoma.

DIAGNOSIS

- Diagnosis is usually clinical.
- Skin lesions are enhanced by a Wood's UV lamp.
- Imaging:
    - **Head CT:** Reveals calcified tubers within the cerebrum in the periventricular area. Lesions may on rare occasion transform into malignant astrocytomas.
    - **ECG:** Evaluate for rhabdomyoma of the heart, especially in the apex of the left ventricle (affects > 50% of patients).
    - **Renal ultrasound:** May reveal angiomyolipomas, cysts, or, rarely, renal cell carcinoma.
    - **Renal CT:** May show angiomyolipomas (these lesions are also thought to be responsible for the cystic or fibrous pulmonary changes sometimes seen in tuberous sclerosis patients).
    - **CXR:** May reveal pulmonary lesions or cardiomegaly 2° to rhabdomyoma.

KEY FACT

If you see infantile spasms in the setting of a hypopigmented lesion on the child's trunk, consider tuberous sclerosis.

TREATMENT

- Treatment should be based on symptoms (eg, cosmetic surgery for adenoma sebaceum).
- Simple partial or complex partial seizures can be controlled with oxcarbazepine or carbamazepine; lamotrigine can be given for generalized seizures. Treat infantile spasms with ACTH or vigabatrin.
- Surgical intervention may be indicated in the setting of ↑ ICP or for seizures associated with an epileptogenic focus or severe developmental delay.

Aphasia

A general term for speech and language disorders. Usually results from insults (eg, strokes, tumors, abscesses) to the "dominant hemisphere" (the left hemisphere in > 95% of right-handed people and 60–80% of left-handed people).

BROCA'S APHASIA

- A disorder of language production, including writing, with intact comprehension. Due to an insult to Broca's area in the **posterior inferior frontal gyrus** (see Figure 2.10-11). Often 2° to a left superior **MCA stroke.** Also known as **motor aphasia.**
- Hx/PE:
  - Presents with **impaired speech production, frustration** with awareness of deficits, arm and facial **hemiparesis,** hemisensory loss, and apraxia of the oral muscles. Speech is described as "telegraphic" and agrammatical with frequent pauses.
  - In true Broca's aphasia, repetition is impaired. If repetition is intact, the deficit is called transcortical motor aphasia (TMA), which is due to a lesion around Broca's area.
- Tx: **Speech therapy** (varying outcomes with intermediate prognosis).

WERNICKE'S APHASIA

- A disorder of language comprehension with intact yet nonsensical production.
- Due to an insult to Wernicke's area in the left posterior superior temporal (perisylvian) gyrus. Often 2° to left **inferior/posterior MCA** embolic stroke (see Figure 2.10-11).
- Hx/PE:
  - Presents with **preserved fluency** of language with impaired repetition and comprehension, leading to **"word salad."** Patients are unable to follow commands; make frequent use of **neologisms** (made-up words) and paraphasic errors (word substitutions); and show **lack of awareness** of deficits.
  - In true Wernicke's aphasia, repetition is impaired. If repetition is intact, the deficit is called transcortical sensory aphasia (TSA), which is due to a lesion around Wernicke's area.
- Tx: Treat the underlying etiology and institute speech therapy.

Coma

A state of unconsciousness marked by a profound suppression of responses to external and internal stimuli (ie, a state of unarousable unresponsiveness). Lesser states of impaired arousal are known as "obtundation" or "stupor." Coma is due to either catastrophic structural CNS injury or diffuse metabolic dysfunction. Coma indicates bilateral dysfunction of both cerebral hemispheres or the brainstem (pons or higher); when structural, coma usually results from bilateral pathology. Causes include the following:

- Diffuse **hypoxic/ischemic encephalopathy** (eg, postcardiac arrest).
- **Diffuse axonal injury** from high-acceleration trauma (eg, motor vehicle accidents).

KEY FACT

So many names, it's a wonder we are talking about aphasias!
- Broca's aphasia = motor aphasia, expressive aphasia, or nonfluent aphasia.
- Wernicke's aphasia = sensory aphasia, fluent aphasia, or receptive aphasia.

KEY FACT

- Broca's aphasia—posterior inferior frontal gyrus.
- Wernicke's aphasia—left posterior superior temporal gyrus.

KEY FACT

BROca's is **BRO**ken and **W**ernicke's is **W**ordy.

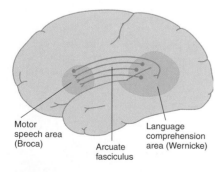

Motor speech area (Broca)
Arcuate fasciculus
Language comprehension area (Wernicke)

FIGURE 2.10-11. Broca's and Wernicke's areas. (Reproduced with permission from Waxman SG. *Clinical Neuroanatomy,* 26th ed. New York: McGraw-Hill, 2010, Fig. 21-1.)

- **Brain herniation** (eg, cerebral mass lesion, SAH with obstructive hydrocephalus).
- **Widespread infection** (eg, viral encephalitis or advanced bacterial meningitis).
- **Massive brainstem hemorrhage or infarction** (eg, pontine myelinolysis).
- **Electrolyte disturbances** (eg, hypoglycemia).
- **Exogenous toxins** (eg, opiates, benzodiazepines, EtOH, other drugs).
- Generalized **seizure** activity or postictal states.
- **Endocrine** (eg, severe hypothyroidism) or **metabolic dysfunction** (eg, thiamine deficiency).

HISTORY/PE

- Obtain a complete medical history from witnesses, including current medications (eg, **sedatives**).
- Conduct thorough medical and neurologic exams, including assessments of mental status, spontaneous motor activity, muscular tone, breathing pattern, funduscopy, pupillary response, eye movements (including the doll's-eye maneuver if the neck has been cleared from fracture), corneal reflex, cold-water caloric testing, gag reflex, and motor or autonomic responses to noxious stimuli applied to the limbs, trunk, and face (eg, retromandibular pressure, nasal tickle).

DIAGNOSIS

- Typically made by a combination of the history/physical and laboratory tests or neuroimaging.
- Check glucose, electrolytes, calcium, a renal panel, LFTs, ABGs, a toxicology screen, and blood and CSF cultures. Other metabolic tests (eg, TSH) may be performed based on the clinical index of suspicion.
- Obtain a **head CT without contrast** before other imaging to evaluate for hemorrhage or structural changes. Imaging should **precede LP** in light of the risk of herniation.
- Obtain an MRI to exclude structural changes and ischemia (eg, brainstem). **EEG** may be both diagnostic and prognostic.
- Rule out catatonia, hysterical or conversion unresponsiveness, **"locked-in" syndrome**, or **persistent vegetative state** (PVS), all of which can be confused with true coma (see Table 2.10-13).
  - **"Locked-in" syndrome:** Patients are awake and alert but can move only their eyes and eyelids. Associated with central pontine myelinolysis, brainstem stroke, and advanced ALS.

TABLE 2.10-13. **Differential Diagnosis of Coma**

VARIABLE	"LOCKED-IN" SYNDROME	PVS	COMA	BRAIN DEATH
Alertness	Wakeful and alert with retained cognitive abilities.	Wakefulness without awareness. Eyes open.	Unconscious; no sleep-wake cycles. Eyes closed.	Unconscious; no sleep-wake cycles.
Most common causes	Central pontine myelinolysis, brainstem stroke, advanced ALS.	Diffuse cortical injury or hypoxic ischemic injury.	See above.	Same as coma.
Voluntary motor ability	Eyes and eyelids.	None.	None.	None.
Respiratory drive	Yes.	Yes.	Yes.	None.

■ **PVS:** Characterized by normal wake-sleep cycles but lack of awareness of self or the environment. The most common causes are trauma with diffuse cortical injury or hypoxic ischemic injury.

TREATMENT

Initial treatment should consist of the following measures:

■ **Stabilize the patient:** Attend to **ABCs.**
■ **Reverse the reversible:** Administer **DONT**—Dextrose, Oxygen, Naloxone, and Thiamine.
■ **Identify and treat the underlying cause** and associated complications.
■ **Prevent further damage.**

KEY FACT

Artificial life support can be discontinued **only** after 2 physicians have declared the patient legally brain dead.

Nutritional Deficiencies

Table 2.10-14 describes neurologic syndromes commonly associated with nutritional deficiencies.

TABLE 2.10-14. Neurologic Syndromes Associated with Nutritional Deficiencies

VITAMIN	SYNDROME	SIGNS/SYMPTOMS	CLASSIC PATIENTS	TREATMENT
Thiamine (vitamin B₁)	Wernicke's encephalopathy	The classic triad consists of **encephalopathy** (disorientation, inattentiveness, confusion, coma), **ophthalmoplegia** (nystagmus, lateral rectus palsy, conjugate gaze palsy, vertical gaze palsy), and **ataxia** (polyneuropathy; cerebellar and vestibular dysfunction leading to problems standing or walking).	**Alcoholics, hyperemesis, starvation, renal dialysis,** AIDS. **Can be brought on or exacerbated by high-dose glucose administration.**	Reversible almost immediately with thiamine administration. Always give thiamine before glucose.
	Korsakoff's dementia	Above plus anterograde and retrograde amnesia, horizontal nystagmus, and confabulations.	Same as above. Usually occurs in the "resolution" phase of Wernicke's syndrome that was treated too late or inadequately.	Irreversible.
Cyano-cobalamin (vitamin B₁₂)ᵃ	Combined system disease (CSD) or subacute combined degeneration of the posterior and lateral columns of the spinal cord; peripheral neuropathy.	Gradual, progressive onset. Symmetric paresthesias, stocking-glove sensory neuropathy, leg stiffness, spasticity, paraplegia, bowel and bladder dysfunction, sore tongue. Dementia.	Patients with pernicious anemia; strict vegetarians; status post gastric or ileal resection; ileal disease (eg, Crohn's); alcoholics or others with malnutrition.	B₁₂ injections or large oral doses.
Folateᵃ	Folate deficiency	Irritability; personality changes without the neurologic symptoms of CSD.	Alcoholics; patients with pernicious anemia.	Reversible if corrected early.

ᵃ Associated with ↑ homocysteine and an ↑ risk of vascular events.

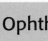

Ophthalmology

VISUAL FIELD DEFECTS

Figure 2.10-12 illustrates common visual field defects and the anatomic areas with which they are associated.

GLAUCOMA

In the eye, aqueous humor is produced by the ciliary body on the iris, travels through the pupil into the anterior chamber, and is then drained via the trabecular meshwork in the angle of the anterior chamber.

- Any process that disrupts this natural flow can ↑ **intraocular pressure (IOP)**, damaging the optic nerve and causing visual field deficits. Glaucoma is the result of such damage to the nerve.
- Open-angle glaucoma is much more common in the United States than closed-angle glaucoma.

Closed-Angle Glaucoma

- Occurs when the iris dilates and pushes against the lens of the eye, disrupting flow of aqueous humor into the anterior chamber. Pressure in the posterior chamber then pushes the peripheral iris forward and blocks the angle.
- Risk factors include family history, older age, Asian ethnicity, hyperopia, prolonged **pupillary dilation** (prolonged time in a dark area, stress, medications), anterior uveitis, and lens dislocation.
- **Hx/PE:**
  - Presents with extreme eye pain, blurred vision, headache, nausea, and vomiting.
  - A hard, red eye is seen (from acute closure of a narrow anterior chamber angle); the pupil is dilated and nonreactive to light.

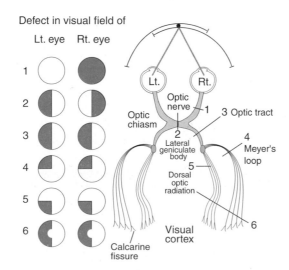

FIGURE 2.10-12. **Visual field defects.** (1) Right anopsia. (2) Bitemporal hemianopsia. (3) Left homonymous hemianopsia. (4) Left upper quadrantic anopsia (right temporal lesion). (5) Left lower quadrantic anopsia (right parietal lesion). (6) Left hemianopsia with macular sparing.

A 45-year-old Caucasian male presents to the ER with sudden-onset headache and a right-sided dilated pupil. His right pupil is nonreactive to light and hard to the touch. What is the most likely diagnosis, and what medications should be avoided in this patient?

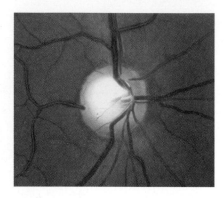

FIGURE 2.10-13. Open-angle glaucoma with an increased cup-to-disk ratio. (Reproduced with permission from USMLERx.com.)

A

Closed-angle glaucoma. Avoid pupil-dilating medications such as atropine, which will ↑ IOP and prevent drainage of aqueous humor.

- If it resolves spontaneously prior to presentation (eg, with pupillary constriction in sunlight), ophthalmologic examination may reveal narrow angles in 1 or both eyes.
- **Dx:** Diagnosis is based on clinical history and examination. Those that resolve may mimic a migraine headache with blurred vision.
- **Tx:** A **medical emergency** that can cause blindness. Treatment to ↓ IOP is as follows:
  - Eyedrops (timolol, pilocarpine, apraclonidine).
  - Systemic medications (oral or IV acetazolamide, IV mannitol).
  - **Laser peripheral iridotomy,** which creates a hole in the peripheral iris, is curative and may be performed prophylactically.
  - Do not give any medications that cause pupillary dilation.

Open-Angle Glaucoma

- Flow of aqueous humor through the trabecular meshwork is limited, increasing IOP. A diseased trabecular meshwork obstructs proper drainage of the eye, leading to a gradual ↑ in pressure and progressive vision loss.
- Risk factors include age > 40 years, **African American ethnicity,** diabetes, and myopia.
- **Hx/PE:**
  - Should be suspected in patients > 35 years of age who need **frequent lens changes** and have mild headaches, visual disturbances, and impaired adaptation to darkness.
  - Usually asymptomatic until late in the clinical course.
  - Characterized by gradual loss of peripheral vision.
  - **Cupping** of the optic nerve head is seen on funduscopic exam (see Figure 2.10-13).
- **Dx:** Tonometry, ophthalmoscopic visualization of the optic nerve, and visual field testing are most important. A diseased trabecular meshwork obstructs proper drainage of the eye, gradually increasing pressure and leading to progressive vision loss.
- **Tx:**
  - Treat with topical β-blockers (timolol, betaxolol) to ↓ aqueous humor production or with pilocarpine to ↑ aqueous outflow.
  - Carbonic anhydrase inhibitors may also be used.
  - If medication fails, laser trabeculoplasty or a trabeculectomy can improve aqueous drainage.

CATARACTS

- Lens opacification resulting in obstructed passage of light. Associated with diabetes, hypertension, advanced age, and exposure to radiation.
- **Hx/PE:** Presents with loss of visual acuity and difficulty with night vision.
- **Tx:** No medical therapy is available. Surgical lens removal and replacement.

AGE-RELATED MACULAR DEGENERATION (AMD)

More common among Caucasians, females, smokers, and those with a family history.

HISTORY/PE

- Presents with **painless loss of central vision.** Early signs include distortion of straight lines.
- **Atrophic ("dry") macular degeneration:** Responsible for 80% of cases. Causes gradual vision loss.

■ **Exudative or neovascular ("wet") macular degeneration:** Much less common, but associated with more rapid and severe vision damage.

DIAGNOSIS

Funduscopy by an ophthalmologist reveals drusen and/or pigmentary changes in patients with atrophic AMD. Hemorrhage and subretinal fluid are suggestive of exudative AMD (see Figure 2.10-14).

TREATMENT

■ **Atrophic AMD:**
  ■ No treatment is currently available, although a combination of vitamins (vitamin C, vitamin E, beta-carotene, and zinc) has been found to slow disease progression.
  ■ An ↑ mortality rate from high doses of vitamin E and an elevated lung cancer incidence among individuals on beta-carotene supplementation may require modification of this regimen for smokers.
■ **Exudative AMD:**
  ■ VEGF inhibitors have been shown to improve vision (ranibizumab, bevacizumab) or slow visual loss (pegaptanib) in patients with exudative AMD.
  ■ Photodynamic therapy with verteporfin, which involves use of a laser to selectively target retinal vessels, may be useful in conjunction with VEGF inhibitors.

KEY FACT

In the United States, macular degeneration is the leading cause of permanent bilateral visual loss in the elderly.

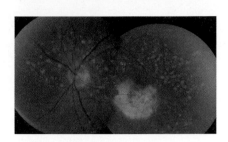

FIGURE 2.10-14. Macular degeneration with evidence of drusen and fibrosis in the macula. (Reproduced with permission from USMLERx.com.)

RETINAL VASCULAR OCCLUSION

■ Occurs in **elderly patients** and is often idiopathic.
■ **Hx/PE:**
  ■ **Central retinal artery occlusion:** Presents with sudden, **painless, unilateral blindness.** The pupil reacts to a near stimulus but is sluggishly reactive to direct light. Patients present with a **cherry-red spot** on the fovea, retinal swelling (whitish appearance to the nerve fiber layer), and retinal arteries that may appear bloodless.
  ■ **Central retinal vein occlusion:** Characterized by rapid, **painless** vision loss of variable severity. Associated with hypertension. A choked, swollen optic disk with hemorrhages, venous stasis retinal hemorrhages, cotton-wool spots, and edema of the macula may be seen on funduscopic exam.
■ **Tx:**
  ■ **Central retinal artery occlusion:** Treatments should be applied immediately before irreversible retinal infarction and permanent blindness ensue.
    ■ **Intra-arterial thrombolysis** of the ophthalmic artery within **8 hours** of onset of symptoms may produce benefit in some patients, although evidence remains controversial.
    ■ Other treatments applied but of unclear benefit include decreasing IOP through drainage of the anterior chamber, ocular massage and high-flow oxygen, or IV acetazolamide.
  ■ **Central retinal vein occlusion:** Laser photocoagulation has variable results.

NOTES

OBSTETRICS

Physiology of Normal Pregnancy

THE BASICS OF PREGNANCY

The following terms and concepts are central to an understanding of the physiologic processes of pregnancy.

- **Gravidity:** The number of times a woman has been pregnant.
- **Parity:**
    - The number of pregnancies that led to a birth beyond 20 weeks' gestational age or an infant weighing > 500 g.
    - In prenatal assessment, **P####** expresses the number of term deliveries, the number of preterm deliveries, the number of abortuses, and the number of living children.
- **Developmental age (DA):** The number of weeks and days since fertilization; usually unknown.
- **Gestational age (GA):** The number of weeks and days measured from the first day of the last menstrual period (LMP). GA can also be determined by:
    - **Fundal height:** Umbilicus – 20 weeks + 2–3 cm/week thereafter.
    - **Fetal heart tones (Doppler):** Typically 10–12 weeks.
    - **Quickening, or appreciation of fetal movement:** Occurs at 17–18 weeks at the earliest.
    - **Ultrasound:**
        - Measures fetal crown-rump length (CRL) at 6–12 weeks.
        - Measures biparietal diameter (BPD), femur length (FL), and abdominal circumference (AC) from 13 weeks.
        - Ultrasound measurement of GA is most reliable during the first trimester.

KEY FACT

A G3P1 woman is one who has had 3 pregnancies but only 1 birth beyond 20 weeks' GA and/or an infant who weighs at least 500 g.

KEY FACT

Get a quantitative β-hCG:
- To diagnose and follow ectopic pregnancy.
- To monitor trophoblastic disease.
- To screen for fetal aneuploidy.

DIAGNOSIS OF PREGNANCY

β-hCG

- The standard for diagnosing pregnancy.
- Produced by the placenta; peaks at 100,000 mIU/mL by 10 weeks' GA.
- ↓ throughout the second trimester; levels off in the third trimester.
- **hCG levels double approximately every 48 hours during early pregnancy.** This is often used to diagnose ectopic pregnancy when doubling is abnormal.

Ultrasound

- Used to confirm an intrauterine pregnancy.
- The gestational sac is visible by:
    - Five weeks' GA.
    - A β-hCG in the range of 1000–1500 IU/mL.

NORMAL PHYSIOLOGY OF PREGNANCY

The normal physiologic changes that occur during pregnancy are graphically illustrated according to system in Figures 2.11-1 and 2.11-2.

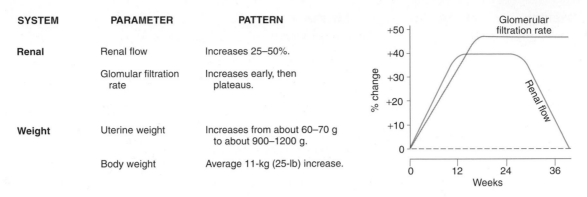

SYSTEM	PARAMETER	PATTERN
Renal	Renal flow	Increases 25–50%.
	Glomular filtration rate	Increases early, then plateaus.
Weight	Uterine weight	Increases from about 60–70 g to about 900–1200 g.
	Body weight	Average 11-kg (25-lb) increase.

FIGURE 2.11-1.   Renal and uterine/body weight changes in normal pregnancy. (Reproduced with permission from Gardner DG, Shoback D. *Greenspan's Basic & Clinical Endocrinology,* 8th ed. New York: McGraw-Hill, 2007, Fig. 17-2A.)

Prenatal Care

The goal of prenatal care is to prevent, diagnose, and treat conditions that can lead to adverse outcomes in pregnancy. Expected weight gain, nutrition, and exercise recommendations are outlined in Table 2.11-1. See Table 2.11-2 for some important factors that can cross the placenta.

TABLE 2.11-1.   Recommendations for Standard Prenatal Care

CATEGORY	RECOMMENDATIONS
Weight gain	Guidelines for weight gain in pregnancy: ▪ **Excessive gain:** > 1.5 kg/mo. ▪ **Inadequate gain:** < 1.0 kg/mo. Guidelines according to prepregnancy body mass index (BMI): ▪ **Underweight** (BMI < 19.8): 12–18 kg. ▪ **Acceptable** (BMI 19.8–26.0): 11–16 kg. ▪ **Overweight** (BMI 26.1–29.0): 7–11 kg. ▪ **Severely overweight** (BMI > 29.0): 7 kg.
Nutrition	Guidelines for nutritional supplementation: ▪ An additional 100–300 kcal/day; 500 kcal/day during breastfeeding. ▪ **Folic acid supplements** (↓ neural tube defects for **all** reproductive-age women): 0.4 mg/day, or 4 mg/day for women with a history of neural tube defects in prior pregnancies. ▪ **Iron:** Starting at the first visit, 30 mg/day of elemental iron (or 150 mg of iron sulfate). ▪ **Calcium:** 1300 mg/day for women < 19 years of age; 1000 mg/day for those > 19 years of age. Additional guidelines for complete vegetarians: ▪ **Vitamin D:** 10 μg or 400 IU/day. ▪ **Vitamin B$_{12}$:** 2 μg/day.
Exercise	Thirty minutes of moderate exercise daily.

SYSTEM	PARAMETER	PATTERN
Cardiovascular	Heart rate	Gradually increases 20%.
	Blood pressure	Gradually decreases 10% by 34 weeks, then increases to prepregnancy values.
	Stroke volume	Increases to maximum at 19 weeks, then plateaus.
	Cardiac output	Rises rapidly by 20%, then gradually increases an additional 10% by 28 weeks.
	Peripheral venous distention	Progressive increase to term.
	Peripheral vascular resistance	Progressive decrease to term.
Pulmonary	Respiratory rate	Unchanged.
	Tidal volume	Increases by 30–40%.
	Expiratory reserve	Gradual decrease.
	Vital capacity	Unchanged.
	Respiratory minute volume	Increases by 40%.
Blood	Volume	Increases by 50% in second trimester.
	Hematocrit	Decreases slightly.
	Fibrinogen	Increases.
	Electrolytes	Unchanged.
Gastrointestinal	Sphincter tone	Decreases.
	Gastric emptying time	Increases.

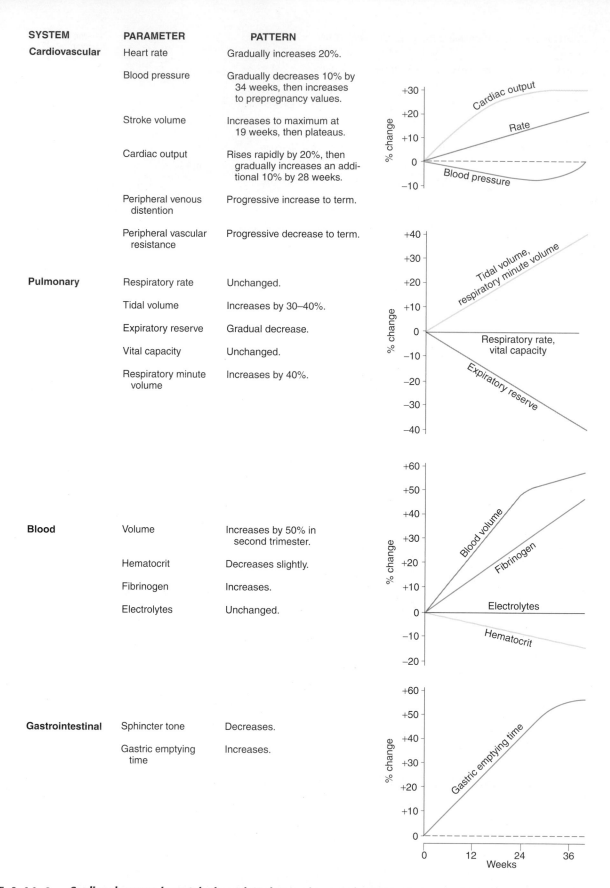

FIGURE 2.11-2. Cardiopulmonary, hematologic, and GI changes in normal pregnancy. (Reproduced with permission from Gardner DG, Shoback D. *Greenspan's Basic & Clinical Endocrinology,* 8th ed. New York: McGraw-Hill, 2007, Fig. 17-2B.)

TABLE 2.11-2.   Factors That Can Cross the Placenta

IMMUNOGLOBULINS	ORGANISMS	DRUGS
IgG	Toxoplasmosis Rubella HIV Parvovirus CMV Enteroviruses *Treponema pallidum* *Listeria monocytogenes* Parvovirus B19	See the teratology discussion below.

Prenatal Diagnostic Testing

Table 2.11-3 outlines a typical prenatal diagnostic testing schedule by week. The sections that follow describe each recommended screening modality.

TABLE 2.11-3.   Prenatal Diagnostic Testing Schedule

WEEKS	PRENATAL DIAGNOSTIC TESTING
Prenatal visits	**Weeks 0–28:** Every 4 weeks. **Weeks 29–35:** Every 2 weeks. **Weeks 36–birth:** Every week.
Initial visit	**Heme:** CBC, Rh factor, type and screen. **Infectious disease:** UA and culture, rubella antibody titer, HBsAg, RPR/VDRL, cervical gonorrhea and chlamydia, PPD, HIV, Pap smear (to check for dysplasia). Consider HCV and varicella based on history. **If indicated:** HbA_{1c}, sickle cell screening. **Discuss genetic screening:** Tay-Sachs disease, cystic fibrosis.
9–14 weeks	Offer PAPP-A + nuchal transparency + free β-hCG +/− chorionic villus sampling (CVS).
15–22 weeks	Offer maternal serum α-fetoprotein (MSAFP) or quad screen (AFP, estriol, β-hCG, and inhibin A) +/− amniocentesis.
18–20 weeks	Ultrasound for full anatomic screen.
24–28 weeks	One-hour glucose challenge test for gestational diabetes screen.
28–30 weeks	RhoGAM for Rh-⊖ women (after antibody screen).
35–40 weeks	Group B strep culture (GBS); repeat CBC.
34–40 weeks	Cervical chlamydia and gonorrhea cultures, HIV, RPR in high-risk patients.

QUAD SCREENING

- **Quad screening** consists of the following 4 elements (see also Table 2.11-4):
  1. MSAFP
  2. Inhibin A
  3. Estriol
  4. β-hCG
- MSAFP is produced by the fetus and enters the maternal circulation. Results are reported as multiples of the median (MoMs).
  - Measurement results depend on accurate gestational dating.
  - MSAFP is rarely tested alone, as quad screening has ↑ sensitivity for detecting chromosomal abnormalities.
- **Elevated MSAFP (> 2.5 MoMs) is associated with:**
  - Open neural tube defects (anencephaly, spina bifida)
  - Abdominal wall defects (gastroschisis, omphalocele)
  - Multiple gestation
  - Incorrect gestational dating
  - Fetal death
  - Placental abnormalities (eg, placental abruption)
- **Reduced MSAFP (< 0.5 MoM) is associated with:**
  - Trisomy 21 and 18
  - Fetal demise
  - Inaccurate gestational dating

PREGNANCY-ASSOCIATED PLASMA PROTEIN A (PAPP-A)

- Recommended at weeks 9–14.
- PAPP-A + nuchal transparency + free β-hCG can detect ~ 91% of cases of Down syndrome and ~ 95% of cases of trisomy 18.
- Advantages:
  - A screen of **low-risk** pregnant women (< 35 years of age).
  - Available earlier than CVS and less invasive than CVS (see below).

CHORIONIC VILLUS SAMPLING (CVS)

Table 2.11-5 outlines the relative advantages and disadvantages of CVS and amniocentesis (see also Figure 2.11-3).

TABLE 2.11-4. Quad Screening

	MSAFP	ESTRIOL	INHIBIN A	β-hCG
Trisomy 18	↓	↓	↓	↓
Trisomy 21	↓	↓	↑	↑

TABLE 2.11-5. **CVS vs. Amniocentesis**

VARIABLE	CVS	AMNIOCENTESIS
GA	10–12 weeks.	15–20 weeks.
Procedure	Transcervical or transabdominal aspiration of placental tissue.	Transabdominal aspiration of amniotic fluid using an ultrasound-guided needle.
Advantages	Genetically diagnostic. Available at an earlier GA.	Genetically diagnostic.
Disadvantages	Risk of fetal loss is 1%. Cannot detect open neural tube defects. Limb defects are associated with CVS at < 9 weeks.	Premature rupture of membranes (PROM), chorioamnionitis, fetal-maternal hemorrhage.

AMNIOCENTESIS

Indicated for the following:

- In women who will be > **35 years of age at the time of delivery.**
- In conjunction with an abnormal quad screen.
- In Rh-sensitized pregnancy to obtain fetal blood type or to detect fetal hemolysis.
- To evaluate fetal lung maturity via a lecithin-to-sphingomyelin ratio ≥ 2.5 or to detect the presence of phosphatidylglycerol (performed during the third trimester).

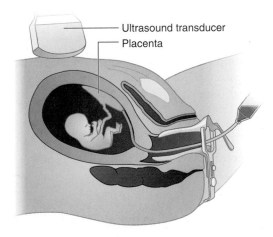

Ultrasound transducer
Placenta

FIGURE 2.11-3. **Chorionic villus sampling.** (Reproduced with permission from Cunningham FG et al. *Williams Obstetrics*, 23rd ed. New York: McGraw-Hill, 2010, Fig. 13-7.)

Teratology

Major defects are apparent in about 3% of births and in roughly 4.5% of children by 5 years of age. Table 2.11-6 outlines common teratogenic agents.

Maternal-Fetal Infections

- May occur at any time during pregnancy, labor, and delivery. Common sequelae include the following:
  - Premature delivery
  - CNS abnormalities
  - Anemia
  - Jaundice
  - Hepatosplenomegaly
  - Growth retardation
- The most common pathogens involved can be remembered through use of the mnemonic **TORCHeS** (see also Table 2.11-7).

MNEMONIC

TORCHeS pathogens:

Toxoplasmosis
Other[a]
Rubella
CMV
Herpes simplex virus
HIV
Syphilis

[a] Parvovirus, varicella, *Listeria*, TB, malaria, fungi.

KEY FACT

Pregnant women should not change the cat's litterbox.

Spontaneous Abortion (SAB)

The loss of POC prior to the 20th week of pregnancy. More than 80% of cases occur in the first trimester. Risk factors are as follows:

- **Chromosomal abnormalities:** A factor in approximately 50% of SABs in the first trimester, 20–30% in second-trimester losses, and 5–10% in third-trimester losses.
- **Maternal factors:**
  - **Inherited thrombophilias:** Factor V Leiden, prothrombin, antithrombin, proteins C and S, methylene tetrahydrofolate reductase (hyperhomocysteinemia).
  - **Immunologic issues:** Antiphospholipid antibodies; alloimmune factors.
  - **Anatomic issues:** Uterine abnormalities, incompetent cervix, cervical conization or loop electrosurgical excision procedure (LEEP), cervical injury, DES exposure, anatomic abnormalities of the cervix.
  - **Endocrinologic issues:** Diabetes mellitus (DM), hypothyroidism, progesterone deficiency.
  - **Other:** Maternal trauma, ↑ maternal age, infection, dietary deficiencies.
- **Environmental factors:** Tobacco, alcohol, caffeine (> 500 mg of caffeine per day), toxins, drugs, radiation.
- **Fetal factors:** Anatomic malformation.

HISTORY/PE
See Table 2.11-8 for types of SAB.

DIAGNOSIS
- ↓ levels of hCG.
- Ultrasound can identify:
  - The gestational sac 5–6 weeks from the LMP.
  - The fetal pole at 6 weeks.
  - Fetal cardiac activity at 6–7 weeks.

TABLE 2.11-6.   Common Teratogenic Agents and Their Associated Defects

DRUGS AND CHEMICALS	DEFECTS
ACEIs	Fetal renal tubular dysplasia and neonatal renal failure, oligohydramnios, intrauterine growth restriction (IUGR), lack of cranial ossification.
Alcohol	Fetal alcohol syndrome (growth restriction before and after birth, mental retardation, midfacial hypoplasia, renal and cardiac defects). Consumption of > 6 drinks per day is associated with a 40% risk of fetal alcohol syndrome.
Androgens	Virilization of females; advanced genital development in males.
Carbamazepine	Neural tube defects, fingernail hypoplasia, microcephaly, developmental delay, IUGR.
Cocaine	Bowel atresias; congenital malformations of the heart, limbs, face, and GU tract; microcephaly; IUGR; cerebral infarctions.
Diethylstilbestrol (DES)	Clear cell adenocarcinoma of the vagina or cervix, vaginal adenosis, abnormalities of the cervix and uterus or testes, possible infertility.
Lead	↑ spontaneous abortion (SAB) rate; stillbirths.
Lithium	Congenital heart disease (Ebstein's anomaly).
Methotrexate	↑ SAB rate.
Organic mercury	Cerebral atrophy, microcephaly, mental retardation, spasticity, seizures, blindness.
Phenytoin	IUGR, mental retardation, microcephaly, dysmorphic craniofacial features, cardiac defects, fingernail hypoplasia.
Radiation	Microcephaly, mental retardation. Medical diagnostic radiation delivering < 0.05 Gy to the fetus has no teratogenic risk.
Streptomycin and kanamycin	Hearing loss; CN VIII damage.
Tetracycline	Permanent yellow-brown discoloration of deciduous teeth; hypoplasia of tooth enamel.
Thalidomide	Bilateral limb deficiencies, anotia and microtia, cardiac and GI anomalies.
Trimethadione and paramethadione	Cleft lip or cleft palate, cardiac defects, microcephaly, mental retardation.
Valproic acid	Neural tube defects (spina bifida); minor craniofacial defects.
Vitamin A and derivatives	↑ SAB rate, microtia, thymic agenesis, cardiovascular defects, craniofacial dysmorphism, microphthalmia, cleft lip or cleft palate, mental retardation.
Warfarin (wages **war** on the fetus)	Nasal hypoplasia and stippled bone epiphyses, developmental delay, IUGR, ophthalmologic abnormalities.

TABLE 2.11-7. **Diagnosis and Treatment of Common Congenital Infections**

DISEASE	TRANSMISSION	SYMPTOMS	DIAGNOSIS	TREATMENT	PREVENTION
Toxoplasmosis	Transplacental; 1° infection via consumption of raw meat or contact with cat feces.	Hydrocephalus Intracranial calcifications Chorioretinitis Ring-enhancing lesions on MRI	Serologic testing.	Pyrimethamine + sulfadiazine.	Avoid exposure to cat feces during pregnancy; spiramycin prophylaxis for the third trimester.
Rubella	Transplacental in the first trimester.	Purpuric "blueberry muffin" rash Cataracts Mental retardation Hearing loss Patent ductus arteriosus (PDA)	Serologic testing.	Symptomatic.	Immunize before pregnancy; vaccinate the mother after delivery if serologic titers remain ⊖.
CMV	Primarily transplacental.	Petechial rash Periventricular calcifications	Urine culture; PCR of amniotic fluid.	Postpartum ganciclovir.	N/A
HSV	Intrapartum transmission if the mother has active lesions; transplacental transmission is rare.	Skin, eye, and mouth infections Life-threatening CNS/systemic infection	Serologic testing.	Acyclovir.	Perform a C-section if lesions are present at delivery.
HIV	In utero, at delivery, or via breast milk.	Often asymptomatic Failure to thrive Bacterial infections ↑ incidence of upper and lower respiratory diseases	ELISA, Western blot.	Highly active antiretroviral therapy (HAART).	AZT or nevirapine in pregnant women with HIV; perform elective C-section if viral load is > 1000. Treat infants with prophylactic AZT; avoid breastfeeding.
Syphilis	Intrapartum; transplacental transmission is possible.	Maculopapular skin rash Lymphadenopathy Hepatomegaly "Snuffles": mucopurulent rhinitis Osteitis Late congenital syphilis: ▪ Saber shins ▪ Saddle nose ▪ CNS involvement ▪ Hutchinson's triad: peg-shaped central incisors, deafness, interstitial keratitis	Dark-field microscopy, VDRL/RPR, FTA-ABS.	Penicillin.	Penicillin in pregnant women who test ⊕.

TABLE 2.11-8.   Types of SAB

TYPE	SYMPTOMS/SIGNS	DIAGNOSIS	TREATMENT
Complete	**POC are expelled.** Pain ceases, but spotting may persist.	**Closed os.** Ultrasound shows an empty uterus.	None.
Incomplete	**Some POC are expelled;** bleeding/ mild cramping. Visible tissue on exam.	**Open os.** Ultrasound shows retained fetal tissue.	Manual uterine aspiration (MUA) or D&C.
Threatened	**No POC are expelled;** uterine bleeding +/− abdominal pain.	**Closed os** + intact membranes + fetal cardiac motion on ultrasound.	Pelvic rest for 24–48 hours and follow-up ultrasound to assess the viability of conceptus.
Inevitable	**No POC are expelled;** uterine bleeding and cramps.	**Open os** +/− rupture of membranes (ROM).	MUA, D&C, misoprostol, or expectant management.
Missed	**No POC are expelled.** No fetal cardiac motion; no uterine bleeding. Brownish vaginal discharge.	**Closed os.** No fetal cardiac activity; retained fetal tissue on ultrasound.	MUA, D&C, or misoprostol.
Septic	Endometritis leading to septicemia. Maternal mortality is 10–15%.	Hypotension, hypothermia, ↑ WBC count.	MUA, D&C, and IV antibiotics.
Intrauterine fetal demise	Absence of fetal cardiac activity.	Uterus small for GA; no fetal heart tones or movement on ultrasound.	Induce labor; evacuate the uterus (D&E) to prevent DIC at GA > 16 weeks.
Recurrent[a]	If early in pregnancy, often due to chromosomal abnormalities. If later in pregnancy, often due to hypercoagulable states (eg, SLE, factor V Leiden, protein S deficiency). Incompetent cervix should be suspected with a history of painless dilation of the cervix and delivery of a normal fetus between 18 and 32 weeks.	Karyotyping of both parents. Hypercoagulability workup of mother. **Evaluate for uterine abnormalities.**	Surgical cerclage procedures to suture the cervix closed until labor or ROM occurs with subsequent removal prior to delivery. Restriction of activities.

[a] Defined as 2 or more consecutive SABs or a total of 3 SABs in 1 year.

Q

A 17-year-old G1P0 female with a history of genital HSV presents at 37 weeks in labor. What is the appropriate management of the patient at delivery?

Abnormal pregnancy is seen as a small, irregular intrauterine sac without a fetal pole on transvaginal ultrasound.
 Administer RhoGAM if the mother is Rh ⊖.

Elective Termination of Pregnancy

It has been estimated that 50% of all pregnancies in the United States are un-intended. Some 25% of all pregnancies end in elective abortion. Options for elective abortion depend on GA and patient preferences (see Table 2.11-9).

Normal Labor and Delivery

OBSTETRIC EXAMINATION

 Leopold's maneuvers are used to determine fetal lie (longitudinal or transverse) and, if possible, fetal presentation (breech or cephalic).
 Cervical examination:
   Evaluate dilation, effacement, station, cervical position, and cervical consistency.
   Confirm or determine fetal presentation.
   Determine fetal position through palpation of the fetal sutures and fontanelles.
   Conduct a sterile speculum exam if ROM is suspected.
   Determine station, or engagement of the fetal head relative to a line through the ischial spines of the maternal pelvis. ⊖ station = fetal head superior to this line; ⊕ station = fetal head inferior to this line.
 Table 2.11-10 depicts the normal stages of labor.

TABLE 2.11-9. Elective Termination of Pregnancy

TRIMESTER	PROCEDURE	TIMING
First (90% therapeutic abortions [TABs])	**Medical management:**	**Up to:**
	■ Oral mifepristone (low dose) + oral/vaginal misoprostol	49 days' GA
	■ IM/oral methotrexate + oral/vaginal misoprostol	49 days' GA
	■ Vaginal or sublingual or buccal misoprostol (high dose), repeated up to 3 times	59 days' GA
	Surgical management:	13 weeks' GA
	■ Manual aspiration	
	■ D&C with vacuum aspiration	
Second (10% TABs)	**Obstetric management:** Induction of labor (typically with prostaglandins, amniotomy, and oxytocin)	13–24 weeks' GA (depending on state laws)
	Surgical management: D&E	Same as above

A

If the patient has any active lesions at the time of delivery, perform a C-section.

TABLE 2.11-10.   Stages of Labor

STAGE	STARTS/ENDS	DURATION		COMMENTS
		PRIMIPAROUS	MULTIPAROUS	
First				
Latent	Onset of labor to 3–4 cm dilation	6–11 hrs	4–8 hrs	Prolongation seen with excessive sedation/hypotonic uterine contractions.
Active	4 cm to complete cervical dilation (10 cm)	4–6 hrs (1.2 cm/hr)	2–3 hrs (1.5 cm/hr)	Prolongation seen with cephalopelvic disproportion.
Second	Complete cervical dilation to delivery of infant	0.5–3.0 hrs	5–30 min	Baby goes through all cardinal movements of delivery.
Third	Delivery of infant to delivery of placenta	0–0.5 hr	0–0.5 hr	Uterus contracts and placenta separates to establish hemostasis.

FETAL HEART RATE (FHR) MONITORING

- Monitoring can be performed with an electrode attached to the fetal scalp (a method that yields more precise results), or external monitoring can be conducted using Doppler ultrasound (a less invasive option).
- Continuous electronic FHR monitoring has not been shown to be more effective than appropriate intermittent monitoring in low-risk patients.

Recommendations for FHR Monitoring

- **Patients without complications:** Review FHR tracings.
  - **First stage of labor:** Every 30 minutes.
  - **Second stage of labor:** Every 15 minutes.
- **Patients with complications:** Review FHR tracings.
  - **First stage of labor:** Every 15 minutes.
  - **Second stage of labor:** Every 5 minutes.

Components of FHR Evaluation

- **Rate** (normal = 110–160 bpm):
  - **FHR < 110 bpm:** Bradycardia. Can be caused by congenital heart malformations or by severe hypoxia (2° to uterine hyperstimulation, cord prolapse, or rapid fetal descent).
  - **FHR > 160 bpm:** Tachycardia. Causes include hypoxia, maternal fever, and fetal anemia.
- **Variability:** See Figures 2.11-4 and 2.11-5.
  - **Undetectable variability:** Indicates severe fetal distress.
  - **Minimal variability:** < 6 bpm. Indicates fetal hypoxia or the effects of opioids, magnesium, or sleep cycle.
  - **Normal variability:** 6–25 bpm.
  - **Marked variability:** > 25 bpm. May indicate fetal hypoxia; may occur before a ↓ in variability.
  - **Sinusoidal variability:** Points to serious fetal anemia; a pseudosinusoidal pattern may also occur during maternal meperidine use.
- **Accelerations:** Onset of an ↑ in FHR to a peak in < 30 seconds. Reassuring because they indicate fetal ability to appropriately respond to the environment.
- **Decelerations:** See Table 2.11-11.

Q

A 23-year-old G1P0 female at 15 weeks' GA presents with abdominal pain and mild bleeding from the cervix. On pelvic examination, some products of conception (POC) are found to be present in the vaginal vault. What test is necessary to determine the next step in management?

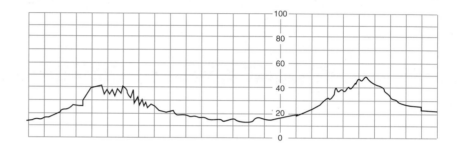

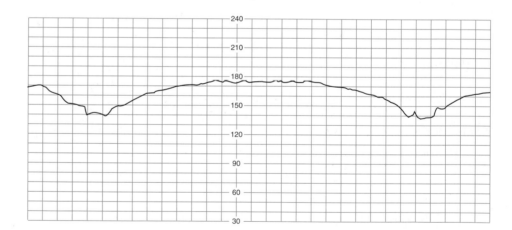

FIGURE 2.11-4. Varying (variable) fetal heart rate decelerations.

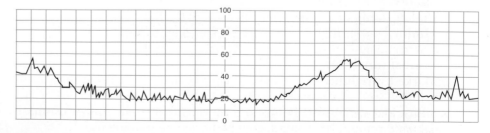

Ultrasound should be performed to determine if all the POC have been expelled (ie, if the uterus is empty). If so, it is a complete abortion and the POC should be sent to pathology to confirm fetal tissue with no other treatment. If POC are retained, it is an incomplete abortion, and manual uterine aspiration or D&C is indicated. Medical management with misoprostol may also be appropriate.

FIGURE 2.11-5. Late fetal heart rate decelerations. Late decelerations due to utero-placental insufficiency resulting from placental abruption. Immediate cesarean delivery was performed. Umbilical artery pH was 7.05 and P_{O_2} was 11 mm Hg. (Adapted with permission from Cunningham FG et al. *Williams Obstetrics,* 23rd ed. New York: McGraw-Hill, 2010, Fig. 18-17.)

TABLE 2.11-11. **Types of Fetal Deceleration**

TYPE	DESCRIPTION	ETIOLOGY	SCHEMATIC
Early	A visually apparent, gradual (onset to nadir in > 30 sec) ↓ in FHR with a return to baseline that mirrors the uterine contraction.	Head compression from the uterine contraction (normal).	
Late	A visually apparent, gradual (onset to nadir in > 30 sec) ↓ in FHR with return to baseline whose onset, nadir, and recovery occur after the beginning, peak, and end of uterine contraction, respectively.	Uteroplacental insufficiency and fetal hypoxemia.	
Variable	An abrupt (onset to nadir in < 30 sec), visually apparent ↓ in FHR below baseline lasting ≥ 15 sec but < 2 min.	Umbilical cord compression.	

(Illustrations reproduced with permission from Cunningham FC et al. *Williams Obstetrics,* 23rd ed. New York: McGraw-Hill, 2010, Figs. 18-14, 18-16, and 18-18.)

ANTEPARTUM FETAL SURVEILLANCE

In general, antepartum fetal surveillance is used in pregnancies in which the risk of antepartum fetal demise is ↑. Testing is initiated in most at-risk patients at 32–34 weeks (or 26–28 weeks if there are multiple worrisome risk factors present). The following assessments are made:

- **Fetal movement assessment:**
    - Assessed by the mother as the number of fetal movements over 1 hour.
    - The average time to obtain 10 movements is 20 minutes.
    - Maternal reports of ↓ fetal movements should be evaluated by means of the tests described below.

- **Nonstress test (NST):**
  - Performed with the mother resting in the lateral tilt position (to prevent supine hypotension).
  - FHR is monitored externally by Doppler along with a tocodynamometer to detect uterine contractions. Acoustic stimulation may be used.
  - **"Reactive" NST (normal response):** Two accelerations ≥ **15 bpm above baseline** (if > 32 weeks GA; ≥ 10 bpm if < 32 weeks GA) **lasting for at least 15 seconds** over a 20-minute period (see Figure 2.11-6).
  - **"Nonreactive" NST:** Fewer than 2 accelerations over a 20-minute period.
    - Perform further tests (eg, a biophysical profile, or BPP).
    - Lack of FHR accelerations may occur with any of the following: GA < 32 weeks, fetal sleeping, fetal CNS anomalies, and maternal sedative or narcotic administration.
- **Contraction stress test (CST):**
  - Performed in the lateral recumbent position.
  - FHR is monitored during spontaneous or induced (via nipple stimulation or oxytocin) contractions.
  - Reactivity is determined from fetal heart monitoring, as with the NST.
  - The procedure is contraindicated in women with preterm membrane rupture or known placenta previa; those with a history of uterine surgery; and those who are at high risk for preterm labor.
  - **"Positive" CST:**
    - Defined by late decelerations following 50% or more of contractions in a 10-minute window.
    - Raises concerns about fetal compromise.
    - Delivery is usually warranted.
  - **"Negative" CST:**
    - Defined as no late or significant variable decelerations within 10 minutes and at least 3 contractions.
    - Highly predictive of fetal well-being in conjunction with a normal NST.
  - **"Equivocal" CST:** Defined by intermittent late decelerations or significant variable decelerations.
- **BPP:** Uses real-time ultrasound to assign a score of 2 (normal) or 0 (abnormal) to 5 parameters: fetal tone, breathing, movement, amniotic fluid volume, and NST. Scoring is as follows:

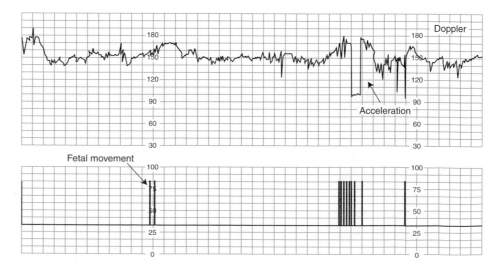

FIGURE 2.11-6. Reactive nonstress test. (Adapted with permission from Cunningham FG et al. *Williams Obstetrics*, 23rd ed. New York: McGraw-Hill, 2010, Fig. 15-7.)

- 8–10: Reassuring for fetal well-being.
- 6: Considered equivocal. Term pregnancies are usually delivered with this profile.
- 0–4: Extremely worrisome for fetal asphyxia; strong consideration should be given to immediate delivery if no other explanation is found.
- **Amniotic fluid index (AFI):** sum of the measurements of the deepest cord-free amniotic fluid measured in each of the abdominal quadrants.
- **Modified biophysical profile (mBPP):**
  - NST + AFI.
  - A normal test consists of a reactive NST and an AFI > 5 cm.
- **Umbilical artery Doppler velocimetry:**
  - Used only when IUGR is suspected.
  - With IUGR, there is a reduction and even a reversal of umbilical artery diastolic flow.
- **Oligohydramnios (AFI < 5 cm) always warrants further workup.**

OBSTETRIC ANALGESIA AND ANESTHESIA

- Uterine contractions and cervical dilation result in visceral pain (T10–L1).
- Descent of the fetal head and pressure on the vagina and perineum result in somatic pain (pudendal nerve, S2–S4).
- In the absence of a medical contraindication, maternal request is a sufficient medical indication for pain relief during labor.
- Absolute contraindications to regional anesthesia (epidural, spinal, or combination) include the following:
  - Refractory maternal hypotension
  - Maternal coagulopathy
  - Maternal use of a once-daily dose of low-molecular-weight heparin within 12 hours
  - Untreated maternal bacteremia
  - Skin infection over the site of needle placement
  - ↑ ICP caused by a mass lesion

Medical Complications of Pregnancy

HYPEREMESIS GRAVIDARUM

Defined as **persistent vomiting** not related to other causes, **acute starvation** (usually large ketonuria), and weight loss (usually at least a 5% ↓ from pre-pregnancy weight).

- More common in first pregnancies, multiple gestations, and molar pregnancies.
- ↑ β-hCG and ↑ estradiol have been implicated in its pathophysiology.

HISTORY/PE

Distinguish from "morning sickness," acid reflux, gastroenteritis, hyperthyroidism, and neurologic conditions.

DIAGNOSIS

- Check β-hCG level and ultrasound to rule out molar pregnancy.
- Evaluate for ketonemia, ketonuria, hyponatremia, and hypokalemic, hypochloremic metabolic alkalosis. Measure liver enzymes, serum bilirubin, and serum amylase/lipase.

KEY FACT

A ⊖ CST is good; a ⊕ one is bad.

MNEMONIC

When performing a BPP, remember to—

Test the Baby, MAN!

Fetal **T**one
Fetal **B**reathing
Fetal **M**ovement
Amniotic fluid volume
Nonstress test

KEY FACT

If "morning sickness" persists after the first trimester, think hyperemesis gravidarum.

KEY FACT

The first step in the diagnosis of hyperemesis gravidarum is to **rule out molar pregnancy** with ultrasound +/− β-hCG.

TREATMENT

- Administer vitamin B$_6$.
- Doxylamine (an antihistamine) PO.
- Promethazine or dimenhydrinate PO/PR.
- **If severe:** Metoclopramide, ondansetron, prochlorperazine, or promethazine IM/PO.
- **If dehydrated:** IV fluids, IV nutritional supplementation, and dimenhydrinate IV.

DIABETES IN PREGNANCY

Diabetes in pregnancy is divided into 2 categories:

- **Gestational:** Onset occurs during pregnancy.
- **Pregestational:** Onset is prior to pregnancy.

Gestational Diabetes Mellitus

Carbohydrate intolerance of variable severity that is first diagnosed during pregnancy. Occurs in 3–5% of all pregnancies, usually in late pregnancy.

HISTORY/PE

- Typically asymptomatic.
- May present with edema, polyhydramnios, or a large-for-GA infant (> 90th percentile).

DIAGNOSIS

- **Conduct a 1-hour 50-g glucose challenge test:**
  - **Venous plasma glucose is measured 1 hour later.**
  - **Performed at 24–28 weeks.**
  - Values ≥ 140 mg/dL are considered abnormal.
- **Confirm with an oral 3-hour (100-g) glucose tolerance test** showing any 2 of the following:
  - **Fasting:** > 95 mg/dL.
  - **One hour:** > 180 mg/dL.
  - **Two hours:** > 155 mg/dL.
  - **Three hours:** > 140 mg/dL.

TREATMENT

- **Mother:**
  - Start with the **ADA diet,** regular exercise, and strict glucose monitoring (4 times a day).
  - Tight maternal glucose control (fasting glucose < 90 mg/dL; 1- to 2-hour postprandial glucose < 140 mg/dL) improves outcomes.
  - Add insulin if dietary control is insufficient.
  - Give intrapartum insulin and dextrose to maintain tight control during delivery.
- **Fetus:**
  - Obtain periodic ultrasound and NSTs to assess fetal growth and well-being.
  - It may be necessary to induce labor at 39–40 weeks if insulin or an oral hypoglycemic agent is necessary for glucose control.

KEY FACT

Keys to the management of gestational diabetes: (1) the ADA diet; (2) insulin if needed; (3) ultrasound for fetal growth; and (4) NST beginning at 30–32 weeks if GDMA2 (requiring insulin or an oral hypoglycemic).

COMPLICATIONS

More than 50% of patients go on to **develop glucose intolerance and/or type 2 DM** later in life.

Pregestational Diabetes and Pregnancy

Observed in 1% of all pregnancies. Insulin requirements may ↑ as much as threefold. Poorly controlled DM is associated with an ↑ **risk of congenital malformations,** fetal loss, and maternal/fetal morbidity during labor and delivery.

TREATMENT

- **Mother:**
  - Renal, ophthalmologic, neural tube, and cardiac evaluation to assess for end-organ damage.
  - Strict glucose control (diet, exercise, insulin therapy, and frequent self-monitoring) to minimize fetal defects.
    - **Fasting morning:** ≤ 90 mg/dL.
    - **Two-hour postprandial:** < 120 mg/dL.
- **Fetus:**
  - **18–20 weeks:**
    - Ultrasound to determine fetal age and growth.
    - Evaluate for cardiac anomalies and polyhydramnios.
    - Quad screen to screen for developmental anomalies.
  - **32–34 weeks:**
    - Close fetal surveillance (eg, NST, CST, BPP).
    - Admit if maternal DM has been poorly controlled or fetal parameters are a concern.
    - Serial ultrasounds for fetal growth.
- **Delivery and postpartum:**
  - Maintain normoglycemia (80–100 mg/dL) during labor with an IV insulin drip and hourly glucose measurements.
  - Consider early delivery in the setting of poor maternal glucose control, preeclampsia, macrosomia, or evidence of fetal lung maturity.
  - Cesarean delivery should be considered in the setting of an estimated fetal weight (EFW) > 4500 g.
  - Encourage breastfeeding with an appropriate ↑ in caloric intake.
  - **Continue glucose monitoring postpartum. Insulin needs rapidly ↓ after delivery.**

COMPLICATIONS

See Table 2.11-12.

KEY FACT

Greater than 8, investigate! If HbA$_{1c}$ is > 8%, look for congenital abnormalities.

KEY FACT

If UA before 20 weeks reveals glycosuria, think pregestational diabetes.

KEY FACT

Hyperglycemia in the first trimester suggests preexisting diabetes and should be managed as pregestational diabetes.

GESTATIONAL AND CHRONIC HYPERTENSION

Defined as follows:

- **Gestational hypertension:**
  - Idiopathic hypertension without significant proteinuria (< 300 mg/L).
  - **Develops at > 20 weeks' GA.**
  - As many as 25% of patients may go on to develop preeclampsia.
- **Chronic hypertension:**
  - Present before conception and at < 20 weeks' GA.
  - May persist for > 12 weeks postpartum.
  - Up to one-third of patients may develop superimposed preeclampsia.

TABLE 2.11-12. **Complications of Pregestational Diabetes Mellitus**

MATERNAL COMPLICATIONS	FETAL COMPLICATIONS
DKA (type 1) or hyperglycemic hyperosmolar nonketotic coma (type 2)	Macrosomia or IUGR
	Cardiac and renal defects
Preeclampsia/eclampsia	Neural tube defects (eg, sacral agenesis)
Cephalopelvic disproportion (from macrosomia) and need for C-section	Hypocalcemia
	Polycythemia
Preterm labor	Hyperbilirubinemia
Infection	Hypoglycemia from hyperinsulinemia
Polyhydramnios	Respiratory distress syndrome (RDS)
Postpartum hemorrhage	Birth injury (eg, shoulder dystocia)
Maternal mortality	Perinatal mortality

TREATMENT

- Monitor BP closely.
- Treat with appropriate antihypertensives (eg, methyldopa, labetalol, nifedipine).
- **Do not give ACEIs or diuretics.**
  - ACEIs are known to lead to uterine ischemia.
  - Diuretics can aggravate low plasma volume to the point of uterine ischemia.

COMPLICATIONS

Similar to those of preeclampsia (see below).

PREECLAMPSIA AND ECLAMPSIA

Distinguished as follows:

- **Preeclampsia:**
  - New-onset hypertension (systolic BP ≥ 140 mm Hg or diastolic BP ≥ 90 mm Hg) **and**
  - Proteinuria (> 300 mg of protein in a 24-hour period) occurring at > 20 weeks' GA.
- **Eclampsia:** New-onset grand mal seizures in women with preeclampsia.
- **HELLP syndrome:** A variant of preeclampsia with a poor prognosis.
  - Consists of hemolytic anemia, elevated liver enzymes, and low platelets (see mnemonic).
  - The etiology is unknown, but clinical manifestations are explained by vasospasm leading to hemorrhage and organ necrosis.
  - Risk factors include nulliparity, African American ethnicity, extremes of age (< 20 or > 35), multiple gestation, molar pregnancy, renal disease (due to SLE or type 1 DM), a family history of preeclampsia, and chronic hypertension.

HISTORY/PE

See Table 2.11-13 for the signs and symptoms of preeclampsia and eclampsia.

MNEMONIC

The classic triad of preeclampsia—

It's not just HyPE

Hypertension
Proteinuria
Edema

MNEMONIC

HELLP syndrome:

Hemolysis
Elevated **L**FTs
Low **P**latelets

TABLE 2.11-13. **Presentation of Preeclampsia and Eclampsia**

DISEASE SEVERITY	SIGNS AND SYMPTOMS
Mild preeclampsia	Usually asymptomatic. BP ≥ **140/90** on 2 occasions > 6 hours apart. Proteinuria (> 300 mg/24 hrs or 1–2 ⊕ urine dipsticks). Edema.
Severe preeclampsia	BP > **160/110** on 2 occasions > 6 hours apart. **Renal: Proteinuria** (> 5 g/24 hrs or 3–4 ⊕ urine dipsticks) or oliguria (< 500 mL/24 hrs). **Cerebral changes: Headache,** somnolence. **Visual changes: Blurred vision,** scotomata. **Other:** Hyperactive reflexes/clonus; **RUQ pain;** hemolysis, elevated liver enzymes, thrombocytopenia (HELLP syndrome).
Eclampsia	The most common signs preceding an eclamptic attack are **headache, visual changes,** and **RUQ/epigastric pain.** Seizures are severe if not controlled with anticonvulsant therapy.

TREATMENT

The only cure for preeclampsia/eclampsia is delivery of the fetus.

- Preeclampsia:
    - **Close to term or worsening preeclampsia:** Induce delivery with IV oxytocin, prostaglandin, or amniotomy.
    - **Far from term:** Treat with modified bed rest and expectant management.
    - Prevent seizures with a **continuous magnesium sulfate drip.**
        - Watch for signs of magnesium toxicity (loss of DTRs, respiratory paralysis, coma).
        - Continue seizure prophylaxis for 24 hours postpartum.
        - Treat magnesium toxicity with IV calcium gluconate.
- Severe preeclampsia:
    - **Control BP** with labetalol and/or hydralazine (goal < 160/110 mm Hg with a diastolic BP of 90–100 mm Hg to maintain fetal blood flow).
    - **Continuous magnesium sulfate drip.**
    - **Deliver** by induction or C-section when the mother is stable.
- Eclampsia:
    - ABCs with supplemental O_2.
    - Seizure control/prophylaxis with **magnesium.**
        - If seizures recur, give IV diazepam.
        - Monitor magnesium blood levels and magnesium toxicity.
        - Monitor fetal status.
        - Control BP (labetalol and/or hydralazine).
        - Limit fluids; Foley catheter for strict I/Os.
    - Initiate delivery if the patient is stable and convulsions are controlled.
    - Postpartum management is the same as that for preeclampsia.
    - Seizures may occur antepartum (25%), intrapartum (50%), or postpartum (25%); most occur within 48 hours after delivery.

KEY FACT

Signs of severe preeclampsia are persistent headache or other cerebral or visual disturbances, persistent epigastric pain, and hyperreactive reflexes.

Q

A 36-year-old G1P0 female with a history of SLE at 36 weeks' GA presents with headache and RUQ pain. She is admitted and found to have a BP of 165/100 and 170/105 mm Hg when tested twice 6 hours apart, as well as 3+ protein on urine dipstick. Once her BP has been controlled with labetalol, what are the next steps in management?

COMPLICATIONS

- **Preeclampsia:** Prematurity, fetal distress, stillbirth, placental abruption, seizure, DIC, cerebral hemorrhage, serous retinal detachment, fetal/maternal death.
- **Eclampsia:** Cerebral hemorrhage, aspiration pneumonia, hypoxic encephalopathy, thromboembolic events, fetal/maternal death.

ANTEPARTUM HEMORRHAGE

- Any bleeding that occurs after 20 weeks' gestation.
- Complicates 3–5% of pregnancies.
- The most common causes are **placental abruption** and **placenta previa** (see Table 2.11-14 and Figure 2.11-7).
- Other causes include other forms of abnormal placentation (eg, placenta accreta), ruptured uterus, genital tract lesions, and trauma.

Obstetric Complications of Pregnancy

ECTOPIC PREGNANCY

Most often tubal, but can be abdominal, ovarian, or cervical.

HISTORY/PE

- Presents with abdominal pain and vaginal spotting/bleeding, although some patients are asymptomatic.
- Associated with etiologies that cause scarring to the fallopian tubes, including a history of PID, pelvic surgery, DES use, or endometriosis.
- The differential includes surgical abdomen, abortion, ovarian torsion, PID, and ruptured ovarian cyst.

DIAGNOSIS

Approach a woman of reproductive age presenting with abdominal pain as a ruptured ectopic pregnancy until proven otherwise.

- Look for a ⊕ pregnancy test and a transvaginal ultrasound showing an empty uterus (see Figure 2.11-8).
- Confirm with a serial hCG without appropriate hCG doubling.

TREATMENT

- Medical treatment (methotrexate) is sufficient for small, unruptured tubal pregnancies.
- Surgical options include salpingectomy or salpingostomy with evacuation (laparoscopy vs. laparotomy).

COMPLICATIONS

Tubal rupture and hemoperitoneum (an obstetric emergency).

INTRAUTERINE GROWTH RESTRICTION (IUGR)

Defined as an EFW less than the 10th percentile for GA.

KEY FACT

With third-trimester bleeding, think anatomically:

- **Vagina:** Bloody show, trauma
- **Cervix:** Cervical cancer, cervical/vaginal lesion
- **Placenta:** Placental abruption, placenta previa
- **Fetus:** Fetal bleeding

MNEMONIC

The classic triad of ectopic pregnancy PAVEs the way for diagnosis:

Pain (abdominal)
Amenorrhea
Vaginal bleeding
Ectopic pregnancy

KEY FACT

Unstable patients or those with signs of peritoneal irritation (eg, rebound tenderness) require emergent surgical intervention.

The patient has severe preeclampsia. Start a magnesium sulfate drip for seizure prophylaxis and deliver by induction or C-section when the mother is stable.

TABLE 2.11-14. Placental Abruption vs. Placenta Previa

Variable	Placental Abruption	Placenta Previa
Pathophysiology	Premature (before delivery) separation of normally implanted placenta.	Abnormal placental implantation: ■ **Total:** The placenta covers the cervical os. ■ **Marginal:** The placenta extends to the margin of the os. ■ **Low lying:** The placenta is in close proximity to the os.
Incidence	1 in 100.	1 in 200.
Risk factors	Hypertension, abdominal/pelvic trauma, tobacco or cocaine use, previous abruption, rapid decompression of an overdistended uterus, excessive stimulation.	Prior C-sections, grand multiparity, advanced maternal age, multiple gestation, prior placenta previa.
Symptoms	**Painful, dark** vaginal bleeding that does not spontaneously cease. Abdominal pain; uterine hypertonicity. Fetal distress.	**Painless, bright red** bleeding that often ceases in 1–2 hours with or without uterine contractions. Usually no fetal distress.
Diagnosis	Primarily clinical. Transabdominal/transvaginal ultrasound sensitivity is only 50%; look for a retroplacental clot. Most useful for ruling out previa.	Transabdominal/transvaginal ultrasound sensitivity is > 95%; look for an abnormally positioned placenta.
Management	Stabilize patients with mild abruption and a premature fetus; **manage expectantly** (hospitalize; start IV and fetal monitoring; type and cross blood; bed rest). **Moderate to severe abruption: Immediate delivery** is indicated (vaginal delivery with amniotomy if mother and fetus are stable and delivery is expected soon; C-section for maternal or fetal distress).	**Do not perform a vaginal exam!** Stabilize patients with a premature fetus; manage expectantly. Give tocolytics. Serial ultrasound to assess fetal growth; resolution of partial previa. Betamethasone to help with fetal lung maturity. **Deliver by C-section.** Indications for delivery include labor, life-threatening bleeding, fetal distress, documented fetal lung maturity, and 36 weeks' GA.
Complications	Hemorrhagic shock. DIC occurs in 10% of patients. Recurrence risk is 5–16% and ↑ to 25% after 2 previous abruptions. Fetal hypoxia.	↑ risk of placenta accreta. Vasa previa (fetal vessels crossing the internal os). Preterm delivery, PROM, IUGR, congenital anomalies. Recurrence risk is 4–8%.

HISTORY/PE

Risk factors include the following:

- Maternal systemic disease leading to uteroplacental insufficiency (intra-uterine infection, hypertension, anemia)
- Maternal substance abuse
- Placenta previa
- Multiple gestations

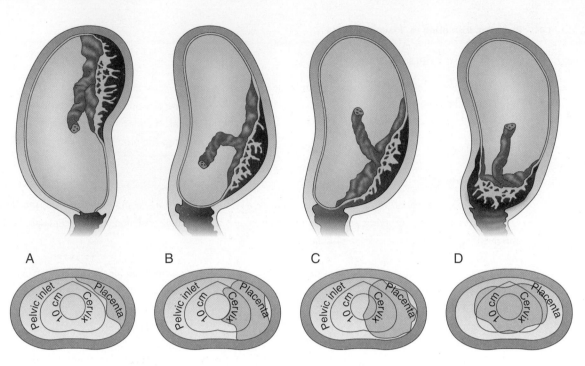

FIGURE 2.11-7. **Placental implantation.** (**A**) Normal placenta. (**B**) Low implantation. (**C**) Partial placenta previa. (**D**) Complete placenta previa. (Adapted with permission from DeCherney AH. *Current Obstetric & Gynecologic Diagnosis & Treatment*, 8th ed. Stamford, CT: Appleton & Lange, 1994: 404.)

DIAGNOSIS

- Confirm serial fundal height measurements with ultrasound.
- Ultrasound the fetus for EFW.

TREATMENT

- Explore the underlying etiology and correct if possible.
- **If the patient is near due date,** administer steroids (eg, betamethasone) to accelerate fetal lung maturity; requires 48 hours prior to delivery.

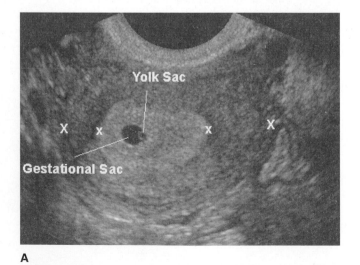

A

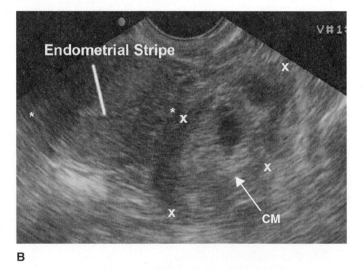

B

FIGURE 2.11-8. **Normal intrauterine pregnancy and ectopic pregnancy.** Transvaginal ultrasound showing (**A**) a normal intrauterine pregnancy with a gestational sac containing a yolk sac within the uterine cavity, and (**B**) a complex mass (CM)/ectopic pregnancy adjacent to an empty uterus. (Reproduced with permission from Tintinalli JE et al. *Tintinalli's Emergency Medicine: A Comprehensive Study Guide*, 6th ed. New York: McGraw-Hill, 2004, Figs. 113-15 and 113-22.)

- Perform fetal monitoring with NST, CST, BPP, and umbilical artery Doppler velocimetry.
- A nonreassuring status near term may prompt delivery.

COMPLICATIONS

↑ perinatal morbidity and mortality.

FETAL MACROSOMIA

- Defined as a birth weight > 95th percentile. A common sequela of gestational diabetes.
- **Dx:** Weigh the newborn at birth (prenatal diagnosis is imprecise).
- **Tx:** Planned cesarean delivery may be considered for an EFW > 5000 g in women without diabetes and for an EFW > 4500 g in women with diabetes.
- **Cx:** ↑ risk of shoulder dystocia (leading to brachial plexus injury and Erb-Duchenne palsy) as birth weight ↑.

POLYHYDRAMNIOS

- An AFI > 20 on ultrasound. May be present in normal pregnancies, but fetal chromosomal developmental abnormalities must be considered. Etiologies include the following:
  - Maternal DM
  - Multiple gestation
  - Isoimmunization
  - Pulmonary abnormalities (eg, cystic lung malformations)
  - Fetal anomalies (eg, duodenal atresia, tracheoesophageal fistula, anencephaly)
  - Twin-twin transfusion syndrome
- **Hx/PE:** Usually asymptomatic.
- **Dx:** Fundal height greater than expected. Evaluation includes ultrasound for fetal anomalies, glucose testing for DM, and Rh screen.
- **Tx:** Etiology specific.
- **Cx:** Preterm labor, fetal malpresentation, cord prolapse.

OLIGOHYDRAMNIOS

- An AFI < 5 on ultrasound. Usually asymptomatic, but IUGR or fetal distress may be present.
- Etiologies include the following:
  - Fetal urinary tract abnormalities (eg, renal agenesis, GU obstruction)
  - Chronic uteroplacental insufficiency
  - ROM
- **Dx:** The sum of the deepest amniotic fluid pocket in all 4 abdominal quadrants on ultrasound.
- **Tx:** Rule out inaccurate gestational dates. Treat the underlying cause if possible.
- **Cx:**
  - Associated with a 40-fold ↑ in perinatal mortality.
  - Other complications include musculoskeletal abnormalities (eg, clubfoot, facial distortion), pulmonary hypoplasia, umbilical cord compression, and IUGR.

Rh ISOIMMUNIZATION

In this condition, fetal RBCs leak into the maternal circulation, and maternal anti-Rh IgG antibodies form that can cross the placenta, leading to hemolysis of fetal Rh RBCs (**erythroblastosis fetalis;** see Figure 2.11-9). There is an ↑ risk among an Rh-⊖ women who have had a previous SAB or TAB as well as among those who have undergone a previous delivery with no RhoGAM given.

DIAGNOSIS

Sensitized Rh-⊖ mothers with titers > 1:16 should be closely monitored with serial ultrasound and amniocentesis for evidence of fetal hemolysis.

TREATMENT

In severe cases, initiate preterm delivery when fetal lungs are mature. Prior to delivery, intrauterine blood transfusions may be given to correct a low fetal hematocrit.

PREVENTION

- If the mother is Rh ⊖ at 28 weeks and the father is Rh ⊕ or unknown, give **RhoGAM** (Rh immune globulin).
- If the baby is Rh ⊕, give the mother RhoGAM postpartum.
- Give RhoGAM to Rh-⊖ mothers who undergo abortion or who have had an ectopic pregnancy, amniocentesis, vaginal bleeding, or placenta previa/placental abruption. **Type and screen is critical;** follow β-hCG closely and prevent pregnancy for 1 year.

COMPLICATIONS

- Hydrops fetalis when fetal hemoglobin is < 7 g/dL.
- Fetal hypoxia and acidosis, kernicterus, prematurity, death.

GESTATIONAL TROPHOBLASTIC DISEASE (GTD)

A range of proliferative trophoblastic abnormalities that can be benign or malignant.

- **Benign GTD:** Includes complete and incomplete molar pregnancies (see Table 2.11-15).
- **Malignant GTD:** Molar pregnancy may progress to malignant GTD, including:
    - **Invasive moles:** 10–15%.
    - **Choriocarcinoma:** 2–5%.

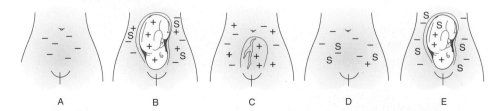

FIGURE 2.11-9. **Rh isoimmunization.** (A) Rh-negative mother prior to pregnancy. (B) Rh-positive fetus in Rh-negative mother. (C) Placental separation. (D) After delivery, the mother develops antibodies (S) to Rh antigen. (E) Rh-positive fetus in the next pregnancy. Maternal antibodies, from Rh isoimmunization at the time of the previous delivery, cross the placenta and cause hemolysis of red blood cells in the fetus. (Reproduced with permission from DeCherney AH, Nathan L. *Current Diagnosis & Treatment Obstetrics & Gynecology,* 10th ed. New York: McGraw-Hill, 2007, Fig. 15-1.)

TABLE 2.11-15.   Complete vs. Incomplete Moles

VARIABLE	COMPLETE	INCOMPLETE
Mechanism	Sperm fertilization of an empty ovum	Normal ovum fertilized by 2 sperm
Karyotype	46,XX	69,XXY
Fetal tissue	No fetal tissue	Contains fetal tissue

- Complications of malignant GTD include pulmonary or CNS metastases and trophoblastic pulmonary emboli.

History/PE

- Presents with first-trimester **uterine bleeding,** hyperemesis gravidarum, preeclampsia/eclampsia at < 24 weeks, and uterine size greater than dates.
- Risk factors include extremes of age (< 20 or > 40 years) and a diet deficient in folate or beta-carotene.

Diagnosis

- No fetal heartbeat is detected.
- Pelvic examination may reveal enlarged ovaries (bilateral theca-lutein cysts) or expulsion of **grapelike molar clusters** into the vagina.
- Labs show markedly ↑ serum β-hCG (**usually > 100,000 mIU/mL).**
- Pelvic ultrasound reveals a "snowstorm" appearance with no gestational sac or fetus present (see Figure 2.11-10).
- CXR may show lung metastases
- D&C reveals **"cluster-of-grapes"** tissue.

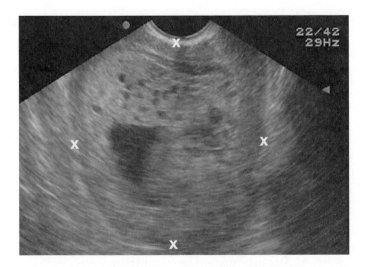

FIGURE 2.11-10.   Molar pregnancy. Transvaginal ultrasound shows a large, complex intrauterine mass with cystic regions that have the characteristic appearance of grapes. (Reproduced with permission from Tintinalli JE et al. *Tintinalli's Emergency Medicine: A Comprehensive Study Guide,* 6th ed. New York: McGraw-Hill, 2004, Fig. 113-27.)

TREATMENT

- Evacuate the uterus and follow with weekly β-hCG.
- Treat malignant disease with chemotherapy (methotrexate or dactinomycin)
- Treat residual uterine disease with hysterectomy
- Chemotherapy and irradiation are highly effective for metastases.

MULTIPLE GESTATIONS

- Affect 3% of all live births.
- Since 1980, the incidence of monozygotic (identical) twins has remained steady, while the incidence of dizygotic (fraternal) and higher-order births has ↑.
- **Hx/PE:** Characterized by rapid uterine growth, excessive maternal weight gain, and palpation of 3 or more large fetal parts on Leopold's maneuvers.
- **Dx:** Ultrasound; hCG, human placental lactogen, and MSAFP are elevated for GA.
- **Tx:**
  - Multifetal reduction and selective fetal termination is an option for higher-order multiple pregnancies.
  - Antepartum fetal surveillance for IUGR.
  - Management by a high-risk specialist is recommended.
- **Cx:**
  - **Maternal:** Patients are 6 times more likely to be hospitalized with complications of pregnancy.
  - **Fetal:** Complications include twin-to-twin transfusion syndrome, IUGR, preterm labor, and a higher incidence of congenital malformations.

Abnormal Labor and Delivery

SHOULDER DYSTOCIA

Affects 0.6–1.4% of all deliveries in the United States. Risk factors include obesity, diabetes, a history of a macrosomic infant, and a history of prior shoulder dystocia.

DIAGNOSIS

Diagnosed by a prolonged second stage of labor, recoil of the perineum ("turtle sign"), and lack of spontaneous restitution.

TREATMENT

In the event of dystocia, be the mother's **HELPER:**

- **H**elp reposition.
- **E**pisiotomy.
- **L**eg elevated (McRoberts' maneuver; see Figure 2.11-11).
- **P**ressure (suprapubic).
- **E**nter the vagina and attempt rotation (Wood's screw).
- **R**each for the fetal arm.

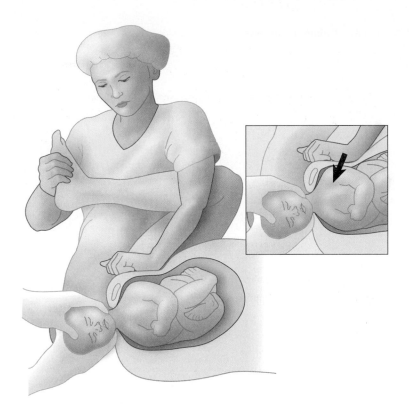

FIGURE 2.11-11. Leg elevation (McRoberts' maneuver). The leg positioning illustrated here can be used to assist in a delivery where the infant is at risk for shoulder dystocia. (Reproduced with permission from Cunningham FG et al. *Williams Obstetrics,* 23rd ed. New York: McGraw-Hill, 2010, Fig. 20-15.)

FAILURE TO PROGRESS

Associated with chorioamnionitis, occiput posterior position, nulliparity, and elevated birth weight.

DIAGNOSIS

- **First-stage protraction or arrest:** Labor that fails to produce adequate rates of progressive cervical change.
- **Prolonged second-stage arrest:** Arrest of fetal descent. See Table 2.11-16 for definitions based on parity and anesthesia.

TREATMENT

See Table 2.11-16.

COMPLICATIONS

- Chorioamnionitis leads to fetal infection, pneumonia, and bacteremia.
- Permanent injury occurs in 10%.
- The risk of postpartum hemorrhage is 11%; that of fourth-degree laceration is 3.8%.

RUPTURE OF MEMBRANES (ROM)

Distinguished as follows:

- **Spontaneous ROM:** Occurs after or at the onset of labor.
- **Premature ROM:** Occurs > 1 hour before onset of labor. May be precipitated by vaginal or cervical infections, abnormal membrane physiology, or cervical incompetence.

TABLE 2.11-16. Failure to Progress

STAGE	DEFINITION	TREATMENT[a]
FIRST STAGE: FAILURE TO HAVE PROGRESSIVE CERVICAL CHANGE		
Latent	• **Prima:** > 20 hrs • **Multi:** > 14 hrs	Therapeutic rest via parenteral analgesia; oxytocin; amniotomy; cervical ripening.
Active	• **Prima:** > 2 hrs • **Multi:** > 2 hrs after reaching 3–4 cm	Amniotomy; oxytocin; C-section if the previous interventions are ineffective.
SECOND STAGE: ARREST OF FETAL DESCENT		
	• **Prima:** > 2 hrs; > 3 hrs with epidural • **Multi:** > 1 hr; > 2 hrs with epidural	Close observation with a ↓ in epidural rate and continued oxytocin. Assisted vaginal delivery (forceps or vacuum). C-section.

[a] Augmentation with oxytocin should be considered when contraction frequency is < 3 in a 10-minute period or intensity of contraction is < 25 mm Hg above baseline.

- **Preterm premature ROM (PPROM):** ROM occurring at < 37 weeks' gestation.
- **Prolonged ROM:** ROM occurring > 18 hours prior to delivery. Risk factors include low socioeconomic status (SES), young maternal age, smoking, and STDs.

HISTORY/PE

Patients often report a **"gush" of clear or blood-tinged amniotic fluid.** Uterine contractions may be present.

DIAGNOSIS

- A **sterile speculum exam** reveals pooling of amniotic fluid in the vaginal vault.
- **Nitrazine paper test** is ⊕ (paper turns blue, indicating alkaline pH of amniotic fluid).
- **Fern test** is ⊕ (a ferning pattern is seen under a microscope after amniotic fluid dries on a glass slide).
- Ultrasound to assess amniotic fluid volume.
- **If the diagnosis is uncertain,** ultrasound-guided transabdominal instillation of indigo carmine dye can be used to check for leakage (unequivocal test).
- Minimize infection risk; do not perform digital vaginal exams on women who are not in labor or for whom labor is not planned immediately.
- Check fetal heart tracing, maternal temperature, WBC count, and uterine tenderness for evidence of chorioamnionitis.

TREATMENT

- Depends on GA and fetal lung maturity.
  - **Term:** First check GBS status and fetal presentation; then labor may be induced or the patient can be observed for 24–72 hours.

KEY FACT

To minimize the risk of infection, do not perform digital vaginal exams on women with PROM.

- > 34–36 weeks' GA: Labor induction may be considered.
- < 32 weeks' GA: Expectant management with bed rest and pelvic rest.
- **Antibiotics:** To prevent infection and to prolong the latency period in the absence of infection.
- **Antenatal corticosteroids:**
  - Give betamethasone or dexamethasone × 48 hours.
  - Promotes fetal lung maturity in the absence of intra-amniotic infection prior to 32 weeks' GA.
- If signs of infection or fetal distress develop, give antibiotics (ampicillin and gentamicin) and induce labor.

COMPLICATIONS

Preterm labor and delivery, chorioamnionitis, placental abruption, cord prolapse.

PRETERM LABOR

Onset of labor between **20 and 37 weeks' gestation.** The 1° cause of neonatal morbidity and mortality.

- Risk factors include multiple gestation, infection, PROM, uterine anomalies, previous preterm labor or delivery, polyhydramnios, placental abruption, poor maternal nutrition, and low SES.
- **Most patients have no identifiable risk factors.**

HISTORY/PE

Presents with menstrual-like cramps, onset of low back pain, pelvic pressure, and new vaginal discharge or bleeding.

DIAGNOSIS

- Requires the following:
  - **Regular uterine contractions** (3 or more contractions of 30 seconds each over a 30-minute period) and
  - **Concurrent cervical change** at < 37 weeks' gestation.
- Assess for contraindications to tocolysis such as infection, nonreassuring fetal testing, or placental abruption.
- **Sterile speculum exam** to rule out PROM.
- **Ultrasound** to rule out fetal or uterine anomalies, verify GA, and assess fetal presentation and amniotic fluid volume.
- Obtain cultures for chlamydia, gonorrhea, and GBS; obtain a UA and urine culture.

TREATMENT

- Hydration and bed rest.
- **Tocolytic therapy** (β-mimetics, $MgSO_4$, CCBs, PGIs) unless contraindicated.
- **Steroids** to accelerate fetal lung maturation.
- **Penicillin or ampicillin for GBS prophylaxis** if preterm delivery is likely.

COMPLICATIONS

RDS, intraventricular hemorrhage, **PDA,** necrotizing enterocolitis, retinopathy of prematurity, bronchopulmonary dysplasia, death.

KEY FACT

Preterm labor = regular uterine contractions + concurrent cervical change at < 37 weeks' gestation.

FETAL MALPRESENTATION

Any presentation other than vertex (ie, head closest to birth canal, chin to chest, occiput anterior). Risk factors include **prematurity,** prior breech delivery, uterine anomalies, poly- or oligohydramnios, multiple gestations, PPROM, hydrocephalus, anencephaly, and placenta previa.

History/PE

Breech presentations are the most common form and involve presentation of the fetal lower extremities or buttocks into the maternal pelvis (see Figure 2.11-12). Subtypes include the following:

- **Frank breech (50–75%):** The thighs are flexed and the knees are extended.
- **Footling breech (20%):** One or both legs are extended below the buttocks.
- **Complete breech (5–10%):** The thighs and knees are flexed.

Treatment

- **Follow:** Up to 75% spontaneously change to vertex by week 38.
- **External version:** If the fetus has not reverted spontaneously, a version may be attempted by applying directed pressure to the maternal abdomen to turn the infant to vertex. The success rate is roughly 50%. Risks of version are placental abruption and cord compression, so be prepared for an emergency C-section if needed.
- **Trial of breech vaginal delivery:** Attempt only if delivery is imminent. Complications include cord prolapse and/or head entrapment.
- **Elective C-section:** Recommended given the lower risk of fetal morbidity.

KEY FACT

Breech presentation is the most common fetal malpresentation.

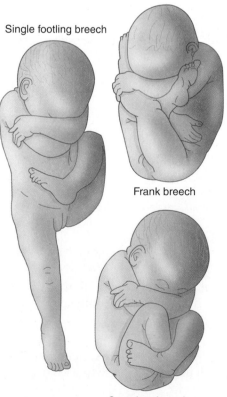

Single footling breech

Frank breech

Complete breech

FIGURE 2.11-12. Types of breech presentations. (Reproduced with permission from DeCherney AH. *Current Obstetric & Gynecologic Diagnosis & Treatment,* 8th ed. Stamford, CT: Appleton & Lange, 1994: 411.)

INDICATIONS FOR CESAREAN SECTION

See Table 2.11-17 for indications. For both elective and indicated cesarean delivery, sodium citrate should be used in the mother to ↓ gastric acidity and prevent acid aspiration syndrome.

EPISIOTOMY

- Surgical extension of the vaginal opening into the perineum.
- Can be **median** (midline) or **mediolateral.**
- Complications include the following:
    - **Extension to the anal sphincter (third degree) or rectum (fourth degree):** More common with midline episiotomy.
    - **Other:** Bleeding, infection, dyspareunia, rectovaginal fistula formation or maternal death (rare).
- **Routine use of episiotomy is not recommended.**

Puerperium

POSTPARTUM HEMORRHAGE

- A loss of **> 500 mL of blood for vaginal delivery** or **> 1000 mL for C-section.**
- May occur before, during, or after delivery of the placenta.
- Table 2.11-18 summarizes common causes.
- Complications include the following:
    - Acute blood loss (potentially fatal).
    - Anemia due to chronic blood loss (predisposes to puerperal infection).
    - Sheehan's syndrome.
- Severe postpartum hemorrhage may be controlled with uterine artery embolization.

POSTPARTUM INFECTIONS

- **A temperature ≥ 38°C for at least 2 of the first 10 postpartum days (not including the first 24 hours).**

KEY FACT

Postpartum endometritis:
- Fever > 38°C within 36 hours
- Uterine tenderness
- Malodorous lochia

TABLE 2.11-17. Indications for Cesarean Section

Maternal Factors	Fetal and Maternal Factors	Fetal Factors
Prior classical C-section (vertical incision predisposes to uterine rupture with vaginal delivery)	Cephalopelvic disproportion (the most common cause of 1° C-section)	Fetal malposition (eg, posterior chin, transverse lie, shoulder presentation)
Active genital herpes infection	Placenta previa/placental abruption	Fetal distress
Cervical carcinoma	Failed operative vaginal delivery	Cord compression/prolapse
Maternal trauma/demise	Postterm pregnancy (relative indication)	Erythroblastosis fetalis (Rh incompatibility)
HIV infection		
Prior transverse C-section (relative indication)		

TABLE 2.11-18. **Common Causes of Postpartum Hemorrhage**

VARIABLE	UTERINE ATONY	GENITAL TRACT TRAUMA	RETAINED PLACENTAL TISSUE
Risk factors	Uterine overdistention (multiple gestation, macrosomia, polyhydramnios). Exhausted myometrium (rapid or prolonged labor, oxytocin stimulation). Uterine infection. Conditions interfering with contractions (anesthesia, myomas, MgSO$_4$).	Precipitous labor. Operative vaginal delivery (forceps, vacuum extraction). Large infant. Inadequate episiotomy repair.	Placenta accreta/increta/percreta. Placenta previa. Uterine leiomyomas. Preterm delivery. Previous C-section/curettage.
Diagnosis	Palpation of a soft, enlarged, "boggy" uterus. The most common cause of postpartum hemorrhage (90%).	Manual and visual inspection of the lower genital tract for any laceration > 2 cm long.	Manual and visual inspection of the placenta and uterine cavity for missing cotyledons. Ultrasound may also be used to inspect the uterus.
Treatment[a]	Bimanual uterine massage (usually successful). Oxytocin infusion. Methergine (methylergonovine) if not hypertensive. Prostaglandin (PGF$_{2a}$).	Surgical repair of the physical defect.	Manual removal of remaining placental tissue. Curettage with suctioning (carries risk of uterine perforation).

[a] For all uterine causes, when bleeding persists after conventional therapy, uterine/internal iliac artery ligation, uterine artery embolization, or hysterectomy can be lifesaving.

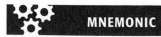

MNEMONIC

The 7 W's of postpartum fever (10 days postdelivery):

Womb (endomyometritis)
Wind (atelectasis, pneumonia)
Water (UTI)
Walk (DVT, pulmonary embolism)
Wound (incision, episiotomy)
Weaning (breast engorgement, abscess, mastitis)
Wonder drugs (drug fever)

- Risk factors for postpartum endometritis include emergent C-section, PROM, prolonged labor, multiple intrapartum vaginal exams, intrauterine manipulations, delivery, low SES, young age, prolonged ruptured membranes, bacterial colonization, and corticosteroid use.
- Tx: Broad-spectrum empiric IV antibiotics (eg, clindamycin and gentamicin) until patients have been afebrile for 48 hours (24 hours for chorioamnionitis). Add ampicillin for complicated cases.
- **Cx: Septic pelvic thrombophlebitis.**
  - Pelvic infection leads to infection of the vein wall and intimal damage, leading in turn to thrombogenesis. The clot is then invaded by microorganisms.
  - Suppuration follows, with liquefaction, **fragmentation, and, finally, septic embolization.**
  - Presents with abdominal and back pain and a "picket-fence" fever curve ("hectic" fevers) with wide swings from normal to as high as 41°C (105.8°F).
  - Diagnose with blood cultures and CT looking for a pelvic abscess.
  - Treat with broad-spectrum antibiotics and **anticoagulation** with heparin × 7–10 days.

SHEEHAN'S SYNDROME (POSTPARTUM PITUITARY NECROSIS)

- Pituitary ischemia and necrosis that lead to anterior pituitary insufficiency 2° to massive obstetric hemorrhage and shock.
- Hx/PE:
  - The 1° cause of anterior pituitary insufficiency in adult females.
  - **The most common presenting syndrome is failure to lactate (due to ↓ prolactin levels).**
  - Other symptoms include weakness, lethargy, cold insensitivity, genital atrophy, and menstrual disorders.
- **Dx:** Provocative hormonal testing and MRI of the pituitary and hypothalamus to rule out tumor or other pathology.
- **Tx:** Replacement of all deficient hormones. Some patients may recover TSH and even gonadotropin function after cortisol replacement alone.

LACTATION AND BREASTFEEDING

- During pregnancy, ↑ estrogen and progesterone result in breast hypertrophy and inhibition of prolactin release.
- After delivery of the placenta, hormone levels ↓ markedly and prolactin is released, stimulating milk production.
- Periodic infant suckling leads to further release of prolactin and oxytocin, which stimulate myoepithelial cell contraction and milk ejection ("letdown reflex").
- Colostrum ("early breast milk") contains protein, fat, **secretory IgA,** and minerals.
- Within 1 week postpartum, mature milk with protein, fat, lactose, and water is produced.
- High IgA levels in colostrum provide passive immunity for the infant and protect against enteric bacteria.
- Other benefits include the following:
  - ↓ incidence of infant allergies.
  - ↓ incidence of early URIs and GI infections.
  - Facilitation of mother-child bonding.
  - Maternal weight loss.
- Patients should use caution, especially if they have bleeding or cracked nipples, as exposure to blood could spread hepatitis. Contraindications to breastfeeding include HIV infection, active TB infection, active alcohol/drug abuse, and use of certain medications (eg, tetracycline, chloramphenicol).

KEY FACT

Breastfeeding is contraindicated in maternal HIV infection, active tuberculosis, drug abuse, use of certain medications, and in babies with galactosemia.

MASTITIS

Cellulitis of the periglandular tissue caused by nipple trauma from breastfeeding coupled with the introduction of bacteria, usually **S aureus,** from the infant's pharynx into the nipple ducts.

HISTORY/PE

- Symptoms often begin 2–4 weeks postpartum.
- Symptoms are **usually unilateral** and include the following:
  - Breast tenderness
  - A palpable mass
  - Erythema, edema, warmth, and possible purulent nipple drainage
- Significant fever, chills, and malaise may also be seen.

DIAGNOSIS

- Differentiate from simple breast swelling.
- Infection is suggested by focal symptoms, an ↑ WBC count, and fever.

TREATMENT

- **Continued breastfeeding** to prevent the accumulation of infected material (or use of a breast pump in patients who are no longer breastfeeding).
- **PO antibiotics** (dicloxacillin, cephalexin, amoxicillin/clavulanate, azithromycin, clindamycin).
- Targeted breast ultrasound to assess for abscess. If present, treat with incision and drainage.

GYNECOLOGY

Menarche and Normal Female Development

- **Thelarche:** Breast development; usually occurs between the ages of 8 and 11.
- **Menarche:** The first menstrual cycle; onset generally occurs between the ages of 10 and 16.
- Figure 2.12-1 graphically illustrates the stages of normal female development.

Normal Menstrual Cycle

The progression of a normal menstrual cycle is as follows (see also Figure 2.12-2):

- **Follicular phase (days 1–13):**
  - May vary, but typically lasts ~ 13 days.
  - ↑ FSH → growth of follicles → ↑ estrogen production.
  - Results in the development of straight glands and thin secretions of the uterine lining (proliferative phase).
- **Ovulation (day 14):**
  - LH and FSH spike, leading to rupture of the ovarian follicle and release of a mature ovum.
  - Ruptured follicular cells involute and create the corpus luteum.
- **Luteal phase (days 15–28):**
  - The length of time (14 days) that the corpus luteum can survive without further LH stimulation.

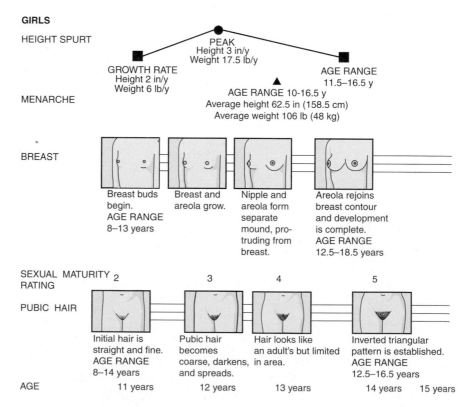

FIGURE 2.12-1. Normal female development. (Reproduced with permission from Hay WW Jr et al. *Current Diagnosis & Treatment: Pediatrics,* 19th ed. New York: McGraw-Hill, 2008, Fig. 3-4.)

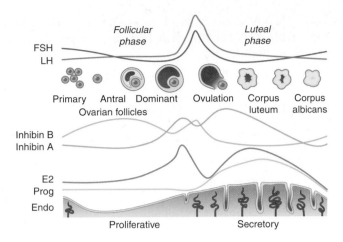

FIGURE 2.12-2. **Normal menstrual cycle.** (Reproduced with permission from Fauci AS et al. *Harrison's Principles of Internal Medicine,* 17th ed. New York: McGraw-Hill, 2008, Fig. 341-8.)

- The corpus luteum produces estrogen and progesterone, allowing the endometrial lining to develop thick endometrial glands with thick secretions (secretory phase).
- In the absence of implantation, the corpus luteum cannot be sustained, and the endometrial lining sloughs off.

Menopause

Cessation of menses for a minimum of 12 months as a result of cessation of follicular development.

HISTORY/PE

- The average age of onset is 51 years.
- Symptoms include hot flashes, vaginal atrophy, insomnia, anxiety/irritability, poor concentration, mood changes, dyspareunia, and loss of libido.
- "Premature menopause" is cessation of menses before age 40.

DIAGNOSIS

- A clinical diagnosis.
- The following studies are not routine but may be helpful:
  - **Labs:** ↑ **FSH;** then ↑ **LH.**
  - **Lipid profile:** ↑ total cholesterol, ↓ HDL.

TREATMENT

- **Vasomotor symptoms:**
  - **Hormone replacement therapy (HRT; combination estrogen and progestin):**
    - May ↑ the incidence of breast cancer.
    - ↑ cardiovascular morbidity and mortality.
    - Contraindications include vaginal bleeding, breast cancer (known or suspected), untreated endometrial cancer, a history of thromboembolism, chronic liver disease, and hypertriglyceridemia.
  - **Non-HRT:** SSRI/SNRIs, clonidine, and/or gabapentin to ↓ the frequency of hot flashes.
- **Vaginal atrophy:** Topical estrogen preparations.

KEY FACT

Currently, HRT is **not** recommended as first-line treatment for menopausal symptoms.

- **Osteoporosis:** DEXA scan is used to measure bone mineral density (BMD). Treat with daily calcium and vitamin D supplementation and exercise +/− bisphosphonates.

Contraception

Eighty-five percent of women who are sexually active with no contraception will become pregnant within 1 year.

- Table 2.12-1 describes the effectiveness of contraceptive methods along with their relative advantages and disadvantages.
- See Table 2.12-2 for contraindications to common methods of contraception.
- Emergency contraception (EC) methods prevent pregnancy after unprotected sex or contraceptive failure. Table 2.12-3 describes the various methods of EC.

Abnormalities of the Menstrual Cycle

1° AMENORRHEA/DELAYED PUBERTY

Defined as the absence of menses by age 16 with 2° sexual development present, or the absence of 2° sexual characteristics by age 14.

HISTORY/PE

- **Absence of 2° sexual characteristics** (no estrogen production): Etiologies are as follows:
    - **Constitutional growth delay:** The most common cause.
    - **1° ovarian insufficiency:** Most commonly Turner's syndrome. Look for a history of radiation and chemotherapy.
    - **Central hypogonadism:** May be caused by a variety of factors, including the following:
        - Undernourishment, stress, hyperprolactinemia, or exercise.
        - CNS tumor or cranial irradiation.
        - Kallmann's syndrome (isolated gonadotropin deficiency) associated with anosmia.
- **Presence of 2° sexual characteristics** (estrogen production but other anatomic or genetic problems): Etiologies include the following:
    - **Müllerian agenesis:** Absence of two-thirds of the vagina; uterine abnormalities.
    - **Imperforate hymen:** Presents with hematocolpos (blood in the vagina) that cannot escape, along with a bulging hymen.
    - **Complete androgen insensitivity:** Patients present with breast development (aromatization of testosterone to estrogen) but are amenorrheic and lack pubic hair.

DIAGNOSIS

- **Get a pregnancy test.**
- Obtain a bone age radiograph (PA left hand) to determine if bone age is consistent with pubertal onset (> 12 years in girls).
    - If the patient is of short stature (bone age < 12 years) with normal growth velocity, **constitutional growth delay** (the most common cause of 1° amenorrhea) is the probable cause.

TABLE 2.12-1.   Contraceptive Methods

METHOD	MECHANISM	ADVANTAGES	DISADVANTAGES
MOST EFFECTIVE: > 99%			
Implanon (progestin-only implant)	Inhibits ovulation; ↑ cervical mucus viscosity.	Effective for up to 3 years. Immediate fertility once removed. Safe with breastfeeding.	Weight gain, depression, irregular periods.
IUD with progestin (Mirena)	Foreign body results in inflammation; progesterone leads to cervical thickening and endometrial decidualization.	Effective for up to 5 years. Immediate fertility once removed. Safe with breastfeeding. Lighter periods; less cramping.	Spotting (up to 6 months), acne. Risk of uterine puncture (1/1000).
Copper T IUD (ParaGard)	Foreign body results in inflammation; copper has a spermicidal effect.	Effective for up to 10 years. Immediate fertility once removed. Safe with breastfeeding.	↑ cramping and bleeding (5–10%). Risk of uterine puncture (1/1000).
Surgical sterilization (vasectomy, tubal ligation)		Permanently effective; safe with breastfeeding.	**Tubal ligation:** Irreversible; ↑ ectopic pregnancy. **Vasectomy:** Most failures are due to not waiting for 2 ⊖ semen samples.
VERY EFFECTIVE: 90–99%			
Depo-Provera (medroxyprogesterone)	IM injection every 3 months.	Lighter or no periods. Each shot works for 3 months. Safe with breastfeeding.	Irregular bleeding and weight gain. Decreases in BMD (reversible). Delayed fertility after discontinuation (up to 10 months).
Ortho Evra ("the patch")	Combined weekly estrogen and progestin dermal patch.	Periods may be more regular. Weekly administration.	Thromboembolism risk (especially in smokers and those > 35 years of age).
NuvaRing ("the ring")	Combined low-dose progestin and estrogen vaginal ring.	Can make periods more regular. Three weeks—continuous; 1 week—no ring. Safe to use continuously.	May ↑ vaginal discharge. Spotting (first 1–2 months).

(continues)

TABLE 2.12-1. **Contraceptive Methods** *(continued)*

METHOD	MECHANISM	ADVANTAGES	DISADVANTAGES
OCPs (combination estrogen and progestin)	Inhibit FSH/LH, suppressing ovulation; thicken cervical mucus; decidualize endometrium.	↓ risk of ovarian and endometrial cancers.[a] Predictable, lighter, less painful menses. Can improve acne. Immediate fertility upon cessation.	Requires daily compliance. Breakthrough bleeding (10–30%). Thromboembolism risk (especially in smokers and those > 35 years of age).
Progestin-only "minipills"	Thicken cervical mucus.	Safe with breastfeeding.	Requires strict compliance with daily timing.
MODERATELY EFFECTIVE: 75–90%			
Male condoms	A latex sheath covers the penis.	The only method that effectively protects against pregnancy and STDs, including HIV.	Possible allergy to latex or spermicides.
Diaphragm with spermicide		Some protection against STDs.	Must be fitted by the provider.
Female condom		Some protection against STDs.	Can be difficult to use.
Fertility awareness methods		No side effects.	Requires the partner's participation. No STD/HIV protection.
LESS EFFECTIVE: 68–74%			
Withdrawal		No side effects.	No STD/HIV protection. Not recommended as a 1° method.
Spermicide		May be used as a 2° method.	Not recommended as a 1° method.

[a] Other combined hormonal methods (eg, patch, ring) may also protect against endometrial and ovarian cancer; however, data are still lacking given their relatively recent introduction.

- If bone age is > 12 years but there are no signs of puberty, obtain **LH/FSH** levels and consider where the problem is on the HPA axis (see Table 2.12-4).
- Ultrasound to evaluate the ovaries.
- **Normal breast development and no uterus:** Obtain a karyotype to evaluate for androgen insensitivity syndrome (XY).
- **Normal breast development and uterus:** Measure prolactin and obtain an MRI to assess the pituitary gland.

TABLE 2.12-2.   Contraindications to Common Methods of Contraception

ESTROGEN-CONTAINING HORMONAL METHODS[a]	IUDs (MIRENA AND COPPER)
Pregnancy	Known or suspected pregnancy
A history of stroke or DVT	Unexplained vaginal bleeding
Breast cancer	Current purulent cervicitis
Undiagnosed abnormal vaginal bleeding	Active (within 3 months) or recurrent PID
Estrogen-dependent cancer	Confirmed symptomatic actinomycosis on culture (but not asymptomatic colonization)
A benign or malignant liver neoplasm	A bicornuate or septate uterus
Current tobacco use **and** age > 35	Cervical or uterine cancer
	A Pap smear with a squamous intraepithelial lesion or 2 atypical Pap smears
	A history of heart valve replacement or artificial joints
	Copper T alone:
	▪ Copper intolerance (allergy to copper, Wilson's disease)
	▪ Severe dysmenorrhea and/or menorrhagia
	Mirena alone:
	▪ Levonorgestrel allergy
	▪ Breast cancer
	▪ Acute liver disease or liver tumor

[a] Includes OCPs, NuvaRing, and Ortho Evra.

TREATMENT

- **Constitutional growth delay:** No treatment is necessary.
- **Hypogonadism:** Begin HRT with estrogen alone at the lowest dose. Twelve to 18 months later, begin cyclic estrogen/progesterone therapy (if the uterus is present).
- **Anatomic:** Generally requires surgical intervention.

2° AMENORRHEA

Defined as the absence of menses for 6 consecutive months in women who have passed menarche.

DIAGNOSIS

- Get a pregnancy test.
- If ⊖, measure TSH and prolactin.
    - ↑ **TSH:** Indicates hypothyroidism.
    - ↑ **prolactin** (inhibits the release of LH and FSH): Points to a pituitary pathology. Order an MRI of the pituitary to look for a prolactin-secreting pituitary adenoma.

Q   1

A 56-year-old female presents with complaints of insomnia, vaginal dryness, and lack of menses for 13 months. What is the most likely diagnosis?

Q   2

A 16-year-old female presents with ↓ appetite, insomnia, and amenorrhea for 3 months. What is the most likely diagnosis, and how will you confirm it?

TABLE 2.12-3. **Emergency Contraceptive Methods**

METHOD	ADVANTAGES	DISADVANTAGES
"Morning-after pill"[a]		
Combined estrogen/ progestin (75% effective)	Available over the counter. Does not disrupt embryo postimplantation. Can be used as bridge contraception. Safe for all women.	Nausea, vomiting, fatigue, headache, dizziness, breast tenderness. No protection against STDs.
Progestin only (80% effective)	Same as above. Fewer nausea/vomiting side effects than combined EC.	Same as above.
Copper T IUD (99% effective)[b]	Can be used as EC and continued for up to 10 years of contraception.	High initial cost of insertion. Must be inserted by the provider. No protection against STDs.

[a] Used within 120 hours of unprotected sex.

[b] Used within 7 days of unprotected sex.

- **Initiate a progestin challenge** (10 days of progestin): See Figure 2.12-3 for an algorithm of the diagnostic workup.
  - ⊕ **progestin challenge (withdrawal bleed):** Indicates anovulation that is likely due to noncyclic gonadotropin secretion, pointing to PCOS or idiopathic anovulation.
  - ⊖ **progestin challenge (no bleed):** Indicates uterine abnormality or estrogen deficiency.
- **Signs of hyperglycemia (polydipsia, polyuria) or hypotension:** Conduct a 1-mg overnight dexamethasone suppression test to distinguish congenital adrenal hyperplasia (CAH), Cushing's syndrome, and Addison's disease.
- **If clinical virilization is present:** Measure testosterone, DHEAS, and 17-hydroxyprogesterone.
  - **Mild pattern:** PCOS, CAH, or Cushing's syndrome.
  - **Moderate to severe pattern:** Look for an ovarian or adrenal tumor.

TREATMENT

- **Hypothalamic:** Reverse the underlying cause and induce ovulation with gonadotropins.
- **Tumors:** Excision; medical therapy for prolactinomas (eg, bromocriptine, cabergoline).
- **Premature ovarian failure (age < 40 years):** If the uterus is present, treat with estrogen plus progestin replacement therapy.

1° DYSMENORRHEA

Menstrual pain associated with ovulatory cycles in the absence of pathologic findings. Caused by uterine vasoconstriction, anoxia, and sustained contractions mediated by an excess of prostaglandin ($PGF_{2\alpha}$).

---

1 **A**

The most likely diagnosis is menopause. As a clinical diagnosis, menopause does not require the ordering of any tests. However, if you are trying to rule it out as a cause of 2° amenorrhea, you may consider ordering an FSH level. Elevation is suggestive of menopause.

2 **A**

The most likely diagnosis is pregnancy. Confirm with a β-hCG.

TABLE 2.12-4. Etiologies of 1° Amenorrhea

	GnRH	LH/FSH	ESTROGEN/ PROGESTERONE	ETIOLOGY
Constitutional growth delay	↓	↓	↓ (prepuberty levels)	Puberty has not started.
Hypogonadotropic hypogonadism	↓	↓	↓	Hypothalamic or pituitary problem.
Hyper-gonadotropic hypogonadism	↑	↑	↓	Ovaries have failed to produce estrogen.
Anovulatory problem	↑	↑	↑	PCOS or a problem with estrogen receptors.
Anatomic problem	Normal	Normal	Normal	Menstrual blood cannot get out.

HISTORY/PE

- Presents with low, midline, spasmodic pelvic pain that often radiates to the back or inner thighs.
- Cramps occur in the first 1–3 days of menstruation and may be associated with nausea, diarrhea, headache, and flushing.
- There are **no pathologic findings on pelvic exam.**

DIAGNOSIS

A diagnosis of exclusion. Rule out 2° dysmenorrhea (see below).

TREATMENT

NSAIDs; topical heat therapy; combined OCPs, Mirena IUD.

2° DYSMENORRHEA

Menstrual pain for which an organic cause exists. Common causes include endometriosis and adenomyosis, fibroids, adhesions, polyps, and PID.

HISTORY/PE

- Patients may have a palpable uterine mass, cervical motion tenderness, adnexal tenderness, a vaginal or cervical discharge, or visible vaginal pathology (mucosal tears, masses, prolapse). However, normal abdominal and pelvic exams do not rule out pathology.
- See Table 2.12-5 for distinguishing features of endometriosis vs. adenomyosis.

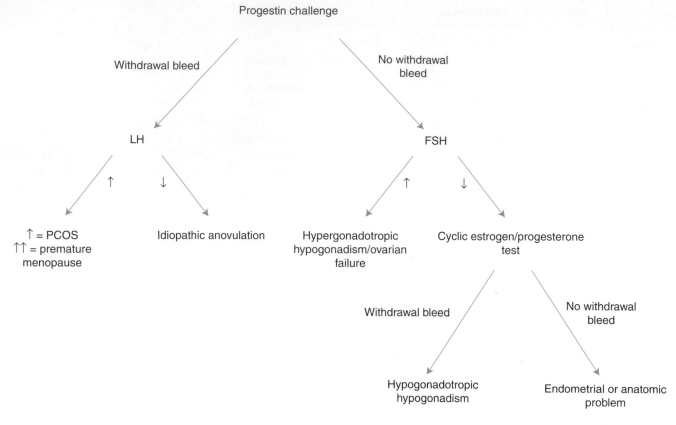

FIGURE 2.12-3. Workup of 2° amenorrhea.

DIAGNOSIS

- Obtain a β-hCG to exclude ectopic pregnancy.
- Order the following:
    - CBC with differential to rule out infection or neoplasm.
    - UA to rule out UTI.
    - Gonococcal/chlamydial swabs to rule out STDs/PID.
- Look for pelvic pathology causing pain (see Table 2.12-5).

TREATMENT

Treatment is etiology specific.

ABNORMAL UTERINE BLEEDING

Normal menstrual bleeding ranges from 2 to 7 days. Dysfunctional uterine bleeding (DUB) is a diagnosis of exclusion that is defined as follows:

- Abnormal uterine bleeding without evidence of an underlying cause.
- May be ovulatory or anovulatory.

HISTORY/PE

- Assess the extent of bleeding:
    - **Oligomenorrhea:** An ↑ length of time between menses (35–90 days between cycles).
    - **Polymenorrhea:** Frequent menstruation (< 21-day cycle); anovular.
    - **Menorrhagia:** ↑ amount of flow (> 80 mL of blood loss per cycle) or prolonged bleeding (flow lasting > 8 days); may lead to anemia.

TABLE 2.12-5. **Endometriosis vs. Adenomyosis**

VARIABLE	ENDOMETRIOSIS	ADENOMYOSIS
Definition	Functional endometrial glands and stroma **outside** the uterus.	Endometrial tissue **in** the myometrium of the uterus.
History/PE	**Cyclical** pelvic and/or rectal pain and dyspareunia.	Classic triad of **noncyclical** pain, menorrhagia, and an enlarged uterus.
Diagnosis	Requires direct visualization by laparoscopy or laparotomy. Classic lesions have a blue-black ("raspberry") or dark brown ("powder-burned") appearance. The ovaries may have endometriomas ("chocolate cysts").	Ultrasound is useful but cannot always distinguish between leiomyoma and adenomyosis. MRI can aid in diagnosis but is costly. Ultimately a pathologic diagnosis.
Treatment	**Pharmacologic:** Inhibit ovulation. Combination OCPs (first line), GnRH analogs (leuprolide), danazol, NSAIDs, or progestins. **Conservative surgical treatment:** Excision, cauterization, or ablation of the lesions and lysis of adhesions. Twenty percent of patients can become pregnant subsequent to treatment. **Definitive surgical treatment:** Total abdominal hysterectomy/bilateral salpingo-oophorectomy (TAH/BSO) +/– lysis of adhesions.	**Pharmacologic:** Largely symptomatic relief. NSAIDs (first line) plus OCPs or progestins. **Conservative surgical treatment:** Endometrial ablation or resection using hysteroscopy. Complete eradication of deep adenomyosis is difficult and results in high treatment failure. **Definitive surgical treatment:** Hysterectomy is the only definitive treatment.
Complications	Infertility (the most common cause among menstruating women > 30 years of age).	Can rarely progress to endometrial carcinoma.

- **Metrorrhagia:** Bleeding between periods.
- **Menometrorrhagia:** Excessive and irregular bleeding.
- On pelvic examination, look for an enlarged uterus, a cervical mass, or polyps to assess for myomas, pregnancy, or cervical cancer.

DIAGNOSIS

- β-hCG: To rule out ectopic pregnancy.
- CBC: To evaluate for anemia.
- **Pap smear:** To rule out cervical cancer.
- **TFTs:** To rule out hyper-/hypothyroidism and hyperprolactinemia.
- **Platelet count, PT/PTT:** To rule out von Willebrand's disease and factor XI deficiency, primarily in adolescent patients.
- **Ultrasound:** To look for uterine masses, polycystic ovaries, and thickness of the endometrium.
- Endometrial biopsy should be performed:
  - If the endometrium is ≥ 4 mm in a **postmenopausal woman, or**
  - If the patient is > 35 years of age with risk factors for endometrial hyperplasia (eg, obesity, diabetes).

TREATMENT

- **Heavy bleeding:**
  - High-dose estrogen IV stabilizes the endometrial lining and typically stops bleeding within 1 hour.

KEY FACT

Pregnancy is the most common cause of abnormal uterine bleeding and amenorrhea. Always check a pregnancy test!

KEY FACT

First-line treatment of abnormal uterine bleeding consists of NSAIDs to ↓ blood loss!

- If bleeding is not controlled within 12–24 hours, a D&C is often indicated.
- **Ovulatory bleeding:**
  - NSAIDs to ↓ blood loss.
  - If the patient is hemodynamically stable, give OCPs or a Mirena IUD.
- **Anovulatory bleeding:**
  - The goal is to convert proliferative endometrium to secretory endometrium (to ↓ the risk of endometrial hyperplasia/cancer).
  - Progestins × 10 days to stimulate withdrawal bleeding.
  - Desmopressin to cause a rapid ↑ in von Willebrand's factor and factor VIII (young patients who may also have a bleeding disorder).
  - OCPs.
  - Mirena IUD.
- If medical management fails:
  - **D&C.**
  - **Hysteroscopy:** To identify endometrial polyps or to perform directed uterine biopsies.
  - **Hysterectomy or endometrial ablation:** Appropriate for the following:
    - Women who fail or do not want hormonal treatment.
    - Women who have symptomatic anemia and/or who experience a disruption in their quality of life from persistent, unscheduled bleeding.

Reproductive Endocrinology

CONGENITAL ADRENAL HYPERPLASIA (CAH)

A deficiency of at least 1 enzyme required for the biochemical synthesis of cortisol from cholesterol (see Figure 2.12-4). Includes the following:

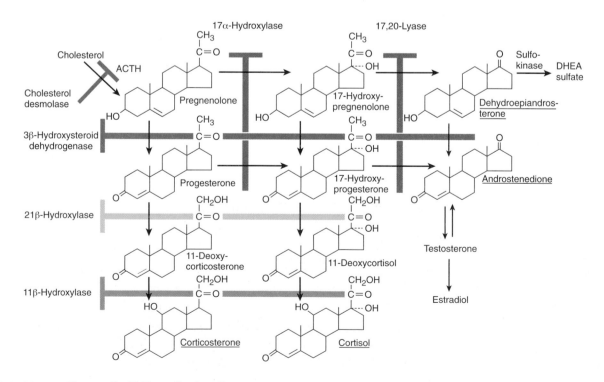

FIGURE 2.12-4. Glucocorticoid biosynthesis pathway. (Reproduced with permission from Barrett KE et al. *Ganong's Review of Medical Physiology,* 23rd ed. New York: McGraw-Hill, 2010, Fig. 22-7.)

- **21-hydroxylase deficiency:** The most severe, classic form; presents as a newborn female infant with ambiguous genitalia and life-threatening salt wasting.
- **11β-hydroxylase deficiency:** A less common cause of adrenal hyperplasia.

HISTORY/PE

Presents with excessive hirsutism, acne, amenorrhea and/or abnormal uterine bleeding, infertility, and, rarely, a palpable pelvic mass.

DIAGNOSIS

- ↑ **androgens (testosterone > 2 ng; DHEAS > 7 µg/mL):** Rule out adrenal or ovarian neoplasm.
- ↑ **serum testosterone:** Suspect an ovarian tumor.
- ↑ **DHEAS:** Suspect an adrenal source (adrenal tumor, Cushing's syndrome, CAH).
- ↑ **17-OH progesterone levels** (either basally or in response to ACTH stimulation).

TREATMENT

- **Glucocorticoids** (eg, prednisone). Medical therapy for adrenal and ovarian disorders prevents new terminal hair growth but does not resolve hirsutism.
- Laser ablation, electrolysis, or conventional hair removal techniques must be used to remove unwanted hair.

POLYCYSTIC OVARIAN SYNDROME (PCOS)

PCOS has a prevalence of 6–10% among U.S. women of reproductive age. Diagnosis requires 2 of the following 3 criteria:

1. Polycystic ovaries
2. Oligo-/anovulation
3. Clinical or biochemical evidence of hyperandrogenism

HISTORY/PE

- Look for a high BP and obesity (BMI > 30).
- Stigmata of hyperandrogenism or insulin resistance include menstrual cycle disturbances, hirsutism, obesity, acne, androgenic alopecia, and acanthosis nigricans.
- Women with PCOS are also at ↑ risk for the following:
  - Type 2 diabetes mellitus (DM)
  - Insulin resistance
  - Infertility
  - Metabolic syndrome—insulin resistance, obesity, atherogenic dyslipidemia, and hypertension

DIAGNOSIS

- **Biochemical hyperandrogenemia:** ↑ testosterone (total +/– free); DHEAS, DHEA.
- **Exclude other causes of hyperandrogenism:**
  - TSH, prolactin.
  - 17-OH progesterone to rule out nonclassical CAH.
  - Consider screening in the setting of clinical signs of Cushing's syndrome (eg, moon facies, buffalo hump, abdominal striae) or acromegaly (eg, ↑ head size).

Q

A 23-year-old female presents with fever and abdominal pain of 2 days' duration. She has a ⊕ chandelier sign. Antibiotics are started. What is the next step in management?

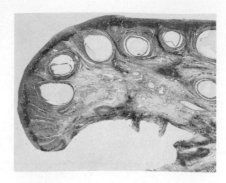

FIGURE 2.12-5. Polycystic ovary with prominent multiple cysts. (Reproduced with permission from DeCherney AH, Nathan R. *Current Diagnosis & Treatment: Obstetrics & Gynecology,* 10th ed. New York: McGraw-Hill, 2007, Fig. 40-3.)

KEY FACT

Combined hormonal contraception or progestin ↓ the risk of endometrial hyperplasia/carcinoma among women with PCOS.

A pelvic ultrasound to rule out tubo-ovarian abscess.

- **Evaluate for metabolic abnormalities:**
  - Two-hour oral glucose tolerance test.
  - Fasting lipid and lipoprotein levels (total cholesterol, HDL, LDL, triglycerides).
- **Optional tests:**
  - **Ultrasound:** Look for > 8 small, subcapsular follicles forming a **"pearl necklace" sign** (see Figure 2.12-5). Seen in roughly two-thirds of women with PCOS.
  - **Gonadotropins:** ↑ LH/FSH ratio (> 2:1).
  - **24-hour urine for free cortisol:** Adult-onset CAH or Cushing's syndrome.

TREATMENT

- **Women who are not attempting to conceive:** Treat with a combination of OCPs, progestin, and metformin (or other insulin-sensitizing agents).
- **Women who are attempting to conceive:** Clomiphene +/− metformin is first-line treatment for ovulatory stimulation.
- **Symptom-specific treatment:**
  - **Hirsutism:** Combination OCPs are first line; antiandrogens (spironolactone, finasteride) and metformin may also be used.
  - **Cardiovascular risk factors and lipid levels:** Diet, weight loss, and exercise plus potentially lipid-controlling medication (eg, statins).

COMPLICATIONS

↑ risk of early-onset type 2 DM; ↑ risk of miscarriages; ↑ long-term risk of breast and endometrial cancer due to unopposed estrogen secretion.

INFERTILITY

- The inability to conceive after 12 months of normal, regular, unprotected sexual activity.
- 1° infertility is characterized by no prior pregnancies; 2° infertility occurs in the setting of at least 1 prior pregnancy. Etiologies are shown in Figure 2.12-6 and Table 2.12-6.

Gynecologic Infections

CYST AND ABSCESS OF BARTHOLIN'S DUCT

Obstruction of the gland leads to pain, swelling, and abscess formation.

HISTORY/PE

- Presents with periodic painful swelling on either side of the introitus along with dyspareunia.
- A fluctuant swelling 1–4 cm in diameter is seen in the inferior portion of either labium minus.
- Tenderness is evidence of active infection.

TREATMENT

- **Asymptomatic cysts:** No therapy +/− warm soaks.
- **Abscess:** Aspiration or incision and drainage with Word catheter insertion to prevent reaccumulation; culture for *Chlamydia* and other pathogens.
- Antibiotics are unnecessary unless cellulitis is present.

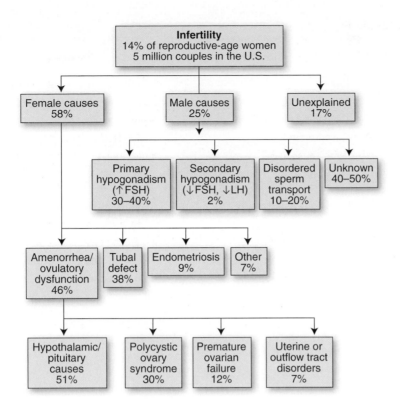

FIGURE 2.12-6. **Causes of infertility.** (Reproduced with permission from Fauci AS et al. *Harrison's Principles of Internal Medicine,* 17th ed. New York: McGraw-Hill, 2008, Fig. 341-9.)

VAGINITIS

A spectrum of conditions that cause vulvovaginal symptoms such as itching, burning, irritation, and abnormal discharge. The most common causes are bacterial vaginosis, vulvovaginal candidiasis, and trichomoniasis (see Table 2.12-7).

HISTORY/PE

- Presents with a change in discharge, malodor, pruritus, irritation, burning, swelling, dyspareunia, and dysuria.
- Normal secretions are as follows:
    - **Midcycle estrogen surge:** Clear, elastic, mucoid secretions.
    - **Luteal phase/pregnancy:** Thick and white secretions; adhere to the vaginal wall.
- Conduct a thorough examination of the vulva, vaginal walls, and cervix.
- If there are many WBCs and no organism on saline smear, suspect *Chlamydia.*

DIAGNOSIS/TREATMENT

- Cervical fluid for vaginal pH, amine (whiff) test, wet mount (with saline), and 10% potassium hydroxide (KOH) microscopy.
- In patients with a purulent discharge, numerous leukocytes on wet prep, cervical friability, and any symptoms of PID, order DNA tests or cultures for *Neisseria gonorrhoeae* or *Chlamydia trachomatis* to rule out cervicitis.
- Treatment is etiology specific (see Table 2.12-7).

> **KEY FACT**
>
> Criteria for the clinical diagnosis of bacterial vaginosis (3 of 4 are required):
> - Abnormal whitish-gray discharge
> - Vaginal pH > 4.5
> - ⊕ amine (whiff) test
> - Clue cells comprise > 20% of epithelial cells on wet mount

TABLE 2.12-6. Infertility Workup

Etiology	History/PE	Diagnosis	Treatment
Male causes	Testicular injury or infection Medications (corticosteroids, cimetidine, spironolactone) Thyroid or liver disease Signs of hypogonadism Varicocele	TSH Prolactin Karyotype (to rule out Klinefelter's syndrome) Semen analysis	Treatment of hormonal deficiency Intrauterine insemination (IUI) Donor insemination In vitro fertilization (IVF) Intracytoplasmic sperm injection
Ovulatory factors	Age (incidence ↑ with age) Symptoms of hyper-/hypothyroidism Galactorrhea Menstrual cycle abnormalities	Basal body temperature Ovulation predictor Midluteal progesterone Early follicular FSH +/− estradiol level (ovarian reserve) TSH, prolactin, androgens Ovarian sonography (antral follicle count) Endometrial biopsy (luteal-phase defect)	Treatment depends on the etiology (eg, levothyroxine, dopamine) Induction of ovulation with **clomiphene**, gonadotropins, and pulsatile GnRH IUI IVF
Tubal/pelvic factors	History of PID, appendicitis, endometriosis, pelvic adhesions, tubal surgery	Hysterosalpingogram Endometrial biopsy	Laparoscopic resection or ablation of endometriomas or fibroids IVF
Cervical factors	Abnormal Pap smears, postcoital bleeding, cryotherapy, conization, or DES exposure in utero	Pap smear Physical examination Antisperm antibodies	IUI with washed sperm IVF

KEY FACT

IUDs do not ↑ PID risk.

CERVICITIS

- **Inflammation of the uterine cervix.** Etiologies are as follows:
  - **Infectious** (most common): *Chlamydia*, gonococcus, *Trichomonas*, HSV, HPV.
  - **Noninfectious:** Trauma, radiation exposure, malignancy.
- **Hx/PE:** Yellow-green mucopurulent discharge; ⊕ cervical motion tenderness; absence of other signs of PID.
- **Dx/Tx:** See the discussion of STDs in the Infectious Disease chapter.

PELVIC INFLAMMATORY DISEASE (PID)

A polymicrobial infection of the upper genital tract. Associated with *N gonorrhoeae* (one-third of cases), *C trachomatis* (one-third of cases), and endogenous aerobes/anaerobes. Risk factors include non-Caucasian ethnicity, douching, smoking, multiple sex partners, and prior STDs and/or PID.

KEY FACT

The chandelier sign is defined as severe cervical motion tenderness that makes the patient "jump for the chandelier" on examination.

History/PE

- Presents with lower abdominal pain, fever and chills, menstrual disturbances, and a purulent cervical discharge.
- Cervical motion tenderness (chandelier sign) and adnexal tenderness are also seen.

TABLE 2.12-7. Causes of Vaginitis

VARIABLE	BACTERIAL VAGINOSIS	TRICHOMONAS	YEAST
Incidence	15–50% (most common).	5–50%.	15–30%.
Etiology	Reflects a shift in vaginal flora.	Protozoal flagellates **(an STD)**.	Usually *Candida albicans*.
Risk factors	Pregnancy, > 1 sexual partner, female sexual partner, frequent douching.	Unprotected sex with multiple partners.	**DM, broad-spectrum antibiotic use, pregnancy, corticosteroids**, HIV, OCP use, ↑ frequency of intercourse.
History	Odor, ↑ discharge.	↑ discharge, odor, pruritus, dysuria.	Pruritus, dysuria, burning, ↑ discharge.
Exam	Mild vulvar irritation.	"Strawberry petechiae" in the upper vagina/cervix.	Erythematous, excoriated vulva/vagina.
Discharge	Homogenous, **grayish-white, fishy/stale** odor.	Profuse, malodorous, **yellow-green, frothy.**	Thick, white, curdy texture without odor.
Wet mount[a]	**"Clue cells"** (epithelial cells coated with bacteria; see Figure 2.12-7); shift in vaginal flora (↑ cocci, ↓ lactobacilli).	**Motile trichomonads** (flagellated organisms that are slightly larger than WBCs).	–
KOH prep	⊕ "whiff" test (fishy smell).	–	Hyphae (see Figure 2.12-7).
Treatment	PO or vaginal metronidazole or vaginal clindamycin.	Single-dose PO metronidazole or tinidazole. Treat partners; test for other STDs.	Topical azole or PO fluconazole.
Complications	Chorioamnionitis/endometritis, infection, preterm delivery, miscarriage, PID.	Same as for bacterial vaginosis.	

[a] If there are many WBCs and no organism on saline smear, suspect *Chlamydia*.

DIAGNOSIS

- Diagnosed by the presence of acute lower abdominal or pelvic pain plus 1 of the following:
  - Uterine tenderness
  - Adnexal tenderness
  - Cervical motion tenderness
- A WBC count > 10,000 cells/μL has **poor positive and negative predictive value** for PID.
- Order a β-hCG to rule out pregnancy.
- Ultrasound may show thickening or dilation of the fallopian tubes, fluid in the cul-de-sac, a multicystic ovary, or tubo-ovarian abscess.

TREATMENT

- Antibiotic treatment should not be delayed while awaiting culture results. All sexual partners should be examined and treated appropriately.

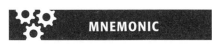

MNEMONIC

Acute causes of pelvic pain—

A ROPE

Appendicitis
Ruptured ovarian cyst
Ovarian torsion/abscess
PID
Ectopic pregnancy

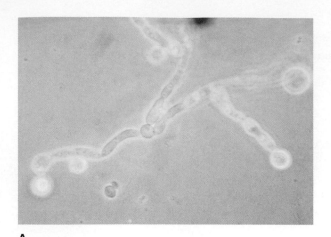
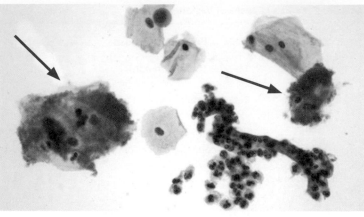

A

B

FIGURE 2.12-7. **Causes of vaginitis.** (A) Candidal vaginitis. *Candida albicans* organisms are evident on KOH wet mount. (B) *Gardnerella vaginalis.* Note the granular epithelial cells ("clue cells") and indistinct cell margins. (Image A reproduced with permission from Wolff K et al. *Fitzpatrick's Color Atlas & Synopsis of Clinical Dermatology,* 5th ed. New York: McGraw-Hill, 2005: 717. Image B reproduced with permission from USMLERx.com.)

- Outpatient regimens:
    - **Regimen A:** Ceftriaxone IM × 1 dose **or** cefoxitin **plus** probenecid **plus** doxycycline × 14 days +/− metronidazole × 14 days.
    - **Regimen B:** Ofloxacin **or** levofloxacin × 14 days +/− metronidazole × 14 days.
- Inpatient antibiotic regimens:
    - Cefoxitin or cefotetan plus doxycycline × 14 days.
    - Clindamycin plus gentamicin × 14 days.
- Surgery:
    - Drainage of a tubo-ovarian/pelvic abscess is appropriate if the mass persists after antibiotic treatment; the abscess is > 4–6 cm; or the mass is in the cul-de-sac in the midline and drainable through the vagina.
    - If the abscess is dissecting the rectovaginal septum and is fixed to the vaginal membrane, colpotomy drainage is appropriate.
    - If the patient's condition deteriorates, perform exploratory laparotomy.
    - Surgery may range from TAH/BSO with lysis of adhesions in severe cases to conservative surgery for women who desire to maintain fertility.

COMPLICATIONS

- Repeated episodes of infection, chronic pelvic pain, dyspareunia, and ectopic pregnancy.
- Infertility (10% after the first episode, 25% after the second episode, and 50% after a third episode).
- Fitz-Hugh–Curtis syndrome (presents with associated perihepatitis, RUQ pain, abnormal liver function, and shoulder pain).

KEY FACT

Mild and subclinical PID is a major cause of tubal factor infertility, ectopic pregnancy, and chronic pelvic pain due to pelvic scarring.

TOXIC SHOCK SYNDROME (TSS)

Caused by preformed *S aureus* toxin (TSST-1); often occurs within 5 days of the onset of a menstrual period in women who have used **tampons.** The incidence in menstruating women is now 6–7:100,000 annually. Nonmenstrual cases are nearly as common as menstrual cases.

HISTORY/PE

- Presents with abrupt onset of fever, vomiting, and watery diarrhea, with a fever of 38.9°C (102°F) or higher.

- A diffuse macular erythematous rash is also seen.
- Nonpurulent conjunctivitis is common.
- Desquamation, especially of the palms and soles, generally occurs during recovery within 1–2 weeks of illness.

DIAGNOSIS

Blood cultures are ⊖ because symptoms result from preformed toxin and are not due to the invasive properties of the organism.

TREATMENT

- **Rapid rehydration.**
- **Antistaphylococcal drugs** (nafcillin, oxacillin); vancomycin for women with penicillin allergy.
- Corticosteroids can reduce the severity of illness and ↓ fever.
- Manage renal or cardiac failure.

COMPLICATIONS

- The mortality rate associated with TSS is 3–6%.
- Three major causes of death are ARDS, intractable hypotension, and hemorrhage 2° to DIC.

KEY FACT

TSS is a rare but potentially fatal reaction to *S aureus* toxin. Diagnosis is clinical because the reaction is to the toxin, not to the bacterium itself. The first steps in treatment are rapid rehydration and antibiotic treatment.

Gynecologic Neoplasms

Gynecologic cancers include uterine, endometrial, ovarian, cervical, and vulvar neoplasms. Ovarian cancer carries the highest mortality.

UTERINE LEIOMYOMA (FIBROIDS)

The most common **benign** neoplasm of the female genital tract. They present as discrete, round, firm, and often multiple tumors composed of smooth muscle and connective tissue.

- Tumors are estrogen and progesterone sensitive, often increasing in size during pregnancy and decreasing after menopause.
- Malignant transformation to leiomyosarcoma is rare (0.1–0.5%).
- Prevalence is 25% among Caucasian women and 50% among African American women.

KEY FACT

Uterine myomas are benign but can cause infertility or menorrhagia.

HISTORY/PE

- The majority of cases are asymptomatic.
- Symptomatic patients may present with the following:
  - **Bleeding:** Longer, heavier periods; anemia.
  - **Pressure:** Pelvic pressure and bloating; constipation and rectal pressure; urinary frequency or retention.
  - **Pain:** 2° dysmenorrhea, dyspareunia.
  - **Pelvic symptoms:** A firm, nontender, irregular enlarged ("lumpy-bumpy"), or cobblestone uterus may be felt on physical examination.

DIAGNOSIS

- **CBC:** To look for anemia.
- **Ultrasound:** To look for uterine myomas; can also exclude ovarian masses.
- **MRI:** Can delineate intramural and submucous myomas.

KEY FACT

If a uterine mass continues to grow after menopause, suspect malignancy.

TREATMENT

- **Pharmacologic:**
    - NSAIDs.
    - Combined hormonal contraception.
    - Medroxyprogesterone acetate or danazol to slow or stop bleeding.
    - GnRH analogs (leuprolide or nafarelin) to ↓ the size of myomas, suppress further growth, and ↓ surrounding vascularity. Also used prior to surgery.
- **Surgery:** Emergent surgery is indicated for torsion of a pedunculated myoma.
    - **Women of childbearing years:** Abdominal or hysteroscopic myomectomy.
    - **Women who have completed childbearing:** Total or subtotal abdominal or vaginal hysterectomy.
    - **Uterine artery embolization** (~ 25% will need further invasive treatment).

COMPLICATIONS

Infertility may be due to a myoma that distorts the uterine cavity and plays a role similar to that of an IUD.

ENDOMETRIAL CANCER

Type I endometrioid adenocarcinomas derive from **atypical endometrial hyperplasia** and are the most common female reproductive cancer in the United States. Type II cancers derive from serous or clear cell histology (see Table 2.12-8). Although Type II cancers tend to be more aggressive, diagnosis and management are similar for both types.

HISTORY/PE

- Vaginal bleeding (early finding).
- Pain (late finding).
- Metabolic syndrome.

TABLE 2.12-8. **Types of Endometrial Cancer**

VARIABLE	TYPE I: ENDOMETRIOID	TYPE II: SEROUS
Epidemiology	75% of endometrial cancers.	25% of endometrial cancers.
Etiology	Unopposed estrogen stimulation (eg, tamoxifen use, exogenous estrogen-only therapy).	Unrelated to estrogen; the p53 mutation is present in 90% of cases.
Precursor lesion	Hyperplasia and atypical hyperplasia.	None.
Mean age at diagnosis	55 years.	67 years.
Prognosis	Favorable.	Poor.

DIAGNOSIS

- Endometrial/endocervical biopsy.
- Pelvic ultrasound shows a thickened endometrium leading to hypertrophy and neoplastic change (see Figure 2.12-8).

TREATMENT

- High-dose progestins for women of childbearing age.
- TAH/BSO +/– radiation for postmenopausal women.
- TAH/BSO with adjuvant chemotherapy for advanced-stage cancer.

CERVICAL CANCER

The upper third of the cervix (endocervix) is composed of columnar cells (similar to the lower uterine segment). The lower two-thirds (ectocervix) is made up of squamous cells (similar to the vagina). The exposure of columnar cells to an acidic vaginal pH results in metaplasia to squamous cells. The normal squamocolumnar junction (transformation zone) is located in the ectocervix and can be exposed to carcinogens, resulting in cervical intraepithelial neoplasia (CIN), an abnormal proliferation or overgrowth of the basal cell layer.

- HPV DNA is found in 99.7% of all cervical carcinomas. HPV 16 is the most prevalent type in squamous cell carcinoma; HPV 18 is most prevalent in adenocarcinoma.
- Additional risk factors for cervical cancer include immunosuppression, infection with HIV or a history of STDs, tobacco use, high parity, and OCPs.
- The Gardasil vaccine may protect against HPV types 6, 11, 16, and 18 and may also prevent the development of cervical cancer.

HISTORY/PE

- Metrorrhagia, postcoital spotting, and cervical ulceration are the most common signs.
- A bloody or purulent, malodorous, nonpruritic discharge may appear after invasion.

KEY FACT

Hormonal contraceptives are protective against endometrial cancer.

KEY FACT

Screening of asymptomatic women for endometrial cancer is not recommended.

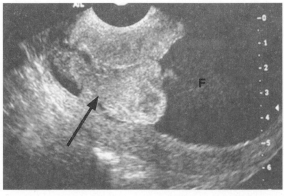

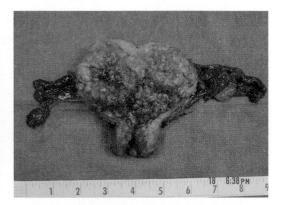

A   B

FIGURE 2.12-8. Endometrial cancer. (A) Sagittal endovaginal ultrasound image demonstrates a mass (arrow) in the lower uterine segment endometrial canal, with fluid (F) distending the canal in the fundus. (B) Gross specimen from a different patient shows a large mass filling the endometrial canal and invading the myometrium. (Image A reproduced with permission from USMLERx.com. Image B reproduced with permission from Schorge JO et al. *Williams Gynecology.* New York: McGraw-Hill, 2008, Fig. 33-16.)

SCREENING

- The American Congress of Obstetricians and Gynecologists (ACOG) currently recommends that screening for cervical cancer begin at age 21.
- ACOG previously recommended that cervical screening begin 3 years after the onset of sexual activity or by age 21, whichever occurred first. More recently, however, it was determined that despite the high incidence of HPV infection among sexually active adolescents, invasive cervical cancer was relatively rare among women < 21 years of age.
- Screening for cervical cancer should consist of the following (see also Table 2.12-9):
    - < 21 years of age: No testing.
    - 21 to 29 years of age: Every 3 years.
    - 30 to 65 years of age: Every 3 years or Pap plus HPV testing every 5 years.
    - > 65 years: Can stop screening if negative so far.

Additional changes to screening guidelines are as follows:

- Women ≥ 30 years of age can be screened once every 5 years with cytology and HPV DNA testing for high-risk strands.
- Screening can be be discontinued for women ≥ 65 years of age who have had adequate screening and are not high risk.
- Women with DES exposure and/or immunocompromised status (including HIV positivity) should continue to be screened as long as they do not have a life-limiting condition.
- Women who have had the HPV vaccine should continue to be screened.

DIAGNOSIS

The diagnosis and follow-up of specific subtypes of cervical lesions should be as follows (these guidelines do not apply to adolescents and pregnant women):

1. **ASC-US:** All nonpregnant women with cervical cytology showing ASC-US should have the following:
    - **HPV DNA testing:**
        - If ⊖: Repeat Pap smear at 12 months.
        - If ⊕: Colposcopy.
      OR

> **KEY FACT**
>
> Fifty percent of women with cervical cancer had not had a Pap smear in the 3 years preceding their diagnosis, and another 10% had not been screened in 5 years.

TABLE 2.12-9. **Classification Systems for Pap Smears**

NUMERICAL	DYSPLASIA	CIN	BETHESDA SYSTEM
1	Benign	Benign	Normal
2	Benign with inflammation	Benign with inflammation	Normal, atypical squamous cells (ASC)
3	Mild dysplasia	CIN I	LSIL
3	Moderate dysplasia	CIN II	HSIL
3	Severe dysplasia	CIN III	HSIL
4	Carcinoma in situ	CIN III	HSIL
5	Invasive cancer	Invasive cancer	Invasive cancer

- **Repeat cytology at 6 and 12 months:**
  - If both Pap smears are ⊖ at 6 and 12 months, return to routine screening.
  - If either Pap smear is ⊕ for ASC-US or higher, proceed to colposcopy. OR
- **Colposcopy.**
2. **ASC-H:** All nonpregnant women with cervical cytology showing ASC-H should have colposcopy.
3. **LSIL:** All nonpregnant, premenopausal women with cervical cytology showing LSIL should have colposcopy and then proceed as follows:
   - **If unsatisfactory or no visible lesion:** Endocervical sampling.
   - **If CIN 2, 3:** See the management of CIN below.
   - **If no CIN 2, 3:** Repeat Pap smear at 6 and 12 months OR conduct HPV testing at 12 months.
   - **Postmenopausal women** should have reflex HPV DNA testing, colposcopy, or a repeat Pap smear at 6 and 12 months.
   - **Pregnant women** should defer colposcopy until 6 weeks postpartum.
4. **AGC:**
   - All women with cervical cytology showing AGC should have colposcopy with endocervical sampling.
   - Women > 35 years of age or those with abnormal bleeding raising concern for endometrial neoplasia should have colposcopy with endocervical **and** endometrial sampling.
5. **HSIL:** All nonpregnant women with cervical cytology showing HSIL should have colposcopy with endocervical sampling and then proceed as follows:
   - **If CIN 2, 3:** Excision or ablation of lesion.
   - **If no CIN 2, 3:** Excision or observation with Pap smear and colposcopy every 6 months for a year OR immediate loop electrosurgical excision (LEEP).
   - Persistent HSIL should be treated with excision.
   - **Pregnant women** should have colposcopy without endocervical curettage.

TREATMENT

For **noninvasive disease,** treatment based on biopsy results for noninvasive lesions (stage 0 disease) is as follows:

- **CIN I:**
  - The mainstay of treatment is **close observation.**
  - For women > 21 years of age, Pap smear screening at 6 and 12 months and/or HPV DNA testing at 12 months is indicated.
  - For women ≤ 21 years of age, **HPV testing is not recommended.**
  - After 2 ⊖ Pap smears or a ⊖ DNA test, patients can be managed with routine annual follow-up.
- **Persistent CIN I:**
  - **Ablation:** Cryotherapy or laser ablation, or
  - **Excision:** LEEP; laser and cold-knife conization.
- **CIN II and III:**
  - **Ablation:** Cryotherapy or laser ablation, or
  - **Excision:** LEEP; laser and cold-knife conization.
  - Hysterectomy is a treatment option for recurrent CIN II or III.
- Postablative or excisional therapy follow-up is as follows:
  - **CIN I, II, or III with ⊖ margins:** Pap smear at 12 months and/or HPV testing.
  - **CIN II or III with ⊕ margins:** Pap smear at 6 months; consider a repeat endocervical curettage.

KEY FACT

Subtypes of cervical lesions:
- **ASC-US:** Atypical squamous cells of undetermined significance
- **ASC-H:** Atypical squamous cells—cannot exclude HSIL
- **LSIL:** Low-grade intraepithelial lesion
- **AGC:** Atypical glandular cells of undetermined significance
- **HSIL:** High-grade squamous intraepithelial lesion

■ If margins are unknown, obtain a Pap smear at 6 months and HPV DNA testing at 12 months.

Treatment based on biopsy results for **invasive disease** is as follows (for staging, see Figure 2.12-9):

■ **Microinvasive carcinoma (stage IA1):** Treat with cone biopsy and close follow-up or simple hysterectomy.
■ **Stages IA2, IB1, IIA:** May be treated either with radical hysterectomy with concomitant radiation and chemotherapy or with radiation plus chemotherapy alone.
■ **Stages IB2, IIB, III, IV:** Treat with radiation therapy plus concurrent cisplatin-based chemotherapy.

PROGNOSIS

■ The overall 5-year relative survival rate for carcinoma of the cervix is 68% in Caucasian women and 55% in African American women.
■ Survival rates are inversely proportionate to the stage of cancer:
  ■ **Stage 0:** 99–100%.
  ■ **Stage IA:** > 95%.
  ■ **Stage IB-IIA:** 80–90%.
  ■ **Stage IIB:** 65%.
  ■ **Stage III:** 40%.
  ■ **Stage IV:** < 20%.
■ Almost two-thirds of patients with untreated carcinoma of the cervix die of uremia when ureteral obstruction is bilateral.

VULVAR CANCER

Risk factors include **HPV (types 16, 18, and 31)**, lichen sclerosus, infrequent medical exams, diabetes, obesity, hypertension, cardiovascular disease, and immunosuppression. Vulvar intraepithelial neoplasia (VIN) is precancerous and is more commonly found in premenopausal women.

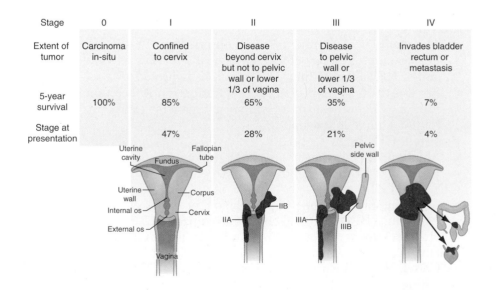

Stage	0	I	II	III	IV
Extent of tumor	Carcinoma in-situ	Confined to cervix	Disease beyond cervix but not to pelvic wall or lower 1/3 of vagina	Disease to pelvic wall or lower 1/3 of vagina	Invades bladder rectum or metastasis
5-year survival	100%	85%	65%	35%	7%
Stage at presentation		47%	28%	21%	4%

FIGURE 2.12-9. Staging of cervical cancer. Anatomic display of the stages of cervix cancer, defined by location, extent of tumor, frequency of presentation, and 5-year survival. (Reproduced with permission from Fauci AS et al. *Harrison's Principles of Internal Medicine,* 17th ed. New York: McGraw-Hill, 2008, Fig. 93-1.)

HISTORY/PE

- Presents with pruritus, pain, or ulceration of the mass.
- Additional symptoms include the following:
  - **Early:** Lesions may appear white, pigmented, raised, thickened, nodular, or ulcerative.
  - **Late:** Presents with a large, cauliflower-like or hard ulcerated area in the vulva.

DIAGNOSIS

Vulvar punch biopsy for any suspicious lesions or persistent vulvar pruritus, especially in postmenopausal women.

TREATMENT

- **High-grade VIN:** Topical chemotherapy, laser ablation, wide local excision, skinning vulvectomy, and simple vulvectomy.
- **Invasive:**
  - Radical vulvectomy and regional lymphadenectomy, or
  - Wide local excision of the 1° tumor with inguinal lymph node dissection +/− preoperative radiation, chemotherapy, or both.

VAGINAL CANCER

Accounts for 1–2% of all gynecologic malignancies. Risk factors include immunosuppression, chronic irritation (eg, long-term pessary use or prolapse of female organs), low socioeconomic status, radiation for cervical cancer, hysterectomy for dysplasia, multiple sexual partners, and DES exposure. Etiologies are as follows:

- **Postmenopausal women:** Usually squamous cell carcinoma.
- **Younger women:** Usually other histologic types (eg, adenocarcinoma, clear cell adenocarcinoma from DES).

HISTORY/PE

- Presents with abnormal vaginal bleeding, an abnormal discharge, or postcoital bleeding.
- Found in the upper third of the vagina in 75% of patients.

DIAGNOSIS

Cytology, colposcopy, and biopsy.

TREATMENT

- Local excision of involved areas when they are few and small.
- Extensive involvement of the vaginal mucosa may require partial or complete vaginectomy.
- Invasive disease requires radiation therapy or radical surgery.

OVARIAN CANCER

Most ovarian tumors are benign, but malignant tumors are the leading cause of death from reproductive tract cancer. Risk factors include the following:

- Age, low parity, ↓ fertility, or delayed childbearing.
- A ⊕ family history. Patients with 1 affected first-degree relative have a 5% lifetime risk. With 2 or more affected first-degree relatives, the risk is 7%.

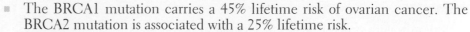

> **KEY FACT**

Frequency of female genital tract cancers: endometrial > ovarian > cervical. Number of deaths: ovarian > endometrial > cervical.

- The BRCA1 mutation carries a 45% lifetime risk of ovarian cancer. The BRCA2 mutation is associated with a 25% lifetime risk.
- Lynch II syndrome, or hereditary nonpolyposis colorectal cancer (HNPCC), is associated with an ↑ risk of colon, ovarian, endometrial, and breast cancer.
- OCPs taken for 5 years or more ↓ risk by 29%.

HISTORY/PE

- Both benign and malignant ovarian neoplasms are generally asymptomatic.
- Mild, nonspecific GI symptoms or pelvic pressure/pain may be seen.
- Early disease is typically not detected on routine pelvic exam.
- Some 75% of woman present with advanced malignant disease, as evidenced by abdominal pain and bloating, a palpable abdominal mass, and ascites.
- Table 2.12-10 differentiates the benign and malignant characteristics of pelvic masses.

DIAGNOSIS

- **Tumor markers** (see Table 2.12-11): ↑ **CA-125** is associated with epithelial cell cancer (90% of ovarian cancers) but is used only as a marker for progression and recurrence.
  - **Premenopausal women:** ↑ CA-125 may point to benign disease such as endometriosis.
  - **Postmenopausal women:** ↑ CA-125 (> 35 units) indicates an ↑ likelihood that the ovarian tumor is malignant.
- **Transvaginal ultrasound:** Used to screen high-risk women and as the first step in the workup of symptomatic women (eg, pelvic fullness, pelvic pain).

> **KEY FACT**

Any palpable ovarian or adnexal mass in a premenarchal or postmenopausal patient is suggestive of an ovarian neoplasm.

TABLE 2.12-10. Benign vs. Malignant Pelvic Masses

FINDING	BENIGN	MALIGNANT
EXAMINATION: PELVIC MASS		
Mobility	Mobile	Fixed
Consistency	Cystic	Solid or firm
Location	Unilateral	Bilateral
Cul-de-sac	Smooth	Nodular
TRANSVAGINAL ULTRASOUND: ADNEXAL MASS		
Size	< 8 cm	> 8 cm
Consistency	Cystic	Solid or cystic and solid
Septations	Unilocular	Multilocular
Location	Unilateral	Bilateral
Other	Calcifications	Ascites

TABLE 2.12-11 **Ovarian Tumor Markers**

Tumor	Marker
Epithelial	CA-125
Endodermal sinus	AFP
Embryonal carcinoma	AFP, hCG
Choriocarcinoma	hCG
Dysgerminoma	LDH
Granulosa cell	Inhibin

TREATMENT

Treatment of **ovarian masses** is as follows:

- **Premenarchal women:** Masses > 2 cm in diameter require close clinical follow-up and often surgical removal.
- **Premenopausal women:**
  - Observation is appropriate for asymptomatic, mobile, unilateral, simple cystic masses < 8–10 cm in diameter. Most resolve spontaneously.
  - Surgically evaluate masses > 8–10 cm in diameter and those that are complex and/or unchanged on repeat pelvic examination and ultrasound.
- **Postmenopausal women:**
  - Closely follow with ultrasound asymptomatic, unilateral simple cysts < 5 cm in diameter with a normal CA-125.
  - Surgically evaluate palpable masses.

Treatment of **ovarian cancer** is as follows:

- **Surgery:**
  - Surgical staging: TAH/BSO with omentectomy and pelvic and para-aortic lymphadenectomy.
  - Benign neoplasms warrant tumor removal or unilateral oophorectomy.
- **Postoperative chemotherapy:** Routine except for women with early-stage or low-grade ovarian cancer.
- **Radiation therapy:** Effective for dysgerminomas.

PREVENTION

- Women with the BRCA1 gene mutation should be screened annually with ultrasound and CA-125 testing. Prophylactic oophorectomy is recommended by age 35 or whenever childbearing is completed.
- OCP use ↓ the risk of ovarian cancer.

Pelvic Organ Prolapse

Risk factors for pelvic organ prolapse include vaginal birth, genetic predisposition, advancing age, prior pelvic surgery, connective tissue disorders, and ↑ intra-abdominal pressure associated with obesity or straining with chronic constipation.

HISTORY/PE

- Presents with the sensation of a bulge or protrusion in the vagina (see Figure 2.12-10).
- Urinary or fecal incontinence, a sense of incomplete bladder emptying, and/or dyspareunia are also seen.

DIAGNOSIS

The degree of prolapse can be evaluated by having the woman perform the Valsalva maneuver while in the lithotomy position.

TREATMENT

- Supportive measures include a high-fiber diet and weight reduction in obese patients and limitation of straining and lifting.
- Pessaries may reduce prolapse and are helpful in women who do not wish to undergo surgery or who are chronically ill.
- The most common surgical procedure is vaginal or abdominal hysterectomy with vaginal vault suspension.

Urinary Incontinence

Defined as the involuntary loss of urine due to either bladder or sphincter dysfunction.

HISTORY/PE

- Table 2.12-12 outlines the types of incontinence along with their distinguishing features and treatment (see also the mnemonic **DIAPPERS**).
- Exclude fistula in cases of total incontinence.
- Look for neurologic abnormalities in cases of urge incontinence (spasticity, flaccidity, rectal sphincter tone) or distended bladder in overflow incontinence.

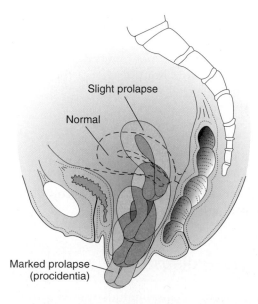

Slight prolapse

Normal

Marked prolapse
(procidentia)

FIGURE 2.12-10. **Uterine prolapse.** Different degrees of uterine prolapse are illustrated.
(Reproduced with permission from DeCherney AH, Nathan L. *Current Diagnosis & Treatment Obstetrics & Gynecology,* 10th ed. New York: McGraw-Hill, 2007, Fig. 44-3.)

TABLE 2.12-12. **Types of Incontinence**

TYPE	HISTORY OF URINE LOSS	MECHANISM	TREATMENT
Total	Uncontrolled loss at all times and in all positions.	Loss of sphincteric efficiency (previous surgery, nerve damage, cancer infiltration). Abnormal connection between the urinary tract and the skin (fistula).	Surgery.
Stress	After ↑ intra-abdominal pressure (coughing, sneezing, lifting).	Urethral sphincteric insufficiency due to laxity of pelvic floor musculature. Common in multiparous women or after pelvic surgery.	Kegel exercises and pessary. Vaginal vault suspension surgery.
Urge[a]	Strong, unexpected urge to void that is unrelated to position or activity.	Detrusor hyperreflexia or sphincter dysfunction due to inflammatory conditions or neurogenic disorders of the bladder.	Anticholinergic medications or TCAs; behavioral training (biofeedback).
Overflow[b]	Chronic urinary retention.	Chronically distended bladder with ↑ intravesical pressure that just exceeds the outlet resistance, allowing a small amount of urine to dribble out.	Placement of urethral catheter in acute settings. Treat underlying diseases. Timed voiding.

[a] Etiologies include inhibited contractions, local irritation (cystitis, stone, tumor), and CNS causes.

[b] Etiologies include physical agents (tumor, stricture), neurologic factors (lesions), and medications.

DIAGNOSIS/TREATMENT

- Obtain a UA and urine culture to exclude UTI.
- Voiding diary.
- Consider urodynamic testing.
- Serum creatinine to exclude renal dysfunction.
- Obtain a cystogram to demonstrate fistula sites and descensus of the bladder neck.
- Table 2.12-12 outlines treatment options according to subtype.

Pediatric Gynecology

PEDIATRIC VAGINAL DISCHARGE

Etiologies of vaginal discharge in pediatric patients include the following:

- **Infectious vulvovaginitis:** May present with a malodorous, yellow-green, purulent discharge. Causes include the following:
  - **Group A streptococcus:** The most common infectious cause.
  - **Candida:** May be associated with diabetes (rare in the pediatric population).
  - **STDs:** May result from sexual abuse.

MNEMONIC

Causes of urinary incontinence without specific urogenital pathology—

DIAPPERS

Delirium/confusional state
Infection
Atrophic urethritis/vaginitis
Pharmaceutical
Psychiatric causes (especially depression)
Excessive urinary output (hyperglycemia, hypercalcemia, CHF)
Restricted mobility
Stool impaction

KEY FACT

Pediatric vaginal discharge may be normal, but STDs resulting from sexual abuse must be ruled out and, if found, reported to Child Protective Services.

- **Noninfectious vulvovaginitis:** Causes include contact dermatitis and eczema.
- **Foreign objects.**
- **Sarcoma botryoides (rhabdomyosarcoma):** A malignancy with lesions that have the appearance of "bunches of grapes" within the vagina.

PRECOCIOUS PUBERTY

Onset of 2° sexual characteristics in a child < 8 years of age. Subtypes are as follows (see also Table 2.12-13):

- **Central precocious puberty:** **Early** activation of hypothalamic GnRH production.
- **Peripheral precocious puberty:** Results from GnRH-independent mechanisms.

HISTORY/PE

- **Signs of estrogen excess** (breast development and possibly vaginal bleeding): Suggest ovarian cysts or tumors.
- **Signs of androgen excess** (pubic and/or axillary hair, enlarged clitoris, and/or acne): Suggest adrenal tumors or CAH.

DIAGNOSIS

Figure 2.12-11 illustrates an algorithm for the workup of precocious puberty.

TREATMENT

- **Central precocious puberty:** Leuprolide is first-line therapy; physical changes regress or cease to progress.
- **Peripheral precocious puberty:** Treat the cause.
  - **Ovarian cysts:** No intervention is necessary, as cysts will usually regress spontaneously.
  - **CAH:** Treat with glucocorticoids. Surgery is not required for the treatment of ambiguous genitalia.
  - **Adrenal or ovarian tumors:** Require surgical resection.
  - **McCune-Albright syndrome:** Antiestrogens (tamoxifen) or estrogen synthesis blockers (ketoconazole or testolactone) may be effective.

KEY FACT

If onset of 2° sexual characteristics is seen by age 8, work up for precocious puberty by determining bone age and conducting a GnRH stimulation test to distinguish central from peripheral precocious puberty.

TABLE 2.12-13. **Causes of Precocious Pubertal Development**

CENTRAL (GnRH DEPENDENT)	PERIPHERAL (GnRH INDEPENDENT)
Constitutional (idiopathic)	CAH
Hypothalamic lesions (hamartomas, tumors, congenital malformations)	Adrenal tumors
Dysgerminomas	McCune-Albright syndrome (polyostotic fibrous dysplasia)
Hydrocephalus	Gonadal tumors
CNS infections	Exogenous estrogen, oral (OCPs) or topical
CNS trauma/irradiation	Ovarian cysts (females)
Pineal tumors (rare)	
Neurofibromatosis with CNS involvement	
Tuberous sclerosis	

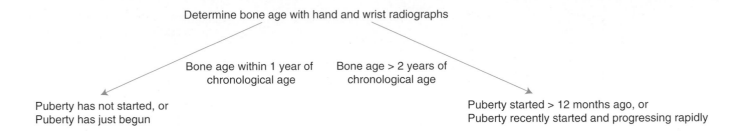

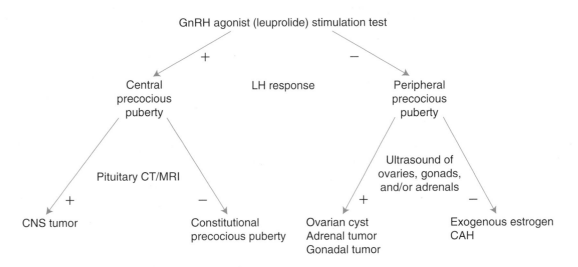

FIGURE 2.12-11. Workup of precocious puberty.

Breast Disorders

FIBROCYSTIC CHANGE

The most common of all benign breast conditions. It involves exaggerated stromal tissue response to hormones and growth factors.

- Findings include cysts (gross and microscopic), papillomatosis, adenosis, fibrosis, and ductal epithelial hyperplasia.
- Primarily affects women 30–50 years of age; rarely found in postmenopausal woman.
- Associated with trauma and caffeine use.

HISTORY/PE

- Cyclic bilateral mastalgia and swelling, with symptoms most prominent just before menstruation.
- Rapid fluctuation in the size of the masses is common.
- Other symptoms include an irregular, bumpy consistency to the breast tissue.

DIAGNOSIS

- See Figure 2.12-12 for an algorithm of a breast mass workup.
- Mammography is of limited use.
- Ultrasound can help differentiate a cystic from a solid mass.

> **KEY FACT**
>
> The differential diagnosis of a breast mass includes fibrocystic disease, fibroadenoma, mastitis/abscess, fat necrosis, and breast cancer.

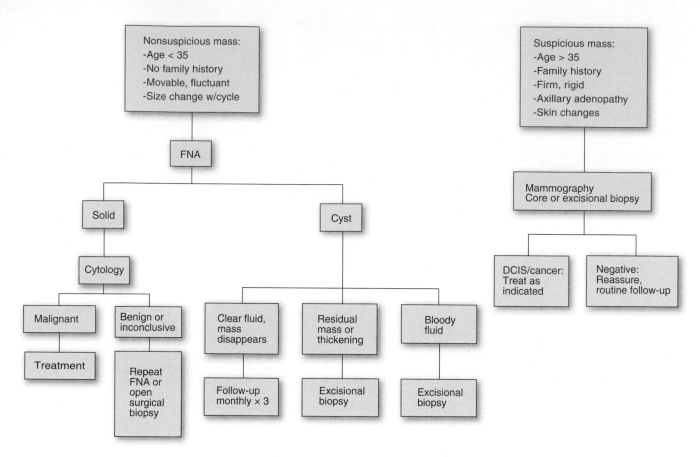

FIGURE 2.12-12. **Workup of a breast mass.**

- Fine-needle aspiration (FNA) of a discrete mass that is suggestive of a cyst is indicated to alleviate pain as well as to confirm the cystic nature of the mass.
- Excisional biopsy is indicated if no fluid is obtained or if the fluid is bloody on aspiration.
- There is an ↑ risk of breast cancer if ductal epithelial hyperplasia or cellular atypia is present.

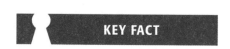

KEY FACT

Intraductal papilloma and mammary duct ectasia are common causes of bloody nipple discharge.

TREATMENT

- Dietary modifications (eg, caffeine restriction).
- Danazol can address severe pain but is rarely used in view of its side effects (acne, hirsutism, edema).
- Consider OCPs, which ↓ hormonal fluctuations.

FIBROADENOMA

A benign, slow-growing breast tumor with epithelial and stromal components. **The most common breast lesion in women < 30 years of age.** Cystosarcoma phyllodes is a large fibroadenoma.

HISTORY/PE

- Presents as a round or ovoid, rubbery, discrete, relatively mobile, non-tender mass 1–3 cm in diameter.
- Masses are usually solitary, although up to 20% of patients develop multiple fibroadenomas.

- Tumors do not change during the menstrual cycle.
- Does not occur after menopause unless the patient is on HRT.

DIAGNOSIS

- Breast ultrasound to differentiate cystic from solid masses.
- Needle biopsy or FNA.
- Excision with pathologic exam if the diagnosis remains uncertain.

TREATMENT

Excision is curative, but recurrence is common.

BREAST CANCER

The most common cancer (affects 1 in 8 women) and the second most common cause of cancer death in women (after lung cancer). **Sixty percent occur in the upper outer quadrant.** Risk factors include the following (**most women have no risk factors**):

- Female gender; older age.
- A personal history of breast cancer.
- Breast cancer in a first-degree relative.
- BRCA1 and BRCA2 mutations (associated with early onset).
- A high-fat and low-fiber diet.
- A history of fibrocystic change with cellular atypia.
- ↑ exposure to estrogen (nulliparity, early menarche, late menopause, first full-term pregnancy after age 35).

KEY FACT

↑ exposure to estrogen (early menarche, late menopause, nulliparity) ↑ the risk of breast cancer.

HISTORY/PE

Ninety percent of breast cancers are found by the patient. Clinical manifestations include the following:

- **Early findings:** May present as a single, nontender, firm-to-hard mass with ill-defined margins or as mammographic abnormalities with no palpable mass.
- **Later findings:** Skin or nipple retraction, axillary lymphadenopathy, breast enlargement, redness, edema, pain, fixation of the mass to the skin or chest wall.
- **Late findings:**
  - Ulceration; supraclavicular lymphadenopathy; edema of the arm; metastases to the bone, lung, and liver.
  - Prolonged unilateral scaling erosion of the nipple with or without discharge (Paget's disease of the nipple).
- **Metastatic disease:**
  - Back or bone pain, jaundice, weight loss.
  - A firm or hard axillary node > 1 cm.
  - Axillary nodes that are matted or fixed to the skin (stage III); ipsilateral supraclavicular or infraclavicular nodes (stage IV).

DIAGNOSIS

- **Screening:**
  - **Postmenopausal women: Mammography.** Look for ↑ density with microcalcifications and irregular borders. Mammography can detect lesions roughly 2 years before they become clinically palpable (see Figure 2.12-13A).
  - **Premenopausal women: Ultrasound** for women < 30 years of age; can distinguish a solid mass from a benign cyst (see Figure 2.12-13B).

Q

A 27-year-old woman palpates a 1 cm × 1cm new breast mass on self-examination. What is the first step in the workup of the mass?

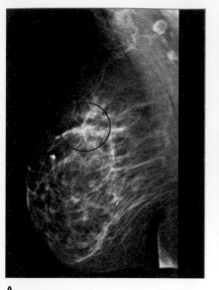
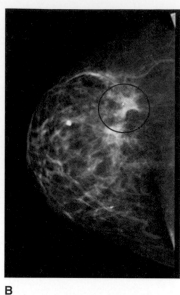
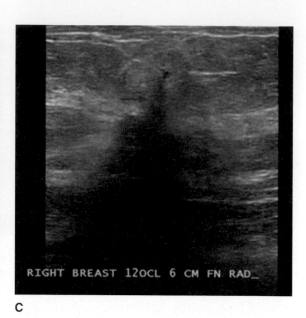

A   B   C

FIGURE 2.12-13. Breast cancer. Mediolateral oblique (**A**) and craniocaudal (**B**) views from a mammogram demonstrate a spiculated mass with a satellite mass (circle) in the central and outer upper right breast. A targeted breast ultrasound (**C**) in a different patient demonstrates a hypoechoic mass (arrow) that is taller than it is wide and demonstrates dense posterior acoustic shadowing. (Reproduced with permission from USMLERx.com.)

KEY FACT

In a postmenopausal woman with a new breast lesion, maintain a high degree of clinical suspicion for breast cancer.

KEY FACT

The first step in the workup of a suspicious mass in postmenopausal women and in those > 30 years of age is a mammogram. For premenopausal women < 30 years of age, get an ultrasound.

■ **Biopsy of suspicious lesions:**
  ■ **FNA:** A good initial biopsy, especially for lesions close to the skin; however, it is a small sample with a high false-⊖ rate. FNA may also be used to follow response to treatment.
  ■ **Core needle biopsy:** A larger sample that allows testing for receptor status.
  ■ **Open biopsy:** Provides tissue for a more accurate diagnosis and allows immediate resection of tumor; however, requires taking the patient to the OR.
■ **Tumor markers for recurrent breast cancer:** Include CEA and CA 15-3 or CA 27-29.
■ **Receptor status of tumor:** Determine estrogen receptor (ER), progesterone receptor (PR), and HER2/neu status.
■ **Metastatic disease:**
  ■ **Labs:** ↑ ESR, ↑ alkaline phosphatase (liver and bone metastases), ↑ calcium.
  ■ **Imaging:** CXR; CT of the chest, abdomen, and pelvis; brain MRI. PET and bone scans can also be useful.

TREATMENT

■ **Pharmacologic:**
  ■ All hormone receptor–⊕ patients should receive **tamoxifen.**
  ■ ER-⊖ patients should receive **chemotherapy.**
  ■ **Trastuzumab,** a monoclonal antibody that binds to HER2/neu receptors on the cancer cell, is highly effective in HER2/neu-expressive cancers.
■ **Surgical options** include the following:
  ■ Partial mastectomy (lumpectomy) plus axillary dissection followed by radiation therapy.
  ■ Modified radical mastectomy (total mastectomy plus axillary dissection).

Ultrasound. The patient is < 30 years of age, so ultrasound is the preferred means of distinguishing a solid mass from a cyst.

- **Contraindications to breast-conserving therapy (lumpectomy)** include large tumor size, subareolar location, multifocal tumors, fixation to the chest wall, prior radiation to the chest wall, or involvement of the nipple or overlying skin.
- **Stage IV disease** should be treated with radiotherapy and hormonal therapy; mastectomy may be required for local symptom control.

PROGNOSIS

- TNM staging (I–IV) is the most reliable indicator of prognosis.
- ER- and PR-⊕ status is associated with a favorable course.
- Cancer localized to the breast has a 75–90% cure rate. With spread to the axilla, the 5-year survival rate is 40–50%.
- Aneuploidy is associated with a poor prognosis.

COMPLICATIONS

Pleural effusion occurs in 50% of patients with metastatic breast cancer; edema of the arm is common.

KEY FACT

Breast cancer stages:
- Stage I: Tumor size < 2 cm.
- Stage II: Tumor size 2–5 cm.
- Stage III: Axillary node involvement.
- Stage IV: Distant metastasis.

Sexual Assault

The most frequently unreported crime in the United States. Physicians are often required to evaluate sexual assault victims and collect evidence. Most rape victims are women; however, men may also be victims of rape.

HISTORY/PE

- Take a full history, including contraceptive use, last time of coitus, condom use prior to the assault, drug or alcohol use, a history of STDs, a description of the assailant, location and time of the assault, circumstances of the assault (eg, penile penetration, use of condoms, extragenital acts, use or display of weapons), and the patient's actions since the assault (eg, douching, bathing, brushing teeth, urination/defecation, changing clothes).
- Conduct a complete physical examination, making note of any signs of trauma, along with a detailed pelvic examination, including a survey of the external genitals, vagina, cervix, and anus.

DIAGNOSIS

- Gonorrhea and chlamydia smear/culture (including rectal if appropriate); serologic testing for HIV, syphilis, HSV, HBV, and CMV.
- Serum pregnancy test.
- Blood alcohol level; urine toxicology screen.

TREATMENT

- STD treatment/prophylaxis (ceftriaxone plus azithromycin).
- HIV risk assessment and possible postexposure prophylaxis.
- EC for pregnancy prevention.
- Refer for psychological counseling.
- Arrange for follow-up with the same physician or with another provider if more appropriate.
- Follow-up should include repeat screening for STDs, repeat screening for pregnancy, and a discussion of coping methods with appropriate referrals for psychiatric care if needed.

NOTES

PEDIATRICS

Child Abuse

Also known as nonaccidental trauma; includes neglect as well as physical, sexual, and psychological maltreatment of children. Suspect abuse if the history is discordant with physical findings or if there is a delay in obtaining appropriate medical care. Certain injuries in children, such as retinal hemorrhages and specific fracture types, are pathognomonic for abuse.

HISTORY/PE

- Suspect abuse if the story is not consistent with the injury pattern or with the child's developmental age. For example, take note if the parents claim that their 2-month-old child "rolled off the couch" (2-month-olds can't roll yet).
- **Risk factors:** Look for parents with a history of alcoholism or drug use, children with mental retardation or a handicap, and repeated hospitalizations.
- **Infants:** Abuse or neglect in infants may present as apnea, seizures, feeding intolerance, excessive irritability, somnolence, or failure to thrive (FTT).
- **Older children:** Neglect in older children may present as poor hygiene or behavioral abnormalities.
- **Examination findings:**
    - **Bruises:**
        - The most common physical sign of abuse.
        - Geometric patterns include belt marks.
        - Found in atypical places such as the face or thighs.
    - **Burns:**
        - A well-demarcated line on the buttocks suggests forced immersion in hot water.
        - Look for cigarette burns, iron-shaped burns, or stocking-glove burns.
    - **Fractures:**
        - **Spiral fractures of the humerus and femur:** Suggest abuse in children < 3 years of age.
        - **Epiphyseal-metaphyseal "bucket fractures":** Suggest shaking or jerking of the child's limbs; highly diagnostic of physical abuse in an infant.
        - **Posterior rib fractures:** Usually caused by squeezing of the chest.

DIAGNOSIS

- Rule out **conditions that mimic abuse**—eg, bleeding disorders or Mongolian spots (resemble bruises; see Figure 2.13-1), osteogenesis imperfecta (may mimic fractures), bullous impetigo (may look like cigarette burns), and "coining" (an alternative treatment in certain cultures).
- An **x-ray skeletal survey** and **bone scan** can show fractures in various stages of healing. X-rays may not show fractures until 1–2 weeks after injury (although they may show evidence of prior trauma in children < 3 years of age); by contrast, bone scans may show fractures within 48 hours.
- If sexual abuse is suspected, test for gonorrhea, syphilis, chlamydia, HIV, and sperm (within 72 hours of assault).
- Rule out shaken baby syndrome (SBS) by performing an ophthalmologic exam for **retinal hemorrhages** and a **noncontrast CT** for subdural hematomas. Infants with SBS often do not exhibit external signs of abuse.
- Consider an **MRI** to visualize white matter changes associated with violent shaking and the extent of intra- and extracranial bleeds.

KEY FACT

Suspect sexual abuse if there is genital trauma, bleeding, or discharge. In females, consider vaginal foreign body as an alternative diagnosis, especially in the setting of a foul-smelling vaginal discharge, bleeding, and pain.

KEY FACT

Neisseria gonorrhoeae isolated on a vaginal culture is definitive evidence of sexual abuse. *Chlamydia trachomatis* is not because it can be acquired from the mother during delivery and can persist for up to 3 years.

KEY FACT

Mongolian spots, which are common in the first few years of life, look like bruises and may be mistaken for abuse.

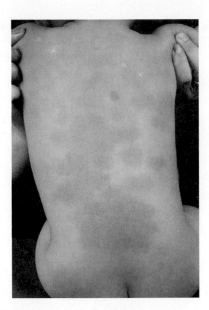

FIGURE 2.13-1.   Mongolian spots. These spots, which are common and are not pathologic in the first few years of life, often resemble bruises. (Reproduced with permission from Wolff K et al. *Fitzpatrick's Dermatology in General Medicine,* 7th ed. New York: McGraw-Hill, 2008, Fig. 73-16.)

TREATMENT

- Document injuries, including location, size, shape, color, and the nature of all lesions, bruises, or burns.
- Notify Child Protective Services for possible removal of the child from the home.
- Hospitalize if necessary to stabilize injuries or to protect the child.

Congenital Heart Disease

Intrauterine risk factors for congenital heart disease include maternal drug use (alcohol, lithium, thalidomide, phenytoin), maternal infections (rubella), and maternal illness (diabetes mellitus [DM], PKU). Disease is classified by the presence or absence of cyanosis:

- **Acyanotic conditions ("pink babies"):** Have **left-to-right shunts** in which oxygenated blood from the lungs is shunted back into the pulmonary circulation.
- **Cyanotic conditions ("blue babies"):** Have **right-to-left shunts** in which deoxygenated blood is shunted into the systemic circulation.

Table 2.13-1 lists common congenital and other pediatric heart conditions along with their disease associations.

VENTRICULAR SEPTAL DEFECT (VSD)

A condition in which an opening in the ventricular septum allows blood to flow between ventricles. VSD is the **most common cause of congenital heart disease.** It is more common among patients with Apert's syndrome (cranial deformities, fusion of the fingers and toes), Down syndrome, fetal alcohol syndrome, TORCH syndrome (toxoplasmosis, other agents, rubella, CMV, HSV), cri du chat syndrome, and trisomies 13 and 18.

MNEMONIC

Cyanotic heart defects—

The 5 T's that have right-to-left shunts

Truncus arteriosus = **ONE** arterial vessel overriding ventricles

Transposition of the great vessels = **TWO** arteries switched

Tricuspid atresia **(THREE)**

Tetralogy of Fallot **(FOUR)**

Total anomalous pulmonary venous return = **FIVE** words

Out of the 5 T's, only **T**ransposition presents with severe cyanosis within the first few hours of life.

MNEMONIC

Noncyanotic heart defects—

The 3 D's

vs**D**

as**D**

p**DA**

TABLE 2.13-1. Pediatric Heart Conditions and Their Disease Associations

CONDITION	DISORDER
ASD and endocardial cushion defects	Down syndrome.
PDA	Congenital rubella.
Coarctation of the aorta	Turner's syndrome (many also have bicuspid aortic valve).
Coronary artery aneurysms	Kawasaki disease.
Congenital heart block	Neonatal lupus.
Supravalvular aortic stenosis	Williams syndrome.
Conotruncal abnormalities	Tetralogy of Fallot (overriding aorta), truncus arteriosus, DiGeorge syndrome (tetralogy), velocardiofacial syndrome.
Ebstein's anomaly	Maternal lithium use during pregnancy.
Heart failure	Neonatal thyrotoxicosis.
Asymmetric septal hypertrophy and transposition of the great vessels	Maternal diabetes.

KEY FACT

VSD is the most common cause of congenital heart disease.

HISTORY/PE

- **Small defects:** Usually asymptomatic at birth, but examination reveals a **harsh holosystolic murmur** heard best at the lower left sternal border.
- **Large defects:**
  - Can present as **frequent respiratory infections, dyspnea, FTT, and CHF.**
  - If present, the holosystolic murmur is softer and more blowing but can be accompanied by a systolic thrill, crackles, hepatomegaly, a narrow S2 with an ↑ P2, and a mid-diastolic apical rumble reflecting ↑ flow across the mitral valve.

DIAGNOSIS

- **Echocardiogram is diagnostic.**
- ECG can demonstrate **LVH** and may show both LVH and RVH with larger VSDs.
- CXR may show **cardiomegaly** and ↑ **pulmonary vascular markings.**

TREATMENT

- Most small VSDs close spontaneously; asymptomatic patients should be monitored via echocardiography. Antibiotic prophylaxis may be considered during procedures but is indicated only if the VSD was previously repaired with prosthetic material.
- Surgical repair is indicated in symptomatic patients who fail medical management, children < 1 year of age with signs of pulmonary hypertension, and older children with large VSDs that have not ↓ in size over time.
- Treat existing CHF with diuretics (initial treatment), inotropes, and ACEIs.

ATRIAL SEPTAL DEFECT (ASD)

A condition in which an opening in the atrial septum allows blood to flow between the atria, leading to left-to-right shunting. Associated with Holt-Oram syndrome (absent radii, ASD, first-degree heart block), fetal alcohol syndrome, and Down syndrome.

History/PE

- Ostium primum defects present in early childhood with findings of a murmur or fatigue with exertion (also seen in Down syndrome). Ostium secundum defects (more common) tend to present in late childhood or early adulthood. Symptom onset and severity depend on the size of the defect.
- Symptoms of easy fatigability, frequent respiratory infections, and FTT may be observed, but patients are **frequently asymptomatic.**
- Examination reveals a right ventricular heave; a **wide and fixed, split S2;** and a systolic ejection murmur at the left upper sternal border (from ↑ flow across the pulmonary valve). There may also be a mid-diastolic rumble at the left lower sternal border.

Diagnosis

- Echocardiogram with color flow Doppler reveals blood flow between the atria (diagnostic), paradoxical ventricular wall motion, and a dilated right ventricle.
- ECG may show RVH and right atrial enlargement. PR prolongation is common.
- CXR reveals cardiomegaly and ↑ pulmonary vascular markings.

Treatment

- Close to 90% of defects close spontaneously, and most do not require treatment.
- Surgical or catheter closure is indicated in infants with CHF and in patients with more than a 2:1 ratio of pulmonary to systemic blood flow. Early correction prevents complications such as arrhythmias, right ventricular dysfunction, and Eisenmenger's syndrome.

PATENT DUCTUS ARTERIOSUS (PDA)

Failure of the ductus arteriosus to close in the first few days of life, leading to an **acyanotic** left-to-right shunt from the aorta to the pulmonary artery. Risk factors include maternal first-trimester **rubella** infection, **prematurity,** and female gender.

History/PE

- Typically asymptomatic; patients with large defects may present with FTT, recurrent lower respiratory tract infections, lower extremity clubbing, and CHF.
- Examination reveals a **continuous "machinery murmur"** at the second left intercostal space at the sternal border, a loud S2, **wide pulse pressure,** and **bounding peripheral pulses.**

Diagnosis

- A color flow Doppler demonstrating blood flow from the aorta into the pulmonary artery is diagnostic.

KEY FACT

ASD has a fixed, widely split S2.

KEY FACT

ASDs and VSDs rarely present at birth. Remember that ASDs, VSDs, and PDAs are acyanotic conditions unless Eisenmenger's syndrome has developed (right-to-left shunt, cyanotic).

KEY FACT

In Eisenmenger's syndrome, left-to-right shunt leads to pulmonary hypertension and shunt reversal.

KEY FACT

In infants presenting in a shocklike state within the first few weeks of life, look for:
1. Sepsis
2. Inborn errors of metabolism
3. Ductal-dependent congenital heart disease, usually left-sided lesions (as the ductus is closing)
4. Congenital adrenal hyperplasia

- With larger PDAs, echocardiography shows left atrial and left ventricular enlargement.
- ECG may show LVH, and CXR may reveal cardiomegaly if lesions are large.

TREATMENT

- Give **indomethacin** unless the PDA is needed for survival (eg, transposition of the great vessels, tetralogy of Fallot, hypoplastic left heart) or if indomethacin is contraindicated (eg, intraventricular hemorrhage).
- If indomethacin fails or if the child is > 6–8 months of age, surgical closure is required.

KEY FACT

Come **IN** and **CLOSE** the door: give **IN**domethacin to **CLOSE** a PDA.

COARCTATION OF THE AORTA

Constriction of a portion of the aorta, leading to ↑ flow proximal to and ↓ flow distal to the coarctation. Occurs just below the left subclavian artery in 98% of patients. The condition is associated with **Turner's** syndrome, berry aneurysms, and male gender. **More than two-thirds of patients have a bicuspid aortic valve.**

HISTORY/PE

- Often presents in childhood with **asymptomatic hypertension (upper extremity hypertension).**
- A murmur may be heard over the back between the scapulae.
- Lower extremity claudication, syncope, epistaxis, and headache may be present.
- The classic physical examination finding is a systolic BP that is higher in the upper extremities; the difference in BP between the left and right arm can indicate the point of coarctation.
- Additional findings include **weak femoral pulses,** radiofemoral delay, a short systolic murmur in the left axilla, and a forceful apical impulse.
- In infancy, critical coarctation requires a patent PDA for survival. Such infants may present in the first few weeks of life in a shocklike state when the PDA closes. Differential cyanosis may be seen with lower O_2 saturation in the left arm and lower extremities (postductal areas) as compared to the right arm (preductal area).

DIAGNOSIS

- Echocardiography and color flow Doppler are diagnostic.
- CXR in young children may demonstrate cardiomegaly and pulmonary congestion.
- In older children, the following compensatory changes may be seen: LVH on ECG; the **"3" sign on CXR** due to pre- and postdilatation of the coarctation segment with aortic wall indentation; and **"rib notching"** due to collateral circulation through the intercostal arteries.

TREATMENT

- If severe coarctation presents in infancy, the ductus arteriosus should be kept open with prostaglandin E_1 (PGE_1).
- Surgical correction or balloon angioplasty is controversial.
- Monitor for restenosis, aneurysm development, and aortic dissection.

KEY FACT

Coarctation of the aorta is associated with Turner's syndrome.

KEY FACT

Coarctation is a cause of 2° hypertension in children.

TRANSPOSITION OF THE GREAT VESSELS

The most common cyanotic congenital heart lesion in the newborn. In this condition, the aorta is connected to the right ventricle and the pulmonary artery to the left ventricle, creating parallel pulmonary and systemic circulations. **Without a septal defect (ASD or VSD) and a PDA, it is incompatible with life.** A PDA alone is usually not sufficient to allow adequate mixing of blood. Risk factors include **diabetic mothers** and, rarely, DiGeorge syndrome.

HISTORY/PE

- Critical illness and **cyanosis typically present within first few hours after birth.** Reverse differential cyanosis may be seen if left ventricular outflow tract obstruction (eg, coarctation, aortic stenosis) is also present.
- Examination reveals tachypnea, progressive hypoxemia, and extreme cyanosis. Some patients have signs of CHF, and a single loud S2 is often present. There may not be a murmur if no VSD is present. If a VSD is present, a systolic murmur may be heard at the left sternal border.

DIAGNOSIS

- Echocardiography.
- CXR may show a narrow heart base, absence of the main pulmonary artery segment, an **"egg-shaped silhouette,"** and ↑ pulmonary vascular markings.

TREATMENT

- Start IV **PGE$_1$** to maintain or open the PDA.
- If surgery is not feasible within the first few days of life or if the PDA cannot be maintained with prostaglandin, perform **balloon atrial septostomy** to create or enlarge an ASD.
- Surgical correction (arterial or atrial switch) is definitive.

TETRALOGY OF FALLOT

Consists of pulmonary stenosis, overriding aorta, RVH, and VSD. **The most common cyanotic congenital heart disease in children.** Early cyanosis results from right-to-left shunting across the VSD. As right-sided pressures ↓ in the weeks after birth, the shunt direction reverses and cyanosis may ↓. If the degree of pulmonary stenosis is severe, the right-sided pressures may remain high and cyanosis may worsen over time. Risk factors include maternal PKU and DiGeorge syndrome.

HISTORY/PE

- Presents in infancy or early childhood with dyspnea and fatigability. Cyanosis is frequently absent at birth but develops over the first 2 years of life; the degree of cyanosis often reflects the extent of pulmonary stenosis.
- Infants are often asymptomatic until 4–6 months of age, when CHF may develop and manifest as diaphoresis with feeding or tachypnea.
- **Children often squat** for relief during hypoxemic episodes called **"tet spells,"** which ↑ systemic vascular resistance.
- Hypoxemia may lead to FTT or mental status changes.
- Examination reveals a systolic ejection murmur at the left upper sternal border (right ventricular outflow obstruction), a right ventricular heave, and a single S2.

KEY FACT

Transposition is the most common congenital heart condition, presenting with cyanosis within the first 24 hours of birth.

MNEMONIC

DiGeorge syndrome—

CATCH 22

Cardiac abnormalities (transposition)
Abnormal facies
Thymic aplasia
Cleft palate
Hypocalcemia
22q11 deletion

KEY FACT

Transposition of the great vessels is the most common cyanotic heart disease of **newborns.** Tetralogy of Fallot is the most common cyanotic heart disease of **childhood.**

A 2-year-old girl is playing on the floor in a squatting position while in the waiting room. The skin around her mouth has a grayish-blue hue, and when she stands up, she suddenly begins to pant and appears cyanotic. When she goes back to a squatting position, she begins to breathe comfortably again. Which 4 anomalies define this patient's condition?

DIAGNOSIS

- Echocardiography and catheterization.
- CXR shows a **"boot-shaped" heart** with ↓ pulmonary vascular markings. Remember that a VSD may result in ↑ pulmonary vascular markings.
- ECG shows right-axis deviation and RVH.

TREATMENT

- Lesions with severe pulmonary stenosis or atresia require immediate PGE₁ to keep the PDA open along with urgent surgical consultation.
- Treat hypercyanotic "tet spells" with O_2, propranolol, phenylephrine, the knee-chest position, fluids, and morphine.
- Temporary palliation can be achieved through the creation of an artificial shunt (eg, balloon atrial septostomy) before definitive surgical correction (Blalock-Taussig shunt).

Development

DEVELOPMENTAL MILESTONES

Table 2.13-2 highlights major developmental milestones, with commonly tested milestones highlighted in bold. Table 2.13-3 summarizes critical milestones in language development.

GROWTH

At each well-child check, height, weight, and head circumference are plotted on growth charts specific for gender and age:

- **Head circumference:** Measured routinely in the first 2 years. ↑ head circumference may indicate hydrocephalus or tumor; ↓ head circumference can point to microcephaly (eg, TORCH infections).
- **Height and weight:** Measured routinely until adulthood. The pattern of growth is more important than the raw numbers. Infants may lose 5–10% of birth weight (BW) over the first few days but should return to their BW by 14 days. Infants can be expected to double their BW by 4–5 months, triple by 1 year, and quadruple by 2 years.
- **FTT:** Persistent weight less than the fifth percentile for age or "falling off the growth curve" (ie, crossing 2 major percentile lines on a growth chart). Classified as follows:
  - **Organic:** Due to an underlying medical condition such as cystic fibrosis, congenital heart disease, celiac sprue, pyloric stenosis, chronic infection (eg, HIV), and GERD.
  - **Nonorganic:** Primarily due to psychosocial factors such as maternal depression, neglect, or abuse.
- A careful dietary history and close observation of maternal-infant interactions (especially preparation of formula and feeding) are critical to diagnosis.
- Children should be hospitalized if there is evidence of neglect or severe malnourishment. Calorie counts and supplemental nutrition (if breastfeeding is inadequate) are mainstays of treatment.

KEY FACT

Both transposition of the great vessels and tetralogy of Fallot are initially treated with PGE₁ but are definitively treated with surgical correction.

KEY FACT

Signs of autism include no babbling and/or gesturing by 12 months, no single words by 16 months, no 2-word phrases by 24 months, failure to make eye contact, and other signs of deficits in language or social skills.

KEY FACT

Newborns can lose up to 10% of their birth weight but will regain the weight by 2 weeks of life.

KEY FACT

Infants with FTT will first fall off of the **weight** curve, then the **height** curve, and finally the **head circumference** curve.

The anomalies included in the mnemonic **PROV**e—**P**ulmonary stenosis, **R**VH, **O**verriding aorta, and **V**SD—define tetralogy of Fallot.

TABLE 2.13-2. **Developmental Milestones**

Age[a]	Gross Motor	Fine Motor	Language	Social/Cognitive
2 months	**Lifts head/chest when prone.**	Tracks past midline.	Alerts to sound; coos.	Recognizes parent; exhibits **social smile.**
4–5 months	**Rolls front to back,** back to front (4 months).	Grasps rattle.	**Laughs and squeals;** orients to voice; begins to make consonant sounds.	Enjoys looking around; laughs.
6 months	**Sits unassisted.**	Transfers objects; demonstrates raking grasp.	**Babbles.**	Demonstrates **stranger anxiety.**
9–10 months	Crawls; pulls to stand.	Uses 3-finger (immature) pincer grasp.	Says "mama/dada" (nonspecific); says first word at 11 months.	Waves bye-bye; plays pat-a-cake.
12 months	**Walks alone;** throws object.	Uses 2-finger (mature) pincer grasp.	Uses **1–3 words; follows 1-step commands.**	Imitates actions; exhibits **separation anxiety.**
2 years	**Walks up/down steps;** jumps.	Builds tower of 6 cubes.	Uses **2-word phrases.**	**Follows 2-step commands;** removes clothes.
3 years	**Rides tricycle;** climbs stairs with alternating feet (3–4 years).	**Copies a circle;** uses utensils.	Uses **3-word sentences.**	Brushes teeth with help; washes/dries hands.
4 years	Hops.	**Copies a cross** (square at 4.5 years).	Knows colors and some numbers.	Exhibits cooperative play; plays board games.
5 years	Skips; walks backward for long distances.	**Copies a triangle;** ties shoelaces; knows left and right; prints letters.	Uses **5-word sentences.**	Exhibits domestic role playing; plays dress-up.

[a]For premature infants < 2 years of age, chronological age must be adjusted for gestational age. For example, an infant born at 7 months' gestation (2 months early) would be expected to perform at the 4-month level at the chronological age of 6 months.

TABLE 2.13-3. **Major Milestones in Language Development**

Age	Milestone
12 months	1 word, 1-step command
15 months	5 words
18 months	8 words
2 years	2-word phrases, 2-step commands
3 years	3-word phrases

■ **Tanner staging:** Performed to assess sexual development in boys and girls (see Figure 2.13-2). Stage 1 is preadolescent; stage 5 is adult. Increasing stages are assigned for testicular and penile growth in boys and breast growth in girls; pubic hair development is used for both stages.
  ■ **Girls:** The average age of puberty is **10.5 years.** The average age of menarche in U.S. girls is 12.5 years.
  ■ **Boys:** The average age of puberty is **11.5 years.**
■ Variants of normal sexual development are as follows (see also Figure 2.13-2):
  ■ **Precocious puberty:** Any sign of 2° sexual maturation in girls < 8 years or boys < 9 years of age. Often idiopathic; may be central or peripheral (see the Gynecology chapter).
  ■ **Delayed puberty:** No testicular enlargement in boys by age 14, or no breast development or pubic hair in girls by age 13.
  ■ **Constitutional growth delay:** A normal variant, and the most common cause of delayed puberty. The growth curve lags behind others of the same age but is consistent. There is often a ⊕ family history, and **children catch up and ultimately achieve target height potential.**
  ■ **Pathological puberty delay:** Rarely, due to systemic disease (eg, IBD), malnutrition (eg, anorexia nervosa), gonadal dysgenesis (eg, Klinefelter's syndrome, Turner's syndrome), or endocrine abnormalities (eg, hypopituitarism, hypothyroidism, Kallmann's syndrome, androgen insensitivity syndrome, Prader-Willi syndrome).

Genetic Disease

Tables 2.13-4 and 2.13-5 outline common genetic diseases and their associated abnormalities.

CYSTIC FIBROSIS (CF)

An **autosomal recessive** disorder caused by mutations in the CFTR gene (chloride channel) on chromosome 7 and characterized by widespread exo-

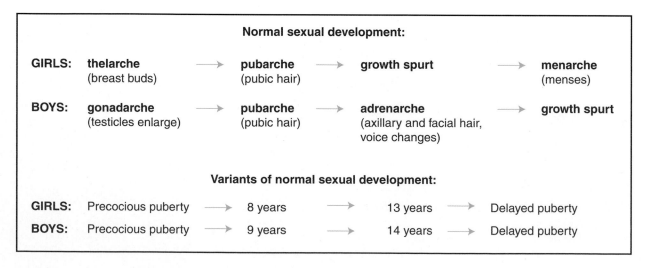

Normal sexual development:

GIRLS:	thelarche (breast buds)	→ pubarche (pubic hair)	→ growth spurt	→ menarche (menses)
BOYS:	gonadarche (testicles enlarge)	→ pubarche (pubic hair)	→ adrenarche (axillary and facial hair, voice changes)	→ growth spurt

Variants of normal sexual development:

GIRLS:	Precocious puberty	→ 8 years	→ 13 years	→ Delayed puberty
BOYS:	Precocious puberty	→ 9 years	→ 14 years	→ Delayed puberty

FIGURE 2.13-2. **Patterns of sexual development in girls vs. boys.**

TABLE 2.13-4. Genetic Diseases

DISEASE	GENETIC ABNORMALITY	COMMON CHARACTERISTICS
Down syndrome	Meiotic nondisjunction (95%), robertsonian translocation (4%), or mosaicism (1%)	The most common chromosomal disorder and cause of mental retardation. Associated with **advanced maternal age.** Presents with mental retardation, a flat facial profile, **upslanted eyes** with epicanthal folds, a **simian crease, general hypotonia,** atlantoaxial instability, and extra neck folds (nuchal folds are sometimes seen on prenatal ultrasound). Associated with **duodenal atresia, Hirschsprung's disease,** and **congenital heart disease.** The most common malformation is AV canal (60%); ASDs, VSDs, and PDAs (20%) and complex congenital heart disease make up the remainder. Also associated with an ↑ risk of **acute lymphocytic leukemia (ALL), hypothyroidism,** and **early-onset Alzheimer's.**
Edwards' syndrome	Trisomy 18	Presents with severe mental retardation, **rocker-bottom feet,** low-set ears, **micrognathia, clenched hands (overlapping fourth and fifth digits),** and a prominent occiput. Associated with congenital heart disease. May have horseshoe kidneys. **Death usually occurs within 1 year of birth.**
Patau's syndrome	Trisomy 13	Presents with severe mental retardation, **microphthalmia, microcephaly,** cleft lip/palate, **holoprosencephaly,** "punched-out" scalp lesions, **polydactyly,** and omphalocele. Associated with congenital heart disease. **Death usually occurs within 1 year of birth.**
Klinefelter's syndrome (male)	47, XXY	Characterized by the presence of an inactivated X chromosome (Barr body). Associated with advanced maternal age. One of the most common causes of **hypogonadism** in males. Presents with **testicular atrophy,** a eunuchoid body shape, **tall stature,** long extremities, **gynecomastia,** and **female hair distribution.** Treat with **testosterone** (prevents gynecomastia; improves 2° sexual characteristics).
Turner's syndrome (female)	45, XO	Missing 1 X chromosome; no Barr body. Not associated with advanced maternal age. The most common cause of **1° amenorrhea;** due to **ovarian dysgenesis** (↓ estrogen). Features include short stature, shield chest, widely spaced nipples, a **webbed neck, coarctation of the aorta** (↓ femoral pulses), and/or bicuspid aortic valve. May present with **lymphedema of the hands and feet in the neonatal period.** May have horseshoe kidney.
Double Y males	47, XYY	Observed with ↑ frequency among inmates of penal institutions. **Phenotypically normal;** patients are very tall with severe acne and antisocial behavior (seen in 1–2% of XYY males).

(continues)

TABLE 2.13-4. Genetic Diseases *(continued)*

DISEASE	GENETIC ABNORMALITY	COMMON CHARACTERISTICS
Phenylketonuria (PKU)	Autosomal recessive; ↓ phenylalanine hydroxylase or ↓ tetrahydrobiopterin cofactor	Tyrosine becomes essential and phenylalanine builds up excess phenyl ketones. Screened for at birth. Normal at birth; presents within the first few months of life. Presents with mental retardation, **fair hair and skin, eczema, blond hair, blue eyes, and a musty urine odor.** Associated with an ↑ risk of heart disease. Modify diet by **decreasing phenylalanine (artificial sweeteners)** and **increasing tyrosine.** A mother with PKU who wants to become pregnant must restrict her diet as above before conception.
Fragile X syndrome	An **X-linked dominant** defect affecting the methylation and expression of the FMR1 gene	The second most common cause of **genetic mental retardation.** Presents with **large jaw, testes, and ears** and with **autistic behaviors.** A triplet repeat disorder that may show genetic anticipation.

crine gland dysfunction. CF is the most common severe genetic disease in the United States and is most frequently found in **Caucasians.**

HISTORY/PE

- Fifty percent of patients present with **FTT** or **chronic sinopulmonary disease.**
- Characterized by **recurrent pulmonary infections** (especially with *Pseudomonas* and *S aureus*) with subsequent cyanosis, **digital clubbing, chronic cough** (the most common pulmonary symptom), dyspnea, bronchiectasis, hemoptysis, chronic sinusitis, rhonchi, rales, hyperresonance to percussion, and **nasal polyposis.**
- Fifteen percent of infants present with **meconium ileus (bilious vomiting in the newborn).** Patients usually have **greasy stools** and flatulence; other prominent GI symptoms include pancreatitis, **rectal prolapse,** hypoproteinemia, biliary cirrhosis, jaundice, and esophageal varices.
- GI symptoms are more prominent in infancy; pulmonary manifestations predominate thereafter.
- Additional symptoms include **type 2 DM, "salty-tasting" skin, male infertility** (agenesis of the vas deferens), and **unexplained hyponatremia.**
- Patients are at risk for **fat-soluble vitamin deficiency** (vitamins A, D, E, and K) 2° to malabsorption and may present with manifestations of these deficiencies.

DIAGNOSIS

- Diagnosed by a **sweat chloride test** > 60 mEq/L in those < 20 years of age and > 80 mEq/L in adults.
- Confirmed by genetic testing.
- ABG shows **hypochloremic alkalosis** in severe cases.
- Most states now perform **mandatory newborn screening,** but occasional false ⊕s occur, so children must be brought in for a sweat test to distinguish disease from a carrier state.

KEY FACT

Almost all cases of meconium ileus are due to CF.

KEY FACT

The sweat chloride test has traditionally been considered the gold standard for the diagnosis of CF, but confirmatory genetic analysis is now routinely done.

TABLE 2.13-5. **Lysosomal Storage Diseases**

Disease	Etiology	Mode of Inheritance/Notes
Fabry's disease	Caused by a deficiency of α-galactosidase A that leads to accumulation of ceramide trihexoside in the heart, brain, and kidneys. The first sign is **severe neuropathic limb pain;** also presents with joint swelling. Skin involvement takes the form of **angiokeratomas and telangiectasias.** Findings include **renal failure and an ↑ risk of stroke and MI (thromboembolic events).**	**X-linked recessive.**
Krabbe's disease	Absence of galactosylceramide and galactoside (due to galactosylceramidase deficiency), leading to the accumulation of galactocerebroside in the brain. Characterized by **progressive CNS degeneration,** optic atrophy, spasticity, and death within the first 3 years of life.	Autosomal recessive.
Gaucher's disease	Caused by a deficiency of **glucocerebrosidase** that leads to the accumulation of glucocerebroside in the brain, liver, spleen, and bone marrow. Gaucher's cells have a characteristic **"crinkled paper"** appearance with enlarged cytoplasm. May present with **anemia and thrombocytopenia.** The infantile form results in early, rapid neurologic decline. The adult form (more common) is compatible with a **normal life span** and does not affect the brain.	Autosomal recessive.
Niemann-Pick disease	A deficiency of **sphingomyelinase** that leads to the buildup of sphingomyelin cholesterol in reticuloendothelial and parenchymal cells and tissues. Patients with type A die by age 3. May present with a **cherry-red spot and hepatosplenomegaly.**	Autosomal recessive. No man **PICKs (Niemann-PICK)** his nose with his **sphinger.**
Tay-Sachs disease	An absence of hexosaminidase that leads to GM_2 ganglioside accumulation. Infants may appear **normal until 3–6 months of age,** when weakness begins and development slows and regresses. An exaggerated startle response may be seen. Death occurs by age 3. Presents with a **cherry-red spot but no hepatosplenomegaly.** The carrier rate is 1 in 30 Jews of European descent (1 in 300 for others).	**Tay-SaX lacks heXosaminidase.**
Metachromatic leukodystrophy	A deficiency of arylsulfatase A that leads to the accumulation of sulfatide in the brain, kidney, liver, and peripheral nerves. **Demyelination leads to progressive ataxia and dementia.**	Autosomal recessive.
Hurler's syndrome	A deficiency of α-L-iduronidase. Leads to **corneal clouding, mental retardation, and gargoylism.**	Autosomal recessive.
Hunter's syndrome	A deficiency of iduronate sulfatase. A mild form of Hurler's syndrome with **no corneal clouding** and mild mental retardation.	**X-linked recessive.** **Hunters** need to **see (no corneal clouding)** to aim for the **X.**

TREATMENT

- Pulmonary manifestations are managed with chest physical therapy, bronchodilators, corticosteroids, antibiotics (**should cover *Pseudomonas***), and DNase.
- Administer **pancreatic enzymes and fat-soluble vitamins** A, D, E, and K for malabsorption.
- Nutritional counseling and support with a high-calorie and high-protein diet are essential for health maintenance.
- Patients who have severe disease but can tolerate surgery may be candidates for lung or pancreas transplants. Life expectancy was once ~ 20 years, but with newer treatments it is increasing to past age 30.

Gastroenterology

INTUSSUSCEPTION

A condition in which a portion of the bowel invaginates or "telescopes" into an adjacent segment, usually proximal to the ileocecal valve (see Figure 2.13-3A). **The most common cause of bowel obstruction in the first 2 years of life (males > females); usually seen between 3 months and 3 years of age.** The cause is often unknown. Risk factors include conditions with potential lead points, including **Meckel's diverticulum**, intestinal lymphoma (> 6 years of age), Henoch-Schönlein purpura, parasites, polyps, adenovirus or rotavirus infection, celiac disease, and CF.

HISTORY/PE

- Presents with abrupt-onset, **colicky abdominal pain** in apparently healthy children, often accompanied by flexed knees and vomiting. The child may appear well in between episodes if intussusception is released.
- The classic triad is **abdominal pain, vomiting, and bloody mucus in stool** ("**currant jelly stool**," a late finding that is hemoccult ⊕).

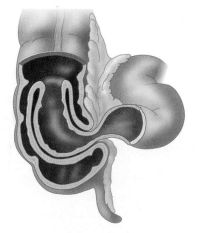
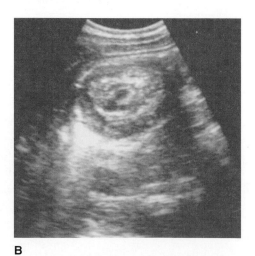

A **B**

FIGURE 2.13-3. **Intussusception.** (**A**) Ileocolic intussusception, the most common location in children. (**B**) Transabdominal ultrasound shows the classic "target sign" of intussusception in cross-section. (Image A reproduced with permission from Doherty GM. *Current Diagnosis & Treatment: Surgery,* 13th ed. New York: McGraw-Hill, 2010, Fig. 43-12. Image B reproduced with permission from Ma OJ et al. *Emergency Ultrasound,* 2nd ed. New York: McGraw-Hill, 2008, Fig. 9-15A.)

- On examination, look for abdominal tenderness, a ⊕ stool guaiac, a palpable **"sausage-shaped" RUQ abdominal mass,** and absence of bowel in the RLQ ("empty" on palpation).

DIAGNOSIS/TREATMENT

- **Abdominal plain films** are often normal early in the disease, but later they may show small bowel obstruction, perforation, or a soft tissue mass. **Ultrasound** is the test of choice and may show a **"target sign"** (see Figure 2.13-3B).
- Correct any volume or electrolyte abnormalities, check CBC for leukocytosis, and consider an NG tube for decompression.
- In the setting of high clinical suspicion, an **air-contrast barium enema** should be performed without delay, as it is diagnostic in > 95% of cases and curative in > 80%. If the child is unstable or has peritoneal signs or if enema reduction is unsuccessful, perform surgical reduction and resection of gangrenous bowel.

KEY FACT

In most cases of intussusception, an air-contrast barium enema is both diagnostic and therapeutic.

PYLORIC STENOSIS

Hypertrophy of the pyloric sphincter, leading to gastric outlet obstruction. More common in **firstborn males;** associated with tracheoesophageal fistula, a maternal history of pyloric stenosis, and **erythromycin** ingestion.

HISTORY/PE

- **Nonbilious** emesis typically begins around **3 weeks of age** and progresses to **projectile emesis** after most or all feedings.
- Babies initially feed well but eventually suffer from malnutrition and dehydration.
- Examination may reveal a **palpable olive-shaped,** mobile, nontender epigastric mass and visible gastric peristaltic waves.

DIAGNOSIS

- **Abdominal ultrasound** is the imaging modality of choice and reveals a hypertrophic pylorus (see Figure 2.13-4).

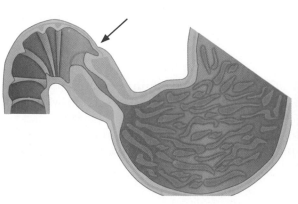
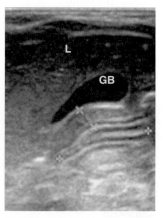

A   **B**

FIGURE 2.13-4.   Hypertrophic pyloric stenosis. (A) Schematic representation of a hypertrophied pylorus. The arrow denotes protrusion of the pylorus into the duodenum. **(B)** Longitudinal ultrasound of the pylorus showing a thickened pyloric musculature (X's) over a long pyloric channel length (plus signs). L = liver; GB = gallbladder. (Image A adapted with permission from Doherty GM. *Current Diagnosis & Treatment: Surgery,* 13th ed. New York: McGraw-Hill, 2010, Fig. 43-9. Image B reproduced with permission from USMLERx.com.)

Q

A newborn presents with lymphedema of the hands and feet, ↓ femoral pulses, a webbed neck, widely spaced nipples, short fourth metacarpals, and nail dysplasia. What form of hormone replacement therapy will the child need in the future?

MNEMONIC

Meckel's rule of 2's:

Most common in children under **2**
2 times more common in males
Contains **2** types of tissue (pancreatic and gastric)
2 inches long
Found within **2** feet of the ileocecal valve
Occurs in **2%** of the population

Estrogen replacement therapy for ovarian dysgenesis. Without exogenous estrogen, this child will be at ↑ risk of delayed puberty and osteoporosis later in life.

- Barium studies show a narrow pyloric channel ("string sign") or a pyloric beak.

TREATMENT

- Correct existing dehydration and acid-base/electrolyte abnormalities.
- Surgical correction with **pyloromyotomy.**

MECKEL'S DIVERTICULUM

Caused by failure of the omphalomesenteric (or vitelline) duct to obliterate. The resulting heterotopic gastric tissue causes ulcers and bleeding. The most common congenital abnormality of the small intestine, affecting up to 2% of children (more common in males). Most frequently occurs in **children < 2 years of age.**

HISTORY/PE

- Typically asymptomatic, and often discovered incidentally.
- Classically presents with **sudden, intermittent, painless rectal bleeding.**
- May result in complications such as intestinal obstruction, diverticulitis (which may mimic acute appendicitis), volvulus, and intussusception.

DIAGNOSIS

- A **Meckel scintigraphy scan** (technetium-99m pertechnetate; detects ectopic gastric tissue) is diagnostic.
- Plain films have limited value but can be useful in diagnosing obstruction or perforation.

TREATMENT

In the presence of active bleeding, treatment is **surgical excision** of the diverticulum together with the adjacent ileal segment (ulcers frequently develop in adjacent ileum).

HIRSCHSPRUNG'S DISEASE

Congenital lack of ganglion cells in the distal colon, leading to uncoordinated peristalsis and ↓ motility. Associated with male gender, **Down syndrome,** Waardenburg's syndrome, and multiple endocrine neoplasia (MEN) type 2.

HISTORY/PE

- Neonates present with **failure to pass meconium within 48 hours of birth,** accompanied by bilious vomiting and FTT; children with less severe lesions may present later in life with chronic constipation.
- Physical examination may reveal abdominal distention and **explosive discharge of stool following a rectal examination;** lack of stool in the rectum; or abnormal sphincter tone.

DIAGNOSIS

- **Barium enema** is the imaging study of choice and reveals a narrowed distal colon with proximal dilation. Plain films reveal distended bowel loops with a paucity of air in the rectum.
- Anorectal manometry detects failure of the internal sphincter to relax after distention of the rectal lumen. It is typically used in atypical presentations or older children.

- **Rectal biopsy** confirms the diagnosis and reveals absence of the myenteric (Auerbach's) plexus and submucosal (Meissner's) plexus along with hypertrophied nerve trunks enhanced with acetylcholinesterase stain.

TREATMENT

Traditionally a **2-stage surgical repair** is used involving the creation of a diverting colostomy at the time of diagnosis, followed several weeks later by a **definitive "pull-through" procedure** connecting the remaining colon to the rectum.

MALROTATION WITH VOLVULUS

Congenital malrotation of the midgut results in abnormal positioning of the small intestine (cecum in the right hypochondrium) and formation of fibrous bands (Ladd's bands). Bands predispose to obstruction and constriction of blood flow.

HISTORY/PE

- Often presents in the **first month of life** with **bilious emesis,** crampy abdominal pain, distention, and passage of blood or mucus in the stool.
- Postsurgical adhesions can lead to obstruction and volvulus at any point in life.

DIAGNOSIS

- AXR may reveal the characteristic **"bird-beak" appearance** and air-fluid levels but may also appear normal.
- If the patient is stable, an **upper GI** is the study of choice and shows an abnormal location of the ligament of Treitz. Ultrasound may be used, but its sensitivity is contingent on the experience of the ultrasonographer.

TREATMENT

- NG tube insertion to decompress the intestine; IV fluid hydration.
- Emergent surgical repair when volvulus is gastric; surgery or endoscopy when volvulus is intestinal.

NECROTIZING ENTEROCOLITIS (NEC)

A condition in which a portion of the bowel undergoes necrosis. The **most common GI emergency in neonates;** most frequently seen in **premature infants,** but can occur in full-term infants as well.

HISTORY/PE

- Symptoms usually present within the **first few days or weeks of life** and are nonspecific, including feeding intolerance, delayed gastric emptying, abdominal distention, and bloody stools.
- Symptoms may rapidly progress to intestinal perforation, peritonitis, abdominal erythema, and shock. Maintain a high index of suspicion.

DIAGNOSIS

- Lab findings are nonspecific and may show hyponatremia, metabolic acidosis, leukopenia or leukocytosis with left shift, thrombocytopenia, and coagulopathy (DIC with prolonged PT/aPTT and a $\oplus$ D-dimer).

KEY FACT

The definitive diagnosis of Hirschsprung's disease requires a rectal biopsy.

- Plain abdominal radiographs may show dilated bowel loops, **pneumatosis intestinalis** (intramural air bubbles representing gas produced by bacteria within the bowel wall; see Figure 2.13-5), portal venous gas, or abdominal free air. Serial abdominal plain films should be taken every 6 hours.
- Ultrasound may also be helpful in discerning free air, areas of loculation or walled-off abscesses, and bowel necrosis.

TREATMENT

- Initiate supportive measures, including NPO, an orogastric tube for gastric decompression, correction of dehydration and electrolyte abnormalities, TPN, and IV antibiotics.
- **Indications for surgery are perforation (free air under the diaphragm) or worsening radiographic signs** on serial abdominal plain films. An ileostomy with mucous fistula is typically performed, with a reanastomosis later.
- Complications include formation of intestinal **strictures** and **short-bowel syndrome.**

Immunology

IMMUNODEFICIENCY DISORDERS

Congenital immunodeficiencies are rare and often present with chronic or recurrent infections (eg, chronic thrush), unusual or opportunistic organisms, incomplete treatment response, or FTT. Categorization is based on the single immune system component that is abnormal (see also Table 2.13-6).

- **B-cell deficiencies:** Most common (50%). Typically present **after 6 months of age** with recurrent sinopulmonary, GI, and urinary tract infections with **encapsulated organisms** (*H influenzae, Streptococcus pneumoniae, Neisseria meningitidis*). **Treat with IVIG (except for IgA deficiencies).**

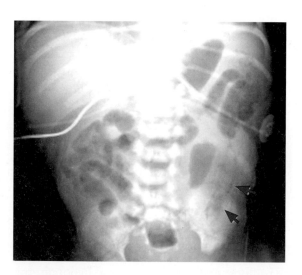

FIGURE 2.13-5. Pneumatosis intestinalis. Short arrows highlight pneumatosis intestinalis on an AXR of a patient with necrotizing enterocolitis. (Reproduced with permission from Brunicardi FC et al. *Schwartz's Principles of Surgery,* 9th ed. New York: McGraw-Hill, 2010, Fig. 39-19.)

TABLE 2.13-6. **Pediatric Immunodeficiencies**

DISORDER	DESCRIPTION	INFECTION RISK/TYPE	DIAGNOSIS/TREATMENT
B-CELL DISORDERS			
Bruton's congenital agammaglobulinemia	An **X-linked recessive B-cell** deficiency found only in **boys.** Symptoms begin **after 6 months of age,** when maternal IgG (transferred transplacentally) is no longer active.	Life threatening; characterized by encapsulated *Pseudomonas, S pneumoniae,* and *Haemophilus* infections after 6 months of age.	Quantitative immunoglobulin levels. If low, confirm with B- and T-cell subsets (B cells are absent; T cells are often high). **Absent tonsils and other lymphoid tissue** may provide a clue. Treat with prophylactic antibiotics and **IVIG.**
Common variable immunodeficiency (CVID)	Usually a combined B- and T-cell defect. **All Ig levels are low** (in the 20s and 30s). **Normal B-cell numbers; ↓ plasma cells.** Symptoms usually present later in life (15–35 years of age).	↑ pyogenic upper and lower respiratory infections. ↑ risk of lymphoma and autoimmune disease.	Quantitative immunoglobulin levels; confirm with B- and T-cell subsets. **Treat with IVIG.**
IgA deficiency	Mild; **the most common immunodeficiency.** ↓ **IgA levels only.**	Usually asymptomatic; patients may develop recurrent respiratory or GI infections (*Giardia*). **Anaphylactic transfusion reaction** due to anti-IgA antibodies is a common presentation.	Quantitative IgA levels; treat infections. **Do not give IVIG,** as it can lead to the production of anti-IgA antibodies.
T-CELL DISORDERS			
Thymic aplasia (DiGeorge syndrome)	See the mnemonic **CATCH 22.** Presents with **tetany** (2° to **hypocalcemia**) in the first days of life.	Variable risk of infection. ↑↑↑ infections with **viruses, fungi, and *Pneumocystis jiroveci* (PCP) pneumonia.** X-ray may show **absent thymic shadow.**	Absolute lymphocyte count; mitogen stimulation response; delayed hypersensitivity skin testing. Treat with bone marrow transplantation and IVIG for antibody deficiency; give PCP prophylaxis. Thymus transplantation is an alternative.

(continues)

TABLE 2.13-6. Pediatric Immunodeficiencies *(continued)*

DISORDER	DESCRIPTION	INFECTION RISK/TYPE	DIAGNOSIS/TREATMENT
	COMBINED DISORDERS		
Ataxia-telangiectasia	Progressive **cerebellar ataxia and oculocutaneous telangiectasias.** Caused by a **DNA repair defect.**	↑ **incidence of malignancies,** including non-Hodgkin's lymphoma, leukemia, and gastric carcinoma.	No specific treatment; may require IVIG depending on the severity of the Ig deficiency.
Severe combined immunodeficiency (SCID)	Severe lack of B and T cells due to a defect in stem cell maturation and ↓ adenosine deaminase. Referred to as "bubble boy disease" because children are confined to an isolated, sterile environment.	Severe, frequent bacterial infections; chronic candidiasis; opportunistic organisms.	Treat with bone marrow or stem cell transplantation and IVIG for antibody deficiency. **Requires PCP prophylaxis.**
Wiskott-Aldrich syndrome	An **X-linked recessive** disorder seen **only in males.** Symptoms usually present at birth. Patients have ↑ IgE/IgA, ↓ **IgM,** and **thrombocytopenia.** The classic presentation involves **bleeding, eczema, and recurrent otitis media.** Remember the mnemonic **WIPE:** **W**iskott-Aldrich **I**nfections **P**urpura (thrombocytopenic) **E**czema	↑↑ risk of atopic disorders, lymphoma/leukemia, and infection from *S pneumoniae, S aureus,* and *H influenzae* type b (**encapsulated organisms;** think back to how IgM functions).	Treatment is supportive (IVIG and antibiotics). **Patients rarely survive to adulthood.** Patients with severe infections may be treated with bone marrow transplantation.
	PHAGOCYTIC DISORDERS		
Chronic granulomatous disease (CGD)	An X-linked (⅔) or autosomal-recessive (⅓) disease with deficient superoxide production by PMNs and macrophages. Anemia, lymphadenopathy, and hypergammaglobulinemia may be present.	Chronic skin, lymph node, pulmonary, GI, and urinary tract infections; osteomyelitis and hepatitis. **Infecting organisms are catalase** ⊕ (*S aureus, E coli, Candida, Klebsiella, Pseudomonas, Aspergillus*). May have granulomas of the skin and GI/GU tracts.	Absolute neutrophil count with neutrophil assays. The **nitroblue tetrazolium test is diagnostic for CGD.** **Treat with daily TMP-SMX;** make judicious use of antibiotics during infections. IFN-γ can ↓ the incidence of serious infection. Bone marrow transplantation and gene therapy are new therapies.
Leukocyte adhesion deficiency	A defect in the chemotaxis of leukocytes.	Recurrent skin, mucosal, and pulmonary infections. May present as **omphalitis in the newborn** period with **delayed separation of the umbilical cords.**	**No pus with minimal inflammation in wounds** (due to a chemotaxis defect). High WBCs in blood. Bone marrow transplantation is curative.

TABLE 2.13-6. Pediatric Immunodeficiencies (continued)

DISORDER	DESCRIPTION	INFECTION RISK/TYPE	DIAGNOSIS/TREATMENT
Chédiak-Higashi syndrome	An autosomal recessive disorder that leads to a defect in neutrophil chemotaxis/ microtubule polymerization. The syndrome includes **partial oculocutaneous albinism, peripheral neuropathy, and neutropenia.**	↑↑ incidence of overwhelming pyogenic infections with *Streptococcus pyogenes, S aureus,* and *Pseudomonas* species.	Look for giant granules in neutrophils. Bone marrow transplantation is the treatment of choice.
Job's syndrome	A defect in neutrophil chemotaxis. Remember the mnemonic **FATED:** Coarse **F**acies **A**bscesses (*S aureus*) Retained primary **T**eeth Hyper-Ig**E** (eosinophilia) **D**ermatologic (severe eczema)	Recurrent *S aureus* infections and abscesses.	Treat with penicillinase-resistant antibiotics and IVIG.
		COMPLEMENT DISORDERS	
C1 esterase deficiency (hereditary angioedema)	An autosomal dominant disorder with **recurrent episodes of angioedema** lasting 2–72 hours and provoked by stress or trauma.	Can lead to life-threatening airway edema.	Total hemolytic complement (CH50) to assess the quantity and function of complement. Purified C1 esterase and FFP can be used prior to surgery.
Terminal complement deficiency (C5–C9)	Inability to form membrane attack complex (MAC).	**Recurrent *Neisseria* infections, meningococcal or gonococcal.** Rarely, lupus or glomerulo-nephritis.	Meningococcal vaccine and appropriate antibiotics.

- Bruton's congenital agammaglobulinemia can be confused with transient hypogammaglobulinemia of infancy (THI), as both are characterized by ↑ susceptibility to infections at ~ 6 months of age, when transplacental maternal IgG is no longer active. B cells are ↓ in Bruton's, whereas those in THI are normal.
- Bruton's and CVID also have similar symptoms, but the former is found in males ~ 6 months of age, whereas CVID is seen in older males and females (15–35 years of age), and its symptoms are less severe.
- **T-cell deficiencies:** Tend to present earlier (1–3 months) with **opportunistic and low-grade fungal, viral, and intracellular bacterial infections** (eg, mycobacteria). 2° B-cell dysfunction may also be seen.
- **Phagocyte deficiencies:** Characterized by mucous membrane infections, abscesses, and poor wound healing. **Infections with catalase-⊕ organisms (eg, *S aureus*), fungi, and gram-⊖ enteric organisms are common.**
- **Complement deficiencies:** Present in children with **congenital asplenia or splenic dysfunction (sickle cell disease).** Characterized by recurrent **bacterial** infections with **encapsulated organisms.**

Q

A 3-month-old infant with a heart murmur has recurrent hospitalizations for fungal and viral infections. A CXR shows no thymic shadow, and the infant's serum calcium level is low. What other defects are common in patients with this disorder?

KEY FACT

Untreated Kawasaki disease can lead to coronary aneurysms and even MI!

MNEMONIC

Kawasaki disease symptoms—

CRASH and BURN

Conjunctivitis
Rash
Adenopathy (unilateral)
Strawberry tongue
Hands and feet (red, swollen, flaky skin)
BURN (fever > 40°C [> 104°F] for ≥ 5 days)

KEY FACT

Kawasaki disease and scarlet fever may both present with "strawberry tongue," rash, desquamation of the hands and feet, and erythema of the mucous membranes. However, children with scarlet fever have normal lips and no conjunctivitis.

This infant has DiGeorge syndrome. Remember the mnemonic **CATCH 22**: **C**ardiac abnormalities, **A**bnormal facies, **T**hymic aplasia, **C**left palate, **H**ypocalcemia, chromosome **22**.

KAWASAKI DISEASE

A multisystemic acute vasculitis that primarily affects young children (80% are < 5 years of age), particularly those of **Asian ancestry.** Divided into acute, subacute, and chronic phases.

DIAGNOSIS

- **Acute phase:** Lasts 1–2 weeks and presents with the following symptoms (**fever plus 4 or more of the criteria below** are required for diagnosis):
  - Fever (usually > 40°C [> 104°F]) for at least **5 days.**
  - Bilateral, nonexudative, painless conjunctivitis sparing the limbus.
  - A polymorphous rash (primarily truncal).
  - Cervical lymphadenopathy (often painful and **unilateral,** with at least 1 node > 1.5 cm).
  - Diffuse mucous membrane erythema (eg, "**strawberry tongue**"); dry, red, chapped lips.
  - Erythema of the palms and soles; indurative edema of the hands and feet; late **desquamation of the fingertips** (in the subacute phase).
  - Other manifestations include sterile pyuria, gallbladder hydrops, hepatitis, and arthritis.
- **Subacute phase:** Begins after the abatement of fever and typically lasts for an additional 2–3 weeks. Manifestations are thrombocytosis and elevated ESR. Untreated children may begin to develop **coronary artery aneurysms** (40%); all patients should be assessed by **echocardiography** at diagnosis.
- **Chronic phase:** Begins when all clinical symptoms have disappeared; lasts until ESR returns to baseline. **Untreated children are at risk of aneurysmal expansion and MI.**

TREATMENT

- High-dose **ASA** (for inflammation and fever) and **IVIG** (to prevent aneurysms).
- Low-dose ASA is then continued, usually for 6 weeks. Children who develop coronary aneurysms may require chronic anticoagulation with ASA or other antiplatelet medications.
- Corticosteroids may be used in IVIG-refractory cases, but **routine use is not recommended.**

JUVENILE IDIOPATHIC ARTHRITIS (JIA)

An autoimmune disorder manifesting as arthritis with "**morning stiffness**" and gradual loss of motion that is present for at least 6 weeks in a patient < 16 **years of age.** Formerly known as juvenile rheumatoid arthritis (JRA).

DIAGNOSIS

- **Pauciarticular (oligoarthritis): Most common;** involves 4 or fewer joints (usually weight-bearing); usually **ANA ⊕ and RF ⊖.** Involves young females; **uveitis** is common and requires **slit-lamp examination** for evaluation. **No systemic symptoms.**
- **Polyarthritis:** Involves 5 or more joints; **symmetric.** RF positivity is rare and indicates severe disease; younger children may be ANA ⊕ with milder disease. Systemic symptoms are rare.
- **Systemic-onset (Still's disease):** May present with recurrent high fever (usually > 39°C [> 102.2°F]), hepatosplenomegaly, and a **salmon-colored macular rash;** usually RF and ANA ⊖.

TREATMENT

- **NSAIDs** and strengthening exercises.
- Corticosteroids (for carditis) and immunosuppressive medications (methotrexate, anti-TNF agents such as etanercept) are second-line agents.

Infectious Disease

ACUTE OTITIS MEDIA

A suppurative infection of the middle ear cavity that is common in children. Up to 75% of children have at least 3 episodes by age 2. Common pathogens include **S pneumoniae, nontypable H influenzae, Moraxella catarrhalis,** and viruses such as influenza A, RSV, and parainfluenza virus.

HISTORY/PE

Symptoms include ear pain, fever, crying, irritability, difficulty feeding or sleeping, vomiting, and diarrhea. Young children may **tug on their ears.**

DIAGNOSIS

Signs on otoscopic exam reveal an erythematous tympanic membrane (TM), bulging or retraction of the TM, loss of TM light reflex, and ↓ TM mobility (test with an insufflator bulb).

TREATMENT

- **High-dose amoxicillin** (80–90 mg/kg/day) × 10 days for empiric therapy. Resistant cases may require amoxicillin/clavulanic acid.
- Complications include TM perforation, mastoiditis, meningitis, cholesteatomas, and chronic otitis media. Recurrent otitis media can cause hearing loss with resultant speech and language delay. Chronic otitis media may require tympanostomy tubes.

BRONCHIOLITIS

An acute inflammatory illness of the small airways in the upper and lower respiratory tracts that primarily affects infants and children < 2 years of age, often in the **fall or winter. RSV is the most common cause;** others include parainfluenza, influenza, and metapneumovirus. Progression to respiratory failure is a potentially fatal complication. For severe RSV, risk factors include age < 6 months, male gender, prematurity, heart or lung disease, and immunodeficiency.

HISTORY/PE

- Presents with low-grade fever, rhinorrhea, cough, and apnea (in young infants).
- Examination reveals **tachypnea, wheezing,** intercostal retractions, **crackles,** prolonged expiration, and hyperresonance to percussion.
- An ↑ **respiratory rate** is the earliest and most sensitive vital sign change.
- Although presentation can be highly variable, symptoms generally **peak on day 3 or 4.**

 KEY FACT

RSV is the most common cause of bronchiolitis. Parainfluenza is the most common cause of croup.

DIAGNOSIS

- Predominantly a clinical diagnosis; routine cases do not need blood work or a CXR.
- A CXR may be obtained to rule out pneumonia and may show hyperinflation of the lungs with flattened diaphragms, interstitial infiltrates, and atelectasis.
- Nasopharyngeal aspirate to test for RSV is highly sensitive and specific but has little effect on management (infants should be treated for bronchiolitis whether RSV is ⊕ or not).

TREATMENT

- Treatment is **primarily supportive;** treat mild disease with outpatient management using fluids and nebulizers if needed. Hospitalize if signs of severe illness are present.
- Treat inpatients with contact isolation, hydration, and O_2. A **trial of aerosolized albuterol** may be attempted; albuterol therapy should be continued only if it is effective.
- **Corticosteroids are not indicated.**
- **Ribavirin** is an antiviral drug that has a controversial role in bronchiolitis treatment. It is sometimes used in high-risk infants with underlying heart, lung, or immune disease.
- **RSV prophylaxis** with injectable poly- or monoclonal antibodies (RespiGam or Synagis) is recommended in winter for high-risk patients ≤ 2 years of age (eg, those with a history of prematurity, chronic lung disease, or congenital heart disease).

CROUP (LARYNGOTRACHEOBRONCHITIS)

An acute viral inflammatory disease of the larynx, primarily within the subglottic space. Pathogens include **parainfluenza** virus type 1 (most common), 2, and 3 as well as RSV, influenza, and adenovirus. Bacterial superinfection may progress to tracheitis.

HISTORY/PE

Prodromal URI symptoms are typically followed by low-grade fever, mild dyspnea, inspiratory stridor that worsens with agitation, a hoarse voice, and the characteristic **barking cough** (usually at night).

DIAGNOSIS

- Diagnosed by clinical impression; often based on the degree of stridor and respiratory distress.
- AP neck film may show the **classic "steeple sign" from subglottic narrowing** (see Figure 2.13-6), but this finding is **neither sensitive nor specific.**
- Table 2.13-7 differentiates croup from epiglottitis and tracheitis.

TREATMENT

- **Mild cases:** Outpatient management with cool mist therapy and fluids.
- **Moderate cases:** May require supplemental O_2, oral or **IM corticosteroids,** and **nebulized racemic epinephrine.**
- **Severe cases** (eg, respiratory distress at rest, inspiratory stridor): Hospitalize and give **nebulized racemic epinephrine.**

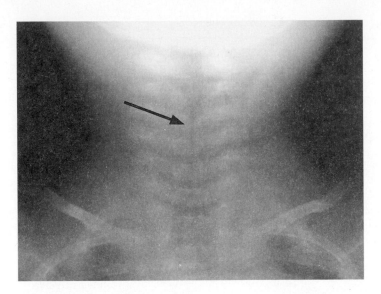

FIGURE 2.13-6. **Croup.** AP radiograph of the neck in this 1-year-old with inspiratory stridor and cough shows the classic "steeple sign" (arrow) consistent with the subglottic narrowing of laryngotracheobronchitis. (Reproduced with permission from Stone CK, Humphries RL. *Current Diagnosis & Treatment: Emergency Medicine,* 6th ed. New York: McGraw-Hill, 2008, Fig. 30-10A.)

EPIGLOTTITIS

A serious and rapidly progressive infection of supraglottic structures (eg, the epiglottis and aryepiglottic folds). Prior to immunization, *H influenzae* type b was the 1° pathogen. Common causes now include *Streptococcus* species, nontypable *H influenzae*, and viral agents.

HISTORY/PE

- Presents with **acute-onset high fever** (39–40°C [102–104°F]), **dysphagia, drooling,** a muffled voice, **inspiratory retractions,** cyanosis, and soft stridor.
- Patients sit with the **neck hyperextended and the chin protruding** ("sniffing dog" position) and **lean forward in a "tripod" position** to maximize air entry.
- Untreated infection can lead to life-threatening airway obstruction and respiratory arrest.

DIAGNOSIS

- Diagnosed by clinical impression. The differential diagnosis must include diffuse and localized causes of airway obstruction (see Tables 2.13-7 and 2.13-8).
- **The airway must be secured before a definitive diagnosis can be made.** In light of potential laryngospasm and airway compromise, **do not examine the throat unless an anesthesiologist or otolaryngologist is present.**
- Definitive diagnosis is made via direct fiberoptic visualization of a cherry-red, swollen epiglottis and arytenoids.
- Lateral x-ray shows a swollen epiglottis obliterating the valleculae (**"thumbprint sign"**; see Figure 2.13-7).

TREATMENT

- This disease is a **true emergency,** so time should not be wasted on ordering an x-ray or examining the throat.

KEY FACT

Epiglottitis is a true emergency and can lead to life-threatening airway obstruction.

TABLE 2.13-7. Characteristics of Croup, Epiglottitis, and Tracheitis

VARIABLE	CROUP	EPIGLOTTITIS	TRACHEITIS
Age group affected	3 months to 3 years	3–7 years	3 months to 2 years
Incidence in children presenting with stridor	**88%**	8%	2%
Pathogen	**Parainfluenza virus**	*H influenzae*	Often *S aureus;* commonly follows viral URI
Onset	Prodrome (1–7 days)	Rapid (4–12 hours)	Prodrome (3 days) leading to acute decompensation (10 hours)
Fever severity	Low grade	**High grade**	Intermediate grade
Associated symptoms	**Barking cough,** inspiratory stridor, hoarseness	**Respiratory distress:** acute decompensation, toxic appearance, inspiratory stridor, muffled voice, drooling	Variable respiratory distress; slower onset than epiglottitis; pseudomembrane
Position preference	None	Seated, neck extended (tripod position)	None
Response to racemic epinephrine	**Stridor improves**	None	None
CXR findings	**"Steeple sign"** on AP film	**"Thumbprint sign"** on lateral film	**Subglottic narrowing**

- Remember the ABCs; **secure the airway first** with endotracheal intubation or tracheostomy, and then give IV antibiotics (ceftriaxone or cefuroxime).

KEY FACT

What are the most common bacteria that cause meningitis in neonates (< 1 month) as opposed to infants and children?
- **Neonates:** GBS, *Listeria, E coli*
- **Infants/children:** *S pneumoniae, N meningitidis, H influenzae*

MENINGITIS

Bacterial meningitis most often occurs in children < 3 years of age; common organisms include **S pneumoniae, N meningitidis, and E coli.** Enteroviruses are the most common agents of viral meningitis and occur in children of all ages. Risk factors include sinofacial infections, trauma, and sepsis.

HISTORY/PE

- Bacterial meningitis classically presents with the triad of **headache, high fever, and nuchal rigidity.**
- Viral meningitis is typically preceded by a prodromal illness that includes fever, sore throat, and fatigue.
- **Kernig's sign** (reluctance of knee extension when the hip is flexed) and **Brudzinski's sign** (pain with passive neck flexion) are nonspecific signs of meningeal irritation.
- Additional physical examination findings may include signs of ↑ ICP (papilledema, cranial nerve palsies) or a **petechial rash** (**N meningitidis**).

TABLE 2.13-8. Retropharyngeal vs. Peritonsillar Abscess

VARIABLE	RETROPHARYNGEAL ABSCESS	PERITONSILLAR ABSCESS
Age group affected	Six months to 6 years of age.	Usually > 10 years of age.
History/PE	**Acute-onset high fever** with sore throat, a muffled **"hot potato" voice**, trismus, drooling, and cervical lymphadenopathy. Usually unilateral; a mass may be seen in the posterior pharyngeal wall on visual inspection.	Sore throat, a muffled **"hot potato" voice**, trismus, drooling, **uvula displaced to opposite side.**
Pathogen	**Group A streptococcus** (most common), *S aureus, Bacteroides* (often polymicrobial).	**Group A streptococcus** (most common), *S aureus, S pneumoniae,* anaerobes.
Preferred position	Supine with the **neck extended** (sitting up or flexing the neck worsens symptoms).	None.
Diagnosis	On **lateral neck x-ray,** the soft tissue plane should be ≤ 50% of the width of the corresponding vertebral body. Contrast CT of the neck helps differentiate abscess from cellulitis.	Usually **clinical.**
Treatment	Aspiration or incision and drainage of abscess; antibiotics.	Incision and drainage +/− tonsillectomy; antibiotics.

Signs in neonates include lethargy, hyper- or hypothermia, **poor tone, a bulging fontanelle, and vomiting.**

DIAGNOSIS

- Obtain a head CT to rule out ↑ ICP (risk of brainstem herniation).
- Perform an LP; send cell count with differential, glucose and protein levels, Gram stain, and culture.

TREATMENT

- **Neonates** should receive **ampicillin and cefotaxime or gentamicin.** Consider **acyclovir** if there is concern for **herpes encephalitis** (eg, if the mother had HSV lesions at the time of the infant's birth).
- **Older children** should receive **ceftriaxone and vancomycin.**

PERTUSSIS (WHOOPING COUGH)

A highly infectious form of bronchitis caused by the gram-⊖ bacillus *Bordetella pertussis.* The DTaP vaccine (given in 5 doses in early childhood) is pro-

KEY FACT

Don't be fooled—neonates and young children rarely have meningeal signs on exam!

KEY FACT

Neonates should not be given ceftriaxone in light of the ↑ risk of biliary sludging and kernicterus.

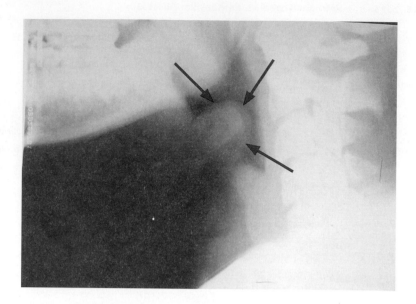

FIGURE 2.13-7. **Epiglottitis.** Lateral radiograph of the neck shows a markedly swollen epiglottis (arrows) demonstrating the classic "thumbprint sign," with near-complete airway obstruction. (Reproduced with permission from Stone CK, Humphries RL. *Current Diagnosis & Treatment: Emergency Medicine,* 6th ed. New York: McGraw-Hill, 2008, Fig. 48-4.)

tective, but immunity wanes by adolescence. Adolescents and young adults serve as the 1° reservoir for pertussis. Transmission is through aerosol droplets. Pertussis can be life threatening for young infants but is generally a milder infection in older children and adults.

HISTORY/PE

- Has **3 stages:** (1) catarrhal (mild URI symptoms; lasts 1–2 weeks), (2) paroxysmal (paroxysms of cough with inspiratory whoop and posttussive emesis; lasts 2–3 months), and (3) convalescent (symptoms wane).
- Patients most often present in the paroxysmal stage but are most contagious in the catarrhal stage.
- The classic presentation is an **infant < 6 months of age with posttussive emesis and apnea.**

DIAGNOSIS

- Labs show an elevated WBC count with lymphocytosis (often ≥ 70%).
- **Culture is the gold standard.**

TREATMENT

- Hospitalize infants < 6 months of age.
- Give **erythromycin × 14 days** to patients and close contacts (including day care contacts). Exposed newborns are at high risk irrespective of their immunization status because they may not be entirely protected by maternal transplacental immunoglobulins.

VIRAL EXANTHEMS

Table 2.13-9 outlines the clinical presentation of common viral exanthems.

TABLE 2.13-9.   Viral Exanthems

Disease	Cause	Characteristics	Complications
Erythema infectiosum (fifth disease)	Parvovirus B19	**Prodrome:** None; fever is often absent or low grade. **Rash:** **"Slapped-cheek,"** pruritic, maculopapular, erythematous rash (see Figure 2.13-8). Starts on the arms and spreads to the trunk and legs. **Worsens with fever and sun exposure.**	**Arthropathy** in children and adults. Congenital infection is associated with fetal hydrops and death. **Aplastic crisis** may be precipitated in children with ↑ RBC turnover (eg, sickle cell anemia, hereditary spherocytosis) or in those with ↓ RBC production (eg, severe iron deficiency anemia).
Measles	Paramyxovirus	**Prodrome:** Low-grade fever with **C**ough, **C**oryza, and **C**onjunctivitis (the **"3 C's"**); **Koplik's spots** (small irregular red spots with central gray specks) appear on the buccal mucosa after 1–2 days. **Rash:** An erythematous **maculopapular rash spreads from head to toe** (see Figure 2.13-9).	**Common:** Otitis media, pneumonia, laryngotracheitis. **Rare:** Subacute sclerosing panencephalitis.
Rubella ("3-day measles")	Rubella virus	**Prodrome:** Asymptomatic or tender, generalized lymphadenopathy (clue: posterior auricular lymphadenopathy). **Rash:** Presents with an erythematous, tender maculopapular rash that **also spreads from head to toe.** **In contrast to measles, children with rubella often have only a low-grade fever and do not appear as ill.** Polyarthritis may be seen in adolescents.	Encephalitis, thrombocytopenia (a rare complication of postnatal infection). Congenital infection is associated with congenital anomalies (PDA, deafness, cataracts, mental retardation).
Roseola infantum	HHV-6 and -7	**Prodrome:** Acute onset of high fever (> 40°C [> 104°F]); no other symptoms for 3–4 days. **Rash:** A maculopapular rash appears as fever breaks (begins on the trunk and quickly spreads to the face and extremities) and often lasts < 24 hours.	**Febrile seizures** may result from rapid fever onset.
Varicella (chickenpox)	Varicella-zoster virus (VZV)	**Prodrome:** Mild fever, anorexia, and malaise precede the rash by 24 hours. **Rash:** Generalized, pruritic, "teardrop" vesicular periphery; lesions are often at **different stages of healing.** Usually appears on the face and spreads to the rest of the body, sparing the palms and soles. Infectious from 24 hours before eruption until lesions crust over.	Progressive varicella with meningoencephalitis, pneumonia, and hepatitis in the immunocompromised. Skin lesions may develop 2° bacterial infections. Reye's syndrome (associated with ASA use).

(continues)

TABLE 2.13-9. Viral Exanthems (continued)

DISEASE	CAUSE	CHARACTERISTICS	COMPLICATIONS
Varicella zoster	VZV	**Prodrome:** Reactivation of varicella infection; starts as pain along an affected sensory nerve. **Rash:** Pruritic "teardrop" vesicular rash in a **dermatomal** distribution. Uncommon unless the patient is **immunocompromised.**	Encephalopathy, aseptic meningitis, pneumonitis, TTP, Guillain-Barré syndrome, cellulitis, arthritis.
Hand-foot-and-mouth disease	Coxsackie A	**Prodrome:** Fever, anorexia, oral pain. **Rash:** Oral ulcers; maculopapular vesicular rash on the hands and feet and sometimes on the buttocks.	None (self-limited).

Neonatology

MNEMONIC

Apgar scoring—

APGAR (0, 1, 2 in each category)

Appearance (blue/pale, pink trunk, all pink)
Pulse (0, < 100, > 100)
Grimace with stimulation (0, grimace, grimace and cough)
Activity (limp, some, active)
Respiratory effort (0, irregular, regular)

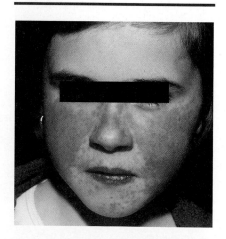

FIGURE 2.13-8. Fifth disease.
Note the classic "slapped-cheek" appearance of fifth disease, which is caused by parvovirus B19. (Reproduced with permission from Wolff K, Johnson RA. *Fitzpatrick's Color Atlas & Synopsis of Clinical Dermatology,* 6th ed. New York: McGraw-Hill, 2009, Fig. 27-24.)

APGAR SCORING

A rapid scoring system that helps evaluate the need for neonatal resuscitation. Each of 5 parameters (see the mnemonic **APGAR**) is assigned a score of 0–2 at 1 and 5 minutes after birth.

- **Scores of 8–10:** Typically reflect good cardiopulmonary adaptation.
- **Scores of 4–7:** Indicate the possible need for resuscitation. Infants should be observed, stimulated, and possibly given ventilatory support.
- **Scores of 0–3:** Indicate the need for immediate resuscitation.

CONGENITAL MALFORMATIONS

Table 2.13-10 describes selected congenital malformations.

NEONATAL JAUNDICE

An elevated serum bilirubin concentration (> 5 mg/dL) due to ↑ hemolysis or ↓ excretion. Subtypes are as follows:

- **Conjugated (direct) hyperbilirubinemia:** Always pathologic.
- **Unconjugated (indirect) hyperbilirubinemia:** May be physiologic or pathologic. See Table 2.13-11 for differentiating characteristics.
- **Kernicterus:** A complication of unconjugated hyperbilirubinemia that results from irreversible bilirubin deposition in the basal ganglia, pons, and cerebellum. It typically occurs at levels of > 25–30 mg/dL and can be fatal. Risk factors include prematurity, asphyxia, and sepsis.

HISTORY/PE

- The differential includes the following:
  - **Conjugated:** Extrahepatic cholestasis (biliary atresia, choledochal cysts), intrahepatic cholestasis (neonatal hepatitis, inborn errors of

metabolism, TPN cholestasis), Dubin-Johnson syndrome, Rotor's syndrome, TORCH infections (see the Infectious Disease chapter).

- **Unconjugated:** Physiologic jaundice, breast milk jaundice, ↑ enterohepatic circulation (eg, GI obstruction), disorders of bilirubin metabolism, hemolysis, sepsis, Crigler-Najjar syndrome, Gilbert's syndrome.
- The history should focus on diet (breast milk or formula), intrauterine drug exposure, and family history (hemoglobinopathies, enzyme deficiencies, RBC defects).
- Physical examination may reveal signs of hepatic or GI dysfunction (abdominal distention, delayed passage of meconium, light-colored stools, dark urine), infection, or hemoglobinopathies (cephalohematomas, bruising, pallor, petechiae, hepatomegaly).
- **Kernicterus** presents with lethargy, poor feeding, a high-pitched cry, hypertonicity, and seizures; jaundice may follow a cephalopedal progression as bilirubin concentrations ↑.

DIAGNOSIS

- CBC with peripheral blood smear; blood typing of mother and infant (for ABO or Rh incompatibility); Coombs' test and bilirubin levels.
- Ultrasound and/or HIDA scan can confirm suspected cholestatic disease.
- For direct hyperbilirubinemia, check LFTs, bile acids, blood cultures, sweat test, and tests for aminoacidopathies and α_1-antitrypsin deficiency.
- A jaundiced neonate who is febrile, hypotensive, and/or tachypneic needs a full sepsis workup and ICU monitoring.

TREATMENT

- Treat underlying causes (eg, infection).
- Treat **unconjugated** hyperbilirubinemia with **phototherapy** (for mild elevations) or **exchange transfusion** (for severe elevations > 20 mg/dL). Start phototherapy earlier (10–15 mg/dL) for preterm infants. **Phototherapy is not indicated for conjugated hyperbilirubinemia** and can lead to skin bronzing.

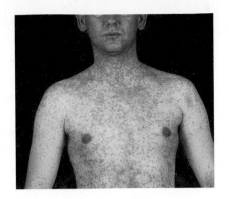

FIGURE 2.13-9. Measles exanthem. A classic morbilliform exanthem is seen, with red papules spreading from the forehead and postauricular area to the neck, trunk, and extremities. (Reproduced with permission from Wolff K et al. *Fitzpatrick's Dermatology in General Medicine*, 7th ed. New York: McGraw-Hill, 2008, Fig. 192-3.)

KEY FACT

Direct (conjugated) hyperbilirubinemia is always pathologic.

RESPIRATORY DISTRESS SYNDROME (RDS)

The most common cause of respiratory failure in **preterm** infants (affects > 70% of infants born at 28–30 weeks' gestation); formerly known as hyaline membrane disease. **Surfactant deficiency** leads to poor lung compliance, alveolar collapse, and atelectasis. Risk factors include maternal DM, male gender, and the second born of twins.

HISTORY/PE

Presents in the **first 48–72 hours of life** with a respiratory rate > 60/min, progressive hypoxemia, cyanosis, nasal flaring, intercostal retractions, and expiratory grunting.

DIAGNOSIS

- Check ABGs, CBC, and blood cultures to rule out infection.
- Diagnosis is clinical and confirmed with characteristic CXR findings:
    - **RDS:** "Ground-glass" appearance, diffuse atelectasis, and **air bronchograms** on CXR.
    - **Transient tachypnea of the newborn:** Retained amniotic fluid results in prominent perihilar streaking in interlobular fissures. Resolves with O_2 administration.

KEY FACT

RDS is the most common cause of respiratory failure in preterm infants.

TABLE 2.13-10. **Selected Congenital Malformations**

MALFORMATION	PRESENTATION/DIAGNOSIS/TREATMENT
Tracheoesophageal fistula	Tract between the trachea and esophagus. Associated with defects such as esophageal atresia and **VACTERL** (**V**ertebral, **A**nal, **C**ardiac, **T**racheal, **E**sophageal, **R**enal, **L**imb) anomalies. **Presentation:** Polyhydramnios in utero, ↑ oral secretions, inability to feed, gagging, aspiration pneumonia, respiratory distress. **Diagnosis:** CXR showing an NG tube coiled in the esophagus identifies esophageal atresia. The presence of air in the GI tract is suggestive; confirm with bronchoscopy. **Treatment:** Surgical repair.
Congenital diaphragmatic hernia	GI tract segments protrude through the diaphragm into the thorax; 90% are posterior left (Bochdalek). **Presentation:** Respiratory distress (from pulmonary hypoplasia and pulmonary hypertension); sunken abdomen; **bowel sounds over the left hemithorax.** **Diagnosis:** Ultrasound in utero; confirmed by postnatal CXR. **Treatment:** High-frequency ventilation or extracorporeal membrane oxygenation to manage pulmonary hypertension; surgical repair.
Gastroschisis	Herniation of the intestine only through the abdominal wall **next to the umbilicus (usually on the right) with no sac (the GI tract is exposed).** **Presentation:** Polyhydramnios in utero; often premature; associated with GI stenoses or atresia. **Treatment:** A **surgical emergency!** Single-stage closure is possible in only 10% of cases.
Omphalocele	Herniation of abdominal viscera through the abdominal wall **at the umbilicus into a sac** covered by peritoneum and amniotic membrane (see Figure 2.13-10). **Presentation/diagnosis:** Polyhydramnios in utero; often premature; associated with other GI and cardiac defects. Seen in **Beckwith-Wiedemann syndrome and trisomies.** **Treatment:** C-section can prevent sac rupture; if the sac is intact, postpone surgical correction until the patient is fully resuscitated. **Keep the sac covered/stable** with petroleum and gauze. Intermittent NG suction to prevent abdominal distention.
Duodenal atresia	Complete or partial failure of the duodenal lumen to recanalize during gestational weeks 8–10. **Presentation:** Polyhydramnios in utero; **bilious emesis within hours after the first feeding.** Associated with **Down syndrome** and other cardiac/GI anomalies (eg, annular pancreas, malrotation, imperforate anus). **Diagnosis:** AXRs show the **"double bubble"** sign (air bubbles in the stomach and duodenum) proximal to the site of the atresia (see Figure 2.13-11). **Treatment:** Surgical repair.

TABLE 2.13-11. **Physiologic vs. Pathologic Jaundice**

PHYSIOLOGIC JAUNDICE	PATHOLOGIC JAUNDICE
Not present until 72 hours after birth.	Present in the first 24 hours of life.
Bilirubin ↑ < 5 mg/dL/day.	Bilirubin ↑ > 0.5 mg/dL/hr.
Bilirubin peaks at < 14–15 mg/dL.	Bilirubin ↑ to > 15 mg/dL.
Direct bilirubin is < 10% of total.	Direct bilirubin is > 10% of total.
Resolves by 1 week in term infants and 2 weeks in preterm infants.	Persists beyond 1 week in term infants and 2 weeks in preterm infants.

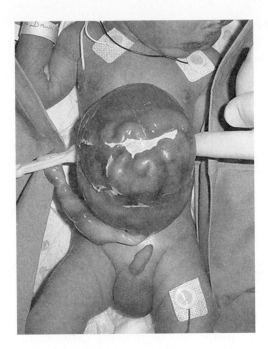

FIGURE 2.13-10. **Giant omphalocele in a newborn male.** Herniation of abdominal viscera through the abdominal wall at the umbilicus into a sac covered by peritoneum and amniotic membrane. (Reproduced with permission from Brunicardi FC et al. *Schwartz's Principles of Surgery,* 9th ed. New York: McGraw-Hill, 2010, Fig. 39-30.)

- **Meconium aspiration:** Coarse, irregular infiltrates; hyperexpansion and pneumothoraces.
- **Congenital pneumonia:** Nonspecific patchy infiltrates; neutropenia, tracheal aspirate, and Gram stain suggest the diagnosis.

TREATMENT

- Continuous positive airway pressure (CPAP) or intubation and mechanical ventilation.

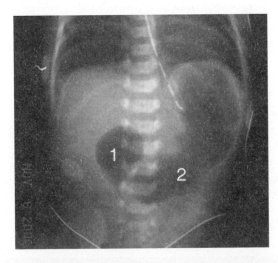

FIGURE 2.13-11. **Duodenal atresia.** Note the characteristic "double bubble" appearance of the duodenal bulb (1) and stomach (2) in a neonate with duodenal atresia presenting with bilious emesis. (Reproduced with permission from Brunicardi FC et al. *Schwartz's Principles of Surgery,* 9th ed. New York: McGraw-Hill, 2010, Fig. 39-13.)

- **Artificial surfactant** administration ↓ mortality.
- Pretreat mothers at risk for preterm delivery (< 30 weeks' gestation) with corticosteroids; if > 30 weeks, monitor fetal lung maturity via a lecithin-to-sphingomyelin (L/S) ratio and the presence of phosphatidylglycerol in amniotic fluid.

COMPLICATIONS

Persistent PDA, **bronchopulmonary dysplasia, retinopathy of prematurity,** barotrauma from positive pressure ventilation, intraventricular hemorrhage, and NEC are complications of treatment.

Neurology

CEREBRAL PALSY

A range of **nonhereditary, nonprogressive disorders of movement and posture;** the most common movement disorder in children. Often results from **perinatal neurologic insult,** but in most cases the cause is unknown. Risk factors include low birth weight, intrauterine exposure to maternal infection, prematurity, perinatal asphyxia, trauma, brain malformation, and neonatal cerebral hemorrhage. Categories include the following:

- **Pyramidal (spastic):** Spastic paresis of any or all limbs. Accounts for 75% of cases. Mental retardation is present in up to 90% of cases.
- **Extrapyramidal (dyskinetic):** A result of damage to extrapyramidal tracts. Subtypes are ataxic (difficulty coordinating purposeful movements), choreoathetoid, and dystonic (uncontrollable jerking, writhing, or posturing). Abnormal movements worsen with stress and disappear during sleep.

HISTORY/PE

- May be associated with seizure disorders, behavioral disorders, hearing or vision impairment, learning disabilities, and speech deficits.
- Affected limbs may show hyperreflexia, pathologic reflexes (eg, Babinski), ↑ tone/contractures, weakness, and/or underdevelopment.
- Toe walking and scissor gait are common. Hip dislocations and scoliosis may be seen.

DIAGNOSIS

Diagnosed by clinical impression. Ultrasound may be useful in infants to identify intracranial hemorrhage or structural malformations. MRI is diagnostic in older children. EEG may be useful in patients with seizures.

TREATMENT

- There is **no cure for cerebral palsy.** Special education, physical therapy, braces, and surgical release of contractures may help.
- Treat spasticity with diazepam, dantrolene, or baclofen. Baclofen pumps and posterior rhizotomy may alleviate severe contractures.

FEBRILE SEIZURES

Usually occur in children between **6 months and 5 years of age** who have no evidence of intracranial infection or other causes. Risk factors include a rapid

↑ in temperature and a history of febrile seizures in a close relative. Febrile seizures recur in approximately 1 in 3 patients.

HISTORY/PE

- Seizures usually **occur during the onset of fever** and may be the first sign of an underlying illness (eg, otitis media, roseola).
- Classified as simple or complex:
    - **Simple:** A **short-duration** (< 15-minute), **generalized** tonic-clonic seizure with 1 seizure in a 24-hour period. A high fever (> 39°C [> 102.2°F]) and fever onset within hours of the seizure are typical.
    - **Complex:** A **long-duration** (> 15-minute) or **focal** seizure, or multiple seizures in a 24-hour period. A low-grade fever for several days before seizure onset may be present.

DIAGNOSIS

- Focus on finding a source of infection. LP is indicated if there are clinical signs of CNS infection (eg, altered consciousness, meningismus, a tense/bulging anterior fontanelle) after ruling out ↑ ICP.
- No workup is necessary for first-time simple febrile seizures, and no lab studies are needed if presentation is consistent with febrile seizures in children > 18 months of age. Infants < 6 months of age need a sepsis workup (CBC, UA, and blood, urine, and CSF culture).
- For atypical presentations, obtain electrolytes, serum glucose, blood cultures, UA, and CBC with differential.

TREATMENT

- Use **antipyretic therapy** (acetaminophen; **avoid ASA in light of the risk of Reye's syndrome**) and treat any underlying illness. Note that antipyretic therapy does not ↓ the recurrence of febrile seizures.
- For complex seizures, perform a thorough neurologic evaluation, including an EEG and an MRI. Chronic anticonvulsant therapy (eg, diazepam or phenobarbital) may be necessary.

COMPLICATIONS

- The risk of recurrence is < 30% and is highest within 1 year of the initial episode. For simple febrile seizures, there is no ↑ risk of developmental abnormalities or epilepsy.
- Risk factors for the development of epilepsy include complex febrile seizures (~ 10% risk), ⊕ family history of epilepsy, an abnormal neurologic exam, and developmental delay.

Oncology

LEUKEMIA

A hematopoietic malignancy of lymphocytic or myeloblastic origin. The most common childhood malignancy; 97% of cases are acute leukemias (ALL > AML). ALL is most common in male Caucasian children between 2 and 5 years of age; AML is seen most frequently in male African American children throughout childhood. Associated with trisomy 21, Fanconi's anemia, prior radiation, SCID, and congenital bone marrow failure states.

KEY FACT

Perform an LP if CNS infection is suspected in a patient with a febrile seizure.

KEY FACT

Simple febrile seizures do **not** cause brain damage, usually do **not** recur, and do **not** lead to an ↑ risk of epilepsy.

KEY FACT

ALL is the most common childhood malignancy, followed by CNS tumors and lymphomas.

HISTORY/PE

- Symptoms are abrupt in onset. They are initially nonspecific (anorexia, fatigue) and are followed by **bone pain with limp or refusal to bear weight, fever (from neutropenia), anemia, ecchymoses, petechiae, and/or hepatosplenomegaly.**
- CNS metastases may be associated with headache, vomiting, and papilledema.
- AML can present with a chloroma, a greenish soft-tissue tumor on the skin or spinal cord.

DIAGNOSIS

- CBC, coagulation studies, and peripheral blood smear, which shows high numbers of blasts (lymphoblasts are found in 90% of cases). **WBC counts can be low, normal, or high.**
- A **bone marrow aspirate** for immunophenotyping (TdT assay and a panel of monoclonal antibodies to T- and B-cell antigens) and genetic analysis help confirm the diagnosis. The diagnosis is made if bone marrow is hypercellular with ↑ lymphoblasts.
- **CXR to rule out a mediastinal mass.**

TREATMENT

- Chemotherapy based, including induction, consolidation, and maintenance phases.
- **Tumor lysis syndrome** (hyperkalemia, hyperphosphatemia, hyperuricemia) is common prior to and during the initiation of treatment. Treat with fluids, diuretics, allopurinol, urine alkalinization, and reduction of phosphate intake. **Corticosteroids are contraindicated** because they can precipitate tumor lysis syndrome.

KEY FACT

Watch for tumor lysis syndrome at the onset of any chemotherapy regimen.

NEUROBLASTOMA

An embryonal tumor of neural crest origin. More than half of patients are **< 2 years of age,** and 70% have distant metastases at presentation. Associated with **neurofibromatosis, Hirschsprung's disease,** and the N-myc oncogene.

HISTORY/PE

- Lesion sites are most commonly abdominal, thoracic, and cervical (in descending order).
- Symptoms may vary with location and may include a **nontender abdominal mass (may cross the midline), Horner's syndrome,** hypertension, or cord compression (from a paraspinal tumor).
- Patients may have anemia, FTT, and fever.
- More than 50% of patients will have metastases at diagnosis. Signs include bone marrow suppression, proptosis, hepatomegaly, subcutaneous nodules, and **opsoclonus/myoclonus.**

DIAGNOSIS

- CT scan; fine-needle aspirate of tumor. Histologically appears as small, round, blue tumor cells with a characteristic rosette pattern.
- **Elevated 24-hour urinary catecholamines (VMA and HVA).**
- Bone scan and bone marrow aspirate.
- CBC, LFTs, coagulation panel, BUN/creatinine.

KEY FACT

Both Wilms' tumor and neuroblastoma are abdominal masses that can cause hypertension. Wilms' tumor is associated with aniridia and hemihypertrophy and does not cross the midline. Neuroblastoma is associated with opsoclonus/myoclonus and may cross the midline.

TREATMENT

Local excision plus postsurgical chemotherapy and/or radiation.

WILMS' TUMOR

A renal tumor of embryonal origin that is most commonly seen in **children 2–5 years** of age. Associated with **Beckwith-Wiedemann syndrome** (hemihypertrophy, macroglossia, visceromegaly), **neurofibromatosis, and WAGR syndrome** (**W**ilms' tumor, **A**niridia, **G**enitourinary abnormalities, mental **R**etardation).

HISTORY/PE

- Presents as an **asymptomatic, nontender,** smooth abdominal mass that **does not usually cross the midline.**
- Abdominal pain, fever, hypertension, and microscopic or gross hematuria are seen.

DIAGNOSIS

- CBC, BUN, creatinine, and UA.
- Abdominal ultrasound.
- CT scans of the chest and abdomen are used to detect metastases.

TREATMENT

Local resection and nephrectomy with postsurgical chemotherapy and radiation depending on stage and histology.

CHILDHOOD BONE TUMORS

It is critical to distinguish between Ewing's sarcoma and osteosarcoma (see Table 2.13-12 and Figure 2.9-5 from the Musculoskeletal chapter).

Preventive Care

ANTICIPATORY GUIDANCE

An important aspect of every well-child visit. Commonly tested advice includes the following:

- Keep the water heater at < 48.8°C (< 120°F).
- Babies should **sleep on their backs** without any stuffed animals or other toys in the crib (to ↓ the risk of SIDS).
- Car safety seats should be **rear facing** and should be placed in the back of the car (seats can face forward if the child is > 2 years of age and weighs > 40 lbs).
- No solid foods should be given before 6 months; they should then be introduced gradually and one at a time. Do not give cow's milk prior to 12 months.
- Syrup of ipecac (an emetic) is no longer routinely recommended for accidental poisoning. Poison control should be contacted immediately for assistance.

TABLE 2.13-12. Ewing's Sarcoma vs. Osteosarcoma

VARIABLE	EWING'S SARCOMA	OSTEOSARCOMA
Origin	Sarcoma (neuroectoderm); associated with chromosome 11:22 translocation.	Osteoblasts (mesenchyme).
Epidemiology	Commonly seen in **Caucasian** male adolescents.	Commonly seen in male adolescents.
History/PE	Local pain and swelling. **Systemic symptoms** (fever, anorexia, fatigue) are common.	Local pain and swelling. Systemic symptoms are rare.
Location	**Midshaft** of long bones (femur, pelvis, fibula, humerus).	**Metaphyses** of long bones (distal femur, proximal tibia, proximal humerus). Metastases to lungs in 20%.
Diagnosis	Leukocytosis, ↑ ESR. Lytic bone lesion with **"onion skin"** periosteal reaction on plain x-ray.	↑ **alkaline phosphatase.** **"Sunburst" lytic bone lesions.** Chest CT to rule out pulmonary metastases.
Treatment	Local excision, chemotherapy, and radiation.	Local excision, chemotherapy.

HEARING AND VISION SCREENING

- Objective hearing screening (otoacoustic emissions and/or auditory brainstem response) for newborns prior to discharge is common.
- Objective hearing screening is indicated for children with a history of meningitis, TORCH infections, measles and mumps, and recurrent otitis media.
- The red reflex should be checked at birth. Leukocoria is the lack of a red reflex.
- **Strabismus** (ocular misalignment) is normal until 3 months of age; beyond 3 months, children should be evaluated by a pediatric ophthalmologist and may require corrective lenses, occlusion, and/or surgery to prevent **amblyopia** (suppression of retinal images in a misaligned eye, leading to permanent vision loss).

KEY FACT

Leukocoria indicates retinoblastoma, congenital cataracts, or retinopathy of prematurity.

CHILDHOOD VACCINATIONS

The Epidemiology chapter summarizes CDC-recommended vaccinations for the pediatric population. Contraindications and precautions in this population are as follows:

- Contraindications:
  - Severe allergy to a vaccine component or a prior dose of vaccine. **Patients who are allergic to eggs may not receive MMR or influenza vaccine.**

- Encephalopathy within 7 days of prior pertussis vaccination.
- Avoid live vaccines (oral polio vaccine, varicella, MMR) in immuno-compromised and pregnant patients (exception: HIV patients may receive MMR and varicella).
- **Precautions:**
  - Current moderate to severe illness (with or without fever).
  - Prior reactions to pertussis vaccine (fever > 40.5°C [> 104.9°F]), a shocklike state, persistent crying for > 3 hours within 48 hours of vaccination, or seizure within 3 days of vaccination).
  - A history of receiving IVIG in the past year.
- The following are **not** contraindications to vaccination:
  - Mild illness and/or low-grade fever.
  - Current antibiotic therapy.
  - Prematurity.
  - Pneumococcal polysaccharide vaccine (PPV) should be administered to high-risk groups (sickle cell disease or splenectomy, immunodeficient).

LEAD POISONING

Most exposure in children is due to lead-contaminated household dust from **leaded paint.** Screening should be routinely performed at 12 and 24 months for patients living in high-risk areas (pre-1950s homes or zip codes with high percentages of elevated blood lead levels); universal screening is not recommended.

HISTORY/PE

- Presents with irritability, headache, hyperactivity or apathy, anorexia, **intermittent abdominal pain,** constipation, intermittent vomiting, and **peripheral neuropathy (wrist or foot drop).**
- Acute encephalopathy (usually with levels > 70 µg/dL) is characterized by ↑ ICP, vomiting, confusion, seizures, and coma.

DIAGNOSIS

- Do a fingerstick test as an initial screen; then obtain serum lead level.
- CBC and peripheral blood smear show **microcytic, hypochromic anemia and basophilic stippling.**

TREATMENT

- **< 45 µg/dL and asymptomatic:** Retest at 1–3 months; remove sources of lead exposure.
- **45–69 µg/dL:** Chelation therapy (inpatient **EDTA** or outpatient oral succimer [**DMSA**]).
- **≥ 70 µg/dL:** Chelation therapy (inpatient **EDTA** + **BAL** [IM dimercaprol]).

KEY FACT

New evidence has shown impaired intelligence and neurodevelopmental outcomes among children exposed to lead levels as low as 10 µg/dL.

NOTES

PSYCHIATRY

Anxiety Disorders

GENERALIZED ANXIETY DISORDER

Uncontrollable, excessive anxiety or worry about multiple activities or events that leads to significant impairment or distress. The male-to-female ratio is 1:2; clinical onset is usually in the early 20s.

HISTORY/PE

Presents with anxiety on most days (**6 or more months**) and with **3 or more somatic symptoms** (restlessness, fatigue, difficulty concentrating, irritability, muscle tension, disturbed sleep).

TREATMENT

- **Short-term therapy:**
    - Benzodiazepines may be used for immediate symptom relief.
    - Taper benzodiazepines as soon as long-term treatment is established (eg, with SSRIs) in view of the high risk of tolerance and dependence.
    - Do not stop benzodiazepines "cold turkey," as patients may develop potentially lethal withdrawal symptoms similar to those of alcohol withdrawal.
- **Long-term therapy:**
    - Lifestyle changes.
    - Psychotherapy.
    - **Medications** (see Table 2.14-1): SSRIs (first-line treatment), venlafaxine, buspirone.
- Patient education is essential.

KEY FACT

Buspirone is another drug, in addition to SSRIs, that should not be used in conjunction with MAOIs.

TABLE 2.14-1. Anxiolytic Medications

DRUG CLASS	INDICATIONS	SIDE EFFECTS
SSRIs (fluoxetine, sertraline, paroxetine, citalopram, escitalopram)	First-line treatment for generalized anxiety disorder, OCD, and PTSD.	Nausea, GI upset, somnolence, sexual dysfunction, agitation.
Buspirone	Generalized anxiety disorder, OCD, PTSD.	Seizures with chronic use. No tolerance, dependence, or withdrawal.
β-blockers	Performance anxiety, PTSD.	Bradycardia, hypotension.
Benzodiazepines	Anxiety, insomnia, alcohol withdrawal, muscle spasm, night terrors, sleepwalking.	↓ sleep duration; risk of abuse, tolerance, and dependence; disinhibition in young or old patients; confusion.
Flumazenil (competitive antagonist at GABA receptor)	Antidote to benzodiazepine intoxication.	Resedation; nausea, dizziness, vomiting, and pain at the injection site.

OBSESSIVE-COMPULSIVE DISORDER (OCD)

Characterized by obsessions and/or compulsions that lead to significant distress and dysfunction in social or personal areas. Typically presents in late adolescence or early adulthood; prevalence is equal in males and females. Often chronic and difficult to treat.

HISTORY/PE

- **Obsessions: Persistent, unwanted, and intrusive ideas, thoughts, impulses, or images** that lead to marked anxiety or distress (eg, fear of contamination, fear of harm to oneself or to loved ones).
- **Compulsions: Repeated mental acts or behaviors** that neutralize anxiety from obsessions (eg, hand washing, elaborate rituals for ordinary tasks, counting, excessive checking).
- Patients **recognize these behaviors as excessive and irrational products of their own minds** (vs. obsessive-compulsive personality disorder, or OCPD; see Table 2.14-2).
- Patients wish they could get rid of the obsessions and/or compulsions.

TREATMENT

- Pharmacotherapy (SSRIs are first-line pharmacologic treatment; see Table 2.14-1).
- Cognitive-behavioral therapy (CBT) using exposure and desensitization relaxation techniques.
- Patient education is imperative.

PANIC DISORDER

Characterized by recurrent, unexpected panic attacks. Two to three times more common in females than in males. **Agoraphobia** is present in 30–50% of cases. The average age of onset is 25, but may occur at any age.

HISTORY/PE

- **Panic attacks** are defined as discrete **periods of intense fear or discomfort** in which at least 4 of the following symptoms develop abruptly and peak within 10 minutes: tachypnea, chest pain, **palpitations, diaphoresis,** nausea, trembling, dizziness, **fear of dying** or "going crazy," depersonalization, or hot flashes.
- Perioral and/or acral paresthesias, when present, are fairly specific to panic attacks, which produce hyperventilation and low O_2 saturation.
- Patients present with **1 or more months** of concern about having additional attacks or significant behavior change as a result of the attacks—eg, avoiding situations that may precipitate attacks.

TABLE 2.14-2.   OCD vs. OCPD

OCD	OCPD
Characterized by obsessions and/or compulsions.	Patients are excessively conscientious and inflexible.
Patients **recognize** the obsessions/compulsions and want to be rid of them (ego dystonic).	Patients **do not recognize** their behavior as problematic (ego syntonic).

- **Determine whether a patient has panic disorder with or without agoraphobia** so that agoraphobia can also be addressed in the treatment plan.

TREATMENT

- **Short-term therapy:** Benzodiazepines (eg, clonazepam) may be used for immediate relief, but long-term use should be avoided in light of the potential for addiction and tolerance (see Table 2.14-1). Taper benzodiazepines as soon as long-term treatment is initiated (eg, SSRIs).
- **Long-term therapy:**
  - CBT.
  - **Medications:** SSRIs (first-line therapy), TCAs.

PHOBIAS (SOCIAL AND SPECIFIC)

Distinguished as follows:

- **Social phobia:** Characterized by marked fear provoked by **social or performance situations** in which embarrassment may occur. It may be specific (eg, public speaking, urinating in public) or general (eg, social interaction) and often begins in adolescence.
- **Specific phobia:** Anxiety is provoked by exposure to a **feared object or situation** (eg, animals, heights, airplanes). Most cases begin in childhood.

HISTORY/PE

Presents with excessive or unreasonable fear and/or avoidance of an object or situation that is persistent and leads to significant distress or impairment in function. **Patients recognize that their fear is excessive.**

TREATMENT

- **Specific phobias:** CBT involving desensitization through incremental exposure to the feared object or situation along with relaxation techniques. Other options include supportive, family, and insight-oriented psychotherapy.
- **Social phobias:** CBT, SSRIs, low-dose benzodiazepines, or β-blockers (for performance anxiety) may be used (see Table 2.14-1).

POSTTRAUMATIC STRESS DISORDER (PTSD)

Follows exposure to an extreme, **life-threatening traumatic event** (eg, assault, combat, witnessing a violent crime) that evoked intense fear, helplessness, or horror.

HISTORY/PE

- Characterized by the following:
  - **Reexperiencing of the event** (eg, nightmares).
  - **Avoidance** of stimuli associated with the trauma.
  - **Numbed responsiveness** (eg, detachment, anhedonia).
  - ↑ **arousal** (eg, hypervigilance, exaggerated startle) that leads to significant distress or impairment in functioning.
- Symptoms must persist for **> 1 month.**
- Survivor guilt, irritability, poor concentration, amnesia, personality change, sleep disturbance, substance abuse, depression, and suicidality may be present.

TREATMENT

- **Short-term therapy:** To target anxiety; includes β-blockers and α_2-agonists (eg, clonidine).
- **Long-term therapy:**
  - **Medications:** SSRIs are first line; buspirone, TCAs, and MAOIs may be helpful (see Table 2.14-1). Benzodiazepines are also used but should be avoided in light of their addictive potential, as there is a high incidence of substance abuse among patients with PTSD.
  - **Psychotherapy** and **support groups** are useful.

Cognitive Disorders

Affect memory, orientation, judgment, and attention.

DEMENTIA

A decline in **cognitive** functioning with **global deficits. Level of consciousness is stable (vs. delirium).** Prevalence is highest among those > 85 years of age. The course is persistent and progressive. The most common causes are **Alzheimer's disease** (65%) and **vascular dementia** (20%). Other causes are outlined in the mnemonic **DEMENTIAS.**

HISTORY/PE

Diagnostic criteria include **memory impairment and 1 or more** of the following:

- **The 4 A's of dementia** (the progression of cognitive impairment follows this order): **A**mnesia (partial or total memory loss), **A**phasia (language impairment), **A**praxia (inability to perform motor activities), **A**gnosia (inability to recognize previously known objects/places/people).
- **Impaired executive function (problems with planning, organizing, and abstracting)** in the presence of a **clear sensorium.**
- Personality, mood, and behavior changes are common (eg, wandering and aggression).
- Patients often can become more confused late in the day and at night (sundowning).

DIAGNOSIS

- A careful history and physical is critical. Serial mini-mental state exams should be performed.
- Rule out treatable causes of dementia; obtain CBC, RPR, CMP, TFTs, HIV, B_{12}/folate, ESR, UA, and a head CT or MRI.
- Table 2.14-3 outlines key characteristics distinguishing dementia from delirium.

TREATMENT

- Provide **environmental cues** and a rigid structure for the patient's daily life.
- **Cholinesterase inhibitors** are used to treat. Low-dose **antipsychotics** may be used for psychotic symptoms and sometimes for agitation, but with the added risk of cardiovascular events in elderly patients. **Avoid benzodiazepines,** which may exacerbate disinhibition and confusion.
- Family, caregiver, and patient education and support are imperative.

MNEMONIC

Causes of dementia—

DEMENTIAS

Degenerative diseases (Parkinson's, Huntington's)
Endocrine (thyroid, parathyroid, pituitary, adrenal)
Metabolic (alcohol, electrolytes, vitamin B_{12} deficiency, glucose, hepatic, renal, Wilson's disease)
Exogenous (heavy metals, carbon monoxide, drugs)
Neoplasia
Trauma (subdural hematoma)
Infection (meningitis, encephalitis, endocarditis, syphilis, HIV, prion diseases, Lyme disease)
Affective disorders (pseudodementia)
Stroke/**S**tructure (vascular dementia, ischemia, vasculitis, normal pressure hydrocephalus)

TABLE 2.14-3. Delirium vs. Dementia

VARIABLE	DELIRIUM	DEMENTIA
Level of attention	Impaired (fluctuating).	Usually alert.
Onset	Acute.	Gradual.
Course	Fluctuating from hour to hour.	Progressive deterioration, "sundowning."
Consciousness	Clouded.	Intact.
Hallucinations	Present (often visual or tactile).	Occur in approximately 30% of patients in highly advanced disease.
Prognosis	Reversible.	Largely irreversible, but up to 15% of cases are due to treatable causes and are reversible.
Treatment	Treat underlying causes. Low-dose antipsychotics; environmental changes.	Cholinesterase inhibitors; low-dose antipsychotics. Environmental changes.

MNEMONIC

Major causes of delirium—

I WATCH DEATH

Infection
Withdrawal
Acute metabolic/substance **A**buse
Trauma
CNS pathology
Hypoxia
Deficiencies
Endocrine
Acute vascular/MI
Toxins/drugs
Heavy metals

KEY FACT

It is common for delirium to be superimposed on dementia.

DELIRIUM

An acute **disturbance of consciousness** with **altered cognition** that develops over a short period of time (usually hours to days). Children, the elderly, and hospitalized patients (eg, **ICU psychosis**) are particularly susceptible. Major causes are outlined in the mnemonic **I WATCH DEATH**. Symptoms are potentially reversible if the underlying cause can be treated.

HISTORY/PE

- Presents with acute onset of **waxing and waning consciousness** with lucid intervals and **perceptual disturbances** (hallucinations, illusions, delusions).
- Patients may be combative, anxious, paranoid, or stuporous.
- Also characterized by a ↓ attention span and short-term memory, and a reversed sleep-wake cycle.

DIAGNOSIS

- Check vitals, pulse oximetry, and glucose; perform physical and neurologic examinations.
- Note recent medications (narcotics, anticholinergics, steroids, or benzodiazepines), substance use, prior episodes, medical problems, signs of organ failure (kidney, liver), and infection (**occult UTI is common in the elderly; check UA**).
- Order lab and radiologic studies to identify a possible underlying cause.

TREATMENT

- **Treat underlying causes** (delirium is often reversible).
- Normalize fluids and electrolytes.

- Optimize the sensory environment, and provide necessary visual and hearing aids.
- Use low-dose **antipsychotics** (eg, haloperidol) for agitation and psychotic symptoms.
- Conservative use of **physical restraints** may be necessary to prevent harm to the patient or others.

Mood Disorders

Also known as **affective disorders.**

MAJOR DEPRESSIVE DISORDER (MDD)

A mood disorder characterized by 1 or more major depressive episodes (MDEs). The male-to-female ratio is 1:2; lifetime prevalence ranges from 15% to 25%. **Onset is usually in the mid-20s;** in the elderly, prevalence ↑ with age. Chronic illness and stress ↑ risk. Approximately 2–9% of patients die by suicide.

HISTORY/PE

Diagnosis requires **depressed mood or anhedonia (loss of interest/pleasure) and 5 or more signs/symptoms** from the **SIG E CAPS** mnemonic for a **2-week period** (you should be sure to learn this mnemonic to ace the MDD questions). Table 2.14-4 outlines the differential diagnosis of conditions that may be mistaken for depression. Selected depression subtypes include the following:

- **Psychotic features:** Typically **mood-congruent** delusions/hallucinations.
- **Postpartum:** Occurs **within 1 month postpartum;** has a 10% incidence and a high risk of recurrence. Psychotic symptoms are common (see Table 2.14-5).
- **Atypical:** Characterized by weight gain, hypersomnia, and rejection sensitivity.
- **Seasonal:** Depressive episodes tend to occur during a particular season, most commonly winter. Responds well to light therapy +/– antidepressants.
- **Double depression:** MDE in a patient with dysthymia. Has a poorer prognosis than MDE alone.

TREATMENT

- **Pharmacotherapy:**
  - Effective in 50–70% of patients.
  - Allow 2–6 weeks to take effect; treat for 6 or more months (see Table 2.14-6).
- **Psychotherapy: Psychotherapy combined with antidepressants is more effective than either treatment alone.**
- **Electroconvulsive therapy (ECT):**
  - Safe, highly effective, and often lifesaving therapy that is reserved for refractory depression or psychotic depression, or if rapid improvement in mood is needed.
  - May also be used for intractable mania and psychosis. Usually requires 6–12 treatments.
  - Adverse effects include postictal confusion, arrhythmias, headache, and **anterograde amnesia.**

MNEMONIC

Symptoms of a depressive episode–

SIG E CAPS

Sleep (hypersomnia or insomnia)
Interest (loss of interest or pleasure in activities)
Guilt (feelings of worthlessness or inappropriate guilt)
Energy (↓) or fatigue
Concentration (↓)
Appetite (↑ or ↓) or weight (↑ or ↓)
Psychomotor agitation or retardation
Suicidal ideation

MNEMONIC

TCA toxicity–

Tri-C's

Convulsions
Coma
Cardiac arrhythmias

A 23-year-old woman complains of difficulty falling asleep and worsening anxiety that began 2 months earlier, after she was involved in a minor biking accident (bike vs. car) in which she did not suffer any injuries. Since the accident, she has refused to participate in any outdoor activities. What is her most likely diagnosis?

TABLE 2.14-4. Differential Diagnosis of Major Depression

DISORDER	DISTINGUISHING FEATURES
Mood disorder due to a medical condition	Hypothyroidism, Parkinson's disease, CNS neoplasm, other neoplasms (eg, pancreatic cancer), stroke (especially ACA stroke), dementias, parathyroid disorders.
Substance-induced mood disorder	Illicit drugs, alcohol, antihypertensives, corticosteroids, OCPs.
Adjustment disorder with depressed mood	A constellation of symptoms that resemble an MDE but do not meet the criteria for MDE. Occurs within 3 months of an identifiable stressor.
Normal bereavement	Occurs after the loss of a loved one. Involves no severe impairment/suicidality. Usually lasts < 6 months; should resolve within 1 year. May lead to MDD that requires treatment. Illusions/hallucinations of the deceased can be normal as long as the person recognizes them as such.
Dysthymia	Milder, chronic depression with depressed mood present most of the time for at least 2 years; often resistant to treatment.

- Contraindications include recent MI/stroke, intracranial mass, and high anesthetic risk (a relative contraindication).
- **Phototherapy:** Effective for patients whose depression has a seasonal pattern.
- **Transcranial magnetic stimulation (TMS):** Now approved for the treatment of major depression. TMS is about as effective as medications for some patients but is not as effective as ECT.

BIPOLAR DISORDER (BPD)

Prevalence is approximately 1% for type I and an additional 3% for type II; males and females are affected equally. A family history of bipolar illness significantly ↑ risk. The average age of onset is 20, and the frequency of mood

TABLE 2.14-5. Differential Diagnosis of Postpartum Disorders

SUBTYPE	TIME OF ONSET	SYMPTOMS
Postpartum "blues"	Within 2 weeks of delivery.	Sadness, moodiness, emotional lability. No thoughts about hurting baby.
Postpartum psychosis	2–3 weeks postdelivery.	Delusions and depression. May have thoughts about hurting baby.
Postpartum depression	1–3 months postdelivery.	Same as above plus sleep disturbances and anxiety. Thoughts about hurting baby.

TABLE 2.14-6. Indications and Side Effects of Common Antidepressants

Drug Class	Examples	Indications	Side Effects
SSRIs	Fluoxetine, sertraline, paroxetine, citalopram, fluvoxamine	Depression, anxiety.	Sexual side effects, GI distress, agitation, insomnia, tremor, diarrhea. **Serotonin syndrome** (fever, myoclonus, mental status changes, cardiovascular collapse) can occur if SSRIs are used with MAOIs, illicit drugs, or herbal medications. Paroxetine can cause pulmonary hypertension in the fetus. Avoid in pregnancy.
Atypicals	Bupropion, mirtazapine, trazodone	Depression, anxiety.	**Bupropion:** ↓ seizure threshold; minimal sexual side effects. Contraindicated in patients with eating disorders as well as in seizure patients. **Mirtazapine:** Weight gain, sedation. **Trazodone:** Highly sedating; priapism.
SNRIs	Venlafaxine, duloxetine	Depression, anxiety, chronic pain.	**Venlafaxine:** Diastolic hypertension.
TCAs	Nortriptyline, desipramine, amitriptyline, imipramine	Depression, anxiety disorder, chronic pain, migraine headaches, enuresis (imipramine).	Lethal with overdose owing to cardiac conduction arrhythmias (eg, prolonged conduction through the AV node, long QRS). Monitor in the ICU for 3–4 days following an OD. Anticholinergic effects (dry mouth, constipation, urinary retention, sedation).
MAOIs	Phenelzine, tranylcypromine, selegiline (a patch form is available)	Depression, especially atypical.	Hypertensive crisis if taken with high-tyramine foods (aged cheese, red wine). Sexual side effects, orthostatic hypotension, weight gain.

episodes tends to ↑ with age. Up to 10–15% of those affected die by suicide. Subtypes are as follows:

- **Bipolar I:** Involves **at least 1 manic or mixed episode** (usually requiring hospitalization).
- **Bipolar II:** Involves **at least 1 MDE and 1 hypomanic episode** (less intense than mania). Patients do not meet the criteria for full manic or mixed episodes.
- **Rapid cycling:** Involves 4 or more episodes (MDE, manic, mixed, or hypomanic) in 1 year.
- **Cyclothymic:** Chronic and less severe, with alternating periods of hypomania and moderate depression for > 2 years.

History/PE

- The mnemonic **DIG FAST** outlines the clinical presentation of mania.
- Patients may report excessive engagement in pleasurable activities (eg, excessive spending or sexual activity), reckless behaviors, and/or psychotic features.
- Antidepressant use may trigger manic episodes.

KEY FACT

SIG E CAPS = MDD. **DIG FAST** = BPD.

MNEMONIC

Symptoms of mania—

DIG FAST

Distractibility
Insomnia (↓ need for sleep)
Grandiosity (↑ self-esteem)/more **G**oal directed
Flight of ideas (or racing thoughts)
Activities/psychomotor **A**gitation
Sexual indiscretions/other pleasurable activities
Talkativeness/pressured speech

DIAGNOSIS

- A manic episode is **1 week or more of persistently elevated, expansive, or irritable mood** plus **3 DIG FAST symptoms. Psychotic symptoms** are common in mania.
- Symptoms are not due to a substance or medical condition and lead to significant impairment socially, occupationally, or familially.
- Hypomania is similar but does not involve marked functional impairment or psychotic symptoms and does not require hospitalization.

TREATMENT

- **Bipolar mania:** Mania is considered a psychiatric emergency owing to impaired judgment and great risk of harm to self and others.
    - **Acute therapy:** Antipsychotics.
    - **Maintenance therapy:** Mood stabilizers (see Table 2.14-7).
    - Use benzodiazepines for refractory agitation.
- **Bipolar depression:** Mood stabilizers +/– antidepressants. **Start mood stabilizers first** (see Table 2.14-7) to avoid inducing mania. ECT may be used to treat refractory cases.
- In patients with **severe depression or bipolar II with predominantly depressive features**, antidepressant treatment can be augmented with low-dose lithium—eg, at blood levels of 0.4–0.6 mEq/L.

MNEMONIC

Characteristics of personality disorders—

MEDIC

Maladaptive
Enduring
Deviate from cultural norms
Inflexible
Cause impairment in social or occupational functioning

Personality Disorders

Personality can be defined as an individual's set of emotional and behavioral traits, which are generally stable and predictable. Personality disorders are de-

TABLE 2.14-7. Mood Stabilizers

DRUG CLASS	INDICATIONS	SIDE EFFECTS
Lithium	First-line mood stabilizer. Used for acute mania (in combination with antipsychotics), for prophylaxis in BPD, and for augmentation in depression treatment.	Thirst, polyuria, diabetes insipidus, tremor, weight gain, hypothyroidism, nausea, diarrhea, seizures, teratogenicity (if used in the first trimester), acne, vomiting. Narrow therapeutic window (but blood level can be monitored). Lithium toxicity: > 1.5 mEq/L; presents with ataxia, dysarthria, delirium, and acute renal failure. Avoid lithium in patients with ↓ renal function.
Carbamazepine	Second-line mood stabilizer; anticonvulsant; trigeminal neuralgia.	Nausea, skin rash, leukopenia, AV block. Rarely, aplastic anemia (monitor CBC biweekly). Stevens-Johnson syndrome (SJS).
Valproic acid	BPD; anticonvulsant.	GI side effects (nausea, vomiting), tremor, sedation, alopecia, weight gain. Rarely, pancreatitis, thrombocytopenia, fatal hepatotoxicity, and agranulocytosis.
Lamotrigine	Second-line mood stabilizer; anticonvulsant.	Blurred vision, GI distress, SJS. ↑ dose slowly to monitor for rashes.

fined when one's traits become chronically rigid and maladaptive and affect most aspects of one's life (see the mnemonic **MEDIC**). Onset occurs by early adulthood. Specific disorders are outlined in Table 2.14-8.

DIAGNOSIS

- Ask about attitudes, mood variability, activities, and reaction to stress.
- Patients have chronic problems dealing with responsibilities, roles, and stressors. They may also deny their behavior, have difficulty changing their behavior patterns, and frequently refuse psychiatric care.

TREATMENT

- **Psychotherapy** is the mainstay of therapy.
- **Pharmacotherapy** is reserved for cases with comorbid mood, anxiety, or psychotic signs/symptoms.

A 22-year-old male frequently washes his hands, refuses to sit on chairs in public places, and will not use public transportation for fear of contracting diseases. He does not think his behaviors are abnormal, nor does he think his behaviors interfere with his daily activities. What is the diagnosis?

TABLE 2.14-8. Signs and Symptoms of Personality Disorders

DISORDER	CHARACTERISTICS	CLINICAL DILEMMA/STRATEGY
CLUSTER A: "WEIRD"		
Paranoid	Distrustful, suspicious; interpret others' motives as malevolent.	Patients are suspicious and distrustful of psychiatrists, making it difficult to form therapeutic relationships between patient and psychiatrist.
Schizoid	Isolated, detached "loners." Restricted emotional expression.	Be clear, honest, noncontrolling, and nondefensive.
Schizotypal	Odd behavior, perceptions, and appearance. **Magical thinking;** ideas of reference.	
CLUSTER B: "WILD"		
Borderline	Unstable mood, relationships, and self-image; feelings of emptiness. Impulsive. History of suicidal ideation or self-harm.	Patients change the rules and demand attention. They are manipulative and demanding and will split staff members.
Histrionic	Excessively emotional and attention seeking. Sexually provocative; theatrical.	Be clear and consistent about boundaries and expectations.
Narcissistic	Grandiose; need admiration; have sense of entitlement. Lack empathy.	
Antisocial	Violate rights of others, social norms, and laws. Impulsive; lack remorse. **Begins in childhood as conduct disorder.**	
CLUSTER C: "WORRIED AND WIMPY"		
Obsessive-compulsive	Preoccupied with perfectionism, order, and control at the expense of efficiency. Inflexible morals and values.	Patients are controlling and may sabotage their treatment. Words may be inconsistent with actions.
Avoidant	Socially inhibited; rejection sensitive. **Fear being disliked or ridiculed.**	Avoid power struggles. Give clear recommendations, but do not push patients into decisions.
Dependent	Submissive, clingy; have a need to be taken care of. Have difficulty making decisions. Feel helpless.	

Obsessive-compulsive personality disorder (OCPD). These patients are perfectionists, are preoccupied with rules and order, and are often inflexible. Patients with OCPD typically are not disturbed by their disease.

KEY FACT

Terms used to describe components of psychosis:

- **Delusion:** A fixed false idiosyncratic belief.
- **Hallucination:** Perception without an existing external stimulus.
- **Illusion:** Misperception of an actual external stimulus.

Psychotic Disorders

SCHIZOPHRENIA

Characterized by hallucinations, delusions, disordered thoughts, behavioral disturbances, and disrupted social functioning with a clear sensorium.

- **Epidemiology:** Prevalence is approximately 1%; males and females are affected equally. **Peak onset is earlier in males (ages 18–25) than in females (ages 25–35),** and has an ↑ incidence in those born in winter or early spring. Schizophrenia in first-degree relatives also ↑ risk. **Ten percent of those affected commit suicide.**
- **Etiology:** Etiologic theories focus on neurotransmitter abnormalities such as dopamine dysregulation (frontal hypoactivity and limbic hyperactivity) and brain abnormalities on CT and MRI (enlarged ventricles and ↓ cortical volume). Subtypes are as follows:
  - **Paranoid:** Delusions (often of persecution of the patient) and/or hallucinations are present. Cognitive function is usually preserved. Associated with the best overall prognosis.
  - **Disorganized:** Speech and behavior patterns are highly disordered and disinhibited with flat affect. The thought disorder is pronounced, and the patient has poor contact with reality. Carries the worst prognosis.
  - **Catatonic:** A rare form characterized by psychomotor disturbance with 2 or more of the following: excessive motor activity, immobility, extreme negativism, mutism, waxy flexibility, echolalia, or echopraxia.

HISTORY/PE

- Two or more of the following are present continuously for **6 or more months** with **social or occupational dysfunction:**
  - **Positive symptoms:** Hallucinations (most often auditory), delusions, disorganized speech, bizarre behavior, and thought disorder.
  - **Negative symptoms:** Flat affect, ↓ emotional reactivity, poverty of speech, lack of purposeful actions, and anhedonia.
- The differential includes the following (see also Table 2.14-9):
  - **Schizophreniform disorder:** Symptoms of schizophrenia with a duration of < 6 months.
  - **Schizoaffective disorder:** Combines the symptoms of schizophrenia with a major affective disorder (MDD or BPD).

TABLE 2.14-9. Differential Diagnosis of the "Schizos"

DISORDER	DURATION/CHARACTERISTICS
Psychotic disorders	**Brief psychotic disorder:** > 1 day and < 1 month.
	Schizophreniform disorder: > 1 month and < 6 months.
	Schizophrenia: > 6 months.
	Schizoaffective disorder: Schizophrenia + major affective disorder.
Personality disorders	**Schizotypal:** "Magical thinking."
	Schizoid: "Loners."

TREATMENT

- **Antipsychotics** (see Table 2.14-10); **long-term follow-up.**
- Supportive psychotherapy, training in social skills, vocational rehabilitation, and illness education may help.
- Negative symptoms may be more difficult to treat than positive symptoms.

Childhood and Adolescent Disorders

ATTENTION-DEFICIT HYPERACTIVITY DISORDER (ADHD)

A persistent pattern of excessive inattention and/or hyperactivity/impulsivity. More common in males; typically presents between ages 3 and 13. Often shows a familial pattern.

HISTORY/PE

Diagnosis requires **6 or more symptoms** from each category listed below for **6 or more months** in **at least 2 settings,** leading to significant social and academic impairment. Some symptoms must be present in patients **before age 7.**

- **Inattention:** Exhibits a **poor attention span** in schoolwork/play; displays poor attention to detail or careless mistakes; does not listen when spoken to; has **difficulty following instructions or finishing tasks;** loses items needed to complete tasks; is forgetful and easily distracted.
- **Hyperactivity/impulsivity:** Fidgets; leaves seat in classroom; runs around inappropriately; cannot play quietly; talks excessively; **does not wait for his or her turn; interrupts others.**

A 26-year-old female has been "hearing voices" and has isolated herself from her friends and family. Within the past 2 months, she has also been sleeping poorly and has reported feeling sad.

 KEY FACT

Children must exhibit ADHD symptoms in 2 or more settings (eg, home and school).

TABLE 2.14-10. Antipsychotic Medications

DRUG CLASS	EXAMPLES	INDICATIONS	SIDE EFFECTS
Typical antipsychotics	Haloperidol, droperidol, fluphenazine, thioridazine, chlorpromazine	Psychotic disorders, acute agitation, acute mania, Tourette's syndrome. Thought to be more effective for positive symptoms of schizophrenia; primarily block D2 dopamine receptors. For patients in whom compliance is a major issue, consider antipsychotics that come in depot forms (eg, haloperidol, fluphenazine).	**Extrapyramidal symptoms** (EPS; see Table 2.14-11), hyperprolactinemia. **Anticholinergic effects** (dry mouth, urinary retention, constipation). Seizures, hypotension, sedation, and QTc prolongation. Irreversible retinal pigmentation (thioridazine). **Neuroleptic malignant syndrome:** Fever, muscle rigidity, autonomic instability, elevated CK, clouded consciousness. **Stop medication;** provide supportive care in the ICU; administer dantrolene or bromocriptine (see Table 2.14-11).
Atypical antipsychotics	Clozapine, risperidone (also available in long-acting depot injection), quetiapine, olanzapine, ziprasidone, aripiprazole	Currently first-line treatment for schizophrenia given fewer EPS and anticholinergic effects. Clozapine is reserved for severe treatment resistance and severe tardive dyskinesia.	Weight gain, type 2 diabetes mellitus, somnolence, sedation, and QTc prolongation. **Agranulocytosis** requiring weekly CBC monitoring (clozapine).

Schizoaffective disorder: symptoms of schizophrenia with mood symptoms, with at least 2 weeks when psychotic symptoms were present without any mood symptoms. Patients often have chronic psychotic symptoms even after mood symptoms have resolved.

MNEMONIC

Evolution of EPS—

4 and A

4 hours: **A**cute dystonia
4 days: **A**kinesia
4 weeks: **A**kathisia
4 months: Tardive dyskinesia (often permanent)

TREATMENT

- Initial treatment may be nonpharmacologic (eg, behavior modification). Sugar and food additives are **not** considered etiologic factors.
- Pharmacologic treatment includes the following:
  - **Psychostimulants: Methylphenidate (Ritalin)**, dextroamphetamine (Dexedrine), mixed salts of dextroamphetamine and amphetamine (Adderall), atomoxetine (Strattera), pemoline (Cylert). Adverse effects include insomnia, irritability, ↓ appetite, tic exacerbation, and ↓ growth velocity (normalizes when medication is stopped).
  - **Antidepressants** (eg, SSRIs, nortriptyline, bupropion) and α₂-agonists (eg, **clonidine**).

PERVASIVE DEVELOPMENTAL DISORDERS (PDD)

A group of disorders (including autistic disorder, Asperger's syndrome, childhood disintegrative disorder, and Rett disorder) associated with delays in socialization, communication, and behavior. More common in males. Symptom severity and IQ vary widely.

HISTORY/PE

- Characterized by abnormal or **impaired social interaction and communication** together with **restricted activities and interests**, evident **before age 3.**
- Patients fail to develop normal social behaviors (eg, social smile, eye contact) and lack interest in relationships.
- Development of spoken language is delayed or absent.
- Children show **stereotyped speech and behavior** (eg, hand flapping) and restricted interests (eg, preoccupation with parts of objects).

TABLE 2.14-11. EPS and Treatment

SUBTYPE	DESCRIPTION	TIME OF ONSET	TREATMENT
Acute dystonia	Prolonged, painful tonic muscle contraction or spasm (eg, torticollis, oculogyric crisis).	Hours	Anticholinergics (benztropine or diphenhydramine) are acute therapy; some patients on antipsychotics who are prone to dystonic reactions may need regular prophylactic dosing (eg, benztropine).
Dyskinesia	Pseudoparkinsonism (eg, shuffling gait, cogwheel rigidity).	Days	Give an anticholinergic (benztropine) or a dopamine agonist (amantadine). ↓ the dose of neuroleptic or discontinue (if tolerated).
Akathisia	Subjective/objective restlessness that is perceived as being distressing.	Weeks	↓ neuroleptic and try β-blockers (propranolol). Benzodiazepines or anticholinergics may help.
Tardive dyskinesia	Stereotypic, involuntary, painless oral-facial movements. Likely from dopamine receptor sensitization from chronic dopamine blockade. Often irreversible (50%).	Months	Discontinue or ↓ the dose of neuroleptic; attempt treatment with more appropriate drugs; and consider changing neuroleptic (eg, to clozapine or risperidone). **Giving anticholinergics or decreasing neuroleptics may initially worsen tardive dyskinesia.**

- Types of PDD include the following:
  - **Autistic disorder: Impaired social interactions and communication with significant language and cognitive delays, together with characteristic repetitive or restricted behaviors.**
  - **Asperger's syndrome:** An autism-like disorder of social impairment and repetitive activities, behaviors, and interests **without marked language or cognitive delays.**
  - **Rett disorder:** A genetic neurodegenerative disorder of females with progressive impairment (eg, language, head growth, coordination) **after 5 months of normal development.**
  - **Childhood disintegrative disorder:** Severe developmental **regression** after > 2 years of normal development (eg, language, motor skills, social skills, bladder/bowel control, play).

TREATMENT

- Intensive special education, **behavioral management,** and symptom-targeted medications (eg, neuroleptics for aggression; SSRIs for stereotyped behavior).
- Family support and counseling are crucial.

DISRUPTIVE BEHAVIORAL DISORDERS

Include conduct disorder and oppositional defiant disorder. More common among males and in patients with a history of abuse.

HISTORY/PE

- **Conduct disorder:** A repetitive, persistent pattern of **violating the basic rights of others** or age-appropriate **societal norms or rules** for **1 year or more.** Behaviors may be aggressive (eg, rape, robbery, animal cruelty) or nonaggressive (eg, stealing, lying, deliberately annoying people). May progress to antisocial personality disorder in adulthood.
- **Oppositional defiant disorder:** A pattern of **negativistic, defiant, disobedient, and hostile behavior** toward authority figures (eg, losing one's temper, arguing) for 6 or more months. **May progress to conduct disorder.**

TREATMENT

Individual and family therapy.

MENTAL RETARDATION

Associated with male gender, chromosomal abnormalities, congenital infections, teratogens, inborn errors of metabolism, and alcohol/illicit substances during pregnancy.

HISTORY/PE

- Patients have significantly subaverage intellectual functioning (**IQ < 70**) with **deficits in adaptive functioning** (eg, hygiene, social skills); onset is before age 18.
- Levels of severity are **mild (IQ 50–70; 85% of cases),** moderate (**IQ 35–49**), severe (**IQ 20–34**), and profound (**IQ < 20**).

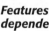

TREATMENT

- 1° prevention consists of educating the general public about possible causes of mental retardation and providing optimal prenatal screening to mothers.
- Treatment measures include family counseling and support; speech and language therapy; occupational/physical therapy; behavioral intervention; educational assistance; and social skills training.

TOURETTE'S SYNDROME

More common in males; shows a genetic predisposition. **Associated with ADHD, learning disorders,** and **OCD.**

HISTORY/PE

- Begins before age 18.
- Characterized by **multiple motor tics** (eg, blinking, grimacing) **and vocal tics** (eg, grunting, coprolalia) occurring many times per day, recurrently, for > 1 year with social or occupational impairment.

TREATMENT

- Treatment includes **dopamine receptor antagonists** (haloperidol, pimozide) or clonidine.
- Behavioral therapy may be of benefit, and counseling can aid in social adjustment and coping. Stimulants can worsen or precipitate tics.

Miscellaneous Disorders

SUBSTANCE ABUSE/DEPENDENCE

Both substance abuse and substance dependence are maladaptive patterns of substance use that lead to clinically significant impairment. They are distinguished as follows:

- **Substance abuse:** Requires 1 or more of the following in 1 year:
  - **Failure to fulfill responsibilities** at work, school, or home.
  - Use of substances in **physically hazardous** situations (eg, driving while intoxicated).
  - **Legal problems** during the time of substance use.
  - Continued substance use despite recurrent social or interpersonal problems 2° to the effects of such use (eg, frequent arguments with spouse over the substance use).
- **Substance dependence:** Requires 3 or more of the following in 1 year:
  - **Tolerance** and use of progressively larger amounts to obtain the same desired effect.
  - **Withdrawal** symptoms when not taking the substance.
  - Failed attempts to cut down use or abstain from the substance.
  - Significant time spent obtaining the substance (eg, visiting many doctors to obtain a prescription for pain pills).
  - Isolation from life activities.
  - Consumption of greater amounts of the substance than intended.
  - Continued substance abuse despite recurrent physical or psychological problems 2° to the effect of the substance use.

DIAGNOSIS/TREATMENT

- Substance use is often denied or underreported, so seek out collateral information from family and friends.
- Check urine and blood toxicology screens, LFTs, and serum EtOH level.
- The management of intoxication for selected drugs is described in Table 2.14-12.

ALCOHOLISM

Occurs more often in **males** (4:1) and in those 21–34 years of age, although the incidence in females is rising. Also associated with a ⊕ family history.

HISTORY/PE

See Table 2.14-12 for the symptoms of intoxication and withdrawal. Look for palmar erythema or telangiectasias as well as for other signs and symptoms of end-organ complications.

DIAGNOSIS

Screen with the **CAGE questionnaire.** Monitor vital signs for evidence of withdrawal. Labs may reveal ↑ LFTs, LDH, and MCV.

TREATMENT

- Rule out medical complications; correct electrolyte abnormalities.
- Start a **benzodiazepine taper** for withdrawal symptoms. Add haloperidol for hallucinations and psychotic symptoms.
- Give **multivitamins and folic acid; administer thiamine before glucose** (which depletes thiamine) to prevent Wernicke's encephalopathy.
- Give anticonvulsants to patients with a seizure history.
- Group therapy, disulfiram, or naltrexone can aid patients with dependence.
- Long-term rehabilitative therapy (eg, Alcoholic Anonymous).

COMPLICATIONS

- **GI bleeding from gastritis, ulcers, varices, or Mallory-Weiss tears.**
- **Pancreatitis, liver disease,** DTs, alcoholic hallucinosis, peripheral neuropathy, Wernicke's encephalopathy, Korsakoff's psychosis, fetal alcohol syndrome, cardiomyopathy, anemia, aspiration pneumonia, ↑ risk of sustaining trauma (eg, subdural hematoma).

ANOREXIA NERVOSA

Risk factors include female gender, low self-esteem, and high socioeconomic status (SES). Also associated with OCD, MDD, anxiety, and careers/hobbies such as modeling, gymnastics, ballet, and running.

HISTORY/PE

Diagnosed as follows (see also Table 2.14-13):

- Body weight is < 85% of that expected.
- Patients present with **refusal to maintain normal body weight,** an intense **fear of weight gain,** a distorted body image (**patients perceive themselves as fat**), and **amenorrhea.**
- Patients **restrict** (eg, severely restricting caloric intake by fasting or by excessively exercising) or **binge and purge** (through vomiting, laxatives, and diuretics).

TABLE 2.14-12. Signs and Symptoms of Substance Abuse

Drug	Intoxication	Withdrawal
Alcohol	Disinhibition, emotional lability, slurred speech, ataxia, aggression, blackouts, hallucinations, memory impairment, impaired judgment, coma.	Tremor, tachycardia, hypertension, malaise, nausea, seizures, DTs, agitation.
Opioids	Euphoria leading to apathy, CNS depression, constipation, **pupillary constriction,** and respiratory depression (life threatening in overdose). Naloxone and naltrexone block opioid receptors and reverse effects, but beware of the antagonist clearing before the opioids, particularly with long-acting opioids such as methadone.	Dysphoria, insomnia, anorexia, myalgias, fever, lacrimation, diaphoresis, dilated pupils, rhinorrhea, piloerection, nausea, vomiting, stomach cramps, diarrhea, yawning. Opioid withdrawal is not life threatening, "hurts all over," and does not cause seizures.
Amphetamines	Psychomotor agitation, impaired judgment, hypertension, **pupillary dilation,** tachycardia, fever, diaphoresis, anxiety, angina, euphoria, prolonged wakefulness/ attention, arrhythmias, delusions, seizures, hallucinations. Haloperidol can be given for severe agitation and symptom-targeted medications (eg, antiemetics, NSAIDs).	Postuse "crash" with anxiety, lethargy, headache, stomach cramps, hunger, fatigue, depression/dysphoria, sleep disturbance, nightmares.
Cocaine	Psychomotor agitation, euphoria, impaired judgment, tachycardia, **pupillary dilation,** hypertension, paranoia, hallucinations, "cocaine bugs" (the feeling of bugs crawling under one's skin), sudden death. ECG changes from ischemia are often seen ("cocaine chest pain"). Treat with haloperidol for severe agitation along with symptom-specific medications (eg, to control hypertension).	Postuse "crash" with hypersomnolence, depression, malaise, severe craving, angina, suicidality, ↑ appetite, nightmares.
Phencyclidine hydrochloride (PCP)	**Assaultiveness,** belligerence, psychosis, violence, impulsiveness, psychomotor agitation, fever, tachycardia, **vertical/horizontal nystagmus,** hypertension, impaired judgment, ataxia, seizures, delirium. Give benzodiazepines or haloperidol for severe symptoms; otherwise reassure. Acidification of urine or gastric lavage can help eliminate the drug.	Recurrence of intoxication symptoms due to reabsorption in the GI tract; sudden onset of severe, random violence.
LSD	Marked anxiety or depression, delusions, visual hallucinations, flashbacks, pupillary dilation, impaired judgment, diaphoresis, tachycardia, hypertension, heightened senses (eg, colors become more intense). Supportive counseling; traditional antipsychotics for psychotic symptoms; benzodiazepines for anxiety.	None.

TABLE 2.14-12.   Signs and Symptoms of Substance Abuse *(continued)*

DRUG	INTOXICATION	WITHDRAWAL
Marijuana	Euphoria, slowed sense of time, impaired judgment, social withdrawal, ↑ appetite, dry mouth, conjunctival injection, hallucinations, anxiety, paranoia, amotivational syndrome.	None.
Barbiturates	Low safety margin; respiratory depression.	Anxiety, seizures, delirium, life-threatening cardiovascular collapse.
Benzodiazepines	Interactions with alcohol, amnesia, ataxia, somnolence, mild respiratory depression. (Avoid using for insomnia in the elderly; can cause paradoxical agitation even in relatively low doses.)	Rebound anxiety, seizures, tremor, insomnia, hypertension, tachycardia, death.
Caffeine	Restlessness, insomnia, diuresis, muscle twitching, arrhythmias, tachycardia, flushed face, psychomotor agitation.	Headache, lethargy, depression, weight gain, irritability, craving.
Nicotine	Restlessness, insomnia, anxiety, arrhythmias.	Irritability, headache, anxiety, weight gain, craving, bradycardia, difficulty concentrating, insomnia.

■ Signs and symptoms include cachexia, a body mass index (BMI) below 18, **lanugo,** dry skin, bradycardia, lethargy, hypotension, cold intolerance, and hypothermia (as low as 35°C [95°F]).

DIAGNOSIS

Measure height and weight; check BMI; check **CBC, electrolytes,** endocrine levels, and **ECG.** Perform a **psychiatric evaluation** to screen patients for co-morbid conditions.

TABLE 2.14-13.   Anorexia vs. Bulimia

VARIABLE	ANOREXIA NERVOSA	BULIMIA NERVOSA
Body image	Disturbed body image; use extensive measures to avoid weight gain (eg, purging, excess exercise).	Same.
Binge eating	May occur.	Same.
Weight	**Patients are underweight** (≥ 15% below expected weight).	Patients are of normal weight or are overweight.
Attitude toward illness	Patients are typically not distressed by their illness and may thus be resistant to treatment.	Patients are typically distressed about their symptoms and are thus easier to treat.
Treatment	Monitor calorie intake and weight gain; hospitalize if necessary. Psychotherapy. Treat comorbidities.	Psychotherapy +/– antidepressants.

TREATMENT

- Initially, monitor caloric intake to restore nutritional status and to stabilize weight; then focus on **weight gain.**
- Hospitalize if necessary to restore nutritional status, rehydrate, and correct electrolyte imbalances.
- Once the patient is medically stable, initiate individual, family, and group **psychotherapy.** Treat comorbid depression and anxiety.

COMPLICATIONS

- Mitral valve prolapse, arrhythmias (2° to electrolyte abnormalities), hypotension, bradycardia, **amenorrhea** (missing 3 consecutive cycles), nephrolithiasis, osteoporosis, multiple stress fractures, pancytopenia, thyroid abnormalities (see Table 2.14-14).
- Mortality from **suicide** or medical complications is **> 10%.**

BULIMIA NERVOSA

More common among women; associated with low self-esteem, mood disorders, and OCD.

HISTORY/PE

Diagnostic criteria are as follows (see also Table 2.14-13):

- **Patients have normal weight or are overweight.** For at least 2 times a week for 3 or more months, patients have episodes of **binge eating and compensatory behaviors** that include **purging** or **fasting.**
- Patients are usually **ashamed** and conceal their behaviors.
- **Signs** include **dental enamel erosion, enlarged parotid glands,** and **scars on the dorsal hand surfaces** (if there is a history of repeated induced vomiting). Patients usually have normal body weight.

TREATMENT

Psychotherapy focuses on behavior modification and body image. **Antidepressants** may be effective for both depressed and nondepressed patients.

COMPLICATIONS

See Table 2.14-14.

KEY FACT

There are 2 types of anorexia nervosa:
- Restricting type
- Binging/purge-eating type

KEY FACT

Bulimic patients tend to be more disturbed by their behavior than anorexics and are more easily engaged in therapy. Anorexic patients deny health risks associated with their behavior, making them resistant to treatment.

KEY FACT

Bupropion should be avoided in the treatment of patients with eating disorders, as it is associated with a ↓ seizure threshold.

TABLE 2.14-14. Medical Complications of Eating Disorders

CONSTITUTIONAL	CARDIAC	GI	GU	OTHER
Cachexia	Arrhythmias	Dental erosions and decay	Amenorrhea	**Dermatologic:** Lanugo
Hypothermia	Sudden death		Nephrolithiasis	**Hematologic:**
Fatigue	Hypotension	Abdominal pain		Leukopenia
Electrolyte abnormalities (hypokalemia, pH abnormalities)	Bradycardia	Delayed gastric emptying		**Neurologic:** Seizures
	Prolonged QT interval			**Musculoskeletal:**
				Osteoporosis, stress fractures

SEXUAL DISORDERS

Sexual Changes With Aging

- Interest in sexual activity usually does not ↓ with aging.
- Men usually require ↑ stimulation of the genitalia for longer periods of time to reach orgasm; intensity of orgasm ↓, and the length of the refractory period before the next orgasm ↑.
- In women, estrogen levels ↓ after menopause, leading to vaginal dryness and thinning, which may result in discomfort during coitus. May be treated with hormone replacement therapy, estrogen vaginal suppositories, or other vaginal creams.

Paraphilias

- Preoccupation with or engagement in unusual sexual fantasies, urges, or behaviors for > 6 months with clinically significant impairment in one's life. Includes criminal sex offenders (eg, pedophilia); see Table 2.14-15. Found almost exclusively in men, and usually begins before or during puberty.
- **Tx:** Treatment includes insight-oriented psychotherapy and behavioral therapy. Antiandrogens (eg, Depo-Provera) have been used for hypersexual paraphilic activity.

Gender Identity Disorders

- **Strong, persistent cross-gender identification** and **discomfort with one's assigned sex or gender role of the assigned sex** in the absence of intersexual disorders. Patients may have a history of dressing like the opposite sex, taking sex hormones, or pursuing surgeries to reassign their sex.
- More common in males than in females. Associated with depression, anxiety, substance abuse, and personality disorders.
- **Tx:** Treatment is complex and includes educating the patient about culturally acceptable behavior patterns and addressing comorbidities. Other options include sex-reassignment surgery or hormonal treatment (eg, estrogen for males, testosterone for females). Supportive psychotherapy is helpful.

TABLE 2.14-15. Features of Common Paraphilias

DISORDER	CLINICAL MANIFESTATIONS
Exhibitionism	Sexual arousal from exposing one's genitals to a stranger.
Pedophilia	Urges or behaviors involving sexual activities with children.
Voyeurism	Observing unsuspecting persons unclothed or involved in sex.
Fetishism	Use of nonliving objects (often clothing) for sexual arousal.
Transvestic fetishism	Cross-dressing for sexual arousal.
Frotteurism	Touching or rubbing one's genitalia against a nonconsenting person (common in subways).
Sexual sadism	Sexual arousal from inflicting suffering on sexual partner.
Sexual masochism	Sexual arousal from being hurt, humiliated, bound, or threatened.

Sexual Dysfunction

- Problems in sexual **arousal, desire, or orgasm, or pain** with sexual intercourse.
- Prevalence is 30%; one-third of cases are attributable to biological factors and another third to psychological factors.
- **Tx:** Treatment depends on the particular condition. Pharmacologic strategies include sildenafil (Viagra) and bupropion (Wellbutrin). Psychotherapeutic strategies include sensate focusing.

SLEEP DISORDERS

Up to one-third of all American adults suffer from some type of sleep disorder during their lives. The term *dyssomnia* describes any condition that leads to a disturbance in the normal rhythm or pattern of sleep. Insomnia is the most common example. **Risk factors** include female gender, the presence of mental and medical disorders, substance abuse, and advanced age.

1° Insomnia

- **Affects up to 30% of the general population;** causes sleep disturbance that is not attributable to physical or mental conditions. Often exacerbated by anxiety, and patients may become preoccupied with getting enough sleep.
- **Dx:** Patients present with a history of **nonrestorative sleep** or **difficulty initiating or maintaining sleep** that is present at least 3 times per week for 1 month.
- **Tx:**
    - First-line therapy includes the initiation of **good sleep hygiene** measures.
    - Pharmacotherapy is considered second-line therapy and should be **initiated with care for short periods of time** (< 2 weeks). Pharmacologic agents include diphenhydramine (Benadryl), zolpidem (Ambien), zaleplon (Sonata), and trazodone (Desyrel).

1° Hypersomnia

- **Dx:** Diagnosed when a patient complains of **excessive daytime sleepiness or nighttime sleep** that occurs for > 1 month. The excessive somnolence cannot be attributable to medical or mental illness, medications, poor sleep hygiene, insufficient sleep, or narcolepsy.
- **Tx:**
    - First-line therapy includes **stimulant drugs** such as amphetamines.
    - Antidepressants such as SSRIs may be useful in some patients.

Narcolepsy

- May affect up to 0.16% of the population. Onset typically occurs by young adulthood, generally before age 30. Some forms of narcolepsy may have a genetic component.
- **Dx:**
    - Manifestations include **excessive daytime somnolence** and ↓ **REM sleep latency** on a daily basis for at least 3 months. **Sleep attacks** are the classic symptom; patients cannot avoid falling asleep.
    - The characteristic excessive sleepiness may be associated with the following:
        - **Cataplexy:** Sudden loss of muscle tone that leads to collapse.
        - **Hypnagogic hallucinations:** Occur as the patient is falling asleep.

KEY FACT

Recommended sleep hygiene measures:

- Establishment of a regular sleep schedule
- Limiting of caffeine intake
- Avoidance of daytime naps
- Warm baths in the evening
- Use of the bedroom for sleep and sexual activity only
- Exercising early in the day
- Relaxation techniques
- Avoidance of large meals near bedtime

- **Hypnopompic hallucinations:** Occur as the patient awakens.
- **Sleep paralysis:** Brief paralysis upon awakening.
- **Tx:** Treat with a regimen of **scheduled daily naps** plus **stimulant drugs** such as amphetamines; give SSRIs for cataplexy.

Sleep Apnea

- Occurs 2° to **disturbances in breathing** during sleep that lead to **excessive daytime somnolence** and **sleep disruption.** Etiologies can be either central or peripheral.
    - **Central sleep apnea (CSA):** A condition in which both airflow and respiratory effort cease. CSA is linked to **morning headaches,** mood changes, and repeated awakenings during the night.
    - **Obstructive sleep apnea (OSA):** A condition in which airflow ceases as a result of obstruction along the respiratory passages. OSA is strongly associated with **snoring.** Risk factors include **male gender, obesity,** prior upper airway surgeries, a deviated nasal septum, a large uvula or tongue, and retrognathia (recession of the mandible).
- In both forms, arousal results in cessation of the apneic event.
- Associated with **sudden death in infants and the elderly,** headaches, depression, ↑ systolic BP, and **pulmonary hypertension.**
- **Dx:** Sleep studies (polysomnography) document the number of arousals, obstructions, and episodes of ↓ O_2 saturation; distinguish OSA from CSA; and identify possible movement disorders, seizures, or other sleep disorders.
- **Tx:**
    - **OSA:** Nasal continuous positive airway pressure (CPAP). Weight loss if obese. In children, most cases are due to tonsillar/adenoidal hypertrophy, which is corrected surgically.
    - **CSA:** Mechanical ventilation (eg, BiPAP) with a backup rate for severe cases.

Circadian Rhythm Sleep Disorder

- A spectrum of disorders characterized by a **misalignment between desired and actual sleep** periods. Subtypes include jet-lag type, shift-work type, delayed sleep-phase type, and unspecified.
- **Tx:**
    - The jet-lag type usually **resolves** within 2–7 days **without specific treatment.**
    - The shift-work type may respond to **light therapy.**
    - Oral melatonin may be useful if given 5½ hours before the desired bedtime.

SOMATOFORM AND FACTITIOUS DISORDERS

Patients often present with **medically unexplained somatic symptoms,** generally with varying etiologies.

- **Somatoform disorders:** Patients have **no conscious control over symptoms.** The 5 main categories are outlined in Table 2.14-16.
- **Factitious disorders: Patients fabricate symptoms or cause self-injury to assume the sick role (1° gain).** More common in females.
- **Munchausen's syndrome:** A form of chronic factitious disorder in which patients fabricate physical signs and symptoms, leading to unnecessary testing or surgery. Common among **health care workers.**
- **Munchausen's syndrome by proxy:** A "caregiver" makes someone else ill and enjoys taking on the role of concerned onlooker.

 KEY FACT

Factitious disorders and malingering are distinct from somatoform disorders in that they involve conscious and intentional processes.

A 57-year-old morbidly obese man presents to his physician with concerns about ↑ daytime sleepiness and ↓ work productivity. He recently received multiple divorce threats from his wife for excessive snoring that sounds like "the snort of a steam engine." What long-term complications are of concern for this patient?

TABLE 2.14-16. **Somatoform Disorders**

DISORDER	CLINICAL PRESENTATION/EPIDEMIOLOGY
Somatization disorder	Multiple, chronic somatic symptoms from different organ systems with multiple GI, sexual, neurologic, and pain complaints. Frequent clinical contacts and/or surgeries; significant functional impairment. The male-to-female ratio is 1:20; onset is usually before age 30. Schedule regular appointments with the identified primary caregiver who maintains communication with consultants and specialists; psychotherapy.
Conversion disorder	Symptoms or deficits of voluntary motor or sensory function (eg, blindness, seizure-like movements, paralysis) incompatible with medical processes. Close temporal relationship to stress or intense emotion. More common in young females and in lower socioeconomic strata and less educated groups. Usually resolves spontaneously, but psychotherapy may help.
Hypochondriasis	Preoccupation with or fear of having a serious disease despite medical reassurance, leading to significant distress/impairment. Often involves a history of prior physical disease. Men and women are equally affected. Onset is in adulthood. Manage with group therapy and schedule regular appointments with the patient's primary caregiver.
Body dysmorphic disorder	Preoccupation with an imagined physical defect or abnormality that leads to significant distress/impairment. Patients often present to dermatologists or plastic surgeons. Has a slight female predominance. May be associated with depression. SSRIs may be of benefit.
Somatoform pain disorder	The intensity or profile of pain symptoms is inconsistent with physiologic processes. Close temporal relationship with psychological factors. More common in females; peak onset is at 40–50 years of age. May be associated with depression. Treatment includes rehabilitation (eg, physical therapy), psychotherapy, and behavioral therapy. Analgesia is usually not helpful. TCAs and SNRIs (venlafaxine and duloxetine) may be therapeutic.

A

This patient has obstructive sleep apnea. Serious consequences include leg swelling, hypertension, cor pulmonale, stroke, and clinical depression.

- **Malingering:** Patients **intentionally cause** or feign symptoms for **2° gain** of **financial benefit** or **housing.**

SEXUAL AND PHYSICAL ABUSE

- Most frequently affects women < 35 years of age who fill the following criteria:
  - Are experiencing marital discord and are substance abusers or have a partner who is a substance abuser; or
  - Are pregnant, are of low SES, or have obtained a restraining order.
- Victims of childhood abuse are more likely to become adult victims of abuse.
- **Hx/PE:**
  - Patients typically have **multiple somatic complaints, frequent ER** visits, and **unexplained injuries** with **delayed medical treatment.** They may also **avoid eye contact** or act afraid or hostile.
  - Children may exhibit precocious sexual behavior, **genital or anal trauma, STDs,** UTIs, and psychiatric problems.
  - Other clues include a partner who answers questions for the patient or refuses to leave the examination room.
- **Tx:** Perform a screening assessment of the patient's safety domestically and in their close personal relationships. Provide **medical care,** emotional **support, and counseling;** educate the patient about **support services** and refer appropriately. **Documentation** is crucial.

SUICIDALITY

- Accounts for 30,000 deaths per year in the United States; the eighth overall cause of death in the United States. One suicide occurs every 17–20 minutes.
- Risk factors include male gender, **age > 45 years,** psychiatric disorders (major depression, presence of psychotic symptoms), a history of an admission to a psychiatric institution, **a previous suicide attempt,** a history of violent behavior, ethanol or substance abuse, recent severe stressors, and a family suicide history (see the mnemonic **SAD PERSONS**).
- Women are more likely to attempt suicide, whereas men are more likely to succeed by virtue of their ↑ use of more lethal methods.
- **Dx:**
  - Perform a comprehensive psychiatric evaluation.
  - Ask about family history, previous attempts, ambivalence toward death, and hopelessness.
  - Ask **directly** about suicidal ideation, intent, and plan, and look for available means.
- **Tx:** A patient who endorses suicidality requires emergent inpatient hospitalization even against his will. Suicide risk may ↑ after antidepressant therapy is initiated because a patient's energy to act on suicidal thoughts can return before the depressed mood lifts.

KEY FACT

In malingering, patients intentionally simulate illness for personal gain.

KEY FACT

Sexual abusers are usually male and are often known to the victim (and are often family members).

MNEMONIC

Risk factors for suicide—

SAD PERSONS

Sex (male)
Age (older)
Depression
Previous attempt
Ethanol/substance abuse
Rational thought
Sickness (chronic illness)
Organized plan/access to weapons
No spouse
Social support lacking

KEY FACT

Suicide is the third leading cause of death (after homicide and accidents) among 15- to 24-year-olds in the United States.

KEY FACT

Emergent inpatient hospitalization is required for patients with suicidal intentions.

NOTES

PULMONARY

Etiologies of obstructive pulmonary disease—

ABCT

Asthma
Bronchiectasis
Cystic fibrosis/**C**OPD
Tracheal or bronchial obstruction

KEY FACT

Beware—all that wheezes is not asthma!

KEY FACT

Asthma should be suspected in children with multiple episodes of croup and URIs associated with dyspnea.

Obstructive Lung Disease

Characterized by airway narrowing, obstructive lung diseases restrict air movement and often cause air trapping. The etiologies of obstructive lung disease are described in the mnemonic **ABCT**. Figure 2.15-1 illustrates the role of lung volume measurements in the diagnosis of lung disease; Table 2.15-1 and Figures 2.15-1 and 2.15-2 contrast obstructive with restrictive lung disease.

ASTHMA

Defined as reversible airway obstruction 2° to bronchial hyperreactivity, airway inflammation, mucous plugging, and smooth muscle hypertrophy.

HISTORY/PE

- Presents with **cough, episodic wheezing,** dyspnea, and/or chest tightness. Symptoms often worsen at night or early in the morning.
- Examination reveals **wheezing, prolonged expiratory duration** (↓ I/E ratio), **accessory muscle use,** tachypnea, tachycardia, hyperresonance, and possible pulsus paradoxus.
- ↓ breath sounds and ↓ O_2 saturation are late signs.

DIAGNOSIS

- **ABGs: Mild hypoxia** and **respiratory alkalosis.** Normalizing P_{CO_2}, respiratory acidosis, and more severe hypoxia may indicate fatigue and impending respiratory failure.

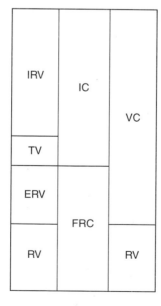
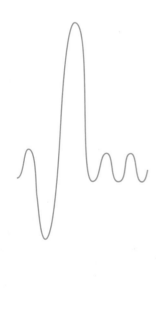

VC = vital capacity
RV = residual volume
FRC = functional residual capacity
TV = tidal volume

ERV = expiratory reserve volume
IRV = inspiratory reserve volume
IC = inspiratory capacity

FIGURE 2.15-1. **Lung volumes in the interpretation of PFTs.** (Reproduced with permission from Gomella LG et al. *Clinician's Pocket Reference,* 11th ed. New York: McGraw-Hill, 2006, Fig. 18-1.)

TABLE 2.15-1.   Obstructive vs. Restrictive Lung Disease[a]

Test	Normal	Mild	Moderate	Severe
Obstructive				
FEV$_1$ (% of FVC)	> 75	60–75	40–60	< 40
RV (% of predicted)	80–120	120–150	150–175	> 200
Restrictive				
FVC (% of predicted)	> 80	60–80	50–60	< 50
FEV$_1$ (% of VC)	> 75	> 75	> 75	> 75
RV (% of predicted)	80–120	80–120	70–80	70

[a] FEV$_1$ = forced expiratory volume in 1 second; FVC = forced vital capacity.

- **Spirometry/PFTs:** ↓ FEV$_1$/FVC; peak flow is diminished acutely; ↑ RV and total lung capacity (TLC). PFTs are often normal between exacerbations.
- **CBC:** Possible eosinophilia.
- **CXR:** Hyperinflation.
- **Methacholine challenge:** Tests for bronchial hyperresponsiveness; useful when PFTs are normal but asthma is still suspected.

TREATMENT

In general, avoid allergens or any potential triggers. Management is as follows (see also Tables 2.15-2 and 2.15-3):

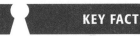
KEY FACT

Asthma triggers include allergens, URIs, cold air, exercise, drugs, and stress.

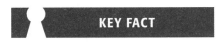
KEY FACT

Corticosteroids are inhaled in a **rush** and can lead to **thrush!**

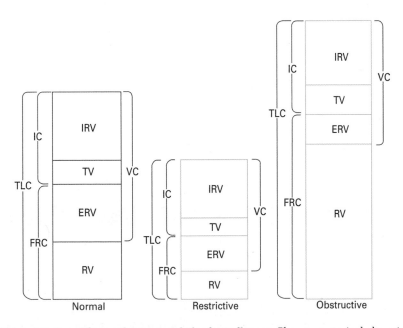

FIGURE 2.15-2.   Obstructive vs. restrictive lung disease. Shown are typical alterations in lung volumes and capacities in restrictive and obstructive diseases. (Reproduced with permission from Levitzky MG. *Pulmonary Physiology,* 7th ed. New York: McGraw-Hill, 2007, Fig. 3-3.)

Q

A 10-year-old with a history of asthma on daily fluticasone has been using an albuterol inhaler once a day for several weeks. What changes should be made to the current regimen?

TABLE 2.15-2. Common Asthma Medications and Their Mechanisms

DRUG	MECHANISM OF ACTION
β_2-agonists	**Albuterol:** Short acting. Relaxes bronchial smooth muscle (β_2-adrenoceptors). **Salmeterol:** Long-acting agent for prophylaxis.
Corticosteroids	**Inhaled corticosteroids** are first-line treatment for long-term control of asthma. **Beclomethasone, prednisone:** Inhibit the synthesis of virtually all cytokines.
Muscarinic antagonists	**Ipratropium:** Competitively blocks muscarinic receptors, preventing bronchoconstriction.
Methylxanthines	**Theophylline:** Likely causes bronchodilation by inhibiting phosphodiesterase, thereby decreasing cAMP hydrolysis and increasing cAMP levels. Usage is limited because of its narrow therapeutic-toxic index (cardiotoxicity, neurotoxicity).
Cromolyn	Prevents the release of vasoactive mediators from mast cells. Useful for exercise-induced bronchospasm. **Effective only for the prophylaxis** of asthma; not effective during an acute attack. Toxicity is rare.
Antileukotrienes	**Zileuton:** A 5-lipoxygenase pathway inhibitor. Blocks conversion of arachidonic acid to leukotrienes. **Montelukast, zafirlukast:** Block leukotriene receptors.

MNEMONIC

Meds for asthma exacerbations—

ASTHMA

Albuterol
Steroids
Theophylline (rare)
Humidified O$_2$
Magnesium (severe exacerbations)
Anticholinergics

- Acute:
  - O$_2$, **bronchodilating agents** (short-acting inhaled β_2-agonists are first-line therapy), **ipratropium** (never used alone for asthma), systemic **corticosteroids,** magnesium (for severe exacerbations).
  - Maintain a low threshold for intubation in severe cases or acutely in patients with a $P_{CO_2} > 50$ mm Hg or a $P_{O_2} < 50$ mm Hg.
- Chronic:
  - Administer long-acting inhaled **bronchodilators** and/or inhaled corticosteroids, systemic **corticosteroids,** cromolyn, or, rarely, theophylline.
  - Montelukast and other leukotriene antagonists are oral adjuncts to inhalant therapy.

BRONCHIECTASIS

A disease caused by cycles of infection and inflammation in the bronchi/bronchioles that lead to fibrosis, remodeling, and **permanent dilation of bronchi** (see Figure 2.15-3).

HISTORY/PE

- Presents with chronic cough accompanied by frequent bouts of yellow or green sputum production, dyspnea, and possible hemoptysis and halitosis.

This is moderate persistent asthma with daily symptoms. The patient will benefit from a long-acting β_2-agonist such as salmeterol for prevention of symptoms.

TABLE 2.15-3. Medications for the Chronic Treatment of Asthma

Type	Symptoms (Day/Night)	FEV₁	Medications
Mild intermittent	≤ 2 days/week ≤ 2 nights/month	≥ 80%	No daily medications. PRN short-acting bronchodilator.

Mild persistent	> 2/week but < 1/day
	> 2 nights/month
		≥ 80%	Daily low-dose inhaled
			  corticosteroids.
			PRN short-acting
			  bronchodilator.

Moderate persistent	Daily
	> 1 night/week
		60–80%	Low- to medium-dose inhaled
			  corticosteroids + long-acting
			  inhaled β₂-agonists.
			PRN short-acting
			  bronchodilator.

Severe persistent	Continual, frequent	≤ 60%	High-dose inhaled
			  corticosteroids + long-acting
			  inhaled β₂-agonists.
			Possible PO corticosteroids.
			PRN short-acting
			  bronchodilator.

- Associated with a history of pulmonary infections, hypersensitivity, cystic fibrosis (CF), immunodeficiency, localized airway obstruction, aspiration, autoimmune disease, or IBD.
- Examination reveals rales, wheezes, rhonchi, purulent mucus, and occasional hemoptysis.

DIAGNOSIS

- **CXR:** Shows ↑ bronchovascular markings and **tram lines** (parallel lines outlining dilated bronchi as a result of peribronchial inflammation and fibrosis).
- **High-resolution CT: Dilated airways** and ballooned cysts are seen at the end of the bronchus (mostly lower lobes).
- Spirometry shows a ↓ FEV₁/FVC ratio consistent with obstruction.

TREATMENT

- Antibiotics for bacterial infections; consider inhaled corticosteroids.
- Maintain bronchopulmonary hygiene (cough control, postural drainage, chest physiotherapy).
- Consider lobectomy for localized disease or lung transplantation for severe disease.

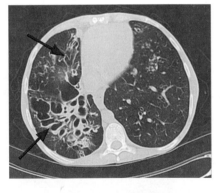

FIGURE 2.15-3. Bronchiectasis. Chest CT demonstrates markedly dilated and thick-walled airways (arrows) consistent with bronchiectasis in this CF patient. (Reproduced with permission from USMLERx.com.)

CHRONIC OBSTRUCTIVE PULMONARY DISEASE (COPD)

A disease with ↓ lung function associated with airflow obstruction. Generally 2° to chronic bronchitis or emphysema, which are distinguished as follows:

■ **Chronic bronchitis:** Productive cough for > 3 months per year for 2 consecutive years.

■ **Emphysema:** Terminal airway destruction and dilation that may be 2° to **smoking** (centrilobular) or to α₁-antitrypsin deficiency (panlobular).

HISTORY/PE

■ Symptoms are minimal or nonspecific until the disease is advanced.

■ The clinical spectrum includes the following (most patients are a combination of the 2 phenotypes):

■ **Emphysema ("pink puffer"): Dyspnea, pursed lips, minimal cough,** ↓ breath sounds, late hypercarbia/hypoxia. Patients often have a thin, wasted appearance. Pure emphysematous patients tend to have few reactive episodes between exacerbations.

■ **Chronic bronchitis ("blue bloater"): Cyanosis with mild dyspnea; productive cough.** Patients are often overweight with peripheral edema, rhonchi, and early signs of hypercarbia/hypoxia.

■ Look for the classic barrel chest, use of accessory chest muscles, JVD, end-expiratory wheezing, and muffled breath sounds.

DIAGNOSIS

■ **CXR: Hyperinflated lungs,** ↓ lung markings with flat diaphragms, and a thin-appearing heart and mediastinum are seen. Parenchymal **bullae** or subpleural **blebs** (pathognomonic of emphysema) are also seen (see Figure 2.15-4).

■ **PFTs:** ↓ **FEV₁/FVC;** normal or ↓ FVC; normal or ↑ TLC (emphysema, asthma); ↓ DL_{CO} (in emphysema).

■ **ABGs:** Hypoxemia with acute or chronic respiratory acidosis (↑ P_{CO_2}).

■ Consider a Gram stain and sputum culture in the setting of fever or productive cough, especially if infiltrate is seen on CXR.

KEY FACT

In COPD patients with chronic hypercapnia, high concentrations of O_2 may suppress patients' hypoxic respiratory drive.

KEY FACT

Supplemental O_2 titrated to > 90% Sao_2 for > 15 hours a day and smoking cessation are the only interventions proven to improve survival in patients with COPD.

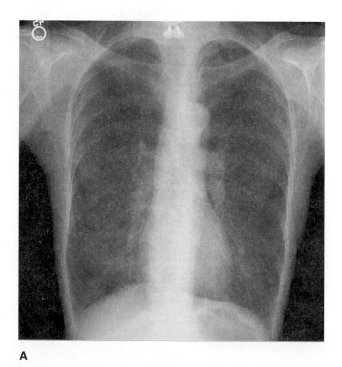

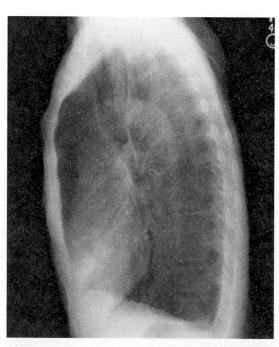

A **B**

FIGURE 2.15-4. **COPD.** PA (A) and lateral (B) radiographs of a patient with emphysema show hyperinflation with large lung volumes, flattening of the diaphragm, and minimal peripheral vascular markings. (Reproduced with permission from USMLERx.com.)

TREATMENT

- **Acute exacerbations:**
  - O_2, inhaled β_2-agonists (albuterol) and **anticholinergics** (ipratropium, tiotropium), IV +/– inhaled **corticosteroids, antibiotics.** Severe cases benefit from noninvasive ventilation with bilevel positive airway pressure (BiPAP).
  - Consider intubation in the setting of severe hypoxemia or hypercapnia, impending respiratory fatigue, or changes in mental status.
- **Chronic:**
  - **Smoking cessation,** inhaled β_2-agonists, anticholinergics (tiotropium), systemic or inhaled corticosteroids.
  - **Supplemental O_2 if resting Pao_2 is $\leq$ 55 mm Hg or Sao_2 is $\leq$ 89%,** or in the setting of cor pulmonale, pulmonary hypertension, a hematocrit > 55%, or nocturnal hypoxia.
  - Give pneumococcal and flu vaccines.

Restrictive Lung Disease

Characterized by a loss of lung compliance, restrictive lung diseases result in ↑ lung stiffness and ↓ lung expansion. Table 2.15-1 and Figure 2.15-2 contrast obstructive with restrictive lung disease. The etiologies of restrictive lung disease are shown in the mnemonic **AIN'T.**

INTERSTITIAL LUNG DISEASE

A heterogeneous group of disorders characterized by **inflammation** and/or **fibrosis** of the **interalveolar septum.** In advanced disease, cystic spaces develop in the lung periphery ("honeycombing"). Causes include idiopathic interstitial pneumonias, collagen vascular disease, granulomatous disorders, drugs, hypersensitivity disorders, pneumoconiosis, and eosinophilic pulmonary syndromes. Idiopathic pulmonary fibrosis (IPF) is also included in this category, although it is a diagnosis of exclusion (as indicated by its name).

HISTORY/PE

- Presents with **shallow, rapid breathing;** dyspnea with exercise; and a nonproductive cough.
- Patients may have cyanosis, inspiratory squeaks, fine or "Velcro-like" crackles, clubbing, or right heart failure.

DIAGNOSIS

- **CXR/CT:** Reticular, nodular, or ground-glass pattern; "**honeycomb**" pattern (severe disease).
- **PFTs:** ↓ **TLC,** ↓ **FVC,** ↓ **DL$_{CO}$** (may be normal if the cause is extrapulmonary), **normal FEV_1/FVC.** Serum markers of connective tissue diseases should be obtained if clinically indicated.
- Surgical biopsy is often indicated to confirm a diagnosis of IPF with evidence of interstitial inflammation and fibrosis (see Figure 2.15-5).

TREATMENT

- **Supportive.** Avoid exposure to causative agents. Some inflammatory diseases respond to **corticosteroids** or other anti-inflammatory/immunosuppressive agents.
- Lung transplantation may be indicated at late stages of IPF.

MNEMONIC

Treatment for COPD—

COPD

Corticosteroids
Oxygen
Prevention (**cigarette-smoking cessation,** pneumococcal and influenza vaccines)
Dilators (β_2-agonists, anticholinergics)

MNEMONIC

If the lungs AIN'T compliant:

Alveolar (edema, hemorrhage, pus)
Interstitial lung disease (idiopathic interstitial pneumonias), **I**nflammatory (sarcoid, cryptogenic organizing pneumonitis), **I**diopathic
Neuromuscular (myasthenia, phrenic nerve palsy, myopathy)
Thoracic wall (kyphoscoliosis, obesity, ascites, pregnancy, ankylosing spondylitis)

KEY FACT

Medications that can cause or contribute to interstitial lung disease include **amiodarone,** busulfan, nitrofurantoin, bleomycin, radiation, and long-term high O_2 concentration (eg, ventilators).

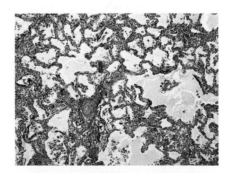

FIGURE 2.15-5. Idiopathic pulmonary fibrosis. Lung biopsy demonstrating increased interstitial fibrosis and nonspecific inflammation with alveolar thickening. (Reproduced with permission from USMLERx.com.)

Learning the features of sarcoid can be—

GRUELING

Granulomas
a**R**thritis
Uveitis
Erythema nodosum
Lymphadenopathy
Interstitial fibrosis
Negative TB test
Gammaglobulinemia

SYSTEMIC SARCOIDOSIS

A multisystem disease of unknown etiology characterized by **noncaseating granulomas**. Most commonly found in **African American females** and Northern European Caucasians; most often arises in the third or fourth decade of life.

HISTORY/PE

- Can present with **fever, cough, malaise,** weight loss, dyspnea, and **arthritis.**
- The lungs, liver, eyes, skin (erythema nodosum, violaceous skin plaques), nervous system, heart, and kidney may be affected.

DIAGNOSIS

- **CXR/CT:** Radiographic findings of **lymphadenopathy** and **nodules** are used to stage the disease.
- **Biopsy:** Lymph node biopsy or transbronchial/video-assisted thoracoscopic lung biopsy reveals noncaseating granulomas.
- **PFTs:** Show a restrictive or obstructive pattern and ↓ diffusion capacity.
- **Other findings:** ↑ **serum ACE levels** (neither sensitive nor specific), **hypercalcemia,** hypercalciuria, ↑ alkaline phosphatase (with liver involvement), lymphopenia, cranial nerve defects, arrhythmias.

TREATMENT

Systemic **corticosteroids** are indicated for deteriorating respiratory function, constitutional symptoms, hypercalcemia, or extrathoracic organ involvement.

HYPERSENSITIVITY PNEUMONITIS

Alveolar thickening and granulomas 2° to environmental exposure.

HISTORY/PE

- **Acute:** Dyspnea, fever, malaise, shivering, and cough starting 4–6 hours after exposure. Gather a job/travel history to determine exposure.
- **Chronic:** Patients present with progressive dyspnea; examination reveals fine bilateral rales.

DIAGNOSIS

The appearance on CXR/CT is variable, but upper lobe fibrosis is a common feature of chronic disease.

TREATMENT

Avoid ongoing exposure to inciting agents; give corticosteroids to ↓ chronic inflammation.

PNEUMOCONIOSIS

Risk factors include prolonged occupational exposure and inhalation of small inorganic dust particles.

HISTORY/PE/DIAGNOSIS

Table 2.15-4 outlines the findings and diagnostic criteria associated with common pneumoconioses.

TABLE 2.15-4. Diagnosis of Pneumoconioses

DISORDER	HISTORY	DIAGNOSIS	COMPLICATIONS
Asbestosis	Work involving the manufacture of tile or brake linings, insulation, construction, demolition, or shipbuilding. Presents 15–20 years after initial exposure.	**CXR: Linear opacities** at lung bases and interstitial fibrosis; calcified pleural plaques are indicative of benign pleural disease.	↑ risk of mesothelioma (rare) and lung cancer; the risk of lung cancer is higher in smokers.
Coal miner's disease	Work in underground coal mines.	**CXR:** Small nodular opacities (< 1 cm) in upper lung zones. **Spirometry:** Consistent with restrictive disease.	**Progressive massive fibrosis.**
Silicosis	Work in mines or quarries or with glass, pottery, or silica.	**CXR:** Small (< 1-cm) nodular opacities in upper lung zones; **eggshell calcifications** (see Figure 2.15-6). **Spirometry:** Consistent with restrictive disease.	↑ **risk of TB;** need annual TB skin test. Progressive massive fibrosis.
Berylliosis	Work in high-technology fields such as **aerospace, nuclear, and electronics plants;** ceramics industries; foundries; plating facilities; dental material sites; and dye manufacturing.	**CXR:** Diffuse infiltrates; hilar adenopathy.	**Requires chronic corticosteroid treatment.**

TREATMENT

Avoid triggers; supportive therapy and supplemental O_2.

EOSINOPHILIC PULMONARY SYNDROMES

A diverse group of disorders characterized by eosinophilic pulmonary infiltrates and peripheral blood eosinophilia. Includes allergic bronchopulmonary aspergillosis, Löffler's syndrome, and acute eosinophilic pneumonia.

HISTORY/PE

Present with dyspnea, cough, and/or fever.

DIAGNOSIS

CBC may reveal peripheral eosinophilia; CXR shows pulmonary infiltrates.

TREATMENT

Removal of the extrinsic cause or treatment of underlying infection if identified. Corticosteroid treatment may be used if no cause is identified.

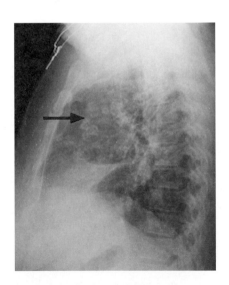

FIGURE 2.15-6. Silicosis. Eggshell calcifications characteristic of silicosis are seen on CXR. (Reproduced with permission from Chen MY et al. *Basic Radiology,* 2nd ed. New York: McGraw-Hill, 2011, Fig. 4-51B.)

Acute Respiratory Failure

HYPOXEMIA

Defined as ↓ P_{O_2}; causes include **ventilation-perfusion (V/Q) mismatch,** right-to-left **shunt, hypoventilation,** low inspired O_2 content (important at altitudes), and **diffusion impairment.**

HISTORY/PE

Findings depend on the etiology. ↓ **HbO_2 saturation,** cyanosis, tachypnea, shortness of breath, pleuritic chest pain, and altered mental status may be seen.

DIAGNOSIS

- **Pulse oximetry:** Demonstrates ↓ HbO_2 saturation.
- **CXR:** To evaluate for an infiltrative process (eg, pneumonia), atelectasis, a large pleural effusion, or pneumothorax and to assess for ARDS.
- **ABGs:** Calculate the **alveolar-arterial (A-a) oxygen gradient:** $[(P_{atm} - 47) \times FI_{O_2} - (Pa_{CO_2}/0.8)] - Pa_{O_2}$.
- An ↑ A-a gradient suggests shunt, V/Q mismatch, or diffusion impairment. Figure 2.15-7 summarizes the approach toward hypoxemic patients.

TREATMENT

- Address the underlying etiology.
- Administer O_2 before initiating evaluation.
- ↑ oxygenation parameters if the patient is on mechanical ventilation (see Table 2.15-5).
- In **hypercapnic patients,** ↑ ventilation to ↑ CO_2 exchange.

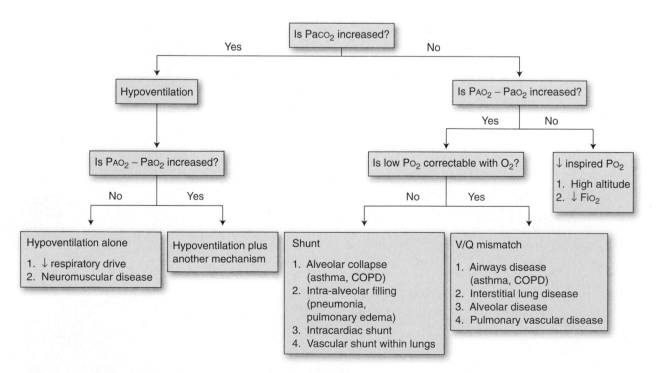

FIGURE 2.15-7. Determination of the mechanism of hypoxia. (Reproduced with permission from Kasper DL et al. *Harrison's Principles of Internal Medicine,* 16th ed. New York: McGraw-Hill, 2005.)

TABLE 2.15-5. **Mechanical Ventilator Parameters Affecting Oxygenation and Ventilation**

↑ OXYGENATION	↑ VENTILATION
↑ Fio_2	↑ respiratory rate
↑ PEEP	↑ tidal volume

ACUTE RESPIRATORY DISTRESS SYNDROME (ARDS)

Respiratory failure with refractory **hypoxemia**, ↓ **lung compliance**, and non-cardiogenic **pulmonary edema** with a Pao_2/Fio_2 ratio ≤ 200. The pathogenesis is thought to be dependent on endothelial injury. Common triggers include sepsis, pneumonia, aspiration, multiple blood transfusions, inhaled/ingested toxins, and trauma. Overall mortality is 30–40%.

HISTORY/PE

Presents with **acute-onset** (12–48 hours) tachypnea, dyspnea, and tachycardia +/– fever, cyanosis, labored breathing, diffuse high-pitched rales, and hypoxemia in the setting of one of the systemic inflammatory causes or exposure. Additional findings are as follows:

- **Phase 1 (acute injury):** Normal physical examination; possible respiratory alkalosis.
- **Phase 2 (6–48 hours):** Hyperventilation, hypocapnia, widening A-a gradient.
- **Phase 3:** Acute respiratory failure, tachypnea, dyspnea, ↓ lung compliance, scattered rales, diffuse chest opacity on CXR (see Figure 2.15-8).
- **Phase 4:** Severe hypoxemia unresponsive to therapy; ↑ intrapulmonary shunting; metabolic and respiratory acidosis.

DIAGNOSIS

The criteria for ARDS diagnosis (according to the American-European Consensus Conference definition) are as follows:

- Acute onset of respiratory distress.
- A Pao_2/Fio_2 ratio ≤ 200.

MNEMONIC

It's not (h)ARDS to diagnose **ARDS:**

Acute onset
Ratio (Pao_2/Fio_2) ≤ 200
Diffuse infiltration
Swan-Ganz wedge pressure < 18 mm Hg

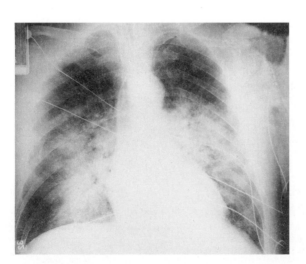

FIGURE 2.15-8. **AP CXR showing a diffuse alveolar filling pattern 2° to ARDS.** (Reproduced with permission from Kasper DL et al. *Harrison's Principles of Internal Medicine,* 16th ed. New York: McGraw-Hill, 2005: 1497.)

Q

A 25-year-old male in the ICU is intubated following an acute asthma exacerbation. A repeat ABG is sent after intubation and shows a pH of 7.6, a $Paco_2$ of 33 mm Hg, and an HCO_3^- of 26 mEq/L. What adjustments, if any, would you make to the ventilator settings?

- Bilateral pulmonary infiltrates on CXR.
- **No evidence of cardiac origin** (capillary wedge pressure < 18 mm Hg or no clinical evidence of elevated left atrial pressure).

TREATMENT

- Mechanical ventilation with low tidal volumes to minimize ventilator-induced lung injury.
- Treat the underlying disease and maintain adequate perfusion to prevent end-organ damage.
- Use PEEP to recruit collapsed alveoli, and titrate PEEP and FiO_2 to achieve adequate oxygenation.
- Goal oxygenation is $PaO_2 > 60$ mm Hg or $SaO_2 > 90\%$ on $FiO_2 \leq 0.6$.
- Slowly wean patients from ventilation, and follow with extubation trials (see Table 2.15-6).

Pulmonary Vascular Disease

PULMONARY HYPERTENSION/COR PULMONALE

Defined as a mean pulmonary arterial pressure of > 25 mm Hg (normal = 15 mm Hg). Five classification categories were defined in 2008:

- Arterial pulmonary hypertension.
- ↑ pulmonary venous pressure from left-sided **heart disease.**
- Hypoxic vasoconstriction 2° to chronic lung disease.
- Chronic thromboembolic disease.
- Pulmonary hypertension with an unclear, multifactorial etiology.

HISTORY/PE

- Presents with dyspnea on exertion, fatigue, lethargy, syncope with exertion, chest pain, and symptoms of right-sided CHF (edema, abdominal distention, JVD).
- Inquire about a history of COPD, interstitial lung disease, heart disease, sickle cell anemia, emphysema, and pulmonary emboli.

KEY FACT

Causes of pulmonary hypertension include left heart failure, mitral valve disease, and ↑ resistance in the pulmonary veins, including hypoxic vasoconstriction.

This patient has an uncompensated respiratory alkalosis due to ↑ ventilation. To ↓ ventilation, tidal volume can be ↓ or respiratory rate can be slowed.

TABLE 2.15-6. Criteria for Extubation from Mechanical Ventilation[a]

PARAMETER	VALUE
Pulmonary mechanics	
Vital capacity	> 10–15 mL/kg
Resting minute ventilation (TV × rate)	> 10 L/min
Spontaneous respiratory rate	< 33 breaths/min
Lung compliance	> 100 mL/cm water
Negative inspiratory force	< –25 cm water
Oxygenation	
A-a gradient	< 300–500 mm Hg
Shunt fraction	< 15%
PO_2 (on 40% FiO_2)	> 70 mm Hg
PCO_2	< 45 mm Hg

[a] Patients who meet these criteria are typically given a weaning (T-piece) trial to determine if they are ready for extubation.

- Examination reveals a loud, palpable S2 (often split), a flow murmur, an S4, or a parasternal heave.

DIAGNOSIS

- CXR shows enlargement of central pulmonary arteries.
- ECG demonstrates RVH.
- Echocardiogram and right heart catheterization may show signs of right ventricular overload and may aid in the diagnosis of the underlying cause.

TREATMENT

Supplemental O_2, anticoagulation, vasodilators, and diuretics if symptoms of right-sided CHF are present. Treat underlying causes of 2° pulmonary hypertension.

PULMONARY THROMBOEMBOLISM

An occlusion of the pulmonary vasculature by a blood clot. **Ninety-five percent of emboli originate from DVTs** in the deep leg veins. Often leads to pulmonary infarction, right heart failure, and hypoxemia.

HISTORY/PE

- Factors predisposing to thromboembolism are summarized by Virchow's triad (see Table 2.15-7).
- Presents with **sudden-onset dyspnea, pleuritic chest pain, low-grade fever,** cough, tachypnea, tachycardia, and, rarely, hemoptysis.
- Hypoxia and hypocarbia are seen with resulting respiratory alkalosis.
- Examination may reveal a loud P2 and prominent jugular A waves with right heart failure.

DIAGNOSIS

- **ABGs:** Respiratory alkalosis (2° hyperventilation) with a $P_{O_2} < 80$ mm Hg.
- **CXR:** Usually normal, but may show atelectasis, pleural effusion, **Hampton's hump** (a wedge-shaped infarct), or **Westermark's sign** (oligemia in the affected lung zone).
- **ECG:** Not diagnostic; most commonly reveals **sinus tachycardia.** The classic triad of **S1Q3T3**—acute right heart strain with an S wave in lead I, a Q wave in lead III, and an inverted T wave in lead III—is uncommon.
- **CT pulmonary angiogram with IV contrast** (spiral CT): Sensitive for pulmonary embolism (PE); see Figure 2.15-9.
- **V/Q scan:** May reveal segmental areas of mismatch. Reported as low, indeterminate, or high probability of PE.

TABLE 2.15-7. Virchow's Triad for Venous Thrombosis

VENOUS STASIS	ENDOTHELIAL INJURY	HYPERCOAGULABILITY
Immobility	Trauma	Pregnancy, postpartum
CHF	Surgery	OCP use
Obesity	Recent fracture	Coagulation disorders
↑ central venous pressure	Previous DVT	(eg, protein C/protein S
		deficiency, factor V Leiden)
		Malignancy
		Severe burns

Q

A 25-year-old African American female presents with painful bumps on her shins, weight loss, and cough. Examination reveals a prominent 1-cm right axillary lymph node. What is the next best step for diagnosis?

KEY FACT

Other etiologies of embolic disease include postpartum status (amniotic fluid emboli), fracture (fat emboli), and cardiac surgery (air emboli).

MNEMONIC

VIRchow's triad:

Vascular trauma
Increased coagulability
Reduced blood flow (stasis)

A

This is presumed sarcoidosis. Biopsy of the right axillary lymph node is the next best step for diagnosis and is less invasive than transbronchial lung biopsy.

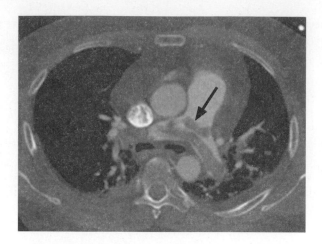

FIGURE 2.15-9. Pulmonary embolus. Axial slice from a CT pulmonary angiogram shows a pulmonary embolus extending from the main pulmonary artery into the right and left pulmonary arteries, consistent with a saddle embolus. (Reproduced with permission from Chen MY et al. *Basic Radiology*, 2nd ed. New York: McGraw-Hill, 2011, Fig. 4-69.)

KEY FACT

Dyspnea, tachycardia, and a normal CXR in a hospitalized and/or bedridden patient should raise suspicion of PE.

- **D-dimer:** Sensitive but not specific in patients at risk for DVT or PE; most useful as a "rule-out" test in patients with low clinical suspicion.
- **Lower extremity venous ultrasound:** Can detect a clot that may have given off the PE.

TREATMENT

- **Anticoagulation:**
  - **Acute:** Bolus followed by weight-based heparin infusion or low-molecular-weight heparin (LMWH) SQ.
  - **Chronic:** Warfarin or LMWH for at least 6 months following the event or as long as predisposition exists (goal INR = 2–3).
- **IVC filter:** Indicated in patients with a documented lower extremity DVT if anticoagulation is contraindicated or if patients experience recurrent emboli while anticoagulated.
- **Thrombolysis:** Indicated only in cases of massive DVT or PE causing right heart failure and hemodynamic instability
- **DVT prophylaxis:** Treat all immobile patients; give SQ heparin or LMWH, intermittent pneumatic compression of the lower extremities (less effective), and **early ambulation (most effective).**

Neoplasms of the Lungs

LUNG NODULES

Commonly found on CXRs. History, physical examination, and imaging features help guide treatment (see Table 2.15-8).

HISTORY/PE

Often asymptomatic, or patients may present with chronic cough, dyspnea, and shortness of breath. Always inquire about smoking and exposure history.

DIAGNOSIS

- **Serial CXRs:** To determine the nodule's location, progression, and extent.
- **Chest CT:** To determine the nature, extent, and infiltrating nature of the nodule.

KEY FACT

Lung nodule clues based on the history:
- Recent immigrant—think TB.
- From the southwestern United States—think coccidioidomycosis.
- From the Ohio River Valley—think histoplasmosis.

TABLE 2.15-8. **Characteristics of Benign and Malignant Lung Nodules**

BENIGN	MALIGNANT
Age < 35	Age > 45–50
Nonsmoker	Smoker
No change from old films	New or enlarging lesions
Central, uniform, or popcorn calcification	Absent or irregular calcification
Smooth margins	Irregular margins
Size < 2 cm	Size > 2 cm

TREATMENT

- **Surgical resection** is indicated for nodules at high risk for malignancy. Low-risk nodules can be followed with **CXR or CT every 3 months** for 1 year and then every 6 months for another year.
- An invasive diagnostic procedure is indicated if the size of the nodule ↑.

LUNG CANCER

The leading cause of **cancer death** in the United States. Risk factors include tobacco smoke (except for bronchoalveolar carcinoma) and radon or asbestos exposure. Types are as follows:

- **Small cell lung cancer (SCLC):**
  - Highly correlated with **cigarette exposure.**
  - Has a central location (see Figure 2.15-10).
  - Has a **neuroendocrine origin;** associated with paraneoplastic syndromes (see Table 2.15-9).
  - Metastases are often found on presentation in intrathoracic and extrathoracic sites such as brain, liver, and bone.
- **Non–small cell lung cancer (NSCLC):** Represents a group of cancers, with the most common types being adenocarcinoma, squamous cell carcinoma (SCC), and large cell carcinoma. These cancers are less likely than SCLC to metastasize at an early stage.
  - **Adenocarcinoma:**
    - The most common lung cancer; has a **peripheral** location.
    - Includes **bronchoalveolar carcinoma,** which is associated with multiple nodules, interstitial infiltration, and prolific sputum production but is **not associated with smoking.**
  - SCC: Has a **central** location; 98% are seen in smokers.
  - **Large cell/neuroendocrine carcinomas:** Least common; associated with a poor prognosis.

HISTORY/PE

- Presents with cough, hemoptysis, dyspnea, wheezing, pneumonia, chest pain, weight loss, and possible abnormalities on respiratory examination (crackles, atelectasis).
- Other findings include the following:
  - **Horner's syndrome** (miosis, ptosis, anhidrosis) in patients with Pancoast's tumor at the apex of the lung.

KEY FACT

Squamous and **S**mall cell cancers are **S**entral lesions.

MNEMONIC

Lung cancer mets are often found in LABBs—

Liver
Adrenals
Brain
Bone

A 65-year-old with a 30-pack-year history presents with a 2-week history of facial swelling. Biopsy reveals a hilar small cell lung cancer (SCLC). What is the next step in treatment?

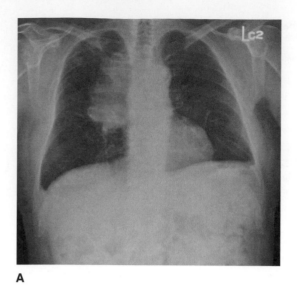

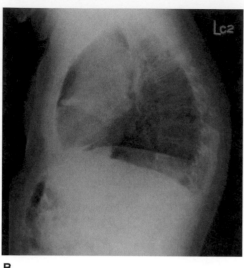

A

B

FIGURE 2.15-10. **Small cell lung cancer.** Note the central location of the tumor in the PA (**A**) and lateral (**B**) CXRs. (Reproduced with permission from Kantarjian HM et al. *MD Anderson Manual of Medical Oncology,* 1st ed. New York: McGraw-Hill, 2006, Fig. 11-2.)

- **SVC syndrome** due to obstruction of the SVC with supraclavicular venous engorgement and facial swelling (see Figure 2.15-11).
- **Hoarseness** 2° to recurrent laryngeal nerve involvement.
- Many **paraneoplastic syndromes** (see Table 2.15-9).

TABLE 2.15-9. **Paraneoplastic Syndromes of Lung Cancer**

CLASSIFICATION	SYNDROME	HISTOLOGIC TYPE
Endocrine/metabolic	Cushing's syndrome (ACTH)	Small cell
	SIADH leading to hyponatremia	Small cell
	Hypercalcemia (PTHrP)	Squamous cell
	Gynecomastia	Large cell
Skeletal	Hypertrophic pulmonary osteoarthropathy	Non–small cell
	Digital clubbing	Non–small cell
Neuromuscular	Peripheral neuropathy	Small cell
	Subacute cerebellar degeneration	Small cell
	Myasthenia (Lambert-Eaton syndrome)	Small cell
	Dermatomyositis	All
Cardiovascular	Thrombophlebitis	Adenocarcinoma
	Nonbacterial verrucous endocarditis	Adenocarcinoma
Hematologic	Anemia	All
	DIC	All
	Eosinophilia	All
	Thrombocytosis	All
	Hypercoagulability	Adenocarcinoma
Cutaneous	Acanthosis nigricans	All

The mainstay of therapy for SCLC is chemotherapy, which yields high rates of response.

DIAGNOSIS

- CXR or chest CT.
- Fine-needle aspiration (CT guided) for peripheral lesions; **bronchoscopy** (biopsy or brushing) for central lesions.

TREATMENT

- **SCLC: Unresectable.** Often responds to radiation and chemotherapy initially but usually recurs; has a low median survival rate.
- **NSCLC: Surgical resection** in early stages. Supplement surgery with radiation or chemotherapy (depending on the stage). Palliative radiation and/or chemotherapy is appropriate for symptomatic but unresectable disease.

Pleural Disease

PLEURAL EFFUSION

An abnormal **accumulation of fluid in the pleural space.** Classified as follows:

- **Transudate:** 2° to ↑ pulmonary capillary wedge pressure (PCWP) or ↓ oncotic pressure.
- **Exudate:** 2° to ↑ pleural vascular permeability.

Table 2.15-10 lists the possible causes of both transudates and exudates.

HISTORY/PE

Presents with **dyspnea,** pleuritic chest pain, and/or cough. Examination reveals **dullness to percussion** and ↓ **breath sounds** over the effusion. A pleural friction rub may be present.

DIAGNOSIS

- CXR shows costophrenic angle blunting. A lateral decubitus view can be used to assess loculation.
- **Thoracentesis** is indicated for new effusions > 1 cm in decubitus view, except with bilateral effusions and other clinical evidence of CHF.
- The effusion is an exudate if it meets **any of Light's criteria** (see Table 2.15-11).

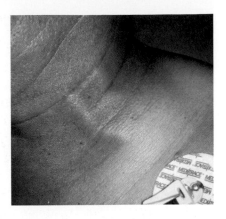

FIGURE 2.15-11.   SVC syndrome. Prominent JVD is seen in SVC syndrome 2° to obstruction of the SVC by a central malignant lesion. (Reproduced with permission from Tintinalli JE et al. *Tintinalli's Emergency Medicine: A Comprehensive Study Guide,* 7th ed. New York: McGraw-Hill, 2011, Fig. 235-1A.)

TABLE 2.15-10.   Causes of Pleural Effusions

TRANSUDATES	EXUDATES
CHF	Pneumonia (parapneumonic effusion)
Cirrhosis	TB
Nephrotic syndrome	Malignancy
	PE
	Collagen vascular disease (rheumatoid arthritis, SLE)
	Pancreatitis
	Trauma

TABLE 2.15-11. Light's Criteria for Pleural Effusions[a]

MEASURE	VALUE
Pleural protein/serum protein	> 0.5.
Pleural LDH/serum LDH	> 0.6.
Pleural fluid LDH	> $\frac{2}{3}$ the upper limit of normal serum LDH.

[a] An effusion is an exudate if **any** of the above criteria are met.

KEY FACT

Complicated parapneumonic effusions necessitate chest tube drainage.

TREATMENT

- Treatment is directed toward the underlying condition causing the effusion.
- Complicated parapneumonic effusions and empyemas require **chest tube drainage** in addition to **antibiotic therapy.**

PNEUMOTHORAX

Defined as a collection of air in the pleural space that can lead to pulmonary collapse. Etiologies include penetrating trauma, infection, and positive-pressure mechanical ventilation. Shock and death result unless the condition is immediately recognized and treated. Subtypes are as follows:

- **1° spontaneous pneumothorax:** 2° to rupture of subpleural apical blebs (usually found in **tall, thin young males**).
- **2° pneumothorax:** 2° to COPD, trauma, infections (TB, *Pneumocystis jiroveci*), and iatrogenic factors (thoracentesis, subclavian line placement, positive-pressure mechanical ventilation, bronchoscopy).
- **Tension pneumothorax:** A pulmonary or chest wall defect acts as a **1-way valve causing air trapping in the pleural space.**

MNEMONIC

Presentation of pneumothorax–

P-THORAX

Pleuritic pain
Tracheal deviation
Hyperresonance
Onset sudden
Reduced breath sounds (and dyspnea)
Absent fremitus (asymmetric chest wall)
X-ray shows collapse

HISTORY/PE

- Presents with acute onset of unilateral pleuritic chest pain and dyspnea.
- Examination reveals tachypnea, diminished or absent breath sounds, hyperresonance, ↓ tactile fremitus, and JVD 2° to compression of the SVC.
- Tension pneumothorax also presents with **tracheal deviation and hemodynamic instability.**

DIAGNOSIS

- The diagnosis of a **tension pneumothorax should be made clinically** and should be followed by immediate treatment.
- CXR shows the presence of a visceral pleural line and/or **lung retraction** from the chest wall (best seen in end-expiratory films; see Figure 2.15-12).

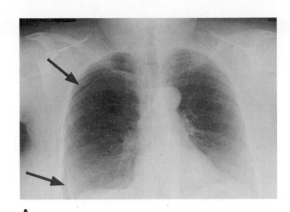 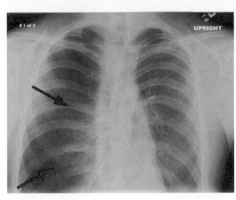

A

B

FIGURE 2.15-12. **Pneumothorax.** (**A**) Small right pneumothorax. (**B**) Right tension pneumothorax with collapse of the right lung and shifting of mediastinal structures to the left. Arrows denote pleural reflections. (Reproduced with permission from USMLERx.com.)

TREATMENT

- Tension pneumothorax requires immediate needle decompression (second intercostal space at the midclavicular line) followed by chest tube placement.
- Small pneumothoraces may resorb spontaneously. Supplemental O_2 is helpful.
- Large, symptomatic pneumothoraces require chest tube placement.

NOTES

RENAL/GENITOURINARY

MNEMONIC

Hypernatremia causes—

The 6 D's

Diuresis
Dehydration
Diabetes insipidus
Docs (iatrogenic)
Diarrhea
Disease (eg, kidney, sickle cell)

Electrolyte Disorders

HYPERNATREMIA

Serum sodium > 145 mEq/L. Usually due to **free water loss** rather than sodium gain.

HISTORY/PE

- Presents with **thirst** (due to hypertonicity) as well as with oliguria or polyuria (depending on the etiology).
- **Neurologic symptoms** include mental status changes, weakness, focal neurologic deficits, and seizures.
- Examination reveals "doughy" skin and signs of volume depletion.

DIAGNOSIS

Assess volume status by conducting a clinical examination and measuring urine volume and osmolality.

- **Hypertonic Na^+ gain:** Due to hypertonic saline/tube feeds or ↑ **aldosterone** (suppresses ADH).
- **Pure water loss:** Due to central or nephrogenic **diabetes insipidus;** characterized by large volumes of dilute urine. Do not neglect dermal and respiratory insensible losses.
- **Hypotonic fluid loss:** Due to ↓ intake, diuretics, intrinsic renal disease, GI losses (**diarrhea**), burns, and osmotic diuresis (mannitol, glucose in diabetic ketoacidosis [DKA], urea with high protein feeds).

TREATMENT

- Treat the underlying causes and replace the free-water deficit depending on volume status:
  - **Hypovolemia:** Use D_5W. If vital signs are unstable, use isotonic sodium chloride solution (0.9% NaCl) before correcting free water deficits.
  - **Euvolemia:** Use hypotonic fluids—eg, D_5W or 0.45% NaCl.
  - **Hypervolemia:** Use a combination of diuretics and D_5W to remove excess sodium.
- Correction of chronic hypernatremia (> 36–48 hours) should be accomplished **gradually over 48–72 hours** (≤ 0.5 mEq/L/hr) to prevent neurologic damage 2° to cerebral edema.

HYPONATREMIA

Serum sodium < 135 mEq/L. Almost always due to ↑ ADH.

HISTORY/PE

- May be asymptomatic or may present with **confusion, lethargy,** muscle cramps, hyporeflexia, and nausea.
- Can progress to seizures, coma, or brainstem herniation.

DIAGNOSIS

Hyponatremia can be categorized according to serum and urine osmolality as well as by volume status (ie, by clinical exam), as seen in Figure 2.16-1. Osmolality is classified as follows:

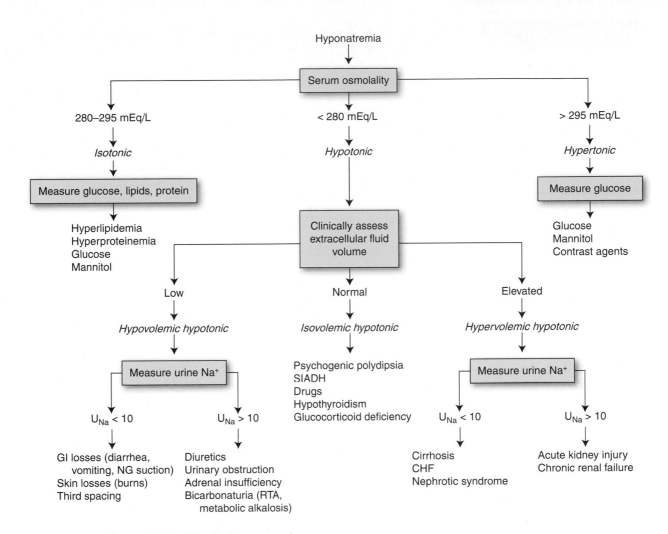

FIGURE 2.16-1. **Diagnostic algorithm for hyponatremia.**

- **High (> 295 mEq/L):** Hyperglycemia, hypertonic infusion (eg, mannitol).
- **Normal (280–295 mEq/L):** Hypertriglyceridemia, paraproteinemia (pseudohyponatremia).
- **Low (< 280 mEq/L):** Applies to the majority of cases. Hypotonic etiologies are listed in Figure 2.16-1.

TREATMENT

- Treat according to volume status:
  - **Hypervolemia:** Water restriction; consider diuretics. Cortisol replacement with adrenal insufficiency; thyroid replacement with hypothyroidism.
  - **Euvolemia:** Water restriction.
  - **Hypovolemia:** Replete volume with normal saline (NS).
- Chronic hyponatremia (> 72 hours' duration) should be corrected slowly (no more than 0.5 mEq/L/hr) in order to prevent central pontine myelinolysis (symptoms include paraparesis/quadriparesis, dysarthria, and coma).

KEY FACT

Consider using hypertonic saline only if a patient has seizures due to hyponatremia, and when serum Na$^+$ is < 120 mEq/L. In most cases, NS is the best replacement fluid.

KEY FACT

What dreaded complication can arise from correcting hyponatremia too rapidly? Central pontine myelinolysis.

HYPERKALEMIA

Serum potassium > 5 mEq/L. Etiologies are as follows:

- **Spurious:** Hemolysis of blood samples, fist clenching during blood draws, delays in sample analysis, extreme leukocytosis or thrombocytosis.

Treatment of hyperkalemia—

C BIG K

Calcium
Bicarbonate
Insulin
Glucose
Kayexalate

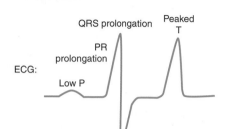

FIGURE 2.16-2. Hyperkalemia on ECG. Electrocardiographic manifestations include peaked T waves, PR prolongation, and a widened QRS complex. (Reproduced with permission from Cogan MG. *Fluid and Electrolytes,* 1st ed. Stamford, CT: Appleton & Lange, 1991: 170.)

KEY FACT

Patients with metabolic alkalosis, hypokalemia, and a normal BP likely have one of the following conditions:

- Surreptitious vomiting
- Diuretic abuse
- Bartter's syndrome
- Gitelman's syndrome

KEY FACT

Hypokalemia is usually due to renal or GI losses.

- ↓ **excretion:** Renal insufficiency, drugs (eg, spironolactone, triamterene, ACEIs, trimethoprim, NSAIDs), hypoaldosteronism, type IV renal tubular acidosis (RTA), calcineurin inhibitors.
- **Cellular shifts:** Cell lysis, tissue injury (rhabdomyolysis), insulin deficiency, acidosis, drugs (eg, succinylcholine, digitalis, arginine, β-blockers), exercise, resorption of blood (hematomas, GI bleeding).
- **Iatrogenic.**

HISTORY/PE

May be asymptomatic or may present with nausea, vomiting, **intestinal colic, areflexia, weakness,** flaccid paralysis, arrhythmias, and paresthesias.

DIAGNOSIS

- Confirm hyperkalemia with a **repeat blood draw.** In the setting of extreme leukocytosis or thrombocytosis, check plasma potassium.
- ECG findings include **tall, peaked T waves;** a wide QRS; PR prolongation; and loss of P waves (see Figure 2.16-2). Can progress to **sine waves,** ventricular fibrillation, and cardiac arrest.

TREATMENT

- Values > 6.5 mEq/L or ECG changes (especially PR prolongation or wide QRS) require emergent treatment.
- The mnemonic **C BIG K** and the steps listed below summarize the treatment of hyperkalemia.
  - The first step is always to give **calcium gluconate** for cardiac cell membrane stabilization (it also has the quickest onset of a few minutes).
  - Give **bicarbonate and/or insulin and glucose** to temporarily shift potassium into cells.
  - β-agonists (eg, albuterol) promote cellular reuptake of potassium.
  - Eliminate potassium from diet and IV fluids.
  - **Kayexalate (sodium polystyrene sulfonate)** to remove potassium from the body. Contraindications include ileus, bowel obstruction, ischemic gut, or pancreatic transplants (can cause bowel necrosis).
- Loop diuretics can be used for increasing urinary excretion of potassium.
- Dialysis is appropriate for patients with renal failure or for severe, refractory cases.

HYPOKALEMIA

Serum potassium < 3.6 mEq/L. Etiologies are as follows:

- **Transcellular shifts:** Insulin, β2-agonists, and alkalosis all cause potassium to shift intracellularly (see Figure 2.16-3).
- **GI losses:** Diarrhea, chronic laxative abuse, vomiting, NG suction.
- **Renal losses: Diuretics** (eg, loop or thiazide), 1° mineralocorticoid excess or 2° hyperaldosteronism, ↓ circulating volume, Bartter's and Gitelman's syndromes, drugs (eg, gentamicin, amphotericin), DKA, **hypomagnesemia,** type I RTA (defective distal H⁺ secretion), polyuria.

HISTORY/PE

Presents with fatigue, **muscle weakness or cramps, ileus,** hypotension, hyporeflexia, paresthesias, rhabdomyolysis, and ascending paralysis.

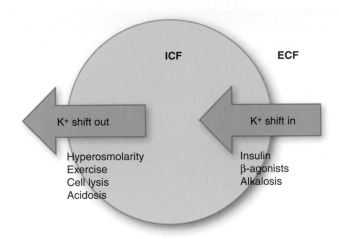

FIGURE 2.16-3. **Causes of transcellular potassium shifts.**

DIAGNOSIS

- Twenty-four-hour or spot urine potassium may distinguish renal from GI losses.
- ECG may show **T-wave flattening, U waves** (an additional wave after the T wave), and ST-segment depression, leading to AV block and subsequent cardiac arrest.
- Consider RTA in the setting of metabolic acidosis.

TREATMENT

- Treat the underlying disorder.
- Oral and/or IV **potassium repletion.** Do not exceed 20 mEq/L/hr.
- Replace magnesium, as this deficiency complicates potassium repletion.
- Monitor ECG and plasma potassium levels frequently during replacement.

HYPERCALCEMIA

Serum calcium > 10.2 mg/dL. The most common causes are **hyperparathyroidism and malignancy** (eg, breast cancer, squamous cell carcinoma, multiple myeloma). Other causes are summarized in the mnemonic **CHIMPANZEES.**

HISTORY/PE

Usually asymptomatic, but may present with **bones** (osteopenia, fractures), **stones** (kidney stones), abdominal **groans** (anorexia, constipation), and **psychiatric overtones** (weakness, fatigue, altered mental status).

DIAGNOSIS

Order a total/ionized calcium, albumin, phosphate, PTH, parathyroid hormone–related peptide (PTHrP), vitamin D, and ECG (may show a **short QT interval**).

TREATMENT

- **IV hydration** followed by **furosemide** to ↑ calcium excretion.
- Calcitonin, bisphosphonates (eg, pamidronate), glucocorticoids, calcimimetics, and dialysis are used for severe or refractory cases. **Avoid thiazide diuretics,** which ↑ tubular reabsorption of calcium.

KEY FACT

Hypokalemia sensitizes the heart to digitalis toxicity because K⁺ and digitalis compete for the same sites on the Na⁺/K⁺ pump. Thus, if a patient is on digitalis, potassium levels must be carefully monitored.

MNEMONIC

Causes of hypercalcemia–

CHIMPANZEES

Calcium supplementation
Hyperparathyroidism/**H**yperthyroidism
Iatrogenic (eg, thiazides, parenteral nutrition)/**I**mmobility (especially in the ICU setting)
Milk-alkali syndrome
Paget's disease
Adrenal insufficiency/**A**cromegaly
Neoplasm
Zollinger-Ellison syndrome (eg, MEN type 1)
Excess vitamin A
Excess vitamin D
Sarcoidosis and other granulomatous disease

KEY FACT

Loops (furosemide) **L**ose calcium.

HYPOCALCEMIA

Serum calcium < 8.5 mg/dL. Etiologies include hypoparathyroidism (post-surgical, idiopathic), malnutrition, hypomagnesemia, acute pancreatitis, vitamin D deficiency, and pseudohypoparathyroidism. In infants, consider DiGeorge's syndrome (tetany shortly after birth; absence of thymic shadow).

HISTORY/PE

- Presents with **abdominal muscle cramps**, dyspnea, **tetany, perioral and acral paresthesias,** and convulsions.
- Facial spasm elicited from tapping of the facial nerve (**Chvostek's sign**) and carpal spasm after arterial occlusion by a BP cuff (**Trousseau's sign**) are classic findings that are most commonly seen in severe hypocalcemia.

DIAGNOSIS

- Order an ionized Ca^{2+}, Mg^+, PTH, albumin, 25-OH vitamin D, and 1,25-OH vitamin D levels. If the patient is postthyroidectomy, review the operative note to determine if there was any potential damage to the parathyroid glands.
- ECG may show a **prolonged QT interval.**

TREATMENT

- Treat the underlying disorder.
- Magnesium repletion.
- Administer oral **calcium supplements;** give oral and IV calcium for severe symptoms.

HYPOMAGNESEMIA

Serum magnesium < 1.5 mEq/L. Etiologies are as follows:

- ↓ **intake:** Malnutrition, malabsorption, short bowel syndrome, TPN.
- ↑ **loss:** Diuretics, diarrhea, vomiting, hypercalcemia, alcoholism.
- **Miscellaneous: DKA,** pancreatitis, extracellular fluid volume expansion.

HISTORY/PE

In severe cases, symptoms may include hyperactive reflexes, tetany, paresthesias, irritability, confusion, lethargy, seizures, and arrhythmias.

DIAGNOSIS

- Labs may show concurrent hypocalcemia and hypokalemia.
- ECG may reveal prolonged PR and QT intervals.

TREATMENT

- IV and oral supplements.
- **Hypokalemia and hypocalcemia will not correct without magnesium correction.**

Acid-Base Disorders

See Figure 2.16-4 for a diagnostic algorithm of acid-base disorders.

KEY FACT

A classic case of hypocalcemia is a patient who develops cramps and tetany following thyroidectomy.

KEY FACT

Serum calcium levels may be falsely low in hypoalbuminemia; check ionized calcium.

KEY FACT

Alcoholics are the most common patient population with hypomagnesemia.

KEY FACT

ASA (salicylate) overdose can cause both a metabolic acidosis and a respiratory alkalosis.

MNEMONIC

Specific treatments for anion-gap causes of metabolic acidosis—

MUDPILES

Methanol: Fomepizole
Uremia: Dialysis
DKA: Insulin, fluids
Paraldehyde, **P**henformin
Iron, **I**NH: GI lavage, charcoal (INH)
Lactic acidosis
Ethylene glycol: Fomepizole
Salicylates: Alkalinize urine

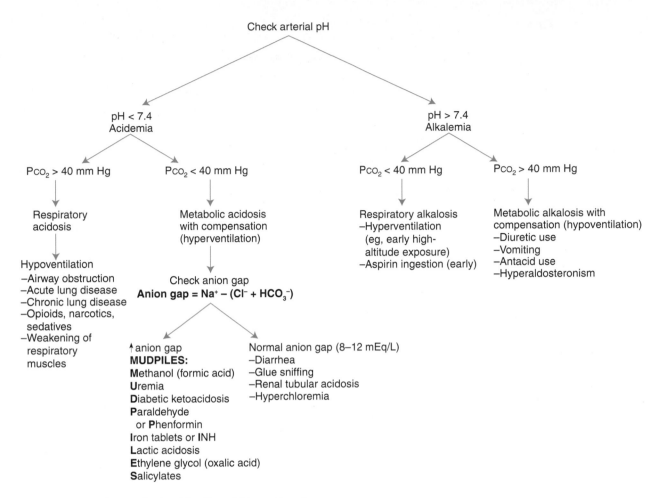

FIGURE 2.16-4. **Diagnostic algorithm for acid-base disorders.**

Renal Tubular Acidosis (RTA)

A net ↓ in either tubular H^+ secretion or HCO_3^- reabsorption that leads to a **non-anion-gap metabolic acidosis.** There are 3 main types of RTA; **type IV (distal)** is the **most common form** (see Table 2.16-1).

Acute Kidney Injury

Formerly known as **acute renal failure.** Defined as an abrupt ↓ in renal function leading to the retention of creatinine and BUN. ↓ urine output (oliguria, defined as < 500 cc/day) is not required for acute kidney injury. Categorized as follows:

- **Prenal:**
    - ↓ renal perfusion.
    - Common causes include **hypovolemia** (hemorrhage, dehydration, burns), cardiogenic shock, **sepsis,** anaphylaxis, drugs (ACEIs, **NSAIDs**), **renal artery stenosis,** ↓ effective circulating volume from hypoalbuminemia (cirrhosis and nephrotic syndrome), abdominal compartment syndrome, and hepatorenal syndrome.

Q 1

A 17-year-old male with a history of asthma presented to the ER with severe shortness of breath. His arterial pH has gone from 7.49 to 7.38 since the time of admission. What is the next best step in management?

Q 2

A 37-year-old homeless man was found unconscious on a park bench. Upon waking, he complains of muscle soreness and dark urine. His urine dipstick is ⊕. What is the likely cause of this finding, and what is the best next step?

TABLE 2.16-1. Types of RTA

VARIABLE	TYPE I (DISTAL)	TYPE II (PROXIMAL)	TYPE IV (DISTAL)
Defect	H$^+$ secretion.	HCO$_3^-$ reabsorption.	Aldosterone deficiency or resistance.
Serum K$^+$	Low.	Low.	**High.**
Urinary pH	> 5.3.	5.3 initially; < 5.3 once serum is acidic.	< 5.3.
Etiologies (most common)	Hereditary, cirrhosis, autoimmune disorders (Sjögren's syndrome, SLE), hypercalciuria, sickle cell disease, drugs (lithium, amphotericin).	Hereditary (Fanconi's syndrome or cystinosis), drugs (carbonic anhydrase inhibitors), multiple myeloma, amyloidosis, heavy metal poisoning, vitamin D deficiency.	1° aldosterone deficiency, hyporeninemic hypoaldosteronism (eg, from kidney disease, ACEIs, NSAIDs), drugs (eg, amiloride, spironolactone, heparin), pseudo-hypoaldosteronism.
Treatment	Replace bicarbonate.	Thiazides, volume depletion to increase reabsorption.	Furosemide, mineralocorticoid +/− glucocorticoid replacement.
Complications	**Nephrolithiasis.**	Rickets, osteomalacia.	Hyperkalemia.

- **Intrinsic:**
    - Injury within the nephron unit.
    - Common causes include ischemic or nephrotoxic **acute tubular necrosis** (ATN), allergic interstitial nephritis, glomerulonephritis, thromboembolism, atheroembolic disease, and rhabdomyolysis.
- **Postrenal:**
    - Urinary outflow obstruction.
    - Common causes include **prostatic disease,** pelvic tumors, intratubular crystalluria causing obstruction (indinavir/acyclovir), retroperitoneal fibrosis, and bilateral nephrolithiasis.

HISTORY/PE

- Symptoms of **uremia** include malaise, fatigue, confusion, oliguria, anorexia, and nausea.
- Examination may show a **pericardial rub, asterixis, hypertension,** ↓ urine output, and an ↑ respiratory rate (compensation of metabolic acidosis or from pulmonary edema 2° to volume overload).
- Category-specific symptoms are as follows:
    - **Prerenal:** Thirst, orthostatic hypotension, tachycardia, ↓ skin turgor, dry mucous membranes.
    - **Intrinsic:** Associated with a history of drug exposure (aminoglycosides, NSAIDs), infection, or exposure to contrast media or toxins (eg, myoglobin, myeloma protein). Hematuria or tea-colored urine, foamy urine (from proteinuria), hypertension, and/or edema may also be present. Other features of systemic diseases that may cause glomerulonephritis include lupus-related hair loss and unilateral peripheral neuropathy of vasculitis.
    - **Atheroemboli:** Subcutaneous nodules, livedo reticularis, digital ischemia.
    - **Postrenal:** Prostatic disease, ↓ urine output leading to suprapubic pain, distended bladder and flank pain.

1 **A**

This is a sign of respiratory muscle fatigue and may require urgent intubation.

2 **A**

This patient likely has rhabdomyolysis, and the urine dipstick is detecting myoglobin. He should be managed with saline hydration, mannitol, bicarbonate, and an ECG to rule out life-threatening hyperkalemia.

DIAGNOSIS

- Check serum electrolytes. Examine the urine for RBCs, WBCs, casts (see Table 2.16-2), and **urine eosinophils.**
- An **$Fe_{Na} < 1\%$, a $U_{Na} < 20$, a urine specific gravity > 1.020, or a BUN/Cr ratio > 20 suggests a prerenal etiology** (see Table 2.16-3).
- A urinary catheter and renal ultrasound can help rule out obstruction. Ultrasound can also identify kidneys that are ↓ in size, as occurs with chronic kidney disease (CKD).
- In patients with oliguria, the Fe_{Na} can help identify prerenal failure and distinguish it from intrinsic renal disease.
- Obtain a renal biopsy only when the cause of intrinsic renal disease is unclear.

TREATMENT

- Balance fluids and electrolytes; avoid nephrotoxic drugs.
- In acute or allergic interstitial nephritis, discontinue offending medications.
- Dialyze if indicated (see the popular mnemonic **AEIOU**) using hemodialysis. Peritoneal dialysis should be considered only for long-term dialysis patients or for patients who are not hemodynamically stable.
- In the setting of postrenal acute kidney injury, treatment often includes an intervention such as nephrostomy tubes, ureteral stents, or a suprapubic catheter.

COMPLICATIONS

- Metabolic acidosis; hyperkalemia leading to arrhythmias.
- Hypertension (from renin hypersecretion).
- Volume overload leading to CHF and pulmonary edema.
- CKD may result, requiring dialysis to prevent the buildup of K^+, H^+, phosphate, and toxic metabolites.

TABLE 2.16-2. Findings on Microscopic Urine Examination in Acute Kidney Injury

URINE SEDIMENT	ETIOLOGY	CLASSIFICATION
Hyaline casts	Normal finding, but an ↑ amount suggests volume depletion.	Prerenal.
Red cell casts, dysmorphic red cells	Glomerulonephritis.	Intrinsic.
White cells, eosinophils	Allergic interstitial nephritis, atheroembolic disease.	Intrinsic.
Granular casts, renal tubular cells, "muddy-brown cast"	ATN.	Intrinsic.
White cells, white cell casts	Pyelonephritis.	Postrenal.

KEY FACT

Acute kidney injury and toxin exposure in the history should lead you to a diagnosis of ATN.

MNEMONIC

Indications for urgent dialysis—

AEIOU

Acidosis
Electrolyte abnormalities (hyperkalemia)
Ingestions (salicylates, theophylline, methanol, barbiturates, lithium, ethylene glycol)
Overload (fluid)
Uremic symptoms (pericarditis, encephalopathy, bleeding, nausea, pruritus, myoclonus)

KEY FACT

Do not give metformin to septic patients or those with renal or hepatic failure because it can worsen the metabolic acidosis.

A 68-year-old female with a history of hepatitis and CKD presents with RUQ abdominal pain. A CT scan identifies liver cirrhosis. Two days later, her creatinine levels have doubled. What is the likely cause, and what could have prevented this outcome?

TABLE 2.16-3. Laboratory Findings in Acute Kidney Injury

TEST	PRERENAL AZOTEMIA	ACUTE TUBULAR NECROSIS
BUN/creatinine	> 20:1	< 20:1
Fractional excretion of sodium (Fe_{Na})	< 1%	> 1%
Urine sodium (U_{Na})	< 20 mEq/L	> 20 mEq/L
Urine osmolality	> 500 mOsm/kg	< 300 mOsm/kg

Chronic Kidney Disease (CKD)

Defined as > 3 months of one of the following: GFR < 60 mL/min, urinary abnormalities (proteinuria/microscopic hematuria), or structural abnormalities. Most commonly due to diabetes mellitus (DM), hypertension, and glomerulonephritis. Another commonly tested etiology is polycystic kidney disease (the autosomal dominant form is more common and is adult onset; the autosomal recessive form is seen in children).

HISTORY/PE

Generally asymptomatic until GFR is < 30 mL/min, but patients gradually experience the signs and symptoms of uremia (anorexia, nausea, vomiting, uremic pericarditis, "uremic frost," delirium, seizures, coma).

DIAGNOSIS

Common metabolic derangements include the following:

- Azotemia (↑ BUN and creatinine).
- Fluid retention (hypertension, edema, CHF, pulmonary edema).
- Metabolic acidosis.
- Hyperkalemia.
- Anemia of chronic disease (↓ erythropoietin production).
- Abnormal hemostasis caused by impaired platelet aggregation.
- Hypocalcemia, hyperphosphatemia (↓ phosphate excretion; impaired vitamin D production leading to renal osteodystrophy).

TREATMENT

- ACEIs/ARBs and hypertension control have been shown to ↓ the progression of CKD.
- Use **desmopressin (DDAVP) in cases of abnormal bleeding.**
- Erythropoietin analogs for anemia of chronic disease.
- Fluid restriction; low Na^+/K^+/phosphate intake.
- Oral phosphate binders and calcitriol (1,25-OH vitamin D) for renal osteodystrophy.
- **Renal replacement therapy** includes hemodialysis, peritoneal dialysis, and renal transplantation.

The patient likely has contrast-induced nephropathy and would have benefited from saline hydration before and during the CT scan. *N*-acetylcysteine and sodium bicarbonate can be used in addition to hydration but are more controversial.

Diuretics

Table 2.16-4 summarizes the mechanisms of action and side effects of commonly used diuretics.

Glomerular Disease

NEPHRITIC SYNDROME

A disorder of glomerular inflammation, also called glomerulonephritis. Proteinuria may be present but is usually < 1.5 g/day. Causes are summarized in Table 2.16-5.

HISTORY/PE

The classic findings are oliguria, macroscopic/microscopic hematuria (tea- or cola-colored urine), hypertension, and **edema.**

DIAGNOSIS

- UA shows hematuria and possibly mild proteinuria.
- Patients have a ↓ GFR with elevated BUN and creatinine. Complement, ANA, ANCA, and anti-GBM antibody levels should be measured to determine the underlying etiology.
- Renal biopsy may be useful for histologic evaluation.

MNEMONIC

Nephritic syndrome findings—

PHAROH

Proteinuria
Hematuria
Azotemia
RBC casts
Oliguria
Hypertension

TABLE 2.16-4. **Mechanism of Action and Side Effects of Diuretics**

TYPE	DRUGS	SITE OF ACTION	MECHANISM OF ACTION	SIDE EFFECTS
Carbonic anhydrase inhibitors	Acetazolamide	Proximal convoluted tubule.	Inhibit carbonic anhydrase, ↑ H^+ reabsorption, block Na^+/H^+ exchange.	Hyperchloremic metabolic acidosis, sulfa allergy.
Osmotic agents	Mannitol, urea	Entire tubule.	↑ tubular fluid osmolarity.	Pulmonary edema due to CHF and anuria.
Loop agents	Furosemide, ethacrynic acid, bumetanide, torsemide	Ascending loop of Henle.	Inhibit $Na^+/K^+/2Cl^-$ transporter.	Water loss, metabolic alkalosis, ↓ K^+, ↓ Ca^{2+}, ototoxicity, sulfa allergy (except ethacrynic acid), hyperuricemia.
Thiazide agents	HCTZ, chlorothiazide	Distal convoluted tubule.	Inhibit Na^+/Cl^- transporter.	Water loss, metabolic alkalosis, ↓ **Na⁺**, ↓ K^+, ↑ glucose, ↑ **Ca²⁺**, ↑ uric acid, sulfa allergy, pancreatitis.
K⁺-sparing agents	Spironolactone, triamterene, amiloride	Cortical collecting tubule.	Aldosterone receptor antagonist (spironolactone); block sodium channel (triamterene, amiloride).	Metabolic acidosis; ↑ K^+; antiandrogenic effects, including gynecomastia (spironolactone).

TABLE 2.16-5. **Causes of Nephritic Syndrome**

DISORDER	DESCRIPTION	HISTORY/PE	LABS/HISTOLOGY	TREATMENT/PROGNOSIS
IMMUNE COMPLEX				
Postinfectious glomerulonephritis	Classically associated with recent group A β-hemolytic **streptococcal infection,** but can be seen with any infection (usually 2–6 weeks prior).	Oliguria, edema, hypertension, tea- or cola-colored urine.	Low serum C3 that normalizes 6–8 weeks after presentation; ↑ **ASO titer; lumpy-bumpy immunofluorescence.**	Supportive with diuretics to prevent fluid overload. Most patients have a complete recovery.
IgA nephropathy (Berger's disease)	The most common type; **typically follows upper respiratory or GI infections.** Commonly seen in young males; may be seen in Henoch-Schönlein purpura.	Episodic gross hematuria or persistent microscopic hematuria.	Normal C3.	Glucocorticoids for select patients; ACEIs in patients with proteinuria. Some 20% of cases progress to end-stage renal disease (ESRD).
PAUCI-IMMUNE				
Wegener's granulomatosis	Granulomatous inflammation of the respiratory tract and kidney with necrotizing vasculitis.	Fever, weight loss, hematuria, hearing disturbances, respiratory and sinus symptoms. Cavitary pulmonary lesions bleed and lead to **hemoptysis.**	Presence of **c-ANCA** (cell-mediated immune response). Renal biopsy shows segmental necrotizing glomerulonephritis with few immunoglobulin deposits on immunofluorescence.	High-dose corticosteroids and cytotoxic agents. Patients tend to have frequent relapses.
ANTI-GBM DISEASE				
Goodpasture's syndrome	Rapidly progressing glomerulonephritis with pulmonary hemorrhage; peak incidence is in males in their mid-20s.	**Hemoptysis,** dyspnea, possible respiratory failure. No upper respiratory tract involvement.	**Linear anti-GBM deposits** on immunofluorescence; iron deficiency anemia; hemosiderin-filled macrophages in sputum; pulmonary infiltrates on CXR.	Plasma exchange therapy; pulsed steroids. May progress to ESRD.
Alport's syndrome	Hereditary glomerulonephritis; presents in boys 5–20 years of age.	Asymptomatic hematuria associated with **sensorineural deafness** and eye disorders.	GBM splitting on electron microscopy (EM).	Progresses to renal failure. Anti-GBM nephritis may recur after transplant.

TREATMENT

- Treat hypertension, fluid overload, and uremia with salt and water restriction, diuretics, and, if necessary, dialysis.
- In some cases, **corticosteroids** are useful in reducing glomerular inflammation.

NEPHROTIC SYNDROME

Defined as **proteinuria (≥ 3.5 g/day), generalized edema, hypoalbuminemia,** and **hyperlipidemia.** Approximately one-third of all cases result from systemic diseases such as DM, SLE, or amyloidosis. Causes are summarized in Table 2.16-6.

TABLE 2.16-6.   Causes of Nephrotic Syndrome

DISORDER	DESCRIPTION	HISTORY/PE	LABS/HISTOLOGY	TREATMENT/PROGNOSIS
Minimal change disease	The most common cause of nephrotic syndrome in **children.** Idiopathic etiology; 2° causes include NSAIDs and hematologic malignancies (eg, Hodgkin's disease).	Tendency toward infections and thrombotic events. Sudden onset of edema.	Light microscopy appears **normal;** EM shows **fusion of epithelial foot processes** with lipid-laden renal cortices.	Steroids; excellent prognosis.
Focal segmental glomerulosclerosis	Idiopathic, **IV drug use, HIV,** obesity.	The typical patient is a young **African American** male with uncontrolled hypertension.	Microscopic hematuria; biopsy shows sclerosis in capillary tufts.	Prednisone, cytotoxic therapy, ACEIs/ARBs to ↓ proteinuria.
Membranous nephropathy	**The most common nephropathy in Caucasian adults.** 2° causes includes solid tumor malignancies (especially in patients > 60 years of age) and immune complex disease.	Associated with HBV, syphilis, malaria, and gold.	**"Spike-and-dome"** appearance due to granular deposits of IgG and C3 at the basement membrane.	Prednisone and cytotoxic therapy for severe disease.
Diabetic nephropathy	Has 2 characteristic forms: diffuse hyalinization and nodular glomerulosclerosis **(Kimmelstiel-Wilson lesions).**	Patients generally have long-standing, poorly controlled DM with evidence of retinopathy or neuropathy.	Thickened GBM; ↑ **mesangial matrix.**	Tight control of blood sugar; ACEIs for type 1 DM and ARBs for type 2 DM.

(continues)

TABLE 2.16-6. Causes of Nephrotic Syndrome *(continued)*

DISORDER	DESCRIPTION	HISTORY/PE	LABS/HISTOLOGY	TREATMENT/PROGNOSIS
Lupus nephritis	Classified as WHO types I–VI. Both nephrotic and nephritic. The severity of renal disease often determines overall prognosis.	Proteinuria or RBCs on UA may be found during evaluation of SLE patients.	Mesangial proliferation; subendothelial and/or subepithelial immune complex deposition.	Prednisone and cytotoxic therapy may slow disease progression.
Renal amyloidosis	1° (plasma cell dyscrasia) and 2° (infectious or inflammatory) are the most common.	Patients may have multiple myeloma or a chronic inflammatory disease (eg, rheumatoid arthritis, TB).	Nodular glomerulosclerosis; EM reveals amyloid fibrils; **apple-green** birefringence with Congo red stain.	Prednisone and melphalan. Bone marrow transplantation may be used for multiple myeloma.
Membranoproliferative nephropathy	Can also be nephritic syndrome. Type I is associated with HCV, cryoglobulinemia, SLE, and subacute bacterial endocarditis.	Idiopathic form is present at 8–30 years of age. Slow progression to renal failure.	**"Tram-track,"** double-layered basement membrane. Type I has subendothelial deposits and mesangial deposits; all 3 types have low serum C3. Type II occurs by way of C3 nephritic factor.	Corticosteroids and cytotoxic agents may help.

HISTORY/PE

- Presents with **generalized edema** and **foamy urine.** In severe cases, dyspnea and ascites may develop.
- Patients have ↑ susceptibility to infection as well as a predisposition to hypercoagulable states with an ↑ risk of venous thrombosis and pulmonary embolism.

DIAGNOSIS

- UA shows **proteinuria** (≥ 3.5 g/day) and lipiduria.
- Blood chemistry shows ↓ **albumin** (< 3 g/dL) and hyperlipidemia.
- Evaluation should include workup for 2° causes.
- Renal biopsy is used to definitively diagnose the underlying etiology.

TREATMENT

- Treat with **protein and salt restriction,** judicious diuretic therapy, and antihyperlipidemics.
- Immunosuppressant medications may be useful for certain etiologies.
- **ACEIs** ↓ proteinuria and diminish the progression of renal disease in patients with renal scarring.
- Vaccinate with 23-polyvalent pneumococcus vaccine (PPV23), as patients are at ↑ risk of *Streptococcus pneumoniae* infection.

Nephrolithiasis

Renal calculi. Stones are most commonly calcium oxalate, but many other types exist (see Table 2.16-7). Risk factors include a ⊕ family history, **low fluid intake,** gout, medications (allopurinol, chemotherapy, loop diuretics), postcolectomy/postileostomy, specific enzyme deficiencies, type I RTA (due to alkaline urinary pH and associated hypocitruria), and hyperparathyroidism. Most common in older males.

HISTORY/PE

- Presents with **acute onset of severe, colicky flank pain** that may **radiate to the testes or vulva** and is associated with nausea and vomiting.
- Patients are unable to get comfortable and shift position frequently (as opposed to those with peritonitis, who lie still).

DIAGNOSIS

- UA may show gross or **microscopic hematuria** (85%) and an **altered urine pH.**
- **Noncontrast abdominal CT scan is the gold standard** for the diagnosis of kidney stones (see Figure 2.16-5). However, plain AXRs are still useful for following the progression/treatment of larger stones.
- **Ultrasound is preferred for pregnant patients and children,** in whom radiation from CT should be avoided.
- KUB (kidney/ureter/bladder radiography) identifies radiopaque stones but will often miss stones that are radiolucent.
- IVP is rarely used.

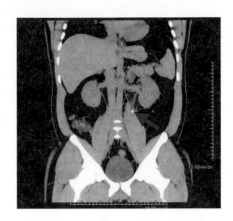

FIGURE 2.16-5. Nephrolithiasis. CT scan shows a dense 1-cm calcification (arrow) in the left ureter, consistent with nephrolithiasis. (Reproduced with permission from Tintinalli JE et al. *Tintinalli's Emergency Medicine: A Comprehensive Study Guide,* 7th ed. New York: McGraw-Hill, 2011, Fig. 97-1A.)

TABLE 2.16-7. Types of Nephrolithiasis

TYPE	FREQUENCY	ETIOLOGY AND CHARACTERISTICS	TREATMENT
Calcium oxalate/calcium phosphate	83%	The most common causes are **idiopathic hypercalciuria** and 1° hyperparathyroidism. Alkaline urine. Radiopaque.	Hydration, dietary sodium and protein restriction, thiazide diuretics. Do not ↓ calcium intake (can lead to hyperoxaluria and an ↑ risk of osteoporosis).
Struvite (Mg-NH_4-PO_4) or "triple phosphate"	9%	Associated with urease-producing organisms (eg, *Proteus*). Form **staghorn calculi.** Alkaline urine. Radiopaque.	Hydration; treat UTI if present; surgical removal of staghorn stone.
Uric acid	7%	Associated with gout, xanthine oxidase deficiency, and high purine turnover states (eg, chemotherapy). Acidic urine (pH < 5.5). **Radiolucent** on plain film, but detectable with CT.	Hydration; alkalinize urine with citrate, which is converted to HCO_3^- in the liver; dietary purine restriction and allopurinol.
Cystine	1%	Due to a defect in renal transport of certain amino acids (COLA—cystine, ornithine, lysine, and arginine). **Hexagonal crystals.** ⊕ **urinary cyanide nitroprusside test.** Radiopaque.	Hydration, dietary sodium restriction, alkalinization of urine, penicillamine.

TREATMENT

- **Hydration and analgesia** are the initial treatment.
- Kidney stones < 5 mm in diameter can pass through the urethra; stones 0.5 cm to 3 cm in diameter can be treated with **extracorporeal shock-wave lithotripsy (ESWL),** percutaneous nephrolithotomy, or retrograde ureteroscopy.
- Preventive measures include **hydration** and dietary changes.
- Dietary changes to prevent calcium stones include ↑ fluid intake (most important), ↑ **calcium intake,** ↓ dietary protein/oxalate intake, and ↓ sodium intake.

Polycystic Kidney Disease (PKD)

Characterized by the presence of progressive cystic dilation of the renal tubules, as well as by cysts in the spleen, liver, and pancreas. The 2 major forms are as follows:

- **Autosomal dominant (ADPKD):**
  - Most common.
  - Usually asymptomatic until patients are > 30 years of age.
  - One-half of ADPKD patients will have ESRD requiring dialysis by age 60.
  - Associated with an ↑ risk of cerebral aneurysm, especially in patients with a ⊕ family history.
- **Autosomal recessive (ARPKD):** Less common but more severe. Presents in infants and young children with renal failure, liver fibrosis, and portal hypertension; may lead to death in the first few years of life.

HISTORY/PE

- **Pain and hematuria** are the most common presenting symptoms. Sharp, localized pain may result from cyst rupture, infection, or passage of renal calculi.
- Additional findings include **hypertension, hepatic cysts, cerebral berry aneurysms,** diverticulosis, and mitral valve prolapse.
- Patients may have large, palpable kidneys on abdominal exam.

DIAGNOSIS

Based on ultrasound (most common) or CT scan (see Figure 2.16-6). Multiple bilateral cysts will be present throughout the renal parenchyma, and renal enlargement will be visualized. Genetic testing by DNA linkage analysis for ADPKD1 and ADPKD2 is available.

TREATMENT

- **Prevent complications and ↓ the rate of progression to ESRD.** Early management of UTIs is critical to prevent renal cyst infection. BP control (ACEIs, ARBs) is necessary to ↓ hypertension-induced renal damage.
- Dialysis and renal transplantation are used to manage patients with ESRD.

Hydronephrosis

Dilation of renal calyces. Usually occurs 2° to obstruction of the urinary tract. In pediatric patients, the obstruction is often at the ureteropelvic junction. In adults, it may be due to BPH, neurogenic bladder (diabetics/spinal cord inju-

KEY FACT

If a patient with known ADPKD develops a sudden-onset, severe headache, you must rule out SAH from a ruptured berry aneurysm!

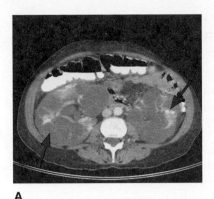 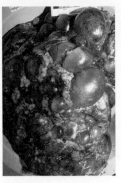

A   **B**

FIGURE 2.16-6. **Autosomal dominant polycystic kidney disease.** (A) Contrast-enhanced CT scan demonstrates bilaterally enlarged kidneys that have been almost entirely replaced by cysts (arrows). (B) Gross specimen of a right kidney from a patient with ADPKD who underwent renal transplantation. (Image A reproduced with permission from Fauci AS et al. *Harrison's Principles of Internal Medicine,* 17th ed. New York: McGraw-Hill, 2008, Fig. 278-1B. Image B reproduced with permission from USMLERx.com.)

ries), tumors, aortic aneurysms, or renal calculi. Can also be caused by high-output urinary flow and vesicoureteral reflux.

HISTORY/PE

May be asymptomatic, or may present with flank/back pain, ↓ urine output, abdominal pain, and UTIs.

DIAGNOSIS

- **Ultrasound** or CT scan to detect dilation of the renal calyces and/or ureter (see Figure 2.16-7).
- ↑ BUN and creatinine provide evidence of 2° renal failure.

TREATMENT

- Surgically correct any anatomic obstruction; use laser or sound wave lithotripsy if calculi are causing obstruction.
- Ureteral stent placement across the obstructed area of the urinary tract and/or percutaneous nephrostomy tube placement to relieve pressure may be appropriate if the urinary outflow tract is not sufficiently cleared of obstruction. Foley or suprapubic catheters may be required for lower urinary tract obstruction (eg, **BPH**).

A 19-year-old male with a history of recurrent kidney stones presents with acute left flank pain. His father also has a history of kidney stones. A urinary cyanide nitroprusside test is ⊕. A CT scan confirms nephrolithiasis. What is the most likely diagnosis?

KEY FACT

Left untreated, hydronephrosis resulting from urinary obstruction leads to hypertension, acute or chronic renal failure, or sepsis and has a very poor prognosis.

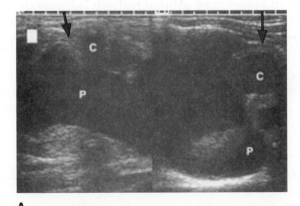 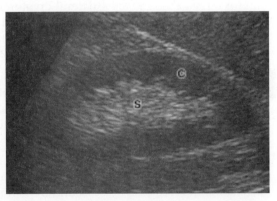

A   **B**

FIGURE 2.16-7. **Hydronephrosis.** (A) Ultrasound of a renal transplant shows severe hydronephrosis, with dilation of the renal pelvis (P) and the renal calyces (C). The overlying renal cortex is severely thinned (arrows). (B) Normal renal ultrasound for comparison. C = cortex; S = sinus fat. (Reproduced with permission from Tanagho EA, McAninch JW. *Smith's General Urology,* 17th ed. New York: McGraw-Hill, 2008, Fig. 6-22.)

Cystinuria. You would also likely see hexagonal crystals on UA.

KEY FACT

Posterior urethral valves are the most common congenital urethral obstruction. Classic findings are a male infant with a distended, palpable bladder and low urine output.

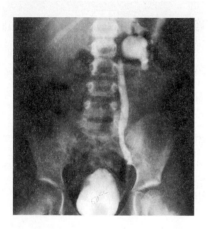

FIGURE 2.16-8. Vesicoureteral reflux. Frontal radiograph from a voiding cystourethrogram shows reflux to the left ureter and intrarenal collecting system with hydronephrosis. Note the absence of reflux on the normal right side. (Reproduced with permission from Doherty GM. *Current Diagnosis & Treatment: Surgery,* 13th ed. New York: McGraw-Hill, 2010, Fig. 38-7.)

KEY FACT

Bringing the testes into the scrotum does **not** ↓ the risk of testicular cancer.

Vesicoureteral Reflux

Retrograde projection of urine from the bladder to the ureters and kidneys. May be due to posterior urethral valves, urethral or meatal stenosis, or a neurogenic bladder. Classified as follows:

- **Mild reflux (grades I–II):** No ureteral or renal pelvic dilation. Often resolves spontaneously.
- **Moderate to severe reflux (grade III–V):** Ureteral dilation with associated caliceal blunting in severe cases.

HISTORY/PE

Patients present with recurrent UTIs, typically in childhood. Prenatal ultrasound may identify hydronephrosis.

DIAGNOSIS

Obtain a **voiding cystourethrogram** (VCUG) to detect abnormalities at ureteral insertion sites and to classify the grade of reflux (see Figure 2.16-8). For children 2 years of age and under with their first febrile UTI, an ultrasound should first be obtained and a VCUG only performed if there is evidence of scarring, hydronephrosis, or other findings suspicious for high-grade VUR.

TREATMENT

- Treat infections aggressively. Treat mild reflux with daily prophylactic antibiotics (amoxicillin if < 2 months of age; otherwise TMP-SMX or nitrofurantoin) until reflux resolves.
- Surgery (ureteral reimplantation) is generally reserved for children with persistent high-grade (III to V) reflux. Inadequate treatment can lead to progressive renal scarring and ESRD.

Cryptorchidism

Failure of 1 or both of the testes to fully descend into the scrotum. **Low birth weight is a risk factor.**

HISTORY/PE

Bilateral cryptorchidism is associated with prematurity, oligospermia, congenital malformation syndromes (Prader-Willi, Noonan syndromes), and infertility. Associated with an ↑ **risk of testicular malignancy.**

DIAGNOSIS

The testes **cannot be manipulated into the scrotal sac** with gentle pressure (vs. retractile testes) and may be palpated anywhere along the inguinal canal or in the abdomen.

TREATMENT

- **Orchiopexy** by 6–12 months of age (most testes will spontaneously descend by 3 months).
- If discovered later, treat with orchiectomy to avoid the risk of testicular cancer.

Scrotal Swelling

Table 2.16-8 outlines the etiologies, presentation, diagnosis, and treatment of scrotal swelling.

TABLE 2.16-8.   Differential Diagnosis of Scrotal Swelling

DISORDER	CAUSE	HISTORY/PE	DIAGNOSIS	TREATMENT
PAINLESS CAUSES				
Hydrocele	Remnant of the processus vaginalis.	Usually asymptomatic; **transilluminates.**	Lab and radiologic workups are rarely indicated. Obtain an ultrasound if there is concern for inguinal hernia or testicular cancer.	**Typically none** unless hernia is present or hydrocele persists beyond 12–18 months of age (indicates patent processus vaginalis, which leads to an ↑ risk for inguinal hernia).
Varicocele	Dilation of the pampiniform venous plexus ("bag of worms").	Asymptomatic or presents with vague, aching scrotal pain. Affects the left testicle more often than the right. May disappear in the supine position. Does **not** transilluminate.	Ultrasound.	If symptomatic or if testis makes up < 40% of total volume, may be treated surgically with a varicocelectomy or ligation, or through embolization via interventional radiology.
PAINFUL CAUSES				
Epididymitis	Infection of the epididymis, usually from STDs, prostatitis, and/or reflux.	Typically affects those > 30 years of age; presents with epididymal tenderness, tender/enlarged testicle(s), fever, scrotal thickening, erythema, and pyuria. Pain may ↓ with scrotal elevation (⊕ Prehn's sign).	UA, culture (pyuria). Culture often shows *Neisseria gonorrhoeae, E coli*, or *Chlamydia*. Doppler ultrasound shows normal to ↑ blood flow to testes.	Antibiotics (tetracycline, fluoroquinolones); NSAIDs; scrotal support for pain.
Testicular torsion	Twisting of the spermatic cord, leading to ischemia and possible testicular infarction.	Typically affects those < 30 years of age; presents with intense, acute-onset scrotal pain that remains the same or ↑ with scrotal elevation (⊖ Prehn's sign). Pain is often accompanied by nausea/vomiting and/or dizziness. Loss of cremasteric reflex is also seen.	Doppler ultrasound shows ↓ blood flow to the testes (see Figure 2.16-9). (If there is a high clinical suspicion for testicular torsion, do not wait for ultrasound and proceed immediately to surgery!)	Attempt manual detorsion. Immediate surgery to salvage testis (the testicle is often unsalvageable after 6 hours of ischemia). Orchiopexy of **both** testes to prevent future torsion.

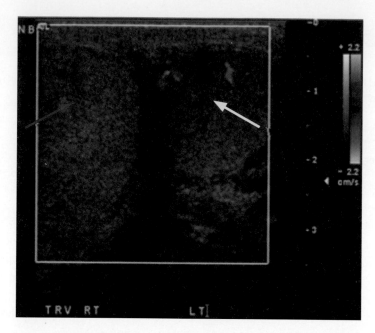

FIGURE 2.16-9. **Testicular torsion.** Transverse Doppler image through the scrotum demonstrates asymmetric swelling and decreased blood flow to the right testis (red arrow) compared to the left testis (yellow arrow) in this patient with acute right testicular pain. (Reproduced with permission from USMLERx.com.)

Erectile Dysfunction (ED)

Found in 10–25% of middle-aged and elderly men. Classified as failure to initiate (eg, psychological, endocrinologic, neurologic), failure to fill (eg, arteriogenic), or failure to store (eg, veno-occlusive dysfunction). Risk factors include **DM, atherosclerosis, medications** (eg, β-blockers, SSRIs, TCAs, diuretics), hypertension, heart disease, surgery or radiation for prostate cancer, and spinal cord injury.

HISTORY/PE

- Ask about risk factors (diabetes, peripheral vascular disease), **medication use,** recent life changes, and psychological stressors.
- The distinction between psychological and organic ED is based on the presence of **nocturnal or early-morning erections** (if present, it is nonorganic) and on **situation dependence** (ie, occurring with only 1 partner).
- Evaluate for **neurologic dysfunction** (eg, anal tone, lower extremity sensation) and for **hypogonadism** (eg, small testes, loss of 2° sexual characteristics).

DIAGNOSIS

- **Testosterone** and **gonadotropin** levels may be abnormal.
- Check prolactin levels, as elevated **prolactin** can result in ↓ androgen activity.

TREATMENT

- Patients with psychological ED may benefit from psychotherapy involving discussion and exercises with the partner.
- Oral **sildenafil (Viagra), vardenafil (Levitra),** and **tadalafil (Cialis)** are phosphodiesterase-5 (PDE5) inhibitors that result in prolonged action of

KEY FACT

"**P**oint and **S**hoot": The **P**arasympathetic nervous system mediates erection; the **S**ympathetic nervous system mediates ejaculation.

- cGMP-mediated smooth muscle relaxation and ↑ blood flow in the corpora cavernosa.
- **Testosterone** is a useful therapy for patients with hypogonadism of testicular or pituitary origin; it is discouraged for patients with normal testosterone levels.
- Vacuum pumps, intracavernosal prostaglandin injections, and surgical implantation of semirigid or inflatable penile prostheses are alternatives for patients who fail PDE5 therapy.

KEY FACT

Which drugs are an absolute contraindication to sildenafil? **Nitrates** (the combined effect of ↓ BP can lead to myocardial ischemia).

Benign Prostatic Hyperplasia (BPH)

Enlargement of the prostate that is a normal part of the aging process and is seen in > **80% of men by age 80.** Most commonly presents in men > **50 years of age.** BPH can result in urinary retention, recurrent UTIs, bladder and renal calculi, hydronephrosis, and kidney damage over time.

HISTORY/PE

- **Obstructive symptoms:** Hesitancy, weak stream, intermittent stream, incomplete emptying, urinary retention, bladder fullness.
- **Irritative symptoms:** Nocturia, daytime frequency, urge incontinence, opening hematuria.
- On digital rectal examination (DRE), the prostate is uniformly enlarged with a rubbery texture. If the prostate is hard or has irregular lesions, cancer should be suspected.

DIAGNOSIS

- Conduct a **DRE** to screen for masses; if findings are suspicious, evaluate for prostate cancer.
- Obtain a **UA and urine culture** to rule out infection and hematuria.
- Measure **creatinine levels** to rule out obstructive uropathy and renal insufficiency.
- PSA testing and cystoscopy are not recommended for longitudinal BPH monitoring.

KEY FACT

BPH most commonly occurs in the central (periurethral) zone of the prostate and may not be detected on DRE.

TREATMENT

- **Medical therapy** includes α-blockers (eg, terazosin), which relax smooth muscle in the prostate and bladder neck, as well as 5α-reductase inhibitors (eg, finasteride), which inhibit the production of dihydrotestosterone.
- Transurethral resection of the prostate (TURP) or open prostatectomy is appropriate for patients with moderate to severe symptoms.

Prostate Cancer

The **most common cancer in men** and the **second leading cause of cancer death** in men (after lung cancer). Risk factors include advanced age and a ⊕ family history.

HISTORY/PE

- Usually **asymptomatic,** but may present with obstructive urinary symptoms (eg, **urinary retention,** a ↓ in the force of the urine stream) as well as with lymphedema due to obstructing metastases, constitutional symptoms, and **back pain due to bone metastases.**

KEY FACT

Leading causes of cancer death in men:
1. Lung cancer
2. Prostate cancer
3. Colorectal cancer
4. Pancreatic cancer
5. Leukemia

- DRE may reveal a **palpable nodule** or an area of induration (see Figure 2.16-10). Early carcinoma is usually not detectable on examination.
- A tender prostate suggests prostatitis.

DIAGNOSIS

- Suggested by clinical findings and/or a markedly ↑ **PSA** (> 4 ng/mL).
- Definitive diagnosis is made with **ultrasound-guided transrectal** biopsy, which typically shows adenocarcinoma.
- Tumors are graded by the **Gleason histologic system,** which sums the scores (from 1 to 5) of the 2 most dysplastic samples (10 is the highest grade).
- Look for metastases with CXR and **bone scan** (metastatic lesions show an **osteoblastic** or ↑ bone density). Fully 40% of patients present with metastatic disease at diagnosis.

TREATMENT

- Treatment is controversial, as many cases of prostate cancer are slow to progress. Treatment choice is based on the aggressiveness of the tumor and the patient's mortality risk.
- **Watchful waiting** may be the best approach for elderly patients with low-grade tumors.
- **Radical prostatectomy** and **radiation therapy** (eg, brachytherapy or external beam) are associated with an ↑ risk of incontinence and/or impotence.
- **PSA,** while controversial as a screening test, is used to follow patients post-treatment to evaluate for disease recurrence.
- Treat metastatic disease with **androgen ablation** (eg, GnRH agonists, orchiectomy, flutamide) and chemotherapy.

PREVENTION

- All males > 50 years of age should have an **annual DRE.** Screening should begin earlier in African American males and in those with a first-degree relative with prostate cancer.
- Screening with PSA is common, but its utility remains controversial.

> **KEY FACT**
>
> An elevated PSA may be due to BPH, prostatitis, UTI, prostatic trauma, or carcinoma.

> **KEY FACT**
>
> An annual DRE after age 50 is the recommended screening method for prostate cancer.

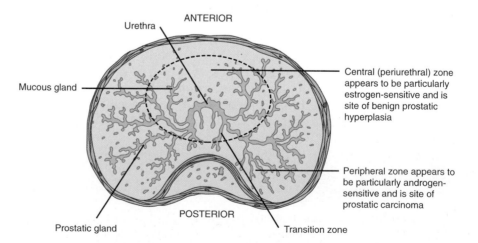

FIGURE 2.16-10. Structure of the prostate. (Adapted with permission from Chandrasoma P, Taylor CE. *Concise Pathology,* 3rd ed. Originally published by Appleton & Lange. Copyright © 1998 by the McGraw-Hill Companies, Inc.)

Bladder Cancer

The second most common urologic cancer and the most frequent malignant tumor of the urinary tract; usually a **transitional cell carcinoma.** Most prevalent in males during the sixth and seventh decades. Risk factors include **smoking,** diets rich in meat and fat, schistosomiasis, chronic treatment with cyclophosphamide, and occupational exposure to **aniline dye.**

History/PE

- **Gross hematuria** is the most common presenting symptom.
- Other urinary symptoms, such as frequency, urgency, and dysuria, may also be seen, but most patients are asymptomatic in the early stages of disease.

Diagnosis

- **Cystoscopy with biopsy is diagnostic** and is recommended in the evaluation of older adults to rule out malignancy.
- **UA** often shows hematuria (macro- or microscopic).
- **Cytology** may show dysplastic cells.
- **MRI, CT,** and bone scan are important tools with which to define invasion and metastases.
- **IVP** can examine the upper urinary tract as well as defects in bladder filling. Seldom used.

Treatment

Treatment depends on the extent of spread beyond the bladder mucosa.

- **Carcinoma in situ:** Intravesicular chemotherapy.
- **Superficial cancers:** Complete transurethral resection or intravesicular chemotherapy with mitomycin-C or BCG (the TB vaccine).
- **Large, high-grade recurrent lesions:** Intravesicular chemotherapy.
- **Invasive cancers without metastases:** Radical cystectomy or radiotherapy for patients who are deemed poor candidates for radical cystectomy as well as for those with unresectable local disease.
- **Invasive cancers with distant metastases:** Chemotherapy alone.

Renal Cell Carcinoma

An adenocarcinoma from tubular epithelial cells (~ 80–90% of all malignant tumors of the kidney). Tumors can spread along the renal vein to the IVC and can metastasize to lung and bone. Risk factors include male **gender, smoking, obesity, acquired cystic kidney disease in ESRD,** and von Hippel–Lindau disease.

History/PE

- Presenting signs include **hematuria, flank pain,** and a **palpable flank mass.** Metastatic disease can present with weight loss and malaise.
- Many patients have **fever** or other constitutional symptoms. Left-sided varicocele may be seen in males (due to tumor blockage of the left gonadal vein, which empties into the left renal vein; the right gonadal vein empties directly into the IVC).
- **Anemia is common at presentation,** but **polycythemia** due to ↑ erythropoietin production may be seen in 5–10% of patients.

MNEMONIC

Differential for hematuria—

I PEE RBCS

Infection (UTI)
Polycystic kidney disease
Exercise
External trauma
Renal glomerular disease
Benign prostatic hyperplasia
Cancer
Stones

KEY FACT

The classic triad of renal cell carcinoma is hematuria, flank pain, and a palpable flank mass, but only 5–10% present with all 3 components of the triad.

DIAGNOSIS

Ultrasound and/or CT (see Figure 2.16-11) to characterize the renal mass (usually complex cysts or solid tumor).

TREATMENT

- **Surgical resection** may be curative in localized disease.
- Response rates from radiation or chemotherapy are only 15–30%. Newer tyrosine kinase inhibitors (sorafenib, sunitinib), which ↓ tumor angiogenesis and cell proliferation, have shown promising results and have recently been approved by the FDA for the treatment of renal cell carcinoma.

Testicular Cancer

A heterogeneous group of neoplasms. Some 95% of testicular tumors derive from **germ cells,** and **virtually all are malignant. Cryptorchidism** is associated with an ↑ risk of neoplasia in both testes. **Klinefelter's syndrome** is also a risk factor. Testicular cancer is the most common malignancy in males 15–34 years of age.

HISTORY/PE

- Patients most often present with **painless enlargement of the testes.**
- Most testicular cancers occur between ages 15 and 30, but seminomas have a peak incidence between 40 and 50 years of age.

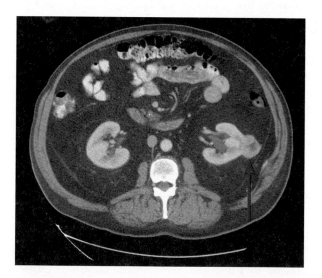

FIGURE 2.16-11. **Renal cell carcinoma.** A contrast-enhanced CT through the abdomen demonstrates an enhancing exophytic mass (arrow) in the left kidney that proved on pathology to be renal cell carcinoma. (Reproduced with permission from Doherty GM. *Current Diagnosis & Treatment: Surgery,* 13th ed. New York: McGraw-Hill, 2010, Fig. 38-12A.)

DIAGNOSIS

- **Testicular** ultrasound.
- **CXR** and abdominal/pelvic CT to evaluate for metastasis.
- **Tumor markers** are useful for diagnosis and in monitoring treatment response.
- β-hCG is always elevated in choriocarcinoma and is elevated in 10% of seminomas.
- α-fetoprotein is often elevated in nonseminomatous germ cell tumors, particularly endodermal sinus (yolk sac) tumors. It is also elevated in hepatocellular carcinoma, hepatoblastoma, and neuroblastoma.

TREATMENT

- Radical orchiectomy.
- Seminomas are **exquisitely radiosensitive** and also respond to chemotherapy.
- Platinum-based chemotherapy is used for nonseminomatous germ cell tumors.

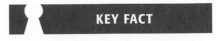

KEY FACT

β-hCG in men = choriocarcinoma.

NOTES

SELECTED TOPICS IN EMERGENCY MEDICINE

1° survey of a trauma patient—

ABCDE

Airway
Breathing
Circulation
Disability
Exposure

KEY FACT

Suspect thermal or inhalational injury to the airway in patients with singed nasal hairs, facial burns, hoarseness, wheezing, soot in the posterior oropharynx, or carbonaceous sputum.

KEY FACT

GCS < 8 = intubate!

KEY FACT

To remember the GCS, think **4**-eyes, Jackson **5,** V**6** engine: 4 points can be assigned for eye response, 5 points for verbal response, and 6 points for motor response.

Trauma Management

The steps underlying the acute management of a trauma patient can be remembered with the mnemonic **ABCDE**. **Establishing and maintaining airway patency takes precedence over all other treatment.** This is followed by maintaining sufficient respiratory support and ensuring adequate circulation for end-organ function.

1° SURVEY

- **Airway:**
  - Visualize the airway. Check for obstruction from secretions, soft tissue, or foreign bodies (broken teeth).
  - Start with supplemental O_2 by nasal cannula or face mask for conscious patients. Use a jaw-thrust maneuver to lift the tongue off the posterior oropharynx in an unconscious patient. A chin-lift maneuver can be further utilized to align the airway, but caution must be taken to avoid hyperextending the neck and moving the potentially unstable C-spine. An oropharyngeal (OP) or nasopharyngeal (NP) airway adjunct can help splint open proximal airways if further respiratory support is needed.
  - Intubate patients with apnea, significantly depressed mental status (Glasgow Coma Scale [GCS] < 8; see Table 2.17-1), or impending airway compromise (eg, significant maxillofacial trauma or inhalation injury in fires).
  - Perform a surgical airway (cricothyroidotomy) in patients who cannot be intubated 2° to upper airway trauma or obstruction.
  - **Maintain cervical spine stabilization/immobilization in trauma patients** until the spine is cleared through examination and radiographic studies. However, **never allow this concern to delay airway management.**
- **Breathing:**
  - Cardiac and pulmonary examinations will identify thoracic causes of immediate death: **tension pneumothorax, open pneumothorax, flail chest and pulmonary contusion, massive hemothorax, cardiac tamponade,** and **airway obstruction.**
  - If tension pneumothorax (absent breath sounds on the affected side in combination with hypotension, distended neck veins, hypoxemia, and

TABLE 2.17-1. GCS Scoring

SCORE	EYE (4)	VERBAL (5)	MOTOR (6)
6			Follows commands
5		Oriented	Localizes pain
4	Spontaneous	Confused speech	Withdraws to pain
3	To command	Inappropriate words	Flexion
2	To pain	Incomprehensible	Extension
1	None	None	None

tracheal deviation) is identified, **immediate needle decompression is warranted.** This should be immediately followed by placement of a thoracostomy tube. Although the diagnosis is clinical, you should be able to recognize it radiographically (see Figure 2.17-1).

- If open pneumothorax is identified, an occlusive dressing must be applied immediately. Secure on 3 sides only to prevent the development of tension pneumothorax. Place a thoracostomy tube as soon as the 1° survey has been completed.
- Massive hemothorax is diagnosed through chest tube placement and is defined as > 1500 cc of immediate blood return. The treatment is volume resuscitation and chest decompression followed by operative management.

- **Circulation:**
  - Apply direct pressure to actively bleeding wounds. Splint any long-bone deformities or suspected fractures to limit blood loss.
  - Place a 16-gauge IV in each antecubital fossa.
  - Isotonic fluids (LR or NS) are repleted in a **3:1 ratio (fluid to blood loss).** Start with a fluid bolus of 1–2 L in adults; then recheck vitals and continue repletion as indicated. If the patient remains unstable (eg, tachycardia, hypotension), consider transfusion with packed RBCs.
  - Patients with chest trauma and shock may have **cardiac tamponade.** The triad of physical examination signs are **JVD, hypotension, and muffled heart sounds.** This can be diagnosed with bedside ultrasound (see Figure 2.17-2). If tamponade is diagnosed, perform an immediate pericardiocentesis.

- **Disability/Exposure:**
  - Disability (CNS dysfunction) is assessed and quantified with the GCS.
  - Exposure requires that the patient be completely disrobed and assessed for injury and temperature status on both the front and back of the body. Hypothermia is a common problem and can worsen bleeding; once the examination is done, the patient should be covered.

KEY FACT

Immediately evaluate trauma patients for open pneumothorax, tension pneumothorax, flail chest, massive hemothorax, cardiac tamponade, and airway obstruction.

KEY FACT

A rough estimate of systolic BP can be made on the basis of palpated pulses. Carotids correspond roughly to an SBP of 60 mm Hg, femorals to an SBP of 70 mm Hg, and radials to an SBP of 80 mm Hg.

2° SURVEY

- After the patient's ABCs are stabilized, conduct a full examination.
- For unstable patients with abdominal pain or suspected hemoperitoneum or cardiac tamponade, do a focused abdominal sonography for trauma

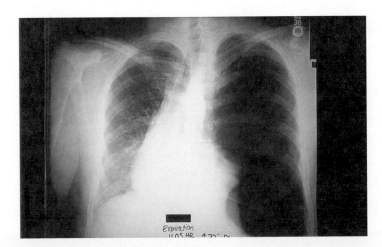

FIGURE 2.17-1.   Tension pneumothorax. Note the hyperlucent left hemithorax, flattening and inferior displacement of the left diaphragm, and rightward shift of the mediastinal structures. These are typical radiographic findings in patients with tension pneumothorax.

Q

A 19-year-old male is brought to the ER after sustaining a gunshot wound to the chest. On arrival, he has a BP of 60/30 mm Hg, ↓ breath sounds on the left side, distended neck veins, and tracheal deviation to the right side. What is the most appropriate next step in management?

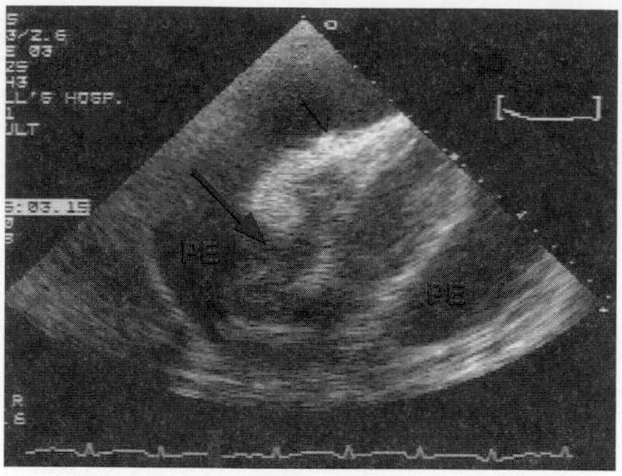

FIGURE 2.17-2. Cardiac tamponade. Echocardiogram in a patient with cardiac tamponade shows a large pericardial effusion (PE) with right atrial (arrow) and right ventricular (arrowhead) collapse. (Reproduced with permission from Hall JB et al. *Principles of Critical Care,* 3rd ed. New York: McGraw-Hill, 2005, Fig. 28-7A.)

KEY FACT

Suspect urethral injury in the presence of blood at the urethral meatus, perineal ecchymosis, blood in the scrotum, a high-riding/nonpalpable prostate, or a pelvic fracture. A retrograde urethrogram can confirm urethral integrity.

(**FAST**) scan. Hemoperitoneum requires immediate surgical consultation for possible operative management; blood in the pericardial sac surrounding the heart warrants immediate pericardiocentesis.

- Radiology studies should be ordered on the basis of the patient assessment. A CXR is needed for all patients with thoracic trauma. A head CT should be ordered for all patients with loss of consciousness or depressed mental status. A C-spine CT is needed for all patients with neck pain or tenderness, neurologic findings, or depressed mental status.
- After urethral injury has been ruled out, place a Foley catheter if it is necessary to monitor urine output (eg, in hemodynamically unstable patients, those receiving fluid resuscitation, or those undergoing major surgery).
- Pertinent labs should be based on the mechanism of injury, suspicion of intoxication or OD, and past medical history.

Penetrating Trauma

The evaluation and treatment of penetrating trauma depend on the location and extent of the injury.

NECK

- Intubate early.
- Immediate surgical exploration is mandatory for patients with shock and active hemorrhage from neck wounds.
- All wounds that violate the platysma are considered true penetrating neck trauma.
- Diagnostic workup depends on the location of the wound, suspected injuries, and the preference of the trauma surgeon. Appropriate tests may include angiography of the aorta and carotid/cerebral arteries, CT scan of the neck with or without CT angiography, Doppler ultrasound, contrast esophagogram, esophagoscopy, or bronchoscopy.

A

Insert a 14-gauge IV angiocatheter into the second intercostal space at the midclavicular line to achieve emergent decompression of the tension pneumothorax. Then place a chest tube.

CHEST

- Unstable patients with penetrating thoracic injuries require immediate **intubation** followed by assessment and treatment of the life-threatening injuries described above. Empiric placement of bilateral chest tubes may be needed if the precise nature of injury is unclear.

- Open thoracotomy may be indicated for patients with penetrating chest trauma leading to cardiac arrest **provided that the patient arrested in the ER or shortly before arrival.**
- Leave any impaled objects in place until the patient is taken to the OR, as such objects may tamponade further blood loss.
- Beware of tension pneumothorax, open pneumothorax, massive hemothorax, flail chest and pulmonary contusion, cardiac tamponade, aortic disruption, diaphragmatic tear, and esophageal injury.
- If a previously stable chest trauma patient suddenly dies, suspect **air embolism.**
- A new diastolic murmur after chest trauma suggests aortic dissection.

ABDOMEN

- The absence of pain does not rule out an abdominal injury.
- Gunshot wounds below the fourth intercostal space (level of the nipple) usually require immediate exploratory laparotomy, although stable patients can be managed conservatively in select cases.
- Stab wounds in a hemodynamically unstable patient or in a patient with peritoneal signs or evisceration require immediate exploratory laparotomy.
- Penetrating stab wounds in a hemodynamically stable patient warrant a CT followed by close inpatient observation.

MUSCULOSKELETAL

- Complete neurovascular assessment is critical; check pulses, motor function, and sensory function.
- Arteriography and surgical management are required for patients with suspected vascular injuries.
- Nerve injuries generally require surgical repair.
- **Early wound irrigation** and **tissue debridement,** not antibiotic therapy, are the most important steps in the treatment of contaminated wounds. However, do administer antibiotics and tetanus prophylaxis.

Blunt and Deceleration Trauma

HEAD

- Look for signs of ↑ intracranial pressure (ICP) such as bradycardia, hypertension, respiratory depression, fixed and dilated pupil(s), vomiting, and/or papilledema. Treat ↑ ICP with head elevation, hyperventilation, and IV mannitol. Consider surgical decompression.
- A rapid-deceleration head injury causes **coup-contrecoup** injuries, in which a bleed is noted both at the site of impact and across from the point of impact.
- Diffuse axonal injury often occurs with rapid-deceleration head injuries. CT characteristically shows blurring and punctate hemorrhaging along the gray–white matter junction. Reduce 2° injury by limiting cerebral edema and increases in ICP.
- **Epidural hematomas:** Lenticular or biconvex in shape on head CT (see Figure 2.17-3A). The bleed is often from the middle meningeal artery (the higher arterial pressure is able to push the dura away from the skull, caus-

Q   **1**

A 25-year-old male walks into the ER holding a blood-soaked towel against his neck after being stabbed by his girlfriend. The patient is calm and his vitals are stable. Physical examination reveals that the knife wound extends through the platysma muscle. What is the next step in management?

Q   **2**

A 10-year-old male is brought to the ER 5 hours after he hit his head on a concrete sidewalk after falling off his skateboard. He briefly lost consciousness at the scene, but his neurologic exam and head CT are normal. What is the next step in ER management?

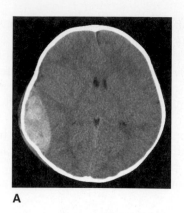
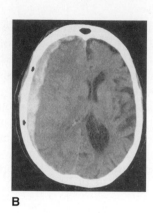

A   **B**

FIGURE 2.17-3. **Acute epidural and acute subdural hematoma.** (**A**) Noncontrast CT showing a right temporal acute epidural hematoma. Note the characteristic **biconvex** shape. (**B**) Noncontrast CT demonstrating a right acute holohemispheric subdural hematoma. Note the characteristic **crescentic** shape. (Image A reproduced with permission from Doherty GM. *Current Diagnosis & Treatment: Surgery,* 13th ed. New York: McGraw-Hill, 2010, Fig. 36-8. Image B reproduced with permission from Chen MY et al. *Basic Radiology,* 1st ed. New York: McGraw-Hill, 2004, Fig. 12-32.)

ing the lens shape on imaging). These bleeds **cannot cross suture lines** but can expand rapidly and cause herniation and death. Patients classically have loss of consciousness immediately after the injury and then have a "lucid interval" after which they become comatose. Examination may show ipsilateral blown pupil and contralateral hemiparesis. Emergent craniotomy is needed.

- **Subdural hematomas:** Follow the curve of the skull and result from damage to the dural bridging veins (see Figure 2.17-3B). These bleeds **can cross suture lines.** They may present acutely (immediate), subacutely (days), or chronically (weeks).

1   **A**

Admit the patient for surgical consultation and possible exploration of the wound. All penetrating trauma that violates the platysma muscle mandates admission and surgical consultation for surgery or further diagnostic evaluation.

2   **A**

Discharge the patient. If the head CT is normal, patients with mild to moderate head injuries can be discharged with instructions to return immediately if neurologic symptoms develop.

CHEST

- Tracheobronchial disruption is most often caused by deceleration shearing forces. Physical findings include respiratory distress, hemoptysis, sternal tenderness, and subcutaneous emphysema. Radiographs may show a large pneumothorax or pneumomediastinum (see Figure 2.17-4).
- Blunt cardiac injury (aka myocardial contusion) may present as a new bundle branch block, dysrhythmia, or hypotension. Serum cardiac biomarkers are often elevated. Intervention is rarely required.
- Pulmonary contusion may lead to hypoxia due to damage to capillaries and leakage of intra- and extravascular fluid. Hypoxia tends to worsen with fluid hydration. Look for patchy alveolar opacities on CXR. Maintain adequate ventilation and control pain. More common in children because of a less rigid, protective chest wall.

Aortic Disruption

The classic cause is a **rapid-deceleration injury** (eg, high-speed motor vehicle accidents, ejection from vehicles, falls from heights). Since complete aortic rupture is rapidly fatal (85% die at the scene), patients with aortic disruption who are seen in the ER usually have a contained hematoma within the adventitia. Laceration is most common just proximal to the ligamentum arteriosum.

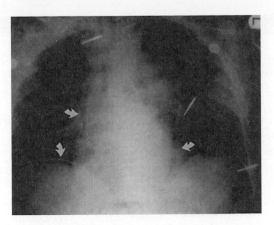

FIGURE 2.17-4.   Pneumomediastinum and pneumoperitoneum. The lucency outlining the heart borders on CXR suggests air in the mediastinum. Also note the air under the right hemidiaphragm, indicating perforated viscus. (Reproduced with permission from Goldfrank LR. *Toxic Emergencies*, 6th ed. Stamford, CT: Appleton & Lange, 1998: 285.)

DIAGNOSIS

- Possible clinical findings include upper extremity hypertension and a hoarse, quiet voice from impingement of the recurrent laryngeal nerve.
- **Immediate CXR** reveals a **widened mediastinum** (> 8 cm), **loss of aortic knob, pleural cap,** deviation of the trachea and esophagus to the right, and depression of the left main stem bronchus.
- CT evaluation and/or transesophageal echocardiography (TEE) prior to surgery.
- **Aortography is the gold standard for evaluation.**

TREATMENT

Basic trauma management (ABCs); emergent surgery for defect repair.

Flail Chest

Three or more adjacent ribs fractured at 2 points, causing paradoxical inward movement of the flail segment with inspiration.

HISTORY/PE

Presents with crepitus and abnormal chest wall movement. Abnormal chest wall movement may not be appreciated if the patient is splinting because of pain.

DIAGNOSIS

Primarily clinical, although CXR and O_2 saturation are helpful.

TREATMENT

- O_2; narcotic analgesia.
- Respiratory support, including intubation and positive-pressure mechanical ventilation, may be needed to treat hypoxemia in severe cases. Surgical fixation of the chest wall is generally needed.

COMPLICATIONS

Respiratory compromise is a complication due to underlying pulmonary contusion.

KEY FACT

Aortic disruption is often associated with first and second rib, scapular, and sternal fractures.

Q   1

A 22-year-old female is brought to the ER after a motor vehicle collision in which she was the restrained driver. She receives 2 L of crystalloid en route and has a BP of 65/40 mm Hg and a heart rate of 135 bpm on arrival. She has ↓ breath sounds on the right, flat neck veins, and dullness to percussion on the right side. What is the most likely diagnosis?

Q   2

A 36-year-old male is brought to the ER following a motor vehicle collision in which he was an unrestrained passenger. X-rays show multiple fractures. Several hours later he develops fever, respiratory distress, and a rash consisting of small red and purple 1- to 2-mm macules covering his arms and shoulders. What is the most likely diagnosis?

Kehr's sign: Referred shoulder pain due to diaphragmatic irritation (classically on the left due to spleen rupture).

KEY FACT

Unstable patients with abdominal trauma should undergo immediate exploratory laparotomy.

MNEMONIC

Possible causes of PEA—

The 5 H's and 5 T's

Hypovolemia
Hypoxia
Hydrogen ion: Acidosis
Hyper/**H**ypo: K+, other metabolic
Hypothermia
Tablets: Drug OD, ingestion
Tamponade: Cardiac
Tension pneumothorax
Thrombosis: Coronary
Thrombosis: Pulmonary embolism

1 **A**

Hemothorax. Three important clues to look for are ↓ or absent breath sounds on the affected side, no chest movement with respiratory effort, and dullness to percussion on the affected side. Each hemithorax can hold 40% of a patient's circulating blood volume, and patients may therefore present in hypovolemic shock.

2 **A**

Fat embolism. The classic presentation of fat embolism is fever, tachypnea, tachycardia, conjunctival hemorrhage, and upper extremity petechiae after a patient suffers long-bone fractures.

ABDOMEN/PELVIS

- The **spleen** and **liver** are the **most commonly injured organs following blunt abdominal trauma.** Symptoms are consistent with signs of blood loss and include hypotension, tachycardia, and peritonitis. Suspect spleen or liver injury when lower rib fractures are present.
- The duodenum is susceptible to compression injury owing to its position in front of the spine. Look for retroperitoneal air on AXR and confirm the diagnosis with CT, which can also rule out a duodenal hematoma.
- Pancreatic injury should be suspected after a direct epigastric blow (handlebar injury).
- **Diaphragmatic rupture** may occur with blunt or penetrating trauma. **Kehr's sign** may be present; radiographs may demonstrate an elevated hemidiaphragm or abdominal viscera in the thorax.
- The **kidneys** are the **most commonly injured GU organ in trauma,** with injuries including renal contusion, laceration, fracture, and pedicle injury.
- In hemodynamically stable patients, abdominal blunt trauma can be diagnosed with FAST scan, CT scan, and serial abdominal exams.
- In hemodynamically unstable patients, abdominal blunt trauma should be treated with immediate exploratory laparotomy to look for organ injury or intra-abdominal bleeding.

Pelvic Fractures

Most commonly occur after high-speed traumas such as motor vehicle accidents or falls from heights. Require prompt stabilization with an external binder and surgical evaluation by a trauma or orthopedic surgeon in light of the potential for life-threatening hemorrhage.

DIAGNOSIS

- May present with an unstable pelvis upon manipulation.
- Pelvic x-rays may confirm the fracture; in a stable patient, a CT scan of the pelvis will better define the extent of injury.
- If hypotension and shock are present, an exsanguinating hemorrhage is likely. An external pelvic binder should be used to splint the fracture and limit blood loss.

TREATMENT

- Consider emergent external pelvic fixation and angiography with embolization of bleeding vessels. Internal pelvic fixation may be considered in a hemodynamically stable patient.
- Give blood early. Hemorrhage results in death in 50% of patients.
- Pelvic injuries can be associated with urethral injury suggested by **blood at the urethral meatus or in the scrotum; a high-riding, "ballotable" prostate;** or a **nonpalpable prostate.**
- If present, a **retrograde urethrogram** must be performed to rule out injury before a Foley catheter is placed.

Cardiac Life Support Basics

Table 2.17-2 summarizes the basic management of cardiac arrhythmias in an acute setting.

TABLE 2.17-2. Management of Cardiac Arrhythmias[a,b]

ARRHYTHMIA	TREATMENT
Asystole or pulseless electrical activity (PEA)	Initiate CPR. Give epinephrine or vasopressin; simultaneously search for the underlying cause (see the **5 H's and 5 T's** mnemonic) and provide empiric treatment.
Ventricular fibrillation or pulseless ventricular tachycardia	Initiate CPR. Defibrillate with 200 J immediately → defibrillate again → epinephrine → defibrillate → amiodarone → defibrillate → epinephrine.
Supraventricular tachycardia (SVT)	If unstable, perform synchronized electrical cardioversion. If stable, control rate with vagal maneuvers (Valsalva maneuver, carotid sinus massage, or cold stimulus). If resistant to maneuvers, give adenosine followed by other AV-nodal blocking agents (calcium channel blockers [CCBs] or β-blockers) if rhythm fails to convert.
Atrial fibrillation(AF)/flutter	If unstable, perform synchronized electrical cardioversion at 120–200 J. If stable, control rate with diltiazem or β-blockers and anticoagulate if duration is > 48 hours. Elective cardioversion may be performed if duration is < 48 hours; otherwise, the clinician must anticoagulate or perform TEE prior to conversion. Do not give nodal blockers if there is evidence of Wolff-Parkinson-White syndrome (δ waves) on ECG. Use procainamide instead.
Bradycardia	If symptomatic, give atropine. If ineffective, use transcutaneous pacing, dopamine, or epinephrine.

[a] In all cases, disruptions of CPR should be minimized. After a shock or administration of a drug, CPR should be resumed immediately, and 5 cycles of CPR should be given before checking for a pulse or rhythm. "→" above represents 5 cycles of CPR followed by a pulse or rhythm check.

[b] Doses of electricity listed above assume a biphasic defibrillator.

Acute Abdomen

Acute-onset abdominal pain has many potential etiologies and may require immediate medical or surgical intervention. Sharp, focal pain with tenderness and guarding generally implies a parietal (peritoneal) etiology; dull, crampy, achy, and midline or diffuse pain is commonly of visceral (organ) origin. Patients with parietal pain generally prefer immobility, whereas those with visceral pain are often unable to lie still. Figure 2.17-5 identifies the common causes of acute abdomen.

Q

A 65-year-old male smoker is brought to the ER for sudden-onset abdominal and back pain. The anxious patient complains of "ripping pain." Physical examination reveals a large pulsatile mass behind the umbilicus. The patient's BP is 80/50 mm Hg and heart rate 125 bpm. You begin crystalloid and blood infusions. What is the most appropriate next step in management?

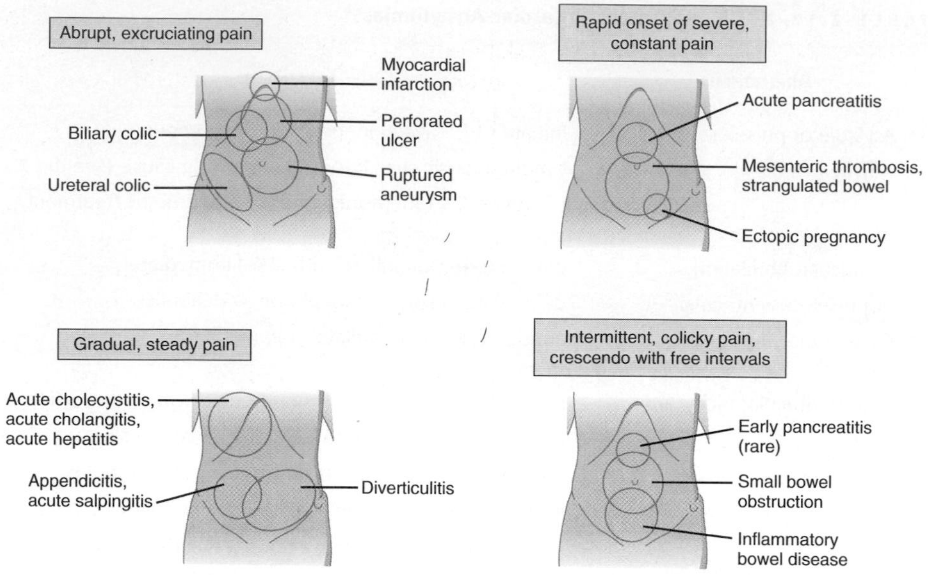

FIGURE 2.17-5. **Acute abdomen.** The location and character of pain are helpful in the differential diagnosis of the acute abdomen. (Reproduced with permission from Doherty GM et al. *Current Diagnosis & Treatment: Surgery,* 13th ed. New York: McGraw-Hill, 2010, Fig. 21-3.)

> **KEY FACT**
>
> A positive β-hCG in the setting of shock is a ruptured ectopic pregnancy until proven otherwise.

> **KEY FACT**
>
> Abdominal pain plus syncope or shock in an older patient is a ruptured abdominal aortic aneurysm (AAA) until proven otherwise.

> **KEY FACT**
>
> Pneumonia can present as right or left upper quadrant abdominal pain.

Immediate laparotomy or endovascular repair. On the basis of the clinical findings of shock, abdominal pain, and a pulsatile mass, the patient has a ruptured AAA, which is a surgical emergency.

HISTORY/PE

- Pay careful attention to the historical features in the acute abdominal presentation.
- Consider the gynecologic history in females (including last menstrual period, pregnancy, and any STD symptoms). If a patient has abdominal pain with cervical motion tenderness, there should be a low threshold to treat for **pelvic inflammatory disease (PID).**
- **Perforation** leads to sudden onset of diffuse, severe pain, usually with abdominal rigidity on exam.
- **Obstruction** leads to acute onset of severe, radiating, colicky pain. Patients may complain of obstipation (failure to pass stool or gas) or bilious emesis. Think of small bowel obstruction in patients with a history of abdominal surgeries.
- **Inflammation** leads to gradual onset (over 10–12 hours) of constant, ill-defined pain.
- **Associated symptoms** include the following:
  - Anorexia, nausea, vomiting, changes in bowel habits, hematochezia, and melena suggest GI etiologies.
  - Fever and cough suggest pneumonia.
  - Hematuria, pyuria, and costovertebral angle tenderness point to a GU etiology.
- If associated with meals, consider mesenteric ischemia (especially in the elderly or those with coronary or peripheral artery disease risk factors), peptic ulcer disease, biliary disease, pancreatitis, or bowel pathology.
- A family history of abdominal pain may indicate familial Mediterranean fever or acute intermittent porphyria.

DIAGNOSIS

- In the presence of peritoneal signs, shock, or impending shock, emergent exploratory laparotomy is necessary.
- If the patient is stable, a complete physical examination—including a **rectal examination** and, in women, a **pelvic examination**—is mandatory.
- Obtain electrolytes, LFTs, lipase, **urine or serum β-hCG,** UA, and a CBC with differential.

- Consider a CXR for suspected perforation or pulmonary pathology. AXR may be useful for obstruction (air-fluid levels, distended loops of bowel) or perforation (free air under the diaphragm; see Figure 2.17-4), but CT is more sensitive and specific.
- CT is used to diagnose appendicitis, diverticulitis, abscess, renal stones, AAA, obstruction, and other pathology.
- Ultrasound is helpful for diagnosing cholecystitis and gynecologic pathology and can diagnose hemoperitoneum and AAA in unstable patients.

TREATMENT

- **Hemodynamically unstable patients must have emergent surgical management.**
- In stable patients, expectant management may include NPO status, NG tube placement (for decompression of bowel in the setting of obstruction or acute pancreatitis), IV fluids, placement of a Foley catheter (to monitor urine output and fluid status), and vital sign monitoring with serial abdominal examinations and serial labs.
- Give broad-spectrum antibiotics to all patients with perforation or signs of sepsis. Antibiotics may also be indicated for patients with infectious processes such as cholecystitis, diverticulitis, and pyelonephritis.
- Type and cross all unstable patients as well as those in whom you suspect potential hemorrhage.

Acute Appendicitis

The inciting event is obstruction of the appendiceal lumen with subsequent inflammation and infection. Rising intraluminal pressure leads to vascular compromise of the appendix, ischemia, necrosis, and possible perforation. Etiologies include hypertrophied lymphoid tissue (55–65%), fecalith (35%), foreign body, tumor (eg, carcinoid tumor), and parasites. Incidence peaks in the early teens (most patients are between 10 and 30 years of age), and the male-to-female ratio is 2:1.

HISTORY/PE

- Classically presents with dull periumbilical pain lasting 1–12 hours that leads to sharp RLQ pain at McBurney's point.
- Can also present with nausea, vomiting, anorexia ("hamburger sign"), and low-grade fever.
- Psoas, obturator, and Rovsing's signs are not sensitive tests, but their presence ↑ the likelihood of appendicitis.
- In **perforated appendix,** partial pain relief is possible, but peritoneal signs (eg, rebound, guarding, hypotension, ↑ WBC count, fever) will ultimately develop.
- Children, the elderly, pregnant women, and those with retrocecal appendices may have atypical presentations that may result in misdiagnosis and ↑ mortality.

DIAGNOSIS

- Diagnosed by clinical impression.
- Look for fever, mild leukocytosis (11,000–15,000 cells/μL) with left shift, and UA with a few RBCs and/or WBCs.
- If the clinical diagnosis is unequivocal, no imaging studies are necessary. Otherwise, studies include the following:

KEY FACT

Think of ischemic colitis in a patient with a history of AF or recent AAA repair, bloody stool, and sudden-onset abdominal pain out of proportion to physical findings.

KEY FACT

Nearly all female patients with an acute abdomen require a pelvic exam and a pregnancy test to look for PID, ectopic pregnancy, and ovarian torsion.

KEY FACT

McBurney's point is located one-third of the distance from the anterior superior iliac spine to the umbilicus.

KEY FACT

- **"Hamburger sign":** If a patient wants to eat, consider a diagnosis other than appendicitis.
- **Psoas sign:** Passive extension of the hip leading to RLQ pain.
- **Obturator sign:** Passive internal rotation of the flexed hip leading to RLQ pain.
- **Rovsing's sign:** Deep palpation of the LLQ leading to RLQ pain.

- **CT scan with PO and IV contrast (95–98% sensitive):** Periappendiceal stranding or fluid; enlarged appendix (see Figure 2.17-6).
- **Ultrasound:** An enlarged, noncompressible appendix. Preferred for children and pregnant women.

TREATMENT

- The patient should be NPO and receive IV hydration, analgesia, antiemetics, and antibiotics with anaerobic and gram-⊖ coverage.
- Immediate open or laparoscopic appendectomy is the definitive treatment. If appendicitis is not found, complete exploration of the abdomen is performed.
- **Perforation:** Administer antibiotics until the patient is afebrile with a normalized WBC count; the wound should be closed by delayed 1° closure.
- **Abscess:** Treat with broad-spectrum antibiotics and percutaneous drainage; an elective appendectomy should be performed 6–8 weeks later.

Burns

The **second leading cause of death in children.** Serious burn patients should be treated in an ICU setting. Burns can be chemical, electrical, or thermal and are categorized by depth of tissue destruction (see Figure 2.17-7):

- **First degree:** Only the epidermis is involved. The area is painful and erythematous, but blisters are not present, and capillary refill is intact. Looks like a sunburn.
- **Second degree:** The epidermis and partial thickness of the dermis are involved. The area is painful, and blisters are present.
- **Third degree:** The epidermis, the full thickness of the dermis, and potentially deeper tissues are involved. The area is painless, white, and charred.

HISTORY/PE

- Patients may present with obvious skin wounds, but significant deep destruction may not be visible, especially with electrical burns.
- Conduct a thorough airway and lung examination to assess for inhalation injury.

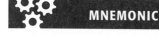

MNEMONIC

Use the "rule of 9's" to estimate % BSA in adults:

Head and each arm = 9%
Back and chest each = 18%
Each leg = 18%
Perineum = 1%

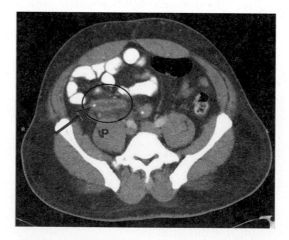

FIGURE 2.17-6. **Acute appendicitis.** Contrast-enhanced CT image through the lower abdomen in a 30-year-old female with RLQ pain demonstrates an enlarged, hyperenhancing appendix (circle) with periappendiceal fat stranding located just anterior to the right psoas muscle (P). An appendicolith (arrow) is noted near the base of the appendix. (Reproduced with permission from USMLERx.com.)

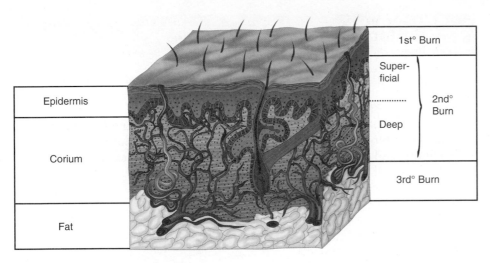

FIGURE 2.17-7. **Depth of burn wounds.** (Reproduced with permission from Strange GR et al. *Pediatric Emergency Medicine*, 3rd ed. New York: McGraw-Hill, 2009, Fig. 138-1.)

- Maintain a high index of suspicion for carbon monoxide poisoning in patients with inhalation injury or involvement in a closed-space fire.
- Consider cyanide poisoning in closed-space fires with burning carpets and textiles.

DIAGNOSIS

- Assess the ABCs. If there is any evidence of thermal or inhalation injury to the upper airway, intubate.
- Be vigilant for shock, inhalation injury, and carbon monoxide poisoning. Obtain a CXR and a carboxyhemoglobin level.
- Evaluate the percentage of body surface area (% BSA) involved (see Figure 2.17-8).

TREATMENT

- Supportive measures; tetanus, stress ulcer prophylaxis, and IV narcotic analgesia.
- For second- and third-degree burns, fluid repletion using the **Parkland formula** is critical; adjust repletion on the basis of additional insensible losses to maintain at least 1 cc/kg/hr of urine output.
- Topical antimicrobials (eg, silver sulfadiazine) may be used prophylactically when the epidermis is no longer intact; however, there is no proven benefit associated with the use of PO/IV antibiotics or corticosteroids.

COMPLICATIONS

- Shock, compartment syndrome, and superinfection (most likely due to *Pseudomonas* or gram-⊕ cocci).
- Criteria for transfer to a burn center include the following:
  - Partial-thickness and full-thickness burns > 10% BSA in patients < 10 years or > 50 years of age.
  - Partial-thickness and full-thickness burns > 20% BSA in other age groups.
  - Any full- or partial-thickness burn over critical areas (face, hands, feet, genitals, perineum, major joints).
  - Circumferential burns; chemical, electrical, or lightning injury; inhalation injury.
  - Any special psychosocial or rehabilitative care needs.

> **KEY FACT**
>
> **Parkland formula:** Fluids for the first 24 hours = 4 × patient's weight in kg × % BSA. Give 50% of fluids over the first 8 hours and the remaining 50% over the following 16 hours.

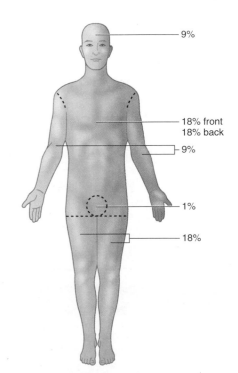

FIGURE 2.17-8. **The rule of 9's in the estimation of BSA.** Estimation of BSA is imperative in the evaluation of burn victims. (Reproduced with permission from Ma OJ et al. *Emergency Medicine Manual*, 6th ed. New York: McGraw-Hill, 2004, Fig. 126-1.)

MNEMONIC

The 6 W's of postoperative fever:

Wind: Atelectasis, pneumonia
Water: UTI
Wounds: Wound infection, abscess
Walking: DVT
Wonder drugs: Drug reaction
Womb: Endometritis

KEY FACT

Heart rate is the first vital sign to change in hemorrhagic shock. BP falls only after the loss of 30–40% of blood volume.

KEY FACT

Avoid pressors in hypovolemic shock.

KEY FACT

Malignant hyperthermia and neuroleptic malignant syndrome (NMS) should be ruled out in any suspected case of hyperthermia. Malignant hyperthermia would be seen after halothane exposure, and NMS after a neuroleptic. Both conditions are treated with dantrolene.

KEY FACT

Following a bite, healthy domestic animals should be observed for 10 days. Skunks, raccoons, foxes, and bats should be euthanized and tested for rabies immediately.

KEY FACT

In carbon monoxide poisoning, the measured O_2 saturation is usually normal. This is because the pulse oximeter recognizes carboxyhemoglobin as a normal saturated hemoglobin molecule, so it does not adequately reflect the low arterial Po_2 levels.

Postoperative Fever

- Occurs in 40% of all postoperative patients. Remember the mnemonic "Wind, Water, Wounds, Walking, and Wonder drugs." Another "W" of postoperative fever is "Womb" in OB/GYN.
- ↓ the risk of postoperative fever with incentive spirometry, pre- and postoperative antibiotics when indicated, short-term Foley catheter use, early ambulation, and DVT prophylaxis (eg, anticoagulation, compression stockings).
- Fevers before postoperative day 3 are unlikely to be infectious unless *Clostridium* or β-hemolytic streptococci are involved.

Shock

Defined as **inadequate tissue-level oxygenation to maintain vital organ function.** The multiple etiologies are differentiated by their cardiovascular effects and treatment options (see Table 2.17-3).

Thermal Dysregulation

HYPOTHERMIA

- A body temperature < 35°C (< 95°F). May be accompanied by mental status and neurologic deficits.
- Remove the patient from the cold or windy environment and remove wet clothing. In mild cases, passively rewarm the patient with blankets or warm water. Also administer warm air and warm IV fluids.
- In more severe cases, the patient may need active rewarming with heating blankets, radiant heat, or warm water immersion. In unstable patients, active core rewarming may be necessary (eg, NG or bladder lavage, pleural lavage, or cardiac bypass). If the patient has frostbite, thaw the affected areas with the same methods. Patients will need narcotic analgesia for thawing.
- Monitor the ECG for arrhythmias such as bradycardia and slow AF, which can be common at < 30°C (< 86°F). The classic sign is the **J wave** (aka Osborn wave). Also monitor electrolytes and acid-base balance.
- Do not stop resuscitation efforts until the patient has been warmed.

HYPERTHERMIA

- A body temperature > 40°C (> 104°F), possibly from heat stroke.
- Cool the patient with cold water, wet blankets, and ice. Give a benzodiazepine to prevent shivering. Rule out causes of fever such as infection or drug reaction.

Bites and Stings

Table 2.17-4 outlines the management of common bites and stings. Table 2.17-5 summarizes the recommended prophylaxis for rabies and tetanus.

TABLE 2.17-3.   Types of Shock

Type	Major Causes	Cardiac Output	PCWP[a]	PVR[b]	Treatment
Hypovolemic	Trauma, blood loss, dehydration with inadequate fluid repletion, third spacing, burns.	↓	↓	↑	Replete with isotonic solution (eg, LR or NS) and blood in a 3:1 (fluid-to-blood) ratio. Initiate blood transfusion for continued blood loss.
Cardiogenic	CHF, arrhythmia, structural heart disease (severe mitral regurgitation, VSD), MI (> 40% of left ventricular function).	↓	↑	↑	Identify the cause and treat if possible. Give inotropic support with pressors such as dopamine (if hypotensive) or dobutamine (if not hypotensive).
Obstructive	Cardiac tamponade, tension pneumothorax, massive pulmonary embolism.	↓	↑	↑	Treat the underlying cause: pericardiocentesis, decompression of pneumothorax, thrombolysis.
Septic	Bacteremia, especially gram-⊖ organisms.	↑	↓	↓	Administer broad-spectrum antibiotics. Measure central venous pressure (CVP) and give fluid until CVP = 8. Pressors (norepinephrine or dopamine) may be needed. If possible, obtain cultures prior to the administration of antibiotics.
Anaphylactic	Bee stings, medication, food allergies.	↑	↓	↓	Administer 1:1000 epinephrine. Consider adjuncts such as H_1/H_2 antagonists and steroids.

[a] PCWP = pulmonary capillary wedge pressure.

[b] PVR = peripheral vascular resistance.

Toxicology

CARBON MONOXIDE POISONING

A **hypoxemic poisoning syndrome** seen in patients who have been exposed to automobile exhaust, smoke inhalation, barbecues, or old appliances in poorly ventilated locations.

HISTORY/PE

- Presents with hypoxemia, **cherry-red skin** (rare), confusion, and **headaches.** Coma or seizures occur in severe cases.
- Chronic low-level exposure may cause **flulike symptoms** with generalized myalgias, nausea, and headaches. Ask about symptoms in others living in the same house.
- **Suspect smoke inhalation** in the presence of **singed nose hairs, facial burns, hoarseness, wheezing,** or **carbonaceous sputum.**

DIAGNOSIS

- Check an ABG and serum carboxyhemoglobin level (normal is < 5% in nonsmokers and < 10% in smokers).

Q

A 44-year-old female is brought to the ER following a motor vehicle collision. On arrival, her BP is 70/35 mm Hg and her heart rate 110 bpm. Physical examination reveals bruises over the chest and abdomen. A pulmonary artery catheter is placed and reveals a PCWP of 16 mm Hg. After resuscitation with 2 L of crystalloid, BP and heart rate measurements are 80/40 mm Hg and 125 bpm. PCWP is now 24 mm Hg. What is the most likely diagnosis?

TABLE 2.17-4. **Management of Bites and Stings**

Source	Potential Complication	Management
Bees and wasps	Anaphylaxis	Antihistamines and steroids; IM epinephrine if anaphylaxis develops.
Spiders	Necrosis, hypocalcemia	Supportive measures; antivenom if available. Surgical resection and skin grafts for severe necrosis.
Scorpions	In severe cases, cranial nerve dysfunction, excessive motor activity, respiratory compromise	Supportive with benzodiazepines and analgesics; atropine for hypersalivation and respiratory distress (not to be used with foreign scorpion stings); IV scorpion-specific antibody.
Snakes	Venom poisoning	Antivenom is the mainstay of treatment. Elevate the affected limb above the heart. Compression bands help, but tourniquets are contraindicated. Suction and incision are dangerous and should not be done.
Dogs and cats	Infection, rabies/tetanus	Amoxicillin/clavulanate for puncture wounds, bites to hands/feet, and high-risk or immunocompromised patients.
Humans	Infection	Amoxicillin/clavulanate unless very minor.
Rodents	Low risk of infection; not known to carry rabies	Local wound care.

TABLE 2.17-5. **Rabies and Tetanus Precautions**

Suspected Pathogen	Exposure	Prophylaxis
Rabies	Bites from dogs, cats, ferrets, skunks, raccoons, **bats**	If an animal displays signs of rabies, administer 1 dose of human rabies immune globulin and 4 doses of rabies vaccine over 14 days if the patient has never been vaccinated. Previously vaccinated patients do not need immune globulin and require only 2 doses of vaccine.
Tetanus	Any wound	Administer tetanus toxoid if the patient had ≤ 3 lifetime toxoids and the last was 10 or more years ago for a minor/clean wound or 5 or more years ago for all other wounds. Administer tetanus immune globulin only if wound is major/dirty and the patient had ≤ 3 lifetime toxoids.

A

Cardiogenic or obstructive shock likely caused by severe blunt trauma to the chest. The patient has signs of shock, and her elevated PCWP suggests either a cardiogenic or an obstructive cause. On the basis of the mechanism of injury, she may have severe myocardial contusion or cardiac tamponade.

- Check an ECG in the elderly and in patients with a history of cardiac disease.

TREATMENT

- Treat with 100% O_2 until the patient is asymptomatic and carboxyhemoglobin falls to normal levels.
- Use **hyperbaric O_2** for pregnant patients, nonresponders, those with signs of CNS or cardiac ischemia, or those with severely ↑ carboxyhemoglobin to facilitate displacement of carbon monoxide from hemoglobin.
- Patients with **airway burns** or **smoke inhalation** may require early intubation, since upper airway edema can rapidly lead to complete obstruction.

COMMON DRUG INTERACTIONS/REACTIONS

Table 2.17-6 outlines drug interactions and reactions that are commonly encountered in a clinical setting.

DRUG OVERDOSE

Table 2.17-7 summarizes antidotes and treatments for substances commonly encountered in overdoses and intoxications. If a patient is unresponsive, it is common to empirically treat with a dose of Narcan.

KEY FACT

Ipecac syrup is an antiquated treatment for poisoning that is rarely if ever used owing to the risks of ↑ damage caused by emesis and the lack of demonstrated patient benefit.

KEY FACT

Orogastric lavage is generally recommended only for life-threatening toxins ≤ 1 hour after ingestion.

KEY FACT

Activated charcoal is indicated for cases of recent isolated ingestion (< 2 hours) of substances known to adsorb to it (not used for lithium, iron, lead, hydrocarbons, or toxic alcohols).

TABLE 2.17-6. Drug Interactions and Reactions

INTERACTION/REACTION	DRUGS
Induction of P-450 enzymes	Quinidine, Barbiturates, St. John's wort, Phenytoin, Rifampin, Griseofulvin, Carbamazepine: "Queen Barb Steals Phen-phen and Refuses Greasy Carbs."
Inhibition of P-450 enzymes	Cimetidine, ketoconazole, INH, grapefruit, erythromycin, sulfonamides.
Metabolism by P-450 enzymes	Benzodiazepines, amide anesthetics, metoprolol, propranolol, nifedipine, phenytoin, quinidine, theophylline, warfarin, barbiturates.
↑ risk of digoxin toxicity	Quinidine, cimetidine, amiodarone, CCBs.
Competition for albumin-binding sites	Warfarin, ASA, phenytoin.
Blood dyscrasias	Ibuprofen, quinidine, methyldopa, chemotherapeutic agents.
Hemolysis in G6PD-deficient patients	Sulfonamides, isoniazid (INH), ASA, ibuprofen, nitrofurantoin, primaquine, pyrimethamine, chloramphenicol.
Gynecomastia	Spironolactone, Estrogens, Digitalis, Cimetidine, chronic Alcohol use, Ketoconazole: "Some Excellent Drugs Create Awesome Knockers."
Stevens-Johnson syndrome	Anticonvulsants, sulfonamides, penicillins.
Photosensitivity	Tetracycline, amiodarone, sulfonamides.
Drug-induced SLE	Procainamide, hydralazine, INH, penicillamine, chlorpromazine, methyldopa, quinidine.

TABLE 2.17-7. **Specific Antidotes**

Toxin	Antidote/Treatment
Acetaminophen	*N*-acetylcysteine.
Acid/alkali ingestion	Upper endoscopy to evaluate for stricture.
Anticholinesterases, organophosphates	Atropine, pralidoxime.
Antimuscarinic/anticholinergic agents	Physostigmine.
Arsenic, mercury, gold	Succimer, dimercaprol.
β-blockers	Glucagon.
Barbiturates (phenobarbital)	Urine alkalinization, dialysis, activated charcoal, supportive care.
Benzodiazepines	Flumazenil (can precipitate withdrawal).
Black widow bite	Calcium gluconate, methocarbamol.
Carbon monoxide	100% O_2, hyperbaric O_2.
Copper, arsenic, lead, gold	Penicillamine.
Cyanide	Hydroxycobalamin, amyl nitrate, sodium nitrate, sodium thiosulfate.
Digitalis	Normalize K^+ but avoid giving Ca^{++}, Mg^{++}, or lidocaine (for torsades); anti-digitalis Fab.
Heparin	Protamine sulfate.
INH	Pyridoxine.
Iron salts	Deferoxamine.
Lead	Succimer, CaEDTA, dimercaprol.
Methanol, ethylene glycol (antifreeze)	EtOH, fomepizole, dialysis, calcium gluconate for ethylene glycol.
Methemoglobin	Methylene blue.
Opioids	Naloxone.
Salicylates	Urine alkalinization, dialysis, activated charcoal.
TCAs	Sodium bicarbonate for QRS prolongation; diazepam or lorazepam for seizures; cardiac monitor for arrhythmias.
Theophylline	Activated charcoal. Consider repeat doses.
tPA, streptokinase	Aminocaproic acid.
Warfarin	Vitamin K, FFP.

MAJOR DRUG SIDE EFFECTS

Table 2.17-8 outlines the major side effects of select drugs.

TABLE 2.17-8. Drug Side Effects

DRUG	SIDE EFFECTS
ACEIs	**Cough,** rash, proteinuria, angioedema, taste changes, teratogenic effects.
Amantadine	Ataxia, **livedo reticularis.**
Aminoglycosides	Ototoxicity, nephrotoxicity (acute tubular necrosis).
Amiodarone	Acute: AV block, hypotension, bradycardia. Chronic: pulmonary fibrosis, peripheral deposition leading to bluish discoloration, arrhythmias, hypo-/hyperthyroidism, corneal deposition.
Amphotericin	Fever/rigors, nephrotoxicity, bone marrow suppression, anemia.
Antipsychotics	Sedation, acute dystonic reaction, akathisia, parkinsonism, tardive dyskinesia, **NMS.**
Azoles (eg, fluconazole)	Inhibition of P-450 enzymes.
AZT	Thrombocytopenia, megaloblastic anemia.
β-blockers	Asthma exacerbation, masking of hypoglycemia, impotence, bradycardia, AV block, CHF.
Benzodiazepines	Sedation, dependence, respiratory depression.
Bile acid resins	GI upset, malabsorption of vitamins and medications.
Carbamazepine	Induction of P-450 enzymes, **agranulocytosis,** aplastic anemia, liver toxicity.
CCBs	Peripheral edema, constipation, cardiac depression.
Chloramphenicol	**Gray baby syndrome,** aplastic anemia.
Cisplatin	Nephrotoxicity, acoustic nerve damage.
Clonidine	Dry mouth; **severe rebound headache and hypertension.**
Clozapine	Agranulocytosis.
Corticosteroids	Mania, hyperglycemia (acute), immunosuppression, bone mineral loss, thinning of skin, easy bruising, myopathy, cataracts (chronic).
Cyclophosphamide	Myelosuppression, **hemorrhagic cystitis.**
Digoxin	GI disturbance, **yellow visual changes, arrhythmias** (eg, junctional tachycardia or SVT).
Doxorubicin	**Cardiotoxicity (cardiomyopathy).**
Ethyl alcohol	Acidosis, renal dysfunction, CNS depression.

(continues)

TABLE 2.17-8. Drug Side Effects *(continued)*

DRUG	SIDE EFFECTS
Fluoroquinolones	Cartilage damage in children; Achilles tendon rupture in adults.
Furosemide	Ototoxicity, hypokalemia, nephritis, gout.
Gemfibrozil	Myositis, reversible ↑ in LFTs.
Halothane	Hepatotoxicity, **malignant hyperthermia.**
HCTZ	Hypokalemia, hyponatremia, hyperuricemia, hyperglycemia, hypercalcemia.
HMG-CoA reductase inhibitors	Myositis, reversible ↑ in LFTs.
Hydralazine	Drug-induced SLE.
Hydroxychloroquine	Retinopathy.
INH	Peripheral neuropathy **(prevent with pyridoxine/vitamin B$_6$),** hepatotoxicity, inhibition of P-450 enzymes, seizures with overdose, hemolysis in G6PD deficiency.
MAOIs	**Hypertensive tyramine reaction, serotonin syndrome** (with meperidine).
Methanol	Blindness, ion-gap metabolic acidosis.
Methotrexate	Hepatic fibrosis, pneumonitis, anemia.
Methyldopa	⊕ Coombs' test, drug-induced SLE.
Metronidazole	Disulfiram reaction, vestibular dysfunction, **metallic taste.**
Niacin	**Cutaneous flushing.**
Nitroglycerin	Hypotension, tachycardia, headache, tolerance.
Penicillamine	Drug-induced SLE.
Penicillin/β-lactams	Hypersensitivity reactions.
Phenytoin	Nystagmus, diplopia, ataxia, arrhythmia (in toxic doses), **gingival hyperplasia,** hirsutism, teratogenic effects.
Prazosin	First-dose hypotension.
Procainamide	Drug-induced SLE.
Propylthiouracil	Agranulocytosis, aplastic anemia.
Quinidine	Cinchonism (headache, tinnitus), thrombocytopenia, arrhythmias (eg, **torsades de pointes**).
Reserpine	Depression.

TABLE 2.17-8.   Drug Side Effects *(continued)*

DRUG	SIDE EFFECTS
Rifampin	Induction of P-450 enzymes; **orange-red body secretions.**
Salicylates	Fever; hyperventilation with **respiratory alkalosis and metabolic acidosis;** dehydration, diaphoresis, hemorrhagic gastritis.
SSRIs	Anxiety, **sexual dysfunction,** serotonin syndrome if taken with MAOIs.
Succinylcholine	**Malignant hyperthermia,** hyperkalemia.
TCAs	Sedation, coma, anticholinergic effects, seizures, **QRS prolongation,** arrhythmias.
Tetracyclines	Tooth discoloration, photosensitivity, Fanconi's syndrome, GI distress.
Trimethoprim	Megaloblastic anemia, leukopenia, granulocytopenia.
Valproic acid	Teratogenicity leads to neural tube defects; rare fatal hepatotoxicity.
Vancomycin	Nephrotoxicity, ototoxicity, **"red man syndrome"** (histamine release; not an allergy).
Vinblastine	Severe myelosuppression.
Vincristine	Peripheral neuropathy, paralytic ileus.

MANAGEMENT OF DRUG WITHDRAWAL

Table 2.17-9 summarizes common drug withdrawal symptoms and treatment.

TABLE 2.17-9.   Symptoms and Treatment of Drug Withdrawal

DRUG	WITHDRAWAL SYMPTOMS	TREATMENT
Alcohol	Tremor (6–12 hours). Tachycardia, hypertension, agitation, seizures (within 48 hours). Hallucinations, **DTs**—severe autonomic instability leading to tachycardia, hypertension, delirium, and possibly death (within 2–7 days). Mortality is 15–20%.	**Benzodiazepines** (can require massive doses); haloperidol for hallucinations; **thiamine,** folate, and multivitamin replacement (do not affect withdrawal, but most alcoholics are deficient).
Barbiturates	Anxiety, seizures, delirium, tremor; tachycardia and hypertension.	**Benzodiazepines.**
Benzodiazepines	Rebound anxiety, seizures, tremor, insomnia.	**Benzodiazepine taper.**
Cocaine/amphetamines	Depression, hyperphagia, hypersomnolence.	Supportive treatment. Avoid pure β-blockers (may lead to unopposed α activity, causing hypertension).
Opioids	Anxiety, insomnia, flulike symptoms, piloerection, fever, rhinorrhea, lacrimation, yawning, nausea, stomach cramps, diarrhea, mydriasis.	Antiemetics, muscle relaxers, and NSAIDs for mild symptoms; clonidine, buprenorphine, or methadone for moderate to severe symptoms.

RECOGNITION OF DRUG INTOXICATION

See the Psychiatry chapter for a summary of common drug intoxication symptoms.

Vitamin Deficiencies

Table 2.17-10 summarizes the signs and symptoms of key vitamin deficiencies.

TABLE 2.17-10.   Vitamin Functions and Deficiencies

VITAMIN	SIGNS/SYMPTOMS OF DEFICIENCY
Vitamin A	Night blindness, dry skin.
Vitamin B$_1$ (thiamine)	Beriberi (polyneuritis, dilated cardiomyopathy, high-output CHF, edema), Wernicke-Korsakoff syndrome.
Vitamin B$_2$ (riboflavin)	Angular stomatitis, cheilosis, corneal vascularization.
Vitamin B$_3$ (niacin)	Pellagra (diarrhea, dermatitis, dementia).
Vitamin B$_5$ (pantothenate)	Dermatitis, enteritis, alopecia, adrenal insufficiency.
Vitamin B$_6$ (pyridoxine)	Convulsions, hyperirritability; required during administration of INH.
Vitamin B$_{12}$ (cobalamin)	Macrocytic, megaloblastic anemia; neurologic symptoms (eg, optic neuropathy, subacute combined degeneration, paresthesias); glossitis.
Vitamin C	Scurvy (eg, swollen gums, bruising, anemia, poor wound healing).
Vitamin D	Rickets in children (bending bones), osteomalacia in adults (soft bones), hypocalcemic tetany.
Vitamin E	↑ fragility of RBCs.
Vitamin K	Neonatal hemorrhage; ↑ PT and aPTT, normal BT.
Biotin	Dermatitis, enteritis. Can be caused by ingestion of **raw eggs** or antibiotic use.
Folic acid	The **most common vitamin deficiency in the United States.** Sprue; macrocytic, megaloblastic anemia without neurologic symptoms.
Magnesium	Weakness, muscle cramps, exacerbation of hypocalcemic tetany, CNS hyperirritability leading to tremors, choreoathetoid movement.
Selenium	Keshan disease (cardiomyopathy).

RAPID REVIEW

CARDIOVASCULAR

Classic ECG finding in atrial flutter.	"Sawtooth" P waves.
Definition of unstable angina.	Angina that is new, is worsening, or occurs at rest.
Antihypertensive for a diabetic patient with proteinuria.	ACEI.
Beck's triad for cardiac tamponade.	Hypotension, distant heart sounds, and JVD.
Drugs that slow heart rate.	β-blockers, calcium channel blockers (CCBs), digoxin, amiodarone.
Hypercholesterolemia treatment that leads to flushing and pruritus.	Niacin.
Murmur—hypertrophic obstructive cardiomyopathy (HOCM).	A systolic ejection murmur heard along the lateral sternal border that ↑ with ↓ preload (Valsalva maneuver).
Murmur—aortic insufficiency.	Austin Flint murmur, a diastolic, decrescendo, low-pitched, blowing murmur that is best heard sitting up; ↑ with ↑ afterload (handgrip maneuver).
Murmur—aortic stenosis.	A systolic crescendo/decrescendo murmur that radiates to the neck; ↑ with ↑ preload (squatting maneuver).
Murmur—mitral regurgitation.	A holosystolic murmur that radiates to the axilla; ↑ with ↑ afterload (handgrip maneuver).
Murmur—mitral stenosis.	A diastolic, mid- to late, low-pitched murmur preceded by an opening snap.
Treatment for atrial fibrillation and atrial flutter.	If unstable, cardiovert. If stable or chronic, rate control with CCBs or β-blockers.
Treatment for ventricular fibrillation.	Immediate cardioversion.
Dressler's syndrome.	An autoimmune reaction with fever, pericarditis, and ↑ ESR occurring 2–4 weeks post-MI.
IV drug use with JVD and a holosystolic murmur at the left sternal border. Treatment?	Treat existing heart failure and replace the tricuspid valve.
Diagnostic test for hypertrophic cardiomyopathy.	Echocardiogram (showing a thickened left ventricular wall and outflow obstruction).
Pulsus paradoxus.	A ↓ in systolic BP of > 10 mm Hg with inspiration; seen in cardiac tamponade.
Classic ECG findings in pericarditis.	Low-voltage, diffuse ST-segment elevation.
Definition of hypertension.	BP > 140/90 mm Hg on 3 separate occasions 2 weeks apart.
Eight surgically correctable causes of hypertension.	Renal artery stenosis, coarctation of the aorta, pheochromocytoma, Conn's syndrome, Cushing's syndrome, unilateral renal parenchymal disease, hyperthyroidism, hyperparathyroidism.

Evaluation of a pulsatile abdominal mass and bruit.	Abdominal ultrasound and CT.
Indications for surgical repair of abdominal aortic aneurysm.	> 5.5 cm, rapidly enlarging, symptomatic, or ruptured.
Treatment for acute coronary syndrome.	ASA, heparin, clopidogrel, morphine, O_2, sublingual nitroglycerin, IV β-blockers.
Metabolic syndrome.	Abdominal obesity, high triglycerides, low HDL, hypertension, insulin resistance, prothrombotic or proinflammatory states.
Appropriate diagnostic test? ■ A 50-year-old man with stable angina can exercise to 85% of maximum predicted heart rate. ■ A 65-year-old woman with left bundle branch block and severe osteoarthritis has unstable angina.	Exercise stress treadmill with ECG. Pharmacologic stress test (eg, dobutamine echo).
Target LDL in a patient with diabetes.	< 70 mg/dL.
Signs of active ischemia during stress testing.	Angina, ST-segment changes on ECG, or ↓ BP.
ECG findings suggesting MI.	ST-segment elevation (depression means ischemia), flattened T waves, and Q waves.
Coronary territories in MI.	Anterior wall (LAD/diagonal), inferior (PDA), posterior (left circumflex/oblique, RCA/marginal), septum (LAD/diagonal).
A young patient with angina at rest and ST-segment elevation with normal cardiac enzymes.	Prinzmetal's angina.
Common symptoms associated with silent MIs.	CHF, shock, and altered mental status.
Diagnostic test for pulmonary embolism (PE).	Spiral CT with contrast.
Protamine.	Reverses the effects of heparin.
Prothrombin time.	The coagulation parameter affected by warfarin.
A young patient with a family history of sudden death collapses and dies while exercising.	Hypertrophic cardiomyopathy.
Endocarditis prophylaxis regimens.	Oral surgery—amoxicillin for certain situations; GI or GU procedures—not recommended.
Virchow's triad.	Stasis, hypercoagulability, endothelial damage.
The most common cause of hypertension in young women.	OCPs.
The most common cause of hypertension in young men.	Excessive EtOH.
Figure 3 sign.	Aortic coarctation.
Water-bottle-shaped heart.	Pericardial effusion. Look for pulsus paradoxus.

DERMATOLOGY

"Stuck-on" appearance.	Seborrheic keratosis.
Red plaques with silvery-white scales and sharp margins.	Psoriasis.
The most common type of skin cancer; the lesion is a pearly-colored papule with a translucent surface and telangiectasias.	Basal cell carcinoma.
Honey-crusted lesions.	Impetigo.
A febrile patient with a history of diabetes presents with a red, swollen, painful lower extremity.	Cellulitis.
⊕ Nikolsky's sign.	Pemphigus vulgaris.
⊖ Nikolsky's sign.	Bullous pemphigoid.
A 55-year-old obese patient presents with dirty, velvety patches on the back of the neck.	Acanthosis nigricans. Check fasting blood glucose to rule out diabetes.
Dermatomal distribution.	Varicella zoster.
Flat-topped papules.	Lichen planus.
Iris-like target lesions.	Erythema multiforme.
A lesion characteristically occurring in a linear pattern in areas where skin comes into contact with clothing or jewelry.	Contact dermatitis.
Presents with a herald patch, Christmas-tree pattern.	Pityriasis rosea.
Pinkish, scaling, flat lesions on the chest and back; KOH prep has a "spaghetti-and-meatballs" appearance.	Tinea (pityriasis) versicolor.
Four characteristics of a nevus suggestive of melanoma.	Asymmetry, border irregularity, color variation, and large diameter.
A premalignant lesion from sun exposure that can lead to squamous cell carcinoma.	Actinic keratosis.
"Dewdrops on a rose petal."	Lesions of 1° varicella.
"Cradle cap."	Seborrheic dermatitis. Treat conservatively with bathing and moisturizing agents.
Associated with *Propionibacterium acnes* and changes in androgen levels.	Acne vulgaris.
A painful, recurrent vesicular eruption of mucocutaneous surfaces.	Herpes simplex.
Inflammation and epithelial thinning of the anogenital area, predominantly in postmenopausal women.	Lichen sclerosus.
Exophytic nodules on the skin with varying degrees of scaling or ulceration; the second most common type of skin cancer.	Squamous cell carcinoma.

ENDOCRINOLOGY

The most common cause of hypothyroidism.	Hashimoto's thyroiditis.
Lab findings in Hashimoto's thyroiditis.	High TSH, low T_4, anti-TPO antibodies.
Exophthalmos, pretibial myxedema, and ↓ TSH.	Graves' disease.
The most common cause of Cushing's syndrome.	Iatrogenic corticosteroid administration. The second most common cause is Cushing's disease.
A patient presents with signs of hypocalcemia, high phosphorus, and low PTH.	Hypoparathyroidism.
"Stones, bones, groans, psychiatric overtones."	Signs and symptoms of hypercalcemia.
A patient complains of headache, weakness, and polyuria; examination reveals hypertension and tetany. Labs show hypernatremia, hypokalemia, and metabolic alkalosis.	1° hyperaldosteronism (due to Conn's syndrome or bilateral adrenal hyperplasia).
A patient presents with tachycardia, wild swings in BP, headache, diaphoresis, altered mental status, and a sense of panic.	Pheochromocytoma.
Which should be used first in treating pheochromocytoma, α- or β-antagonists?	α-antagonists (phentolamine and phenoxybenzamine).
A patient with a history of lithium use presents with copious amounts of dilute urine.	Nephrogenic diabetes insipidus (DI).
Treatment of central DI.	Administration of DDAVP and free-water restriction.
A postoperative patient with significant pain presents with hyponatremia and normal volume status.	SIADH due to stress.
An antidiabetic agent associated with lactic acidosis.	Metformin.
A patient presents with weakness, nausea, vomiting, weight loss, and new skin pigmentation. Labs show hyponatremia and hyperkalemia. Treatment?	1° adrenal insufficiency (Addison's disease). Treat with glucocorticoids, mineralocorticoids, and IV fluids.
Goal HbA_{1c} for a patient with diabetes mellitus (DM).	< 7.0.
Treatment of DKA.	Fluids, insulin, and electrolyte repletion (eg, K^+).
Why are β-blockers contraindicated in diabetics?	They can mask symptoms of hypoglycemia.

EPIDEMIOLOGY

How do you interpret the following 95% confidence interval (CI) for a relative risk (RR) of 0.582: 95% CI 0.502, 0.673?	These data are consistent with RRs ranging from 0.502 to 0.673 with 95% confidence (ie, we are confident that the true RR will be between 0.502 and 0.673 95 out of 100 times).
Bias introduced into a study when a clinician is aware of the patient's treatment type.	Observational bias.
Bias introduced when screening detects a disease earlier and thus lengthens the time from diagnosis to death.	Lead-time bias.
If you want to know if geographical location affects infant mortality rate but most variation in infant mortality is predicted by socioeconomic status, then socioeconomic status is a _____.	Confounding variable.
The proportion of people who have the disease and test $\oplus$ is the _____.	Sensitivity.
Sensitive tests have few false $\ominus$s and are used to rule _____ a disease.	Out.
PPD reactivity is used as a screening test because most people with TB (except those who are anergic) will have a $\oplus$ PPD. Highly sensitive or specific?	Highly sensitive for TB. Screening tests with high sensitivity are good for diseases with low prevalence.
Chronic diseases such as SLE—higher prevalence or incidence?	Higher prevalence.
Epidemics such as influenza—higher prevalence or incidence?	Higher incidence.
What is the difference between incidence and prevalence?	Prevalence is the percentage of cases of disease in a population at 1 snapshot in time. Incidence is the percentage of new cases of disease that develop over a given time period among the total population at risk.
Cross-sectional survey—incidence or prevalence?	Prevalence.
Cohort study—incidence or prevalence?	Incidence and prevalence.
Case-control study—incidence or prevalence?	Neither.
Describe a test that consistently gives identical results, but the results are wrong.	High reliability (precision), low validity (accuracy).
Difference between a cohort and a case-control study.	Cohort studies can be used to calculate RR, incidence, and/or odds ratio (OR). Case-control studies can be used to calculate an OR, which is an estimate of RR when the disease prevalence is low.
Attributable risk?	The difference in risk in the exposed and unexposed groups (ie, the risk that is attributable to the exposure).
Relative risk?	Incidence in the exposed group divided by the incidence in the nonexposed group.

The results of a hypothetical study found an association between ASA intake and risk of heart disease. How do you interpret an RR of 1.5?	In patients who took ASA, the risk of heart disease was 1.5 times that of patients who did not take ASA.
Odds ratio?	In cohort studies, the odds of *developing* the disease in the exposed group divided by the odds of *developing* the disease in the nonexposed group. In case-control studies, the odds that the cases were exposed divided by the odds that the controls were exposed. In cross-sectional studies, the odds that the exposed group has the disease divided by the odds that the nonexposed group has the disease.
The results of a hypothetical study found an association between ASA intake and risk of heart disease. How do you interpret an OR of 1.5?	In patients who took ASA, the odds of acquiring heart disease were 1.5 times those of patients who did not take ASA.
In which patients do you initiate colorectal cancer screening early?	Patients with IBD; those with familial adenomatous polyposis (FAP)/hereditary nonpolyposis colorectal cancer (HNPCC); and those who have first-degree relatives with adenomatous polyps (< 60 years of age) or colorectal cancer.
The most common cancer in men and the most common cause of death from cancer in men.	Prostate cancer is the most common cancer in men, but lung cancer causes more deaths.
The percentage of cases within 1 SD of the mean? Two SDs? Three SDs?	68%, 95.4%, 99.7%.
Birth rate?	Number of live births per 1000 population in 1 year.
Mortality rate?	Number of deaths per 1000 population in 1 year.
Neonatal mortality rate?	Number of deaths from birth to 28 days per 1000 live births in 1 year.
Infant mortality rate?	Number of deaths from birth to 1 year of age per 1000 live births (neonatal + postnatal mortality) in 1 year.
Maternal mortality rate?	Number of deaths during pregnancy to 90 days postpartum per 100,000 live births in 1 year.

ETHICS

True or false: Once patients sign a statement giving consent, they must continue treatment.	False. Patients may change their minds at any time. Exceptions to the requirement of informed consent include emergency situations and patients without decision-making capacity.
A 15-year-old pregnant girl requires hospitalization for preeclampsia. Is parental consent required?	No. Parental consent is not necessary for the medical treatment of pregnant minors.
A doctor refers a patient for an MRI at a facility he/she owns.	Conflict of interest.

Involuntary psychiatric hospitalization can be undertaken for which 3 reasons?	The patient is a danger to self, a danger to others, or gravely disabled (unable to provide for basic needs).
True or false: It is more difficult to justify the withdrawal of futile care than to have withheld the treatment in the first place.	False. Withdrawing a nonbeneficial treatment is ethically similar to withholding a nonindicated one.
A mother refuses to allow her child to be vaccinated.	A parent has the right to refuse treatment for his/her child as long as it does not pose a serious threat to the well-being of the child.
When can a physician refuse to continue treating a patient on the grounds of futility?	When there is no rationale for treatment, maximal intervention is failing, a given intervention has already failed, and treatment will not achieve the goals of care.
An 8-year-old child is in a serious accident. She requires emergent transfusion, but her parents are not present.	Treat immediately. Consent is implied in emergency situations.
A 15-year-old girl seeking treatment for an STD asks that her parents not be told about her condition.	Minors may consent to care for STDs without parental consent or knowledge.
Conditions in which confidentiality must be overridden.	Real threat of harm to third parties; suicidal intentions; certain contagious diseases; elder and child abuse.
Involuntary commitment or isolation for medical treatment may be undertaken for what reason?	When treatment noncompliance represents a serious danger to public health (eg, active TB).
A 10-year-old child presents in status epilepticus, but her parents refuse treatment on religious grounds.	Treat because the disease represents an immediate threat to the child's life. Then seek a court order.
A son asks that his mother not be told about her recently discovered cancer.	A physician can withhold information from the patient only in the rare case of therapeutic privilege or if the patient requests not to be told. A patient's family cannot require the physician to withhold information from the patient.

GASTROINTESTINAL

A patient presents with sudden onset of severe, diffuse abdominal pain. Examination reveals peritoneal signs, and AXR reveals free air under the diaphragm. Management?	Emergent laparotomy to repair a perforated viscus.
The most likely cause of acute lower GI bleed in patients > 40 years of age.	Diverticulosis.
Diagnostic modality used when ultrasound is equivocal for cholecystitis.	HIDA scan.
Risk factors for cholelithiasis.	Fat, female, fertile, forty, flatulent.
Inspiratory arrest during palpation of the RUQ.	Murphy's sign, seen in acute cholecystitis.
The most common cause of small bowel obstruction (SBO) in patients with no history of abdominal surgery.	Hernia.

The most common cause of SBO in patients with a history of abdominal surgery.	Adhesions.
Identify key organisms causing diarrhea: ▪ Most common organism ▪ Recent antibiotic use ▪ Camping ▪ Traveler's diarrhea ▪ Church picnics/mayonnaise ▪ Uncooked hamburgers ▪ Fried rice ▪ Poultry/eggs ▪ Raw seafood ▪ AIDS ▪ Pseudoappendicitis	 *Campylobacter* *Clostridium difficile* *Giardia* ETEC *S aureus* *E coli* O157:H7 *Bacillus cereus* *Salmonella* *Vibrio*, HAV *Isospora, Cryptosporidium, Mycobacterium avium* complex (MAC) *Yersinia*
A 25-year-old Jewish man presents with pain and watery diarrhea after meals. Examination shows fistulas between the bowel and skin and nodular lesions on his tibias.	Crohn's disease.
Inflammatory disease of the colon with an ↑ risk of colon cancer.	Ulcerative colitis (greater risk than Crohn's).
Extraintestinal manifestations of IBD.	Uveitis, ankylosing spondylitis, pyoderma gangrenosum, erythema nodosum, 1° sclerosing cholangitis.
Medical treatment for IBD.	5-ASA agents and steroids during acute exacerbations.
Difference between Mallory-Weiss and Boerhaave tears.	Mallory-Weiss—superficial tear in the esophageal mucosa; Boerhaave—full-thickness esophageal rupture.
Charcot's triad.	RUQ pain, jaundice, and fever/chills—signs of ascending cholangitis.
Reynolds' pentad.	Charcot's triad plus shock and mental status changes—signs of suppurative ascending cholangitis.
Medical treatment for hepatic encephalopathy.	↓ protein intake, lactulose, rifaximin.
The first step in the management of a patient with an acute GI bleed.	Manage ABCs.
A 4-year-old child presents with oliguria, petechiae, and jaundice following an illness with bloody diarrhea. Most likely diagnosis and cause?	Hemolytic-uremic syndrome (HUS) due to *E coli* O157:H7.
Post-HBV exposure treatment.	HBV immunoglobulin.
Classic causes of drug-induced hepatitis.	TB medications (INH, rifampin, pyrazinamide), acetaminophen, and tetracycline.
A 40-year-old obese woman with elevated alkaline phosphatase, elevated bilirubin, pruritus, dark urine, and clay-colored stools.	Biliary tract obstruction.

Hernia with highest risk of incarceration—indirect, direct, or femoral?	Femoral hernia.
A 50-year-old man with a history of alcohol abuse presents with boring epigastric pain that radiates to the back and is relieved by sitting forward. Management?	Confirm the diagnosis of acute pancreatitis with elevated amylase and lipase. Make the patient NPO and give IV fluids, O_2, analgesia, and "tincture of time."

HEMATOLOGY/ONCOLOGY

Four causes of microcytic anemia.	**TICS**–**T**halassemia, **I**ron deficiency, anemia of **C**hronic disease, and **S**ideroblastic anemia.
An elderly man with hypochromic, microcytic anemia is asymptomatic. Diagnostic tests?	Fecal occult blood test and sigmoidoscopy; suspect colorectal cancer.
Precipitants of hemolytic crisis in patients with G6PD deficiency.	Sulfonamides, antimalarial drugs, fava beans.
The most common inherited cause of hypercoagulability.	Factor V Leiden mutation.
The most common inherited bleeding disorder.	von Willebrand's disease.
The most common inherited hemolytic anemia.	Hereditary spherocytosis.
Diagnostic test for hereditary spherocytosis.	Osmotic fragility test.
Pure RBC aplasia.	Diamond-Blackfan anemia.
Anemia associated with absent radii and thumbs, diffuse hyperpigmentation, café au lait spots, microcephaly, and pancytopenia.	Fanconi's anemia.
Medications and viruses that lead to aplastic anemia.	Chloramphenicol, sulfonamides, radiation, HIV, chemotherapeutic agents, hepatitis, parvovirus B19, EBV.
How to distinguish polycythemia vera from 2° polycythemia.	Both have ↑ hematocrit and RBC mass, but polycythemia vera should have normal O_2 saturation and low erythropoietin levels.
Thrombotic thrombocytopenic purpura (TTP) pentad?	**"FAT RN"**: **F**ever, **A**nemia, **T**hrombocytopenia, **R**enal dysfunction, **N**eurologic abnormalities.
HUS triad?	Anemia, thrombocytopenia, and acute renal failure.
Treatment for TTP.	Emergent large-volume plasmapheresis, corticosteroids, antiplatelet drugs. Platelet transfusion is contraindicated!
Treatment for idiopathic thrombocytopenic purpura (ITP) in children.	Usually resolves spontaneously; may require IVIG and/or corticosteroids.
Which of the following are ↑ in DIC: fibrin split products, D-dimer, fibrinogen, platelets, and hematocrit.	Fibrin split products and D-dimer are elevated; platelets, fibrinogen, and hematocrit are ↓.

An 8-year-old boy presents with hemarthrosis and ↑ PTT with normal PT and bleeding time. Diagnosis? Treatment?	Hemophilia A or B; consider desmopressin (for hemophilia A) or factor VIII or IX supplements.
A 14-year-old girl presents with prolonged bleeding after dental surgery and with menses, normal PT, normal or ↑ PTT, and ↑ bleeding time. Diagnosis? Treatment?	von Willebrand's disease; treat with desmopressin, FFP, or cryoprecipitate.
A 60-year-old African American man presents with bone pain. What might a workup for multiple myeloma reveal?	Monoclonal gammopathy, Bence Jones proteinuria, and "punched-out" lesions on x-ray of the skull and long bones.
Reed-Sternberg cells.	Hodgkin's lymphoma.
A 10-year-old boy presents with fever, weight loss, and night sweats. Examination shows an anterior mediastinal mass. Suspected diagnosis?	Non-Hodgkin's lymphoma.
Microcytic anemia with ↓ serum iron, ↓ total iron-binding capacity (TIBC), and normal or ↑ ferritin.	Anemia of chronic disease.
Microcytic anemia with ↓ serum iron, ↓ ferritin, and ↑ TIBC.	Iron deficiency anemia.
An 80-year-old man presents with fatigue, lymphadenopathy, splenomegaly, and isolated lymphocytosis. What is the suspected diagnosis?	Chronic lymphocytic leukemia (CLL).
The lymphoma equivalent of CLL.	Small lymphocytic lymphoma.
A late, life-threatening complication of chronic myelogenous leukemia (CML).	Blast crisis (fever, bone pain, splenomegaly, pancytopenia).
Auer rods on blood smear.	Acute myelogenous leukemia (AML).
AML subtype associated with DIC. Treatment?	M3. Retinoic acid.
Electrolyte changes in tumor lysis syndrome.	↓ Ca^{2+}, ↑ K^+, ↑ phosphate, ↑ uric acid.
A 50-year-old man presents with early satiety, splenomegaly, and bleeding. Cytogenetics show t(9,22). Diagnosis?	CML.
Heinz bodies.	Intracellular inclusions seen in thalassemia, G6PD deficiency, and postsplenectomy.
Virus associated with aplastic anemia in patients with sickle cell anemia.	Parvovirus B19.
A 25-year-old African American man with sickle cell anemia has sudden onset of bone pain. Management of pain crisis?	O_2, analgesia, hydration, and, if severe, transfusion.
A significant cause of morbidity in thalassemia patients. Treatment?	Iron overload; use deferoxamine.

INFECTIOUS DISEASE

The 3 most common causes of fever of unknown origin (FUO).	Infection, cancer, and autoimmune disease.
Four signs and symptoms of streptococcal pharyngitis.	Fever, pharyngeal erythema, tonsillar exudate, lack of cough.
A nonsuppurative complication of streptococcal infection that is not altered by treatment of 1° infection.	Postinfectious glomerulonephritis.
The most common predisposing factor for acute sinusitis.	Viral URI.
Asplenic patients are particularly susceptible to these organisms.	Encapsulated organisms—pneumococcus, meningococcus, *Haemophilus influenzae, Klebsiella*.
The number of bacteria needed on a clean-catch specimen to diagnose a UTI.	10^5 bacteria/mL.
Which healthy population is susceptible to UTIs?	Pregnant women. Treat this group aggressively because of potential complications.
A patient from California or Arizona presents with fever, malaise, cough, and night sweats. Diagnosis? Treatment?	Coccidioidomycosis; amphotericin B.
Nonpainful chancre.	1° syphilis.
A "blueberry muffin" rash is characteristic of what congenital infection?	Rubella.
Meningitis in neonates. Causes? Treatment?	Group B strep (GBS), *E coli, Listeria*. Treat with gentamicin and ampicillin.
Meningitis in infants. Causes? Treatment?	Pneumococcus, meningococcus, *H influenzae*. Treat with cefotaxime and vancomycin.
What should always be done prior to LP?	Check for ↑ ICP; look for papilledema.
CSF findings: ■ Low glucose, PMN predominance ■ Normal glucose, lymphocytic predominance ■ Numerous RBCs in serial CSF samples ■ ↑ gamma globulins	 Bacterial meningitis Aseptic (viral) meningitis Subarachnoid hemorrhage (SAH) MS
Initially presents with a pruritic papule with regional lymphadenopathy; evolves into a black eschar after 7–10 days. Treatment?	Cutaneous anthrax. Treat with penicillin G or ciprofloxacin.
Findings in 3° syphilis.	Tabes dorsalis, general paresis, gummas, Argyll Robertson pupil, aortitis, aortic root aneurysms.
Characteristics of 2° Lyme disease.	Arthralgias, migratory polyarthropathies, Bell's palsy, myocarditis.
Cold agglutinins.	*Mycoplasma*.
A 24-year-old man presents with soft white plaques on his tongue and the back of his throat. Diagnosis? Workup? Treatment?	Candidal thrush. Workup should include an HIV test. Treat with nystatin oral suspension.

At what CD4 count should *Pneumocystis jiroveci* pneumonia prophylaxis be initiated in an HIV-⊕ patient? *Mycobacterium avium–intracellulare* (MAI) prophylaxis?	≤ 200 for *P jiroveci* (with TMP-SMX); ≤ 50–100 for MAI (with clarithromycin/azithromycin).
Risk factors for pyelonephritis.	Pregnancy, vesicoureteral reflux, anatomic anomalies, indwelling catheters, kidney stones.
Neutropenic nadir postchemotherapy.	7–10 days.
Erythema migrans.	Lesion of 1° Lyme disease.
Classic physical findings for endocarditis.	Fever, heart murmur, Osler's nodes, splinter hemorrhages, Janeway lesions, Roth's spots.
Aplastic crisis in sickle cell disease.	Parvovirus B19.
Ring-enhancing brain lesion on CT with seizures.	*Taenia solium* (cysticercosis).

Name the organism:	
▪ Branching rods in oral infection	*Actinomyces israelii*
▪ Weakly gram-⊕, partially acid-fast in lung infection	*Nocardia asteroides*
▪ Painful chancroid	*Haemophilus ducreyi*
▪ Dog or cat bite	*Pasteurella multocida*
▪ Gardener	*Sporothrix schenckii*
▪ Raw pork and skeletal muscle cysts	*Trichinella spiralis*
▪ Sheepherders with liver cysts	*Echinococcus granulosus*
▪ Perianal itching	*Enterobius vermicularis*
▪ Pregnant women with pets	*Toxoplasma gondii*
▪ Meningitis in adults	*Neisseria meningitidis*
▪ Meningitis in elderly	*Streptococcus pneumoniae*
▪ Meningoencephalitis in AIDS patients	*Cryptococcus neoformans*
▪ Alcoholic with pneumonia	*Klebsiella*
▪ "Currant jelly" sputum	*Klebsiella*
▪ Malignant external otitis	*Pseudomonas*
▪ Infection in burn victims	*Pseudomonas*
▪ Osteomyelitis from a foot wound puncture	*Pseudomonas*
▪ Osteomyelitis in a sickle cell patient	*Salmonella*

A 55-year-old man who is a smoker and a heavy drinker presents with a new cough and flulike symptoms. Gram stain shows no organisms; silver stain of sputum shows gram-⊖ rods. What is the diagnosis?	*Legionella* pneumonia.
A middle-aged man presents with acute-onset monoarticular joint pain and bilateral Bell's palsy. What is the likely diagnosis, and how did he get it? Treatment?	Lyme disease, *Ixodes* tick, doxycycline.
A patient develops endocarditis 3 weeks after receiving a prosthetic heart valve. What organism is suspected?	*S aureus* or *Staphylococcus epidermidis*.
A patient develops endocarditis in a native valve after having a dental cleaning.	*Streptococcus viridans*.

MUSCULOSKELETAL

Back pain that is exacerbated by standing and walking and relieved with sitting and hyperflexion of the hips.	Spinal stenosis.
Joints in the hand affected in rheumatoid arthritis.	MCP and PIP joints; DIP joints are spared.
Joint pain and stiffness that worsen over the course of the day and are relieved by rest.	Osteoarthritis.
A genetic disorder that is associated with multiple fractures and blue sclerae and is commonly mistaken for child abuse.	Osteogenesis imperfecta.
Hip and back pain along with stiffness that improves with activity over the course of the day and worsens at rest. Diagnostic test?	Suspect ankylosing spondylitis. Check HLA-B27.
Arthritis, conjunctivitis, and urethritis in young men. Associated organisms?	Reactive (Reiter's) arthritis. Most commonly associated with *Chlamydia.* Also consider *Campylobacter, Shigella, Salmonella,* and *Ureaplasma.*
A 55-year-old man has sudden, excruciating first MTP joint pain after a night of drinking red wine. Diagnosis, workup, and chronic treatment?	Gout. Needle-shaped, negatively birefringent crystals are seen on joint fluid aspirate. Chronic treatment with allopurinol or probenecid.
Rhomboid-shaped, positively birefringent crystals on joint fluid aspirate.	Pseudogout.
An elderly woman presents with pain and stiffness of the shoulders and hips; she cannot lift her arms above her head. Labs show anemia and ↑ ESR.	Polymyalgia rheumatica.
An active 13-year-old boy has anterior knee pain. Diagnosis?	Osgood-Schlatter disease.
Bone is fractured in a fall on an outstretched hand.	Distal radius (Colles' fracture).
A complication of scaphoid fracture.	Avascular necrosis.
Signs suggesting radial nerve damage with humeral fracture.	Wrist drop, loss of thumb abduction.
A young child presents with proximal muscle weakness, waddling gait, and pronounced calf muscles.	Duchenne muscular dystrophy.
A first-born female who was born in breech position is found to have asymmetric skin folds on newborn exam. Diagnosis? Treatment?	Developmental dysplasia of the hip. If severe, consider a Pavlik harness to maintain abduction.
An 11-year-old obese African American boy presents with sudden onset of limp. Diagnosis? Workup?	Slipped capital femoral epiphysis. AP and frog-leg lateral x-rays.
The most common 1° malignant tumor of bone.	Multiple myeloma.

NEUROLOGY

Unilateral, severe periorbital headache with tearing and conjunctival erythema.	Cluster headache.
Prophylactic treatment for migraine.	Antihypertensives, antidepressants, anticonvulsants, dietary changes.
The most common pituitary tumor. Treatment?	Prolactinoma. Dopamine agonists (eg, bromocriptine).
A 55-year-old patient presents with acute "broken speech." What type of aphasia? What lobe and vascular distribution?	Broca's aphasia. Frontal lobe, left MCA distribution.
The most common cause of SAH.	Trauma; the second most common is berry aneurysm.
A crescent-shaped hyperdensity on CT that does not cross the midline.	Subdural hematoma—bridging veins torn.
A history significant for initial altered mental status with an intervening lucid interval. Diagnosis? Most likely source? Treatment?	Epidural hematoma. Middle meningeal artery. Neurosurgical evacuation.
CSF findings with SAH.	Elevated ICP, RBCs, xanthochromia.
Albuminocytologic dissociation.	Guillain-Barré syndrome ($\uparrow$ protein in CSF without a significant $\uparrow$ in cell count).
Cold water is flushed into a patient's ear, and the fast phase of the nystagmus is toward the opposite side. Normal or pathologic?	Normal.
The most common 1° sources of metastases to the brain.	Lung, breast, skin (melanoma), kidney, GI tract.
May be seen in children who are accused of inattention in class and confused with ADHD.	Absence seizures.
The most frequent presentation of intracranial neoplasm.	Headache. 1° neoplasms are much less common than brain metastases.
The most common cause of seizures in children (2–10 years).	Infection, febrile seizures, trauma, idiopathic.
The most common cause of seizures in young adults (18–35 years).	Trauma, alcohol withdrawal, brain tumor.
First-line medication for status epilepticus.	IV benzodiazepine.
Confusion, confabulation, ophthalmoplegia, ataxia.	Wernicke's encephalopathy due to a deficiency of thiamine.
What % lesion is an indication for carotid endarterectomy?	Seventy percent if the stenosis is symptomatic.
The most common causes of dementia.	Alzheimer's and multi-infarct.
A combined UMN and LMN disorder.	ALS.
Rigidity and stiffness with unilateral resting tremor and masked facies.	Parkinson's disease.
The mainstay of Parkinson's therapy.	Levodopa/carbidopa.

Treatment for Guillain-Barré syndrome.	IVIG or plasmapheresis. Avoid steroids.
Rigidity and stiffness that progress to choreiform movements, accompanied by moodiness and altered behavior.	Huntington's disease.
A 6-year-old girl presents with a port-wine stain in the V_1 distribution as well as with mental retardation, seizures, and ipsilateral leptomeningeal angioma.	Sturge-Weber syndrome. Treat symptomatically. Possible focal cerebral resection of the affected lobe.
Multiple café au lait spots on skin.	Neurofibromatosis type 1.
Hyperphagia, hypersexuality, hyperorality, and hyperdocility.	Klüver-Bucy syndrome (amygdala).
May be administered to a symptomatic patient to diagnose myasthenia gravis.	Edrophonium.

OBSTETRICS

1° causes of third-trimester bleeding.	Placental abruption and placenta previa.
Classic ultrasound and gross appearance of complete hydatidiform mole.	Snowstorm on ultrasound. "Cluster-of-grapes" appearance on gross examination.
Chromosomal pattern of a complete mole.	46,XX.
Molar pregnancy containing fetal tissue.	Partial mole.
Symptoms of placental abruption.	Continuous, painful vaginal bleeding.
Symptoms of placenta previa.	Self-limited, painless vaginal bleeding.
When should a vaginal exam be performed with suspected placenta previa?	Never.
Antibiotics with teratogenic effects.	Tetracycline, fluoroquinolones, aminoglycosides, sulfonamides.
Medication given to accelerate fetal lung maturity.	Betamethasone or dexamethasone × 48 hours.
The most common cause of postpartum hemorrhage.	Uterine atony.
Treatment for postpartum hemorrhage.	Uterine massage; if that fails, give oxytocin.
Typical antibiotics for GBS prophylaxis.	IV penicillin or ampicillin.
A patient fails to lactate after an emergency C-section with marked blood loss.	Sheehan's syndrome (postpartum pituitary necrosis).
Uterine bleeding at 18 weeks' gestation; no products expelled; cervical os open.	Inevitable abortion.
Uterine bleeding at 18 weeks' gestation; no products expelled; cervical os closed.	Threatened abortion.

GYNECOLOGY

The first test to perform when a woman presents with amenorrhea.	β-hCG; the most common cause of amenorrhea is pregnancy.
Term for heavy bleeding during and between menstrual periods.	Menometrorrhagia.
Cause of amenorrhea with normal prolactin, no response to estrogen-progesterone challenge, and a history of D&C.	Asherman's syndrome.
Therapy for polycystic ovarian syndrome.	Weight loss and OCPs. Consider metformin.
Medication used to induce ovulation.	Clomiphene citrate.
Diagnostic step required in a postmenopausal woman who presents with vaginal bleeding.	Endometrial biopsy.
Indications for medical treatment of ectopic pregnancy.	Patient stable; unruptured ectopic pregnancy of < 3.5 cm at < 6 weeks' gestation.
Medical options for endometriosis.	OCPs, danazol, GnRH agonists.
Laparoscopic findings in endometriosis.	Powder burns, "chocolate cysts."
The most common location for an ectopic pregnancy.	Ampulla of the oviduct.
How to diagnose and follow a leiomyoma.	Ultrasound.
Natural history of a leiomyoma.	Regresses after menopause.
A patient has ↑ vaginal discharge and petechial patches in the upper vagina and cervix.	Trichomonal vaginitis.
Treatment for bacterial vaginosis.	Oral or topical metronidazole.
The most common cause of bloody nipple discharge.	Intraductal papilloma.
Contraceptive methods that protect against PID.	OCPs and barrier contraception.
Unopposed estrogen is contraindicated in which cancers?	Endometrial or estrogen receptor–⊕ breast cancer.
A patient presents with recent PID with RUQ pain.	Consider Fitz-Hugh–Curtis syndrome.
Breast malignancy presenting as itching, burning, and erosion of the nipple.	Paget's disease.
Annual screening for women with a strong family history of ovarian cancer.	CA-125 and transvaginal ultrasound.
A 50-year-old woman leaks urine when laughing or coughing. Nonsurgical options?	Kegel exercises, estrogen, pessaries for stress incontinence.
A 30-year-old woman has unpredictable urine loss. Examination is normal. Medical options?	Anticholinergics (oxybutynin) or β-adrenergics (metaproterenol) for urge incontinence.

Lab values suggestive of menopause.	↑ serum FSH.
The most common cause of female infertility.	Endometriosis.
Two consecutive findings of atypical squamous cells of undetermined significance (ASCUS) on Pap smear. Follow-up evaluation?	Colposcopy and endocervical curettage.
Breast cancer type that ↑ the future risk of invasive carcinoma in both breasts.	Lobular carcinoma in situ.

PEDIATRICS

Nontender abdominal mass associated with elevated VMA and HVA.	Neuroblastoma.
The most common type of tracheoesophageal fistula (TEF). Diagnosis?	Esophageal atresia with distal TEF (85%). Unable to pass NG tube.
Not contraindications to vaccination.	Mild illness and/or low-grade fever, current antibiotic therapy, and prematurity.
Tests to rule out shaken baby syndrome.	Ophthalmologic exam, CT, and MRI.
A neonate has meconium ileus.	Cystic fibrosis (Hirschsprung's disease is associated with failure to pass meconium for 48 hours).
Bilious emesis within hours after the first feeding.	Duodenal atresia.
A 2-month-old baby presents with nonbilious projectile emesis. Diagnosis? What are the appropriate steps in management?	Pyloric stenosis. Correct metabolic abnormalities; then correct pyloric stenosis with pyloromyotomy.
The most common 1° immunodeficiency.	Selective IgA deficiency.
An infant has a high fever and onset of rash as fever breaks. What is he at risk for?	Febrile seizures (due to roseola infantum).
What is the immunodeficiency? ■ A boy has chronic respiratory infections. Nitroblue tetrazolium test is ⊖. ■ A child has eczema, thrombocytopenia, and high levels of IgA. ■ A 4-month-old boy has life-threatening *Pseudomonas* infection.	Chronic granulomatous disease Wiskott-Aldrich syndrome Bruton's X-linked agammaglobulinemia
Acute-phase treatment for Kawasaki disease.	High-dose ASA for inflammation and fever; IVIG to prevent coronary artery aneurysms.
Treatment for mild and severe unconjugated hyperbilirubinemia.	Phototherapy (mild) or exchange transfusion (severe). (Do not use phototherapy for conjugated hyperbilirubinemia.)
Sudden onset of mental status changes, emesis, and liver dysfunction after ASA intake.	Reye's syndrome.

A child has loss of red light reflex (white pupil). Diagnosis? The child has an ↑ risk of what cancer?	Suspect retinoblastoma. Osteosarcoma.
Vaccinations at a 6-month well-child visit.	HBV, DTaP, Hib, IPV, PCV, rotavirus.
Tanner stage 3 in a 6-year-old girl.	Precocious puberty.
Infection of small airways with epidemics in winter and spring.	RSV bronchiolitis.
Cause of neonatal RDS.	Surfactant deficiency.
A condition associated with red "currant-jelly" stools, colicky abdominal pain, bilious vomiting, and a sausage-shaped mass in the RUQ.	Intussusception.
A congenital heart disease that causes 2° hypertension. What would you find on physical examination?	Coarctation of the aorta; ↓ femoral pulses.
First-line treatment for otitis media.	Amoxicillin × 10 days.
The most common pathogen causing croup.	Parainfluenza virus type 1.
A homeless child is small for his age and has peeling skin and a swollen belly.	Kwashiorkor (protein malnutrition).
Defect in an X-linked syndrome with mental retardation, gout, self-mutilation, and choreoathetosis.	Lesch-Nyhan syndrome (purine salvage problem with HGPRTase deficiency).
A newborn girl has a continuous "machinery murmur." What drug would you give?	Patent ductus arteriosus (PDA). Indomethacin is given to close the PDA.
A newborn with a posterior neck mass and swelling of the hands.	Turner's syndrome.

PSYCHIATRY

First-line pharmacotherapy for depression.	SSRIs.
Antidepressants associated with hypertensive crisis.	MAOIs.
Galactorrhea, impotence, menstrual dysfunction, and ↓ libido.	Dopamine antagonists.
A 17-year-old girl has left arm paralysis after her boyfriend dies in a car crash. No medical cause is found.	Conversion disorder.
Name the defense mechanism: ▪ A mother who is angry at her husband yells at her child. ▪ A pedophile enters a monastery. ▪ A woman calmly describes a grisly murder. ▪ A hospitalized 10-year-old begins to wet his bed.	Displacement Reaction formation Isolation Regression
Life-threatening muscle rigidity, high fever, and rhabdomyolysis.	Neuroleptic malignant syndrome.

Amenorrhea, low body weight (< 85%), bradycardia, and abnormal body image in a young woman.	Anorexia.
A 35-year-old man has recurrent episodes of palpitations, diaphoresis, and fear of going crazy.	Panic disorder.
The most serious side effect of clozapine.	Agranulocytosis.
A 21-year-old man has 3 months of social withdrawal, worsening grades, flattened affect, and concrete thinking.	Schizophreniform disorder (a diagnosis of schizophrenia requires ≥ 6 months of symptoms).
Key side effects of atypical antipsychotics.	Weight gain, type 2 DM, QT-segment prolongation.
A young weight lifter receives IV haloperidol and complains that his eyes are deviated sideways. Diagnosis? Treatment?	Acute dystonia (oculogyric crisis). Treat with benztropine or diphenhydramine.
Medication to avoid in patients with a history of alcohol withdrawal seizures.	Neuroleptics.
A 13-year-old boy has a history of theft, vandalism, and violence toward family pets.	Conduct disorder. Associated with antisocial personality disorder in adults.
A 5-month-old girl has ↓ head growth, truncal discoordination, and ↓ social interaction.	Rett's disorder. Loss of milestones is commonly described.
A patient hasn't slept for days, lost $20,000 gambling, is agitated, and has pressured speech. Diagnosis? Treatment?	Acute mania. Start a mood stabilizer (eg, lithium).
After a minor "fender bender," a man wears a neck brace and requests permanent disability.	Malingering.
A nurse presents with severe hypoglycemia; blood analysis reveals no elevation in C-peptide.	Factitious disorder (Munchausen syndrome).
A patient continues to use cocaine after being in jail, losing his job, and not paying child support.	Substance abuse.
Medication to avoid in patients with PTSD.	Benzodiazepines (have high addiction potential). Patients commonly have a history of substance abuse.
A violent patient has vertical and horizontal nystagmus.	Phencyclidine hydrochloride (PCP) intoxication.
A woman who was abused as a child frequently feels outside of or detached from her body.	Depersonalization disorder.
A schizophrenic patient takes haloperidol for 1 year and develops uncontrollable tongue movements. Diagnosis? Treatment?	Tardive dyskinesia. ↓ or discontinue haloperidol and consider another antipsychotic (eg, risperidone, clozapine).
A man with major depressive disorder is counseled to avoid tyramine-rich foods with his new medication.	MAOIs.

PULMONARY

Risk factors for DVT.	Stasis, endothelial injury, and hypercoagulability (Virchow's triad).
Criteria for exudative effusion.	Pleural/serum protein > 0.5; pleural/serum LDH > 0.6.
Causes of exudative effusion.	Think of leaky capillaries. Malignancy, TB, bacterial or viral infection, PE with infarct, and pancreatitis.
Causes of transudative effusion.	Think of intact capillaries. CHF, liver or kidney disease, and protein-losing enteropathy.
Normalizing P_{CO_2} in a patient having an asthma exacerbation may indicate?	Fatigue and impending respiratory failure.
Sarcoidosis.	Dyspnea, lateral hilar lymphadenopathy on CXR, noncaseating granulomas, ↑ ACE, and hypercalcemia.
PFTs of obstructive pulmonary disease.	↓ FEV_1/FVC.
PFTs of restrictive pulmonary disease.	↑ FEV_1/FVC, ↓ TLC.
Honeycomb pattern on CXR. Treatment?	Diffuse interstitial pulmonary fibrosis. Supportive care; steroids may help.
Treatment for SVC syndrome.	Radiation.
Treatment for mild persistent asthma.	Inhaled β-agonists and inhaled corticosteroids.
Treatment for COPD exacerbation.	O_2, bronchodilators, antibiotics, corticosteroids with taper, smoking cessation.
Treatment for chronic COPD.	Smoking cessation, home O_2, β-agonists, anticholinergics, systemic or inhaled corticosteroids, flu and pneumococcal vaccines.
Acid-base disorder in PE.	Respiratory alkalosis with hypoxia and hypocarbia.
Non–small cell lung cancer (NSCLC) associated with hypercalcemia.	Squamous cell carcinoma.
Lung cancer associated with SIADH.	Small cell lung cancer (SCLC).
Lung cancer highly related to cigarette exposure.	SCLC.
A tall Caucasian man presents with acute shortness of breath. Diagnosis? Treatment?	Spontaneous pneumothorax. Spontaneous regression; supplemental O_2 may be helpful.
Treatment of tension pneumothorax.	Immediate needle thoracostomy.
Characteristics favoring carcinoma in an isolated pulmonary nodule.	Age > 45–50; lesions new or larger in comparison to old films; absence of calcification or irregular calcification; size > 2 cm; irregular margins.
ARDS.	Hypoxemia and pulmonary edema with normal pulmonary capillary wedge pressure (PCWP).

Sequelae of asbestos exposure.	Pulmonary fibrosis, pleural plaques, bronchogenic carcinoma (mass in lung field), mesothelioma (pleural mass).
↑ risk of what infection with silicosis?	*Mycobacterium tuberculosis.*
Causes of hypoxemia.	Right-to-left shunt, hypoventilation, low inspired O_2 tension, diffusion defect, V/Q mismatch.
Classic CXR findings for pulmonary edema.	Cardiomegaly, prominent pulmonary vessels, Kerley B lines, "bat's-wing" appearance of hilar shadows, and perivascular and peribronchial cuffing.
Westermark's sign and Hampton's hump.	CXR findings suggestive of PE.

RENAL/GENITOURINARY

Renal tubular acidosis (RTA) associated with abnormal H^+ secretion and nephrolithiasis.	Type I (distal) RTA.
RTA associated with abnormal HCO_3^- and rickets.	Type II (proximal) RTA.
RTA associated with aldosterone defect.	Type IV (distal) RTA.
"Doughy" skin.	Hypernatremia.
Differential of hypervolemic hyponatremia.	Cirrhosis, CHF, nephritic syndrome.
Chvostek's and Trousseau's signs.	Hypocalcemia.
The most common causes of hypercalcemia.	Malignancy and hyperparathyroidism.
T-wave flattening and U waves.	Hypokalemia.
Peaked T waves and widened QRS.	Hyperkalemia.
First-line treatment for moderate hypercalcemia.	IV hydration and loop diuretics (furosemide).
Type of ARF in a patient with $Fe_{Na} < 1\%$.	Prerenal.
A 49-year-old man presents with acute-onset flank pain and hematuria.	Nephrolithiasis.
The most common type of nephrolithiasis.	Calcium oxalate.
A 20-year-old man presents with a palpable flank mass and hematuria. Ultrasound shows bilateral enlarged kidneys with cysts. Associated brain anomaly?	Cerebral berry aneurysms (autosomal dominant PCKD).
Hematuria, hypertension, and oliguria.	Nephritic syndrome.
Proteinuria, hypoalbuminemia, hyperlipidemia, hyperlipiduria, and edema.	Nephrotic syndrome.
The most common form of nephrotic syndrome.	Membranous glomerulonephritis.

The most common form of glomerulonephritis.	IgA nephropathy (Berger's disease).
Glomerulonephritis with deafness.	Alport's syndrome.
Glomerulonephritis with hemoptysis.	Wegener's granulomatosis and Goodpasture's syndrome.
Presence of red cell casts in urine sediment.	Glomerulonephritis/nephritic syndrome.
Eosinophils in urine sediment.	Allergic interstitial nephritis.
Waxy casts in urine sediment and Maltese crosses (seen with lipiduria).	Nephrotic syndrome.
Drowsiness, asterixis, nausea, and a pericardial friction rub.	Uremic syndrome seen in patients with renal failure.
A 55-year-old man is diagnosed with prostate cancer. Treatment options?	Wait, surgical resection, radiation and/or androgen suppression.
Low urine specific gravity in the presence of high serum osmolality.	DI.
Treatment of SIADH.	Fluid restriction, demeclocycline.
Hematuria, flank pain, and palpable flank mass.	Renal cell carcinoma (RCC).
Testicular cancer associated with β-hCG, AFP.	Choriocarcinoma.
The most common type of testicular cancer.	Seminoma, a type of germ cell tumor.
The most common histology of bladder cancer.	Transitional cell carcinoma.
Complication of overly rapid correction of hyponatremia.	Central pontine myelinolysis.
Salicylate ingestion causes what type of acid-base disorder?	Anion gap acidosis and 1° respiratory alkalosis due to central respiratory stimulation.
Acid-base disturbance commonly seen in pregnant women.	Respiratory alkalosis.
Three systemic diseases that lead to nephrotic syndrome.	DM, SLE, and amyloidosis.
Elevated erythropoietin level, elevated hematocrit, and normal O_2 saturation suggest?	RCC or other erythropoietin-producing tumor; evaluate with CT scan.
A 55-year-old man presents with irritative and obstructive urinary symptoms. Treatment options?	Likely BPH. Options include no treatment, terazosin, finasteride, or surgical intervention (TURP).

SELECTED TOPICS IN EMERGENCY MEDICINE

Class of drugs that may cause syndrome of muscle rigidity, hyperthermia, autonomic instability, and extrapyramidal symptoms.	Antipsychotics (neuroleptic malignant syndrome).
Side effects of corticosteroids.	Acute mania, immunosuppression, thin skin, osteoporosis, easy bruising, myopathies.
Treatment for DTs.	Benzodiazepines.

Treatment for acetaminophen overdose.	*N*-acetylcysteine.
Treatment for opioid overdose.	Naloxone.
Treatment for benzodiazepine overdose.	Flumazenil.
Treatment for neuroleptic malignant syndrome and malignant hyperthermia.	Dantrolene.
Treatment for malignant hypertension.	Nitroprusside.
Treatment of atrial fibrillation.	Rate control, rhythm conversion, and anticoagulation.
Treatment of supraventricular tachycardia.	If stable, rate control with carotid massage or other vagal stimulation; if unsuccessful, consider adenosine.
Causes of drug-induced SLE.	INH, penicillamine, hydralazine, procainamide, chlorpromazine, methyldopa, quinidine.
Macrocytic, megaloblastic anemia with neurologic symptoms.	B_{12} deficiency.
Macrocytic, megaloblastic anemia without neurologic symptoms.	Folate deficiency.
A burn patient presents with cherry-red, flushed skin and coma. Sao_2 is normal, but carboxyhemoglobin is elevated. Treatment?	Treat CO poisoning with 100% O_2 or with hyperbaric O_2 if poisoning is severe or the patient is pregnant.
Blood in the urethral meatus or high-riding prostate.	Bladder rupture or urethral injury.
Test to rule out urethral injury.	Retrograde cystourethrogram.
Radiographic evidence of aortic disruption or dissection.	Widened mediastinum (> 8 cm), loss of aortic knob, pleural cap, tracheal deviation to the right, depression of left main stem bronchus.
Radiographic indications for surgery in patients with acute abdomen.	Free air under the diaphragm, extravasation of contrast, severe bowel distention, space-occupying lesion (CT), mesenteric occlusion (angiography).
The most common organism in burn-related infections.	*Pseudomonas*.
Method of calculating fluid repletion in burn patients.	Parkland formula: 24-hour fluids = 4 × kg × % BSA.
Acceptable urine output in a trauma patient.	50 cc/hr.
Acceptable urine output in a stable patient.	30 cc/hr.
Signs of neurogenic shock.	Hypotension and bradycardia.
Signs of ↑ ICP (Cushing's triad).	Hypertension, bradycardia, and abnormal respirations.
↓ CO, ↓ PCWP, ↑ peripheral vascular resistance (PVR).	Hypovolemic shock.
↓ CO, ↑ PCWP, ↑ PVR.	Cardiogenic (or obstructive) shock.

↑ CO, ↓ PCWP, ↓ PVR.	Septic or anaphylactic shock.
Treatment of septic shock.	Fluids and antibiotics.
Treatment of cardiogenic shock.	Identify cause; pressors (eg, dopamine).
Treatment of hypovolemic shock.	Identify cause; fluid and blood repletion.
Treatment of anaphylactic shock.	Diphenhydramine or epinephrine 1:1000.
Supportive treatment for ARDS.	Continuous positive airway pressure.
Signs of air embolism.	A patient with chest trauma who was previously stable suddenly dies.
Signs of cardiac tamponade.	Distended neck veins, hypotension, diminished heart sounds (Beck's triad); pulsus paradoxus.
Absent breath sounds, dullness to percussion, shock, flat neck veins.	Massive hemothorax.
Absent breath sounds, tracheal deviation, shock, distended neck veins.	Tension pneumothorax.
Treatment for blunt or penetrating abdominal trauma in hemodynamically unstable patients.	Immediate exploratory laparotomy.
↑ ICP in alcoholics or the elderly following head trauma. Can be acute or chronic; crescent shape on CT.	Subdural hematoma.
Head trauma with immediate loss of consciousness followed by a lucid interval and then rapid deterioration. Convex shape on CT.	Epidural hematoma.

TOP-RATED REVIEW RESOURCES

HOW TO USE THE DATABASE

This section is a database of recommended clinical science review books, sample examination books, and commercial review courses marketed to medical students studying for the USMLE Step 2 CK. For each book, we list the **Title** of the book, the **First Author** (or editor), the **Current Publisher,** the **Copyright Year,** the **Edition,** the **Number of Pages,** the **ISBN Code,** the **Approximate List Price,** the **Format** of the book, and the **Number of Test Questions.** Most entries also include Summary Comments that describe the style and utility of each book for studying. Finally, each book receives a **Rating.** The books are sorted into a comprehensive section as well as into sections corresponding to the 6 clinical disciplines (internal medicine, neurology, OB/GYN, pediatrics, psychiatry, and surgery). Within each section, books are arranged first by Rating, then by Author, and finally by Title.

For this eighth edition of *First Aid for the USMLE Step 2 CK*, the database of review books has been completely revised, with in-depth summary comments on more than 100 books and software. A letter rating scale with 6 different grades reflects the detailed student evaluations. Each book receives a rating as follows:

A+	Excellent for boards review.
A	Very good for boards review; choose among the group.
A–	
B+	
B	Good, but use only after exhausting better sources.
B–	

The **Rating** is meant to reflect the overall usefulness of the book in preparing for the USMLE Step 2 CK exam. This is based on a number of factors, including:

- The cost of the book
- The readability of the text
- The appropriateness and accuracy of the book
- The quality and number of sample questions
- The quality of written answers to sample questions
- The quality and appropriateness of the illustrations (eg, graphs, diagrams, photographs)
- The length of the text (longer is not necessarily better)
- The quality and number of other books available in the same discipline
- The importance of the discipline on the USMLE Step 2 CK exam

Please note that **the rating does not reflect the quality of the book for purposes other than reviewing for the USMLE Step 2 CK exam.** Many books with low ratings are well written and informative but are not ideal for USMLE preparation. We have also avoided listing or commenting on the wide variety of general textbooks available in the clinical sciences.

Evaluations are based on the cumulative results of formal and informal surveys of hundreds of medical students from medical schools across the country. The summary comments and overall ratings represent a consensus opinion, but there may have been a large range of opinions or limited student feedback on any particular book.

Please note that the data listed are subject to change because:

- Publishers' prices change frequently.
- Individual bookstores often charge an additional markup.
- New editions come out frequently, and the quality of updating varies.
- The same book may be reissued through another publisher.

We actively encourage medical students and faculty to submit their opinions and ratings of these clinical science review books so that we may update our database (see "How to Contribute," p. xiii). In addition, we ask that publishers and authors submit review copies of clinical science review books, including new editions and books not included in our database, for evaluation. We also solicit reviews of new books or suggestions for alternate modes of study that may be useful in preparing for the examination, such as flash cards, computer-based tutorials, commercial review courses, and Internet Web sites.

DISCLAIMER/CONFLICT-OF-INTEREST STATEMENT

No material in this book, including the ratings, reflects the opinion or influence of the publisher. All errors and omissions will gladly be corrected if brought to the attention of the authors through the publisher.

COMPREHENSIVE

USMLE Step 2 Secrets
O'CONNELL

$39.95   Review

Elsevier, 2010, 3rd ed., 357 pages, ISBN 9780323057134

A review book presented in Secrets-series question-and-answer format. **Pros:** Identifies and tests key facts across all major subjects. **Cons:** Several subject areas are not discussed in sufficient detail; few images and diagrams are included. Questions are not in Step 2 CK format. **Summary:** A great resource for reviewing key concepts closer to test time, but may not be of benefit early in the review process.

Boards & Wards
AYALA

$46.50   Review

Lippincott Williams & Wilkins, 2009, 4th ed., 578 pages, ISBN 9780781787437

A concise book presented in outline format, packed with key information across the various fields of medicine. **Pros:** Very high yield, and makes good use of tables and charts. Good for quick study and last-minute review. Useful on the wards as well, and fits in a pocket. **Cons:** Small print. Not tremendously detailed, but covers many topics. More detailed books are required for further explanation. **Summary:** A good, comprehensive review, but lacks some detail.

Crush Step 2
BROCHERT

$43.95   Review

Elsevier, 2007, 3rd ed., 341 pages, ISBN 9781416029762

A good review of many high-yield topics, organized by specialty. **Pros:** Places good emphasis on key points, and the conversational style is easy to read. Makes good use of charts and diagrams. Covers surgical topics in more depth than similar books. **Cons:** Not comprehensive; contains no practice questions or vignettes. Not sufficiently detailed to be used alone for Step 2 CK preparation. **Summary:** A solid review of key points and frequently tested topics. Should probably be supplemented with other review material and practice tests.

USMLE Step 2 Mock Exam
BROCHERT

$36.95   Test/750 q

Hanley & Belfus, 2004, 2nd ed., 348 pages, ISBN 9781560536109

Includes 750 vignette-style questions in 15 test blocks. **Pros:** Questions are case based and offer a good approximation of real boards questions. Questions cover high-yield topics, and explanations are terse but adequate. Many questions also include images and associated laboratory findings. **Cons:** Explanations may not be adequate for those who require an in-depth review of certain topics. Has not been recently revised. **Summary:** Excellent vignette-type questions in mock exam format.

NMS Review for USMLE Step 2 CK
IBSEN

$50.50   Review/Test/
900 q

Lippincott Williams & Wilkins, 2007, 3rd ed., 634 pages, ISBN 9780781765220

A comprehensive review book in question-and-answer format. **Pros:** Offers clear, concise, and broad coverage of high-yield topics, presented in a format similar to that of the actual Step 2 CK exam. Includes complete explanations. **Cons:** Questions are more detailed than needed for the boards. Lacks illustrations or images. **Summary:** A good source of Step 2 CK–style questions with appropriate format and content, but questions may be more detailed than those on the actual exam.

First Aid Cases for the USMLE Step 2 CK
LE

$45.95   Review

McGraw-Hill, 2010, 2nd ed., 550 pages, ISBN 9780071625708

A review of high-yield clinical vignettes for the Step 2 CK exam. **Pros:** Cases provide detailed answers to high-yield topics and are arranged in an easy-to-follow format. Emphasizes the most likely diagnosis, the next step, and initial management answers. **Cons:** Some topics either are not covered or are given only brief treatment. **Summary:** A good review with emphasis on vignette-style case presentations and boards-relevant answers, but not sufficient as a stand-alone text for review.

First Aid Q&A for the USMLE Step 2 CK
LE

$45.95   Review/Test/
1000 q

McGraw-Hill, 2010, 2nd ed., 741 pages, ISBN 9780071625715

A question book associated with the First Aid series. **Pros:** Features more than 1000 Step 2 CK–style questions with images to facilitate learning. **Cons:** Does not simulate the computer testing program. **Summary:** A great resource to supplement the First Aid text and to provide additional question practice.

Step-Up to USMLE Step 2
VAN KLEUNEN

$44.50   Review

Lippincott Williams & Wilkins, 2008, 2nd ed., 322 pages, ISBN 9780781771566

A Step 2 CK test review typical of the Step-Up series format, organized by system. **Pros:** A concise Step 2 CK review resource featuring many tables that organize the information and quick facts isolated in the page margins. **Cons:** Not very detailed, but covers most exam topics and serves as a good source of study organization. **Summary:** A good, comprehensive review for the Step 2 CK exam with many quick-study features.

Lange Q&A: USMLE Step 2
CHAN

$46.95   Test/1000+ q

McGraw-Hill, 2008, 6th ed., 425 pages, ISBN 9780071494007

Review questions organized by specialty along with several comprehensive practice exams. **Pros:** Overall question content is good, with broad coverage of high-yield topics. Well illustrated. **Cons:** Vignettes are very brief, and explanations are short. Some questions are more detailed than actual Step 2 CK questions. **Summary:** Well suited to focused specialty review by virtue of overall review questions on high-yield topics.

Lange Practice Tests: USMLE Step 2
GOLDBERG

$45.95   Test/900 q

McGraw-Hill, 2006, 3rd ed., 283 pages, ISBN 9780071446167

Comprehensive test questions. **Pros:** A great source of high-yield questions covering all topics. Many questions include clinically relevant radiographs and photographs of pathology. Offers adequate explanations. **Cons:** Some questions are not vignette style and do not reflect USMLE format. **Summary:** A good compilation of test questions that focus on high-yield material, but some questions still do not reflect USMLE style. A good source of supplemental questions.

B+ | **Clinical Vignettes for the USMLE Step 2 CK: PreTest Self-Assessment & Review** | **$32.00** Test/368 q
McGraw-Hill

McGraw-Hill, 2009, 5th ed., 284 pages, ISBN 9780071604635

A volume presented in question-and-answer format. **Pros:** Consists of 8 blocks covering all major topics on the Step 2 CK exam. Features good black-and-white images. **Cons:** Includes a limited number of practice questions, and sections are not organized in related topics. Some questions are much shorter than those of the USMLE. **Summary:** A great resource for additional quick practice before the test.

B+ | **Images from the Wards: Diagnosis and Treatment** | **$54.95** Review
Studdiford

Elsevier, 2010, 1st ed., 305 pages, ISBN 9781416063834

A review book that uses images from real patients to teach and test common exam topics. **Pros:** Includes excellent, high-quality color images and quick facts associated with each case. Good organization and discussion of major topics. **Cons:** Does not go into topics in great detail, and does not cover all aspects of the exam. **Summary:** A great resource to supplement studying, especially for visual learners.

B | **Physical Diagnosis: PreTest Self-Assessment & Review** | **$32.00** Test/500 q
Bernstein

McGraw-Hill, 2011, 7th ed., 442 pages, ISBN 9780071633017

A volume presented in question-and-answer format. **Pros:** Includes 500 questions related to USMLE Step 2 CK topics. **Cons:** Test questions are brief, and some answers are too detailed. **Summary:** A good review source to supplement physical diagnosis study.

B | **Review 2 Rounds: Visual Review and Clinical Reference** | **$30.95** Review
Gallardo

Elsevier, 2010, 1st ed., 452 pages, ISBN 9781437701692

A spiral-bound book designed to serve as both a clinical reference guide and a study guide. **Pros:** Covers all major topics in a 2-color tabular format. **Cons:** Includes no questions and limited text. Consists mainly of review charts and tables for various topics. **Summary:** A great resource for review before the exam, but should not be used alone or early in the review process.

B | **Underground Clinical Vignettes: Step 2 Bundle** | **$174.95** Review
Kim

Lippincott Williams & Wilkins, 2007, 4th ed., 256 pages, ISBN 9780781763639

A set containing clinical case scenarios of the various specialties, including OB/GYN, neurology, internal medicine, surgery, emergency medicine, psychiatry, and pediatrics, along with an extensive color atlas supplement. **Pros:** Well organized by focus points: pathogenesis, epidemiology, management, complications, and associated diseases. Texts are small and portable. **Cons:** Not comprehensive; best used as a supplement for review. Not recently revised. **Summary:** Organized and easy-to-read clinical vignettes. Excellent as a supplement to studying, but not sufficient by itself. More economical to purchase the 9-volume set than individual volumes.

B

Déjà Review: USMLE Step 2 CK   *$25.95*   Review
NAHEEDY
McGraw-Hill, 2010, 2nd ed., 330 pages, ISBN 9780071627160

A review book organized in a recall design focusing on key word associations. **Pros:** Covers most subject areas found on the exam. **Cons:** Contains no images, diagrams, or vignette questions. **Summary:** A good resource for testing quick recall of single facts.

B−

Lange Outline Review: USMLE Step 2   *$42.95*   Review
GOLDBERG
McGraw-Hill, 2006, 5th ed., 568 pages, ISBN 9780071451925

A comprehensive review book with chapters organized by clinical discipline. **Pros:** A comprehensive review source with extensive coverage of clinical topics and an organized, in-depth review of each. **Cons:** Covers some low-yield topics. Includes relatively few images, figures, or tables. Not recently revised. **Summary:** A solid, single-source, comprehensive review for the Step 2 CK exam.

QUESTION BANKS

USMLEWorld Q-bank
USMLEWORLD
www.usmleworld.com

$99–$399

A test bank with more than 2000 questions. Similar to the Kaplan test bank. Questions are written by physicians. **Pros:** Features well-written questions with explanations; cheaper than Kaplan. Questions tend to be more difficult than those on the actual exam, but many students find this an advantage during preparation. **Cons:** Some questions are highly detailed and focus on very specific concepts that are not likely to be tested. Explanations can also be long. **Summary:** A great source of questions; highly recommended by students.

USMLERx Qmax
MEDIQ LEARNING
www.usmlerx.com

$99–$199

A test bank with more than 2600 top-rated USMLE questions. The questions are presented in the same online format as the actual Step 2 CK exam. **Pros:** Questions are written by students who have done very well on the Step 2 CK exam. All questions are reviewed by faculty experts. The question bank offers highly comprehensive explanations of all subject areas covered on the Step 2 CK exam. **Cons:** A newer resource that is still evolving. **Summary:** An excellent, cost-effective question bank source. Newer, but feedback from students has been excellent thus far.

USMLE Consult's Step 2 CK Question Bank
ELSEVIER
www.usmleconsult.com

$75–$395

A question bank consisting of more than 2300 questions written by Elsevier physicians. Questions are intended to be of varying difficulty similar to the NBME exams. The online exam layout is designed in the same format as that of the Step 2 CK. Online features are similar to those of the other programs already discussed. **Pros:** Uses Elsevier's numerous publications in the design and explanation of questions. There is an additional option for a Robbins Pathology Qbank and a Rapid Review Qbank. **Cons:** Some questions are too detailed for the Step 2 CK exam. **Summary:** An excellent review resource supported by many medical texts. Also well priced in comparison to other online review resources.

Kaplan QBank
KAPLAN
www.kaplanmedical.com

$99–$199

A large online question bank with more than 2250 questions. There is an optional bank with 750 internal medicine questions available for an additional cost. **Pros:** Questions can be arranged randomly or by topic to simulate the real exam. The bank includes an extensive number of questions in vignette format. The content level of questions reflects that of the Step 2 CK exam. **Cons:** Some questions are overly detailed or difficult. **Summary:** A good, cost-effective source of questions with thorough explanations.

B

USMLEasy   *$39–$169*
McGraw-Hill
www.usmleasy.com

A comprehensive test bank with more than 3300 questions and explanations. Similar in style to the Kaplan question bank described above. **Pros:** Features a large number of questions. Cheaper than Kaplan. Access is often free through medical libraries. **Cons:** Questions can be more obscure than those appearing on the actual exam. Questions overlap with those of the PreTest series of review books. **Summary:** A fair source of questions that may be good for supplemental review, especially in preparation for clerkship shelf exams.

Case Files: Emergency Medicine
$34.95 Review

Toy

McGraw-Hill, 2009, 3rd ed., 542 pages, 9780071598996

A review of emergency medicine in case format. **Pros:** A well-organized review featuring 50 cases that focus on high-yield material. **Cons:** Review questions are much easier than those on the Step 2 CK exam, and few images are included. **Summary:** A great text for the USMLE and for the wards.

Step-Up to Medicine
$46.50 Review

Agabegi

Lippincott Williams & Wilkins, 2008, 2nd ed., 537 pages, ISBN 9780781771535

A comprehensive review of commonly tested diseases and topics in internal medicine, organized in an outline format. Includes a color atlas and an appendix on interpreting x-rays, ECGs, and physical exam findings. **Pros:** Highly comprehensive, with informative tables and diagrams to help synthesize information. Includes occasional clinical vignettes that correlate with the topic being discussed. Quick facts to remember are included in the margins of each page. **Cons:** Very lengthy; geared more toward clerkship preparation than Step 2 CK review. **Summary:** A good book that is packed with useful information for the wards, but may be too lengthy and detailed for the Step 2 CK exam.

First Aid for the Medicine Clerkship
$46.95 Review

Kaufman

McGraw-Hill, 2010, 3rd ed., 420 pages, ISBN 9780071633826

A high-yield review of symptoms and diseases. **Pros:** A comprehensive review that is well organized by symptom with good illustrations, scenarios, diagrams, algorithms, and mnemonics. **Cons:** May not be suited to readers who prefer information arranged in text form. May be too basic for certain topics. **Summary:** An excellent, concise review of medicine for those who prefer its format.

High-Yield Internal Medicine
$30.95 Review

Nirula

Lippincott Williams & Wilkins, 2007, 3rd ed., 219 pages, ISBN 9780781781695

A core review of internal medicine in outline format. **Pros:** Focuses on high-yield diseases and symptoms. A quick and easy read. **Cons:** Not comprehensive; lacks many illustrations and has no index. **Summary:** A good, fast review presented in a format that allows for quick and repetitive reading. Best used as a supplement, not as a primary study source.

Emergency Medicine: PreTest Self-Assessment & Review
$32.00 Test/500 q

Rosh

McGraw-Hill, 2009, 2nd ed., 570 pages, ISBN 9780071598613

A question-and-answer review of emergency medicine, organized by presenting symptoms. **Pros:** Well organized for this material, and covers many topics encountered on the Step 2 CK exam. **Cons:** Includes few images or diagrams, and questions are not in Step 2 CK format. **Summary:** A great review of common emergency medicine topics.

A−   ***USMLE Road Map: Emergency Medicine***   ***$33.95***   Review
SHERMAN

McGraw-Hill, 2008, 1st ed., 542 pages, ISBN 9780071463881

A review book that uses an outline format to teach high-yield facts. **Pros:** Features clear explanations and good organization of material. **Cons:** Offers only a general overview of emergency medicine. **Summary:** A solid overview of emergency medicine topics.

A−   ***First Aid for the Emergency Medicine Clerkship***   ***$46.95***   Review
STEAD

McGraw-Hill, 2011, 3rd ed., 542 pages, ISBN 9780071739061

A high-yield review of symptoms and diseases. **Pros:** A comprehensive review; well organized by symptom with good illustrations, scenarios, diagrams, algorithms, and mnemonics. **Cons:** May not be suited to the reader who prefers information arranged in text form. **Summary:** An excellent review of emergency medicine and a nice presentation of high-yield topics for Step 2 CK preparation, but not sufficient for stand-alone review for the Step 2 CK exam.

B+   ***Medical Secrets***   ***$39.95***   Review
HARWARD

Elsevier, 2012, 5th ed., 624 pages, ISBN 9780323063982

A review book presented in Secrets-series question-and-answer format. **Pros:** Covers a great deal of clinically relevant information. Concise answers are given with pearls, tips, and memory aids. **Cons:** Too lengthy and detailed for USMLE review. **Summary:** Not a focused review. May be more appropriate for wards use.

B+   ***Family Medicine: PreTest Self-Assessment & Review***   ***$32.00***   Test/500 q
KNUTSON

McGraw-Hill, 2009, 2nd ed., 303 pages, 9780071598880

A question-and-answer review of family medicine. **Pros:** Well organized, and covers many topics encountered on the Step 2 CK exam. **Cons:** Includes few images or diagrams. **Summary:** A great review of family medicine, but very detailed compared to the material on the Step 2 CK exam. The preventive medicine section is especially high yield.

B+   ***Case Files: Family Medicine***   ***$34.95***   Review
TOY

McGraw-Hill, 2010, 2nd ed., 608 pages, ISBN 9780071600231

A review of family medicine in case format. **Pros:** A well-organized review featuring 55 cases that focus on high-yield material. **Cons:** Review questions are much easier than those of the Step 2 CK exam, and few images are included. **Summary:** Better for the wards than for the Step 2 CK.

B+   ***Case Files: Internal Medicine***   ***$34.95***   Review
TOY

McGraw-Hill, 2009, 3rd ed., 580 pages, ISBN 9780071613644

A review of internal medicine in case format. **Pros:** A well-organized review featuring 60 cases that focus on high-yield material. Includes numerous charts and diagrams to facilitate learning. **Cons:** Review questions are much easier than those of the Step 2 CK exam, and it is difficult to offer a good overview of this subject in just 60 cases. **Summary:** A great supplement for the Step 2 CK exam; also good for the clerkship.

B

Medicine Recall
BERGIN

$42.95 Review

Lippincott Williams & Wilkins, 2011, 4th ed., 809 pages, ISBN 9781605476759

A review book presented in standard Recall-series question-and-answer format, organized by medical specialty. **Pros:** Addresses a broad range of high-yield clinical topics. Presented in a format that is good for self-quizzing. Appropriate level of detail. **Cons:** Contains no vignettes or images; requires significant time commitment. The style simulates questions asked on rounds, not those on the Step 2 CK exam. **Summary:** Written in a style that may be more conducive to wards than to USMLE preparation. Best used as a supplement to other resources.

B

In A Page Emergency Medicine
CATERINO

$43.50 Review

Lippincott Williams & Wilkins, 2003, 1st ed., 316 pages, ISBN 9781405103572

A collection of short, 1-page summaries of 250 medical emergencies discussed in terms of etiology, differential diagnosis, presentation, diagnostic tests, treatment, and disposition. **Pros:** Concise and high yield. Covers a wide variety of emergencies seen in the ER. **Cons:** The text is crowded and somewhat confusing. Contains no images or diagrams. **Summary:** Good for use during the emergency medicine clerkship, but may not be appropriate for Step 2 CK review.

B

Underground Clinical Vignettes Step 2: Emergency Medicine
KIM

$30.95 Review

Lippincott Williams & Wilkins, 2007, 4th ed., 200 pages, ISBN 9780781768344

A clinical vignette–based review of emergency medicine topics. **Pros:** Well organized by focus points: pathogenesis, epidemiology, management, complications, and associated diseases. Well illustrated, and includes high-yield "minicases" and links to the Underground Clinical Vignettes' Clinical and Basic Science Color Atlases. **Cons:** Not comprehensive; best used as a supplement. **Summary:** A well-organized and easy-to-read supplement to studying.

B

Underground Clinical Vignettes Step 2: Internal Medicine, Vols. I and II
KIM

$29.95 each Review

Lippincott Williams & Wilkins, 2007, 4th ed., 190 pages each, ISBN 9780781768351, 9780781768368

A clinical vignette–based review of common topics in internal medicine. **Pros:** Well organized by focus points: pathogenesis, epidemiology, management, complications, and associated diseases. Vignettes mirror the boards-style presentation of questions. **Cons:** Not comprehensive; best used as a supplement. **Summary:** An organized and easy-to-read supplement to studying.

B

Blueprints Clinical Cases in Medicine
LI

$36.95 Test/200 q

Lippincott Williams & Wilkins, 2007, 2nd ed., 418 pages, ISBN 9781405104913

A compendium of vignette-type cases arranged by symptom, followed by related questions and answers. **Pros:** An excellent companion to the Blueprints series. Focuses on high-yield cases. Easy to read with nice illustrations and a good review of management. **Cons:** Not comprehensive; use as a supplement for review. Better suited to clerkship preparation than to the Step 2 CK exam. Not recently revised. **Summary:** An organized and easy-to-read supplement. Adds clinical correlates to the Blueprints series. Best used with the Blueprints text.

B | ***Lange Q&A: Internal Medicine*** | ***$43.95*** Test/1000+ q
PATEL

McGraw-Hill, 2007, 4th ed., 318 pages, ISBN 9780071473644

A question book covering all major topics in internal medicine. Includes a comprehensive practice test at the end of the book. **Pros:** Offers a diverse and comprehensive set of questions. **Cons:** Questions are not in Step 2 CK format, and the text has only a limited number of black-and-white images. **Summary:** A good source of additional questions for students who do not want an online question bank.

B | ***Déjà Review: Family Medicine*** | ***$19.95*** Review
PEREZ

McGraw-Hill, 2008, 1st ed., 253 pages, ISBN 9780071485685

A review book that follows the Déjà Review style for rapid recall of facts using a quick question-and-answer format. **Pros:** A comprehensive and detailed review of common topics in family medicine. **Cons:** Questions are not in Step 2 CK format, and there are no images in the text. **Summary:** Best used for clerkships and for last-minute review.

B | ***Déjà Review: Internal Medicine*** | ***$19.95*** Review
SAADAT

McGraw-Hill, 2008, 1st ed., 208 pages, ISBN 9780071477161

A review book that follows the Déjà Review style for rapid recall of facts using a quick question-and-answer format. **Pros:** A comprehensive and detailed review of common topics in internal medicine. **Cons:** Questions are not in Step 2 CK format, and the text includes very few images. **Summary:** Best used for clerkships and for last-minute USMLE review.

B | ***Medicine: PreTest Self-Assessment & Review*** | ***$32.00*** Test/500 q
URBAN

McGraw-Hill, 2009, 12th ed., 421 pages, ISBN 9780071601627

A question-and-answer format organized by medical subspecialty. **Pros:** Organization by subspecialty helps readers pinpoint weak areas. Offers a substantial number of vignette-style questions with detailed explanations. **Cons:** Many questions are more detailed than needed for the boards and are geared more toward the shelf exam. Includes few illustrations. **Summary:** A solid source of challenging review questions.

B | ***Blueprints in Medicine*** | ***$43.50*** Review/
YOUNG | Test/100 q

Lippincott Williams & Wilkins, 2010, 5th ed., 381 pages, ISBN 9780781788700

A text review of internal medicine, organized by common diseases and common symptoms. Includes a question-and-answer section with explanations. **Pros:** A well-organized, concise review that makes for easy reading. Differential diagnoses for symptoms are helpful. Contains good charts and diagrams. **Cons:** Offers few illustrations. Contains some superfluous details, and some areas are too broad and simplistic to be useful for testing purposes. **Summary:** Poorly illustrated, but a good primary boards review for internal medicine.

Blueprints Clinical Cases in Family Medicine
CHANG
$36.95 Test/200 q

Lippincott Williams & Wilkins, 2007, 2nd ed., 437 pages, ISBN 9781405104951

A compendium of vignette-type cases arranged by symptom, followed by related questions and answers. **Pros:** An excellent companion to the Blueprints series. Focuses on high-yield cases. Easy to read with nice illustrations and a good review of management. **Cons:** Not comprehensive; best used as a supplement for review. Not recently revised. **Summary:** An organized and easy-to-read supplement. Adds clinical correlates to the Blueprints series. Best if used with the Blueprints text.

Déjà Review: Emergency Medicine
JANG
$19.95 Review

McGraw-Hill, 2008, 1st ed., 369 pages, ISBN 9780071476256

A review book that follows the Déjà Review style for rapid recall of facts using a quick question-and-answer format. **Pros:** Offers a quick and detailed review of common topics in emergency medicine. **Cons:** The text is not comprehensive, and questions are not in Step 2 CK format. There are no images in the text. **Summary:** Best for last-minute review.

NEUROLOGY

A−

Blueprints in Neurology   **$43.50**   Review/Test/
DRISLANE   100 q
Lippincott Williams & Wilkins, 2009, 3rd ed., 219 pages, ISBN 9780781796859

A review of neurology by disease and symptom with a brief exam. **Pros:** Reviews high-yield topics of a complex discipline while remaining easy to follow. Makes good use of tables, images, and diagrams. Questions in the exam are similar to those found on both the shelf exam and the Step 2 CK. **Cons:** Lengthy. **Summary:** An excellent review of high-yield material for the wards and the Step 2 CK exam.

B+

Neurology: PreTest Self-Assessment & Review   **$32.00**   Test/500 q
ANSCHEL
McGraw-Hill, 2009, 7th ed., 355 pages, ISBN 9780071597920

A question-and-answer review of neurology. **Pros:** Offers thorough coverage of neurology topics with a substantial number of clinical vignettes. Places appropriate emphasis on common topics and thorough explanations of answers. Good practice for interpreting common head CTs/MRIs that might be tested. **Cons:** Some questions may be more detailed than needed for the boards. **Summary:** A good source of test questions for rapid review of neurology, but may be too detailed for boards review.

B

Underground Clinical Vignettes Step 2: Neurology   **$29.95**   Review
KIM
Lippincott Williams & Wilkins, 2007, 4th ed., 186 pages, ISBN 9780781768375

A clinical vignette–based review of high-yield topics in neurology. **Pros:** Well organized by focus points: pathogenesis, epidemiology, management, complications, and associated diseases. Well illustrated, and includes "minicases," links to a color atlas supplement, and updated treatments. **Cons:** Not comprehensive; best used as a supplement for review. Not recently revised. **Summary:** An organized and easy-to-read supplement to studying. Lengthy for a dedicated review of neurology.

B

Neurology Secrets   **$49.95**   Review
ROLAK
Elsevier, 2010, 5th ed., 470 pages, ISBN 9780323057127

A review book presented in Secrets-series question-and-answer format. **Pros:** A concise review of many high-yield topics. Makes good use of clinical images. **Cons:** Contains no clinical vignettes, but offers lists of questions that might be posed on the wards. Lacks a structured format, and leaves out important information. Relatively expensive and lengthy. Not a reference book. **Summary:** Overall, good content for self-quizzing and study, but does not substitute for a formal review or practice tests. More appropriate for clerkship than for boards review.

B

Blueprints Clinical Cases in Neurology   **$36.95**   Test/200 q
SHETH
Lippincott Williams & Wilkins, 2007, 2nd ed., 390 pages, ISBN 9781405104944

Vignette-type cases organized by symptom, followed by related question and answers. **Pros:** An excellent companion to the Blueprints subspecialty series. Focuses on high-yield cases. Easy to read, with nice illustrations and a good review of management. **Cons:** Not comprehensive; best used as a supplement. Offers few illustrations. Not recently revised. **Summary:** Organized and easy to read. Adds clinical correlates to the Blueprints series.

B− *Neurology Recall* $45.50 Review
MILLER
Lippincott Williams & Wilkins, 2003, 2nd ed., 377 pages, ISBN 9780781745888

Brief question-and-answer format. **Pros:** Reviews many important facts, making it useful for self-quizzing. **Cons:** Not a comprehensive review. Lengthy and lacks illustrations. Concepts are not integrated. Not recently revised. **Summary:** Good for review of some high-yield concepts, but not a stand-alone resource for this topic.

OB/GYN

A− ***Blueprints in Obstetrics and Gynecology***   *$40.95*   Review/Test/
CALLAHAN   100 q
Lippincott Williams & Wilkins, 2009, 5th ed., 401 pages, ISBN 9780781782494

A text review with tables and illustrations. Includes a short exam with explanations. **Pros:** Places strong emphasis on high-yield topics with concise text, clear diagrams, and many classic illustrations. Makes for easy reading. Appropriate for both clinical clerkship and Step 2 CK preparation. **Cons:** Some topics are overly detailed, while others are not detailed enough. **Summary:** Overall, a good choice for boards and wards preparation.

A− ***Underground Clinical Vignettes Step 2: OB/GYN***   *$29.95*   Review
KIM
Lippincott Williams & Wilkins, 2008, 4th ed., 184 pages, ISBN 9780781768405

A clinical vignette–style review of frequently tested diseases in obstetrics and gynecology. **Pros:** Well organized by focus points: pathogenesis, epidemiology, management, complications, and associated diseases. Well illustrated. An easy read that stresses high-yield facts. **Cons:** Not comprehensive; best used as a supplement. **Summary:** Well-organized and easy-to-read practice vignettes.

B+ ***First Aid for the Obstetrics & Gynecology Clerkship***   *$46.95*   Review
KAUFMAN
McGraw-Hill, 2011, 3rd ed., 400 pages, ISBN 9780071634199

A high-yield review of symptoms and diseases. **Pros:** A comprehensive review with nice charts, algorithms, and mnemonics. **Cons:** A lengthy review with fewer images and diagrams than other First Aid books. **Summary:** An excellent review of OB/GYN, but too lengthy in some sections for USMLE review.

B+ ***NMS Obstetrics and Gynecology***   *$45.95*   Review/Test/
PFEIFER   500 q
Lippincott Williams & Wilkins, 2008, 6th ed., 469 pages, ISBN 9780781770712

A detailed outline of OB/GYN with few tables and diagrams. **Pros:** A comprehensive review for both wards and boards. The final exam is relatively good and offers complete explanations. **Cons:** The OB/GYN review is dense and lengthy. Many questions do not reflect the Step 2 CK format. Lacks illustrations. **Summary:** A complete review with questions and discussions. Better for clerkship studying than for USMLE review.

B+ ***Obstetrics and Gynecology: PreTest Assessment & Review***   *$32.00*   Test/500 q
SCHNEIDER
McGraw-Hill, 2009, 12th ed., 335 pages, ISBN 9780071599795

A question-and-answer review with detailed explanations for OB/GYN. **Pros:** Organization by subtopic may be useful for studying weak areas. Good content emphasis. Generally well illustrated. **Cons:** Some questions are too difficult or detailed. Vignette-based questions are shorter and more simplistic than those on the Step 2 CK exam. **Summary:** A decent source of questions to supplement topic study, especially for addressing specific areas of weakness.

B+   ***Case Files: Obstetrics and Gynecology***   *$34.95*   Review
Toy

McGraw-Hill, 2009, 3rd ed., 508 pages, ISBN 9780071605809

A review of OB/GYN in case format with questions and answers following each vignette. **Pros:** Cases reflect high-yield topics and are arranged in an easy-to-follow format. **Cons:** Some topics either are not covered or are given only brief treatment. Contains few diagrams and images. Lengthy and time-consuming. Explanations are terse. **Summary:** A good review of the subject in clinical vignette format, but may be too detailed for Step 2 CK review.

B+   ***Blueprints Q & A Step 2 Obstetrics & Gynecology***   *$19.95*   Test/100 q
Tran

Lippincott Williams & Wilkins, 2005, 2nd ed., 153 pages, ISBN 9781405103909

One hundred vignette-style questions. **Pros:** A nice companion to the Blueprints series. Focuses on high-yield topics. Explanations are easy to follow. **Cons:** Not comprehensive; best used as a supplement for review. Sparse images. Some questions are esoteric and not boards-like. **Summary:** A well-organized and easy-to-read supplement. Adds clinical correlates to the Blueprints series.

B   ***Blueprints Clinical Cases in Obstetrics and Gynecology***   *$36.95*   Test/200 q
Caughey

Lippincott Williams & Wilkins, 2007, 2nd ed., 418 pages, ISBN 9781405104906

Vignette-type cases arranged by symptom, followed by related questions and answers. **Pros:** An excellent companion to the Blueprints series. Focuses on high-yield cases. Easy to read, with nice illustrations and a good review of management. **Cons:** Not comprehensive; best used as a supplement. Not recently revised. **Summary:** An organized and easy-to-read supplement. Adds clinical correlates to the Blueprints series.

B   ***Déjà Review: Obstetrics and Gynecology***   *$19.95*   Review
Lee

McGraw-Hill, 2008, 1st ed., 490 pages, ISBN 9780071481229

A review book that follows the Déjà Review style for rapid recall of facts using a quick question-and-answer format. **Pros:** A comprehensive and detailed review of common topics in OB/GYN. **Cons:** Questions are not in Step 2 CK format, and the text includes very few images. **Summary:** Best for last-minute USMLE review and for studying difficult concepts in OB/GYN.

B   ***High-Yield Obstetrics and Gynecology***   *$30.95*   Review
Sakala

Lippincott Williams & Wilkins, 2006, 2nd ed., 194 pages, ISBN 9780781796309

A review of high-yield topics in outline format. Clinical scenarios at the end of each chapter highlight key points. **Pros:** Easy to read, with a good discussion of high-yield topics. Not recently revised. **Cons:** Lacks depth and contains no practice questions. Not recently revised. **Summary:** A quick but superficial review.

B−   ***Obstetrics and Gynecology Secrets***   *$39.95*   Review
Bader

Elsevier, 2005, 3rd ed., 428 pages, ISBN 9780323034159

A review book presented in Secrets-series question-and-answer format, organized by topic within OB/GYN. **Pros:** Offers good coverage of many high-yield, clinically relevant topics. Not recently revised. **Cons:** Too detailed to be useful for rapid review. Contains no vignettes and few illustrations or images. **Summary:** Good clinical content, but does not serve as a formal topic review. Better for use during clerkship than for Step 2 CK preparation.

B– ***Obstetrics and Gynecology Recall***   *$45.50*   Review
BOURGEOIS
Lippincott Williams & Wilkins, 2008, 3rd ed., 673 pages, ISBN 9780781770699

A review book presented in standard Recall-series question-and-answer style. **Pros:** The 2-column format makes the text useful for self-quizzing. Reviews many high-yield concepts and facts. **Cons:** Questions emphasize individual facts but do not integrate concepts. Contains no vignettes or images. Coverage of some topics is spotty. **Summary:** Useful for review of selected concepts, but not a comprehensive source for Step 2 CK preparation. More appropriate for clerkship than for boards.

B– ***Lange Q&A: Obstetrics and Gynecology***   *$43.95*   Test/1000+ q
VONTVER
McGraw-Hill, 2006, 8th ed., 388 pages, ISBN 9780071461399

A question book covering major topics in OB/GYN. **Pros:** Offers good organization and short, clear explanations. **Cons:** Questions are not in Step 2 CK format, and the text has only a limited number of black-and-white images. **Summary:** A good source of additional questions in a book format.

PEDIATRICS

A−

First Aid for the Pediatrics Clerkship   **$45.00** Review
STEAD

McGraw-Hill, 2011, 3rd ed., 616 pages, ISBN 9780071664035

A comprehensive review of key topics and concepts in pediatrics. **Pros:** The outline format allows for quick high-yield review, and the mnemonics and key points are very useful. **Cons:** Some chapters are overly detailed. **Summary:** A great review of pediatrics that is well suited to the clerkship, but may be too detailed for Step 2 CK review.

A−

Pediatrics: PreTest Self-Assessment & Review   **$32.00** Test/500 q
YETMAN

McGraw-Hill, 2009, 12th ed., 403 pages, ISBN 9780071597906

A question-and-answer review with detailed discussions. **Pros:** Organization by organ system is useful for pinpointing weaknesses. Gives strong, thorough explanations, and includes a fair number of vignette-style questions. Well illustrated. **Cons:** Some questions are too detailed or emphasize low-yield topics. **Summary:** A great source of pediatric questions. Offers solid content with good illustrations, although not entirely in Step 2 CK format.

B+

Déjà Review: Pediatrics   **$19.95** Review
DAVEY

McGraw-Hill, 2008, 1st ed., 217 pages, ISBN 9780071477826

A review book that follows the Déjà Review style for rapid recall of facts using a quick question-and-answer format. **Pros:** A highly comprehensive and detailed review of common topics in pediatrics. **Cons:** Questions are not in Step 2 CK format, and the text includes very few images. **Summary:** Best used for last-minute USMLE review and studying for the clerkship.

B+

In A Page Pediatrics   **$40.95** Review
KAHAN

Lippincott Williams & Wilkins, 2008, 2nd ed., 455 pages, ISBN 9780781770453

One-page reviews of 228 diseases/topics discussed by etiology, epidemiology, signs/symptoms, differential diagnosis, diagnostic tests, treatment, and prognosis. **Pros:** A fast and concise review of high-yield information on common diseases. **Cons:** Each topic is crowded onto 1 page without any images or diagrams. Includes low-yield topics. **Summary:** Useful for quick study on the wards, but too time intensive for Step 2 CK review.

B+

Underground Clinical Vignettes Step 2: Pediatrics   **$29.95** Review
KIM

Lippincott Williams & Wilkins, 2007, 4th ed., 256 pages, ISBN 9780781768443

A clinical vignette review of frequently tested topics in pediatrics. **Pros:** Well organized by focus points: pathogenesis, epidemiology, management, complications, and associated diseases. Well illustrated, and the current edition includes "minicases" to broaden subject material and present more high-yield information. Not recently revised. **Cons:** Not comprehensive; best used as a supplement to text review. **Summary:** Well organized and easy to read, but intended as a supplement for review.

B+ ***Case Files: Pediatrics***   *$34.95* Review
Toy
McGraw-Hill, 2010, 3rd ed., 497 pages, ISBN 9780071598675

A review of pediatrics in case format with questions and answers following each vignette. **Pros:** Cases reflect high-yield topics and are arranged in an easy-to-follow format. Emphasizes the next step and the most likely diagnosis. **Cons:** Not suited for high-yield, rapid review. **Summary:** An excellent review with emphasis on vignette-style case presentation and important boards-type answers, but may be too detailed for a stand-alone boards review book. Excellent for clerkship preparation.

B ***Lange Q&A: Pediatrics***   *$44.95* Test/1000 q
Jackson
McGraw-Hill, 2010, 7th ed., 326 pages, ISBN 9780071475686

A question book covering major topics in pediatrics. **Pros:** Offers good organization and short, clear explanations. **Cons:** Questions are not in Step 2 CK format, and the text has only a limited number of black-and-white images. **Summary:** A good source of additional questions in a book format.

B ***Blueprints Clinical Cases in Pediatrics***   *$36.95* Test/200 q
Londhe
Lippincott Williams & Wilkins, 2007, 2nd ed., 410 pages, ISBN 9781405104920

Vignette-type cases arranged by symptom followed by related questions and answers. **Pros:** An excellent companion to the Blueprints series. Focuses on high-yield cases. Easy to read with nice illustrations and a good review of management. **Cons:** Not comprehensive; best used as a supplement for review. **Summary:** An organized and easy-to-read supplement. Adds clinical correlates to the Blueprints series.

B ***Blueprints in Pediatrics***   *$43.50* Review/Test/ 100 q
Marino
Lippincott Williams & Wilkins, 2009, 5th ed., 364 pages, ISBN 9780781782517

A text review of pediatrics with tables and diagrams. Includes a question-and-answer section with explanations. **Pros:** Appropriate focus on high-yield topics. **Cons:** A relatively dense text with few illustrations. Overly detailed. **Summary:** Good for a more comprehensive review.

B ***Pediatric Secrets***   *$39.95* Review
Polin
Elsevier, 2011, 5th ed., 739 pages, ISBN 9780323065610

A review book presented in Secrets-series question-and-answer format, organized by pediatric subspecialty. **Pros:** Includes a thorough discussion of a wide variety of clinical topics. **Cons:** The detailed content is geared toward the wards and requires significant time commitment. Contains no images or illustrations. **Summary:** Too detailed for USMLE review; better suited to clerkship.

B– ***NMS Pediatrics***   *$46.50* Review/Test/ 100+ q
Dworkin
Lippincott Williams & Wilkins, 2009, 5th ed., 470 pages, ISBN 9780781770750

A general review of pediatrics in outline format. Includes questions at the end of each chapter. **Pros:** A thorough, detailed review of pediatrics. Boldfacing highlights key points. Case studies and a comprehensive exam at the end of the book (also provided on CD-ROM) are helpful. Includes a good discussion. **Cons:** A dense, lengthy text. Lacks good illustrations of any kind. **Summary:** A thorough review, but more appropriate for clerkships than for Step 2 CK review, in large part because of its depth.

B– ***Blueprints Q & A Step 2 Pediatrics*** $19.95 Test/100 q
FOTI

Lippincott Williams & Wilkins, 2004, 2nd ed., 159 pages, ISBN 9781405103916

Vignette-style questions. **Pros:** A nice companion to the Blueprints series. Focuses on high-yield topics. Explanations are easy to follow. **Cons:** Not comprehensive; best used as a supplement for review. Sparse images. Not recently updated. **Summary:** An organized and easy-to-read supplement. Adds clinical correlates to the Blueprints series.

B– ***Pediatrics Recall*** $40.95 Review
McGAHREN

Lippincott Williams & Wilkins, 2011, 4th ed., 542 pages, ISBN 9781605476766

A review book presented in a concise question-and-answer format typical of the Recall series. **Pros:** The 2-column format makes self-quizzing easy. Emphasis is placed on diagnosis and management. **Cons:** Requires time commitment, and not all topics are covered thoroughly. Contains no vignettes. **Summary:** Contains useful material, but does not provide a systematic review or a substitute for practice tests. Better suited to clerkship review.

PSYCHIATRY

Blueprints in Psychiatry
MURPHY

Lippincott Williams & Wilkins, 2009, 5th ed., 154 pages, ISBN 9780781782531

$43.50   Review/Test/
100 q

A brief text review of psychiatry with DSM-IV criteria. Includes a brief question-and-answer section at the end of the book. **Pros:** A clear, concise review of psychiatry with helpful tables. Offers good coverage of high-yield topics, including pharmacology. A quick read. **Cons:** Too general in certain areas; requires some supplementation. **Summary:** A rapid review with appropriate coverage of high-yield topics.

Psychiatry: PreTest Self-Assessment & Review
KLAMEN

McGraw-Hill, 2009, 12th ed., 302 pages, ISBN 9780071598309

$32.00   Test/500 q

A question-and-answer review of topics in psychiatry. **Pros:** Questions are well written and organized. Most questions have an appropriate content level. Offers good explanations. **Cons:** Includes too few vignette-type questions. Some questions are too detailed for Step 2 CK review. **Summary:** A good source of questions and review for psychiatry and the Step 2 CK exam, although the format may not reflect the actual test.

First Aid for the Psychiatry Clerkship
STEAD

McGraw-Hill, 2011, 3rd ed., 230 pages, ISBN 9780071739238

$45.00   Review

A high-yield review of symptoms and diseases. **Pros:** A comprehensive review that includes DSM-IV criteria with nice mnemonics and scenarios. Includes high-yield tear-out cards. **Cons:** May not appeal to readers who prefer information in text format. **Summary:** A good review of high-yield topics in psychiatry, but better suited to clerkship than to Step 2 CK study.

Blueprints Clinical Cases in Psychiatry
HOBLYN

Lippincott Williams & Wilkins, 2008, 2nd ed., 499 pages, ISBN 9781405104968

$38.95   Test/200 q

Vignette-type cases arranged by symptom, followed by related questions and answers. **Pros:** An excellent companion to the Blueprints series. Focuses on high-yield cases. Easy to read with nice illustrations and a good review of management. **Cons:** Not comprehensive; best used as a supplement for review. **Summary:** An organized and easy-to-read supplement. Adds clinical correlates to the Blueprints series.

Underground Clinical Vignettes Step 2: Psychiatry
KIM

Lippincott Williams & Wilkins, 2007, 4th ed., 189 pages, ISBN 9780781768467

$30.95   Review

A clinical vignette–based review of frequently tested topics in psychiatry. **Pros:** Well organized by focus points: pathogenesis, epidemiology, management, and associated diseases. Well illustrated, and includes "minicases" that present high-yield information. **Cons:** Not comprehensive; best used as a supplement. Not recently revised. **Summary:** Offers organized and easy-to-read practice vignettes.

B+ ***Case Files: Psychiatry***   *$34.95*   Review
Toy
McGraw-Hill, 2010, 3rd ed., 493 pages, ISBN 9780071598651

A review of psychology in case format with questions and answers following each vignette. **Pros:** Cases reflect high-yield topics and are arranged in an easy-to-follow format. Emphasizes the next step, the most likely diagnosis, and the best initial treatment. **Cons:** Not suited to high-yield rapid review, and may be too detailed for Step 2 CK review. **Summary:** An excellent subject review that places emphasis on vignette-style case presentation and important boards-type answers. Great for the wards, and a good supplement for the boards.

B ***High-Yield Psychiatry***   *$30.95*   Review
Fadem
Lippincott Williams & Wilkins, 2003, 2nd ed., 150 pages, ISBN 9780781742689

A brief outline-format review of psychiatry. **Pros:** A quick read, with clinical vignettes scattered throughout. Offers concise tables. **Cons:** Not sufficiently detailed for in-depth review. Not recently revised. **Summary:** An excellent, quick review of psychiatry for use as an additional study source. Similar to *High-Yield Behavioral Sciences* by the same author.

B ***A&L's Review of Psychiatry***   *$39.95*   Test/900+ q
Oransky
McGraw-Hill, 2003, 7th ed., 304 pages, ISBN 9780071402538

A general review of psychiatry with questions and answers. **Pros:** Includes 114 vignette-style questions appropriate for boards review. Appropriate content emphasis; thorough explanations. **Cons:** Questions are shorter and more straightforward than those of the boards. Not recently revised. **Summary:** A decent source of boards review for psychiatry, but does not reflect boards format.

B ***Lange Q&A: Psychiatry***   *$43.95*   Test/750+ q
Oransky
McGraw-Hill, 2007, 9th ed., 273 pages, ISBN 9780071475679

A question book covering major topics in psychiatry. **Pros:** Offers good organization and short, clear explanations. Includes 2 practice tests. **Cons:** Questions are not in Step 2 CK format, and there are no images in the text. Not recently revised. **Summary:** A good source for additional questions in a book format.

B ***NMS Psychiatry***   *$47.95*   Review/Test/
Thornhill   500 q
Lippincott Williams & Wilkins, 2011, 6th ed., 303 pages, ISBN 9781608315741

A general review of topics in outline format with questions at the end of each chapter and a comprehensive final exam. **Pros:** A well-written text with concise disease discussions. Includes an expanded pharmacology section. Questions test appropriate content and have complete explanations, and the new edition offers more vignette-style questions. A good companion text for the clerkship. **Cons:** Lengthy for purposes of boards review. **Summary:** A detailed review that requires time commitment. A good single choice for clerkship study, but may be too long for Step 2 CK review.

B–

Déjà Review: Psychiatry — $19.95 Review
GOPAL

McGraw-Hill, 2008, 1st ed., 230 pages, ISBN 9780071488327

A review book that follows the Déjà Review style for rapid recall of facts using a quick question-and-answer format. **Pros:** Offers a good overview of key facts associated with many common conditions. **Cons:** Questions are not in Step 2 CK format, and there are no images in the text. **Summary:** Best for last-minute USMLE review of specific topics.

B–

Blueprints Q & A Step 2 Psychiatry — $19.95 Test/200 q
McLOONE

Lippincott Williams & Wilkins, 2005, 2nd ed., 85 pages, ISBN 9781405103923

Vignette-style questions. **Pros:** A nice companion to the Blueprints series. Focuses on high-yield topics. Explanations are easy to follow. **Cons:** Not comprehensive; best used as a supplement for review. Sparse images. Some questions are esoteric and not boards-like. Not recently revised. **Summary:** An organized and easy-to-read supplement. Adds clinical correlates to the Blueprints series.

A–

Case Files: Surgery
TOY
McGraw-Hill, 2009, 3rd ed., 510 pages, ISBN 9780071598972

$34.95 Review

A review of surgery in case format with questions and answers following each vignette. **Pros:** Cases reflect high-yield topics and are arranged in an easy-to-follow format. Emphasizes the next step and the most likely diagnosis. **Cons:** Not suited to high-yield rapid review, and may be too detailed for Step 2 CK preparation. **Summary:** An excellent review with emphasis on vignette-style case presentation and important boards-type answers. Great for clerkship study, and a good supplement for USMLE study.

B+

Surgery: PreTest Self-Assessment & Review
KAO
McGraw-Hill, 2009, 12th ed., 373 pages, ISBN 9780071598637

$32.00 Test/500 q

A review of topics in general surgery in question-and-answer format. **Pros:** Predominantly case based. Well organized by subspecialty. **Cons:** Many questions are too detailed or esoteric and do not reflect boards style. Some explanations are overly detailed. **Summary:** A thorough review, but questions may be beyond the level needed for Step 2 CK preparation.

B+

First Aid for the Surgery Clerkship
KAUFMAN
McGraw-Hill, 2009, 2nd ed., 543 pages, ISBN 9780071448710

$46.95 Review

A comprehensive review of key topics and concepts in surgery using the First Aid outline format. **Pros:** The outline format allows for quick high-yield review. The mnemonics and key points are also very useful. **Cons:** The text can be very detailed in some chapters, and there could be more images. **Summary:** A great review of surgery that is very well suited to the surgical clerkship and could also serve as a supplement for Step 2 CK review.

B+

Underground Clinical Vignettes Step 2: Surgery
KIM
Lippincott Williams & Wilkins, 2007, 4th ed., 185 pages, ISBN 9780781768474

$29.95 Review

A clinical vignette–based review of frequently tested surgical topics. **Pros:** Well organized by focus points: pathogenesis, epidemiology, management, complications, and associated diseases. Well illustrated and includes "minicases" that present high-yield information. **Cons:** Not comprehensive; best used as a supplement to review. Not recently updated. **Summary:** Well-organized and easy-to-read practice vignettes.

B

Surgical Recall
BLACKBOURNE
Lippincott Williams & Wilkins, 2011, 6th ed., 824 pages, ISBN 9781608314218

$49.95 Review

A review book presented in standard Recall-series question-and-answer format. **Pros:** Questions emphasize important, high-yield clinical concepts. Columns allow for self-testing. Fast review. Good preparation for "pimping" on rounds. **Cons:** Does not feature boards-type questions. Poorly organized. Coverage of some topics is spotty. **Summary:** A useful adjunct to a more organized topic review. Much more appropriate for clerkships than for USMLE review.

B

NMS Surgery   **$46.50**   Review/Test/
Jarrell   350 q
Lippincott Williams & Wilkins, 2008, 5th ed., 647 pages, ISBN 9780781759014

An outline review of general surgery and surgical subspecialties. **Pros:** Well organized and thorough. Vignette-style questions are included after each chapter with good explanations. **Cons:** Dense, detailed text. Few tables or illustrations. **Summary:** A comprehensive surgery review, but very time consuming. More appropriate for clerkship than for boards review.

B

Blueprints in Surgery   **$43.50**   Review/Test/
Karp   100 q
Lippincott Williams & Wilkins, 2008, 5th ed., 253 pages, ISBN 9780781788687

A short text review of general surgery with tables and diagrams. A brief question-and-answer section is included. **Pros:** Well organized. Easy to read, with a strong focus on high-yield topics. Includes clear diagrams. **Cons:** Some sections are overly detailed (eg, anatomy), while others are occasionally too simplistic. Too few illustrations. **Summary:** A good review of surgery, but not ideal for Step 2 CK preparation.

B

Déjà Review: Surgery   **$19.95**   Review
Tevar
McGraw-Hill, 2008, 1st ed., 415 pages, ISBN 9780071481144

A rapid recall of facts using a quick question-and-answer format. **Pros:** Offers a quick overview of key facts associated with many common procedures. Features more illustrations than other books in the series. **Cons:** Questions are not in Step 2 CK format. Not as comprehensive as other recall books. **Summary:** Best for last-minute USMLE review of specific topics.

B–

Lange Q&A: Surgery   **$44.95**   Test/1000+ q
Cayten
McGraw-Hill, 2007, 5th ed., ISBN 9780071475662

A question book covering major topics in surgery. **Pros:** Offers good organization and short, clear explanations along with good images. **Cons:** Questions are not in Step 2 CK format, and some questions are too detailed for Step 2 CK review. Not recently revised. **Summary:** A good source of additional questions in book format for students who need more practice in surgery.

B–

Abernathy's Surgical Secrets   **$54.95**   Review
Harken
Elsevier, 2009, 6th ed., 517 pages, ISBN 9780323057110

A review book presented in a question-and-answer format typical of the Secrets series. **Pros:** Discussions are up to date and thorough. **Cons:** Too detailed for the purposes of the Step 2 CK, yet not comprehensive. **Summary:** Not a well-organized review. Better suited to clerkships than to USMLE preparation.

B–

In A Page Surgery   **$40.95**   Review
Kahan
Lippincott Williams & Wilkins, 2004, 1st ed., 206 pages, ISBN 9781405103657

One-page reviews of diseases/topics discussed by etiology, epidemiology, signs/symptoms, differential diagnosis, diagnostic tests, treatment, and prognosis. **Pros:** A fast and concise review of high-yield information on common diseases. **Cons:** Text is crowded onto 1 page without any images or diagrams. Includes low-yield topics. Not recently revised. **Summary:** Useful for quick study on the wards, but too time intensive for Step 2 CK review.

B−   *Blueprints Clinical Cases in Surgery*   **$36.95**   Test/200 q
Li

Lippincott Williams & Wilkins, 2007, 2nd ed., 415 pages, ISBN 9781405104937

Vignette-type cases arranged by symptom followed by related questions and answers. **Pros:** A excellent companion to the Blueprints series. Focuses on high-yield cases. Easy to read with nice illustrations and a good review of management. **Cons:** Not comprehensive; best used as a supplement for review. Not recently revised. **Summary:** An organized and easy-to-read supplement. Adds clinical correlates to the Blueprints series.

B−   *High-Yield Surgery*   **$26.95**   Review
NIRULA

Lippincott Williams & Wilkins, 2006, 2nd ed., 149 pages, ISBN 9780781776561

An outline review of most common general surgery topics. **Pros:** Concise; useful for quick topic review. Well organized. **Cons:** Information can be superficial. Some topics are omitted. Offers no practice questions. Not recently revised. **Summary:** A lean text for rapid review.

B−   *A&L's Review of Surgery*   **$39.95**   Test/1000+ q
WAPNICK

McGraw-Hill, 2003, 4th ed., 297 pages, ISBN 9780071378147

A general review of surgery with questions and answers. **Pros:** Good clinical emphasis. Includes many vignette-style questions. Explanations are thorough. **Cons:** Some questions are too short, and the style does not reflect that of the Step 2 CK exam. Questions are highly variable in difficulty and are often far too detailed. Offers few illustrations. Not recently revised. **Summary:** Good content for the exam, but much too detailed for clerkship and Step 2 CK review.

COMMERCIAL REVIEW COURSES

Although commercial preparation courses can be helpful for some students, such courses are typically costly and require significant time commitment. They are usually most effective as an organizing tool for students who feel overwhelmed by the sheer volume of material involved in Step 2 CK preparation. Note, too, that multiweek courses may be quite intense and may thus leave limited time for independent study. Also note that some commercial courses are designed for first-time test takers while others focus on students who are repeating the exam. In addition, some courses are geared toward IMGs who want to take all 3 Steps in a limited amount of time.

Student experience and satisfaction with review courses are highly variable. We suggest that you discuss options with recent graduates of the review courses you are considering. In addition, course content and structure can change rapidly. Some student opinions can be found in discussion groups on the World Wide Web. Listed below is contact information for some Step 2 CK commercial review courses.

Falcon Physician Reviews
440 Wrangler Drive, Suite 100
Coppell, TX 75019
(888)516-9991
Fax: (214) 292-8568
info@falconreviews.com
www.falconreviews.com

Kaplan Medical
700 South Flower Street, Suite 2900
Los Angeles, CA 90017
(800) KAP-TEST (800-527-8378)
www.kaptest.com

Northwestern Medical Review
P.O. Box 22174
East Lansing, MI 48909-2174
(866) MedPass (866-633-7277)
Fax: (517) 347-7005
contactus@northwesternmedicalreview.com
http://northwesternmedicalreview.com

PASS Program
2302 Moreland Blvd.
Champaign, IL 61822
(217) 378-8018
Fax: (217) 378-7809
www.passprogram.net

Postgraduate Medical Review Education (PMRE)
1909 Tyler Street, Suite 305
Hollywood, FL 33020
(877) 662-2005
Fax: (954) 926-3333
sales@pmre.com
www.pmre.com

Youel's Prep, Inc.
P.O. Box 31479
Palm Beach Gardens, FL 33420
(800) 645-3985
Fax: (561) 622-4858
info@youelsprep.com
http://youelsprep.net

ABBREVIATIONS AND SYMBOLS

Abbreviation	Meaning
A-a	alveolar-arterial (oxygen gradient)
AAA	abdominal aortic aneurysm
AAMC	Association of American Medical Colleges
ABG	arterial blood gas
ABI	ankle-brachial index
AC	abdominal circumference
ACA	anterior cerebral artery
ACE	angiotensin-converting enzyme
ACEI	angiotensin-converting enzyme inhibitor
ACh	acetylcholine
ACL	anterior cruciate ligament
ACLS	advanced cardiac life support (protocol)
ACTH	adrenocorticotropic hormone
AD	Alzheimer's disease
ADA	American Diabetes Association, Americans with Disabilities Act
ADH	antidiuretic hormone
ADHD	attention-deficit hyperactivity disorder
ADPKD	autosomal-dominant polycystic kidney disease
AF	atrial fibrillation
AFI	amniotic fluid index
AFP	α-fetoprotein
AGC	atypical glandular cell
AHA	American Heart Association
AI	adrenal insufficiency
AICA	anterior inferior cerebellar artery
AIDS	acquired immunodeficiency syndrome
ALL	acute lymphocytic leukemia
ALS	amyotrophic lateral sclerosis
ALT	alanine aminotransferase
AMD	age-related macular degeneration
AML	acute myelogenous leukemia
ANA	antinuclear antibody
ANC	absolute neutrophil count
ANCA	antineutrophil cytoplasmic antibody
AP	anteroposterior
APC	activated protein C
APL	acute promyelocytic leukemia
aPTT	activated partial thromboplastin time
ARB	angiotensin receptor blocker
ARDS	acute respiratory distress syndrome
ARF	acute renal failure

Abbreviation	Meaning
ARPKD	autosomal-recessive polycystic kidney disease
5-ASA	5-aminosalicylic acid
ASA	acetylsalicylic acid
ASC	atypical squamous cells
ASC-H	atypical squamous cells suspicious of high-grade dysplasia
ASC-US	atypical squamous cells of undetermined significance
ASD	atrial septal defect
ASO	antistreptolysin O
AST	aspartate aminotransferase
ATN	acute tubular necrosis
ATRA	all-*trans* retinoic acid
AV	atrioventricular
AVM	arteriovenous malformation
AVN	avascular necrosis
AVNRT	atrioventricular nodal reentry tachycardia
AVRT	atrioventricular reciprocating tachycardia
AXR	abdominal x-ray
AZT	azidothymidine (zidovudine)
BAL	British anti-Lewisite (dimercaprol), bronchoalveolar lavage
BCC	basal cell carcinoma
BCG	bacille Calmette-Guérin
β-hCG	β-human chorionic gonadotropin
BID	twice a day
BMD	bone mineral density
BMI	body mass index
BP	blood pressure
BPD	biparietal diameter, bipolar disorder
BPH	benign prostatic hyperplasia
bpm	beats per minute
BPP	biophysical profile
BPPV	benign paroxysmal positional vertigo
BSA	body surface area
BUN	blood urea nitrogen
BW	birth weight
CABG	coronary artery bypass graft
CAD	coronary artery disease
CaEDTA	calcium disodium edetate
CAH	congenital adrenal hyperplasia
cAMP	cyclic adenosine monophosphate

Abbreviation	Meaning
c-ANCA	cytoplasmic antineutrophil cytoplasmic antibody
CBC	complete blood count
CBT	cognitive-behavioral therapy, computer-based testing
CCB	calcium channel blocker
CCP	cyclic citrullinated peptide
CCS	computer-based case simulation
CCSSA	Comprehensive Clinical Science Self-Assessment (test)
CD	cluster of differentiation
CEA	carcinoembryonic antigen
CF	cystic fibrosis
CFU	colony-forming unit
CGD	chronic granulomatous disease
cGMP	cyclic guanosine monophosphate
CHF	congestive heart failure
CI	confidence interval
CIN	candidate identification number, cervical intraepithelial neoplasia
CJD	Creutzfeldt-Jakob disease
CK	clinical knowledge, creatine kinase
CKD	chronic kidney disease
CK-MB	creatine kinase, MB fraction
CLL	chronic lymphocytic leukemia
CML	chronic myelogenous leukemia
CMP	comprehensive metabolic panel
CMV	cytomegalovirus
CN	cranial nerve
CNS	central nervous system
COMT	catechol-O-methyltransferase
COPD	chronic obstructive pulmonary disease
CPAP	continuous positive airway pressure
CPPD	calcium pyrophosphate deposition (disease)
CPR	cardiopulmonary resuscitation
Cr	creatinine
CRL	crown-rump length
CRP	C-reactive protein
CS	clinical skills
CSA	central sleep apnea
CSF	cerebrospinal fluid
CST	contraction stress test
CT	computed tomography
CTS	carpal tunnel syndrome
CVA	cerebrovascular accident
CVID	common variable immunodeficiency
CVP	central venous pressure
CVS	chorionic villus sampling
CXR	chest x-ray
D&C	dilation and curettage
D&E	dilation and evacuation
DA	developmental age
DDAVP	desmopressin acetate
DES	diethylstilbestrol
DEXA	dual-energy x-ray absorptiometry

Abbreviation	Meaning
DFA	direct fluorescent antibody
DHEA	dehydroepiandrosterone
DHEAS	dehydroepiandrosterone sulfate
DI	diabetes insipidus
DIC	disseminated intravascular coagulation
DIP	distal interphalangeal (joint)
DKA	diabetic ketoacidosis
DL_{CO}	diffusion capacity of carbon monoxide
DM	diabetes mellitus
DMARD	disease-modifying antirheumatic drug
DMD	Duchenne muscular dystrophy
DMSA	dimercaptosuccinic acid (succimer)
DNA	deoxyribonucleic acid
DNI	do not intubate
DNR	do not resuscitate
DPOAHC	durable power of attorney for health care
DRE	digital rectal exam
dsDNA	double-stranded deoxyribonucleic acid
DTaP	diphtheria, tetanus, acellular pertussis (vaccine)
DTRs	deep tendon reflexes
DTs	delirium tremens
DVT	deep venous thrombosis
EBV	Epstein-Barr virus
EC	emergency contraception
ECFMG	Educational Commission for Foreign Medical Graduates
ECG	electrocardiography
ECT	electroconvulsive therapy
ED	erectile dysfunction
EEG	electroencephalography
EF	ejection fraction
EFW	estimated fetal weight
EGD	esophagogastroduodenoscopy
ELISA	enzyme-linked immunosorbent assay
EM	electron microscopy, erythema multiforme
EMG	electromyography
EOM	extraocular movement
EPS	extrapyramidal symptoms
ER	emergency room, estrogen receptor
ERAS	Electronic Residency Application Service
ERCP	endoscopic retrograde cholangiopancreatography
ERV	expiratory reserve volume
ESR	erythrocyte sedimentation rate
ESRD	end-stage renal disease
ESWL	extracorporeal shock-wave lithotripsy
EtOH	ethanol
FAP	familial adenomatous polyposis
FAST	focused abdominal sonography for trauma (scan)
Fe_{Na}	fractional excretion of sodium
FEV_1	forced expiratory volume in 1 second
FFP	fresh frozen plasma
FHH	familial hypocalciuric hypercalcemia
FHR	fetal heart rate

Abbreviation	Meaning
FiO$_2$	fraction of inspired oxygen
FISH	fluorescence in situ hybridization
FL	femur length
FLAIR	fluid-attenuated inversion recovery (imaging)
FMG	foreign medical graduate
FNA	fine-needle aspiration
FOBT	fecal occult blood test
FRC	functional residual capacity
FSH	follicle-stimulating hormone
FSMB	Federation of State Medical Boards
FTA-ABS	fluorescent treponemal antibody absorption (test)
FTT	failure to thrive
5-FU	5-fluorouracil
FUO	fever of unknown origin
FVC	forced vital capacity
G6PD	glucose-6-phosphate dehydrogenase
GA	gestational age
GABA	gamma-aminobutyric acid
GAF	global assessment of functioning
GAS	group A streptococcus
GBM	glioblastoma multiforme, glomerular basement membrane
GBS	group B streptococcus
GCS	Glasgow Coma Scale
G-CSF	granulocyte colony-stimulating factor
GDMA2	gestational diabetes mellitus, insulin controlled
GERD	gastroesophageal reflux disease
GFR	glomerular filtration rate
GGT	gamma-glutamyl transferase
GH	growth hormone
GI	gastrointestinal
GLP	glucagon-like peptide
GM-CSF	granulocyte-macrophage colony-stimulating factor
GNR	gram-negative rod
GnRH	gonadotropin-releasing hormone
GTD	gestational trophoblastic disease
GU	genitourinary
HAART	highly active antiretroviral therapy
HAV	hepatitis A virus
HbA$_{1c}$	hemoglobin A$_{1c}$
HBcAb	hepatitis B core antibody
HBcAg	hepatitis B core antigen
HBeAb	hepatitis E core antibody
HBeAg	hepatitis E core antigen
HBsAb	hepatitis B surface antibody
HBsAg	hepatitis B surface antigen
HBV	hepatitis B virus
hCG	human chorionic gonadotropin
HCL	hairy cell leukemia
HCTZ	hydrochlorothiazide
HCV	hepatitis C virus
HD	Huntington's disease, Hodgkin's disease

Abbreviation	Meaning
HDL	high-density lipoprotein
HDV	hepatitis D virus
HES	hypereosinophilic syndrome
HEV	hepatitis E virus
HGPRT	hypoxanthine-guanine phosphoribosyltransferase
HHV	human herpesvirus
5-HIAA	5-hydroxyindoleacetic acid
Hib	*Haemophilus influenzae* type b
HIDA	hepato-iminodiacetic acid (scan)
HIT	heparin-induced thrombocytopenia
HIV	human immunodeficiency virus
HLA	human leukocyte antigen
HMG-CoA	hydroxymethylglutaryl coenzyme A
HNPCC	hereditary nonpolyposis colorectal cancer
HOCM	hypertrophic obstructive cardiomyopathy
HPA	human placental antigen, hypothalamic-pituitary-adrenal (axis)
hpf	high-power field
HPV	human papillomavirus
HR	heart rate
HRT	hormone replacement therapy
HSIL	high-grade squamous intraepithelial lesion
HSV	herpesvirus
HTLV	human T-cell lymphotropic virus
HUS	hemolytic-uremic syndrome
HVA	homovanillic acid
IBD	inflammatory bowel disease
IBS	irritable bowel syndrome
IC	inspiratory capacity
ICD	implantable cardiac defibrillator
ICP	intracranial pressure
ICU	intensive care unit
I/E	inspiratory to expiratory (ratio)
IFN-α	α-interferon
Ig	immunoglobulin
IGF	insulin-like growth factor
IM	intramuscular
IMED	International Medical Education Directory
IMG	international medical graduate
INH	isoniazid
INR	International Normalized Ratio
I/O	intake and output
IOP	intraocular pressure
IPV	inactivated polio vaccine
IRV	inspiratory reserve volume
ITP	idiopathic thrombocytopenic purpura
IUD	intrauterine device
IUGR	intrauterine growth restriction
IUI	intrauterine insemination
IV	intravenous
IVC	inferior vena cava
IVF	in vitro fertilization
IVIG	intravenous immunoglobulin
IVP	intravenous pyelography
JIA	juvenile idiopathic arthritis

Abbreviation	Meaning
JNC	Joint National Committee on Prevention, Detection, Evaluation, and Treatment of High Blood Pressure
JRA	juvenile rheumatoid arthritis
JVD	jugular venous distention
JVP	jugular venous pulse
KOH	potassium hydroxide
KS	Kaposi's sarcoma
KSHV	Kaposi's sarcoma–associated herpesvirus
KUB	kidney, ureter, bladder
LAD	left anterior descending (artery)
LAE	left atrial enlargement
LAP	leukocyte alkaline phosphatase
LBBB	left bundle branch block
LBO	large bowel obstruction
LBP	low back pain
LCL	lateral collateral ligament
LDH	lactate dehydrogenase
LDL	low-density lipoprotein
LEEP	loop electrosurgical excision procedure
LES	lower esophageal sphincter
LFT	liver function test
LGV	lymphogranuloma venereum
LH	luteinizing hormone
LLQ	left lower quadrant
LMN	lower motor neuron
LMP	last menstrual period
LMWH	low-molecular-weight heparin
LP	lumbar puncture
LR	lactated Ringer's, likelihood ratio
LSIL	low-grade squamous intraepithelial lesion
LTBI	latent tuberculosis infection
LUQ	left upper quadrant
LVH	left ventricular hypertrophy
MAC	membrane attack complex, *Mycobacterium avium* complex
MALT	mucosa-associated lymphoid tissue
MAOI	monoamine oxidase inhibitor
mBPP	modified biophysical profile
MCA	middle cerebral artery
MCL	medial collateral ligament
MCP	metacarpophalangeal (joint)
MCV	mean corpuscular volume, meningococcal vaccine
MDD	major depressive disorder
MDE	major depressive episode
MEN	multiple endocrine neoplasia
MGUS	monoclonal gammopathy of undetermined significance
MHA-TP	microhemagglutination assay–*Treponema pallidum*
MI	myocardial infarction
MIBG	metaiodobenzylguanidine (scan)
MMA	methylmalonic acid
MMF	mycophenolate mofetil
MMR	measles, mumps, rubella (vaccine)
MoM	multiple of the median

Abbreviation	Meaning
MRA	magnetic resonance angiography
MRCP	magnetic resonance cholangiopancreatography
MRI	magnetic resonance imaging
MRSA	methicillin-resistant *S aureus*
MS	multiple sclerosis
MSAFP	maternal serum α-fetoprotein
MTP	metatarsophalangeal (joint)
MUA	manual uterine aspiration
MuSK	muscle-specific kinase
NBME	National Board of Medical Examiners
NEC	necrotizing enterocolitis
NF	neurofibromatosis
NG	nasogastric
NHL	non-Hodgkin's lymphoma
NK	natural killer (cell)
NMS	neuroleptic malignant syndrome
NNRTI	non-nucleoside reverse transcriptase inhibitor
NP	nasopharyngeal
NPH	normal pressure hydrocephalus
NPO	nil per os (nothing by mouth)
NPV	negative predictive value
NRTI	nucleoside/nucleotide reverse transcriptase inhibitor
NS	normal saline
NSAID	nonsteroidal anti-inflammatory drug
NSCLC	non–small cell lung cancer
NST	nonstress test
NSTEMI	non-ST-elevation myocardial infarction
NYHA	New York Heart Association
O&P	ova and parasites
OA	osteoarthritis
OCD	obsessive-compulsive disorder
OCPD	obsessive-compulsive personality disorder
OCPs	oral contraceptive pills
OD	overdose
OP	oropharyngeal
OR	odds ratio, operating room
ORIF	open reduction and internal fixation
OSA	obstructive sleep apnea
OTC	over the counter
PA	posteroanterior
$PaCO_2$	partial pressure of carbon dioxide in arterial blood
p-ANCA	perinuclear antineutrophil cytoplasmic antibody
PaO_2	partial pressure of oxygen in arterial blood
PAPP-A	pregnancy-associated plasma protein A
PAS	period acid–Schiff
PCA	posterior cerebral artery
PCI	percutaneous coronary intervention
PCL	posterior cruciate ligament
PcO_2	partial pressure of carbon dioxide
PCOS	polycystic ovarian syndrome

Abbreviation	Meaning
PCP	phencyclidine hydrochloride, *Pneumocystis carinii* (now *jiroveci*) pneumonia
PCR	polymerase chain reaction
PCV	polycythemia vera, pneumococcal vaccine
PCWP	pulmonary capillary wedge pressure
PDA	patent ductus arteriosus, posterior descending artery
PDD	pervasive developmental disorder
PDE	phosphodiesterase
PE	pulmonary embolism
PEA	pulseless electrical activity
PEEP	positive end-expiratory pressure
PET	positron emission tomography
PFT	pulmonary function test
PG	prostaglandin
PICA	posterior inferior cerebellar artery
PID	pelvic inflammatory disease
PIP	proximal interphalangeal (joint)
PKD	polycystic kidney disease
PKU	phenylketonuria
PMI	point of maximal impulse
PML	promyelocytic leukemia
PMN	polymorphonuclear (leukocyte)
PND	paroxysmal nocturnal dyspnea
PO	per os (by mouth)
Po_2	partial pressure of oxygen
POC	product of conception
PPD	purified protein derivative (of tuberculin)
PPI	proton pump inhibitor
PPROM	preterm premature rupture of membranes
PPV	pneumococcal polysaccharide vaccine, positive predictive value
PR	per rectum, progesterone receptor
PRN	pro re nata (as needed)
PROM	premature rupture of membranes
PSA	prostate-specific antigen
PT	prothrombin time
PTH	parathyroid hormone
PTHrP	parathyroid hormone–related protein
PTSD	post-traumatic stress disorder
PTT	partial thromboplastin time
PUD	peptic ulcer disease
PUVA	psoralen plus ultraviolet A
PVC	premature ventricular contraction
PVR	peripheral vascular resistance
PVS	persistent vegetative state
RA	rheumatoid arthritis
RAI	radioactive iodine
RBBB	right bundle branch block
RBC	red blood cell
RCA	right coronary artery
RCC	renal cell carcinoma
RCT	randomized controlled trial
RDS	respiratory distress syndrome
RDW	red cell distribution width
REM	rapid eye movement

Abbreviation	Meaning
RF	rheumatoid factor
RLQ	right lower quadrant
ROM	range of motion, rupture of membranes
RPR	rapid plasma reagin
RR	relative risk
RS	Reed-Sternberg (cell)
RSV	respiratory syncytial virus
RTA	renal tubular acidosis
RTI	reverse transcriptase inhibitor
RUQ	right upper quadrant
RV	residual volume
RVH	right ventricular hypertrophy
SAAG	serum-ascites albumin gradient
SAB	spontaneous abortion
SAH	subarachnoid hemorrhage
Sao_2	oxygen saturation in arterial blood
SARS	severe acute respiratory syndrome
SBO	small bowel obstruction
SBS	shaken baby syndrome
SCC	squamous cell carcinoma
SCD	sickle cell disease
SCFE	slipped capital femoral epiphysis
SCID	severe combined immunodeficiency
SCLC	small cell lung cancer
SD	standard deviation
SES	socioeconomic status
SIADH	syndrome of inappropriate secretion of antidiuretic hormone
SIDS	sudden infant death syndrome
SIRS	systemic inflammatory response syndrome
SJS	Stevens-Johnson syndrome
SLE	systemic lupus erythematosus
SMA	superior mesenteric artery
SNRI	serotonin-norepinephrine reuptake inhibitor
SQ	subcutaneous
SRP	sponsoring residency program
SSRI	selective serotonin reuptake inhibitor
SSSS	staphylococcal scalded-skin syndrome
STD	sexually transmitted disease
STEMI	ST-elevation myocardial infarction
SVC	superior vena cava
SVT	supraventricular tachycardia
T_3	triiodothyronine
T_4	thyroxine
TAB	therapeutic abortion
TAH/BSO	total abdominal hysterectomy/bilateral salpingo-oophorectomy
TB	tuberculosis
TBG	thyroxine-binding globulin
TCA	tricyclic antidepressant
TEE	transesophageal echocardiography
TEF	tracheoesophageal fistula
TEN	toxic epidermal necrolysis
TFT	thyroid function test
TIA	transient ischemic attack

Abbreviation	Meaning
TIBC	total iron-binding capacity
TID	three times a day
TIMI	Thrombosis in Myocardial Infarction (study)
TLC	total lung capacity
TM	tympanic membrane
TMA	transcortical motor aphasia
TMJ	temporomandibular joint
TMP-SMX	trimethoprim-sulfamethoxazole
TMS	transcranial magnetic stimulation
TNF	tumor necrosis factor
TNM	tumor, node, metastasis (staging)
TOEFL	Test of English as a Foreign Language
tPA	tissue plasminogen activator
TP-EIA	*Treponema pallidum* enzyme immunoassay
TPN	total parenteral nutrition
TPO	thyroid peroxidase
TP-PA	*Treponema pallidum* particle agglutination (test)
TRAP	tartrate-resistant acid phosphatase
TSA	transcortical sensory aphasia
TSH	thyroid-stimulating hormone
TSS	toxic shock syndrome
TSST	toxic shock syndrome toxin (*S aureus* toxin)
TTP	thrombotic thrombocytopenic purpura
TURP	transurethral resection of the prostate
TV	tidal volume
UA	urinalysis

Abbreviation	Meaning
UMN	upper motor neuron
URI	upper respiratory infection
USMLE	United States Medical Licensing Examination
USPSTF	United States Preventive Services Task Force
UTI	urinary tract infection
UV	ultraviolet
VA	Department of Veterans Affairs
VC	vital capacity
VCUG	voiding cystourethrography
VDRL	Venereal Disease Research Laboratory
VF	ventricular fibrillation
VIN	vulvar intraepithelial neoplasia
VLDL	very low density lipoprotein
VMA	vanillylmandelic acid
VOC	vaso-occlusive crisis
VOR	vestibulo-ocular reflex
VP	ventriculoperitoneal
V/Q	ventilation/perfusion (scan)
VRSA	vancomycin-resistant *S aureus*
VSD	ventricular septal defect
VT	ventricular tachycardia
vWD	von Willebrand's disease
vWF	von Willebrand factor
VZV	varicella-zoster virus
WBC	white blood cell
WPW	Wolff-Parkinson-White (syndrome)

COMMON LABORATORY VALUES

* = Included in the Biochemical Profile (SMA-12)

Blood, Plasma, Serum	Reference Range	SI Reference Intervals
* Alanine aminotransferase (ALT, GPT at 30°C)	8–20 U/L	8–20 U/L
Amylase, serum	25–125 U/L	25–125 U/L
* Aspartate aminotransferase (AST, GOT at 30°C)	8–20 U/L	8–20 U/L
Bilirubin, serum (adult)		
Total // Direct	0.1–1.0 mg/dL // 0.0–0.3 mg/dL	2–17 µmol/L // 0–5 µmol/L
* Calcium, serum (Total)	8.4–10.2 mg/dL	2.1–2.8 mmol/L
* Cholesterol, serum	140–250 mg/dL	3.6–6.5 mmol/L
* Creatinine, serum (Total)	0.6–1.2 mg/dL	53–106 µmol/L
Electrolytes, serum		
Sodium	135–147 mEq/L	135–147 mmol/L
Chloride	95–105 mEq/L	95–105 mmol/L
* Potassium	3.5–5.0 mEq/L	3.5–5.0 mmol/L
Bicarbonate	22–28 mEq/L	22–28 mmol/L
Gases, arterial blood (room air)		
P_{O_2}	75–105 mmHg	10.0–14.0 kPa
P_{CO_2}	33–44 mmHg	4.4–5.9 kPa
pH	7.35–7.45	[H+] 36–44 nmol/L
* Glucose, serum	Fasting: 70–110 mg/dL	3.8–6.1 mmol/L
	2-h postprandial: < 120 mg/dL	< 6.6 mmol/L
Growth hormone - arginine stimulation	Fasting: < 5 ng/mL	< 5 µg/L
	provocative stimuli: > 7 ng/mL	> 7 µg/L
Osmolality, serum	275–295 mOsm/kg	275–295 mOsm/kg
* Phosphatase (alkaline), serum (p-NPP at 30°C)	20–70 U/L	20–70 U/L
* Phosphorus (inorganic), serum	3.0–4.5 mg/dL	1.0–1.5 mmol/L
* Proteins, serum		
Total (recumbent)	6.0–7.8 g/dL	60–78 g/L
Albumin	3.5–5.5 g/dL	35–55 g/L
Globulins	2.3–3.5 g/dL	23–35 g/L
* Urea nitrogen, serum (BUN)	7–18 mg/dL	1.2–3.0 mmol urea/L
* Uric acid, serum	3.0–8.2 mg/dL	0.18–0.48 mmol/L
Cerebrospinal Fluid		
Glucose	40–70 mg/dL	2.2–3.9 mmol/L
Hematologic		
Erythrocyte count	Male: 4.3–5.9 million/mm³	4.3–5.9 × 10¹²/L
	Female: 3.5–5.5 million/mm³	3.5–5.5 × 10¹²/L
Hematocrit	Male: 41–53%	0.41–0.53
	Female: 36–46%	0.36–0.46
Hemoglobin, blood	Male: 13.5–17.5 g/dL	2.09–2.71 mmol/L
	Female: 12.0–16.0 g/dL	1.86–2.48 mmol/L

(continues)

Hematologic (continued)

Hemoglobin, plasma	1–4 mg/dL	0.16–0.62 µmol/L
Leukocyte count and differential		
Leukocyte count	4500–11,000/mm³	4.5–11.0 × 10⁹/L
Segmented neutrophils	54–62%	0.54–0.62
Band forms	3–5%	0.03–0.05
Eosinophils	1–3%	0.01–0.03
Basophils	0–0.75%	0–0.0075
Lymphocytes	25–33%	0.25–0.33
Monocytes	3–7%	0.03–0.07
Mean corpuscular hemoglobin	25.4–34.6 pg/cell	0.39–0.54 fmol/cell
Platelet count	150,000–400,000/mm³	150–400 × 10⁹/L
Prothrombin time	11–15 seconds	11–15 seconds
Reticulocyte count	0.5–1.5% of red cells	0.005–0.015
Sedimentation rate, erythrocyte	Male: 0–15 mm/h	0–15 mm/h
(Westergren)	Female: 0–20 mm/h	0–20 mm/h
Proteins, total	< 150 mg/24 h	< 0.15 g/24 h

Index

NOTES

NOTES

NOTES

NOTES

NOTES

NOTES

NOTES

About the Authors

Tao Le, MD, MHS

Tao developed a passion for medical education while still a medical student. He currently edits over 15 titles in the *First Aid* series. In addition, he is the founder of the *USMLERx* online video and test bank series as well as a cofounder of the *Underground Clinical Vignettes* series. As a medical student, he was editor-in-chief of the University of California, San Francisco (UCSF) *Synapse,* a university newspaper with a weekly circulation of 9000. Tao earned his medical degree from UCSF in 1996 and completed his residency training in internal medicine at Yale University and fellowship training at Johns Hopkins University. At Yale, he was a regular guest lecturer on the USMLE review courses and an adviser to the Yale University School of Medicine curriculum committee. Dr. Le subsequently went on to cofound Medsn, a medical education technology venture, and served as its chief medical officer. He is currently conducting research in asthma education at the University of Louisville.

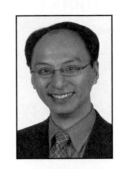

Vikas Bhushan, MD

Vikas is an author, editor, entrepreneur, and teleradiologist. In 1990 he conceived and authored the original *First Aid for the USMLE Step 1.* His entrepreneurial adventures include a successful software company, a medical publishing enterprise (S2S), an e-learning company (Medsn), and an ER teleradiology service (24/7 Radiology). His eclectic interests include medical informatics, independent film, humanism, Urdu poetry, world music, South Asian diasporic culture, and avoiding a day job. A dilettante at heart, he coproduced a music documentary on qawwali music and coproduced and edited *Shabash 2.0: The Hip Guide to All Things South Asian in North America.* Vikas completed a bachelor's degree in biochemistry from the University of California, Berkeley; an MD with thesis from the University of California, San Francisco; and a radiology residency from the University of California, Los Angeles.

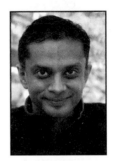

Nathan William Skelley, MD

Nathan is an orthopaedic surgery resident at Washington University in St. Louis. He has always had an interest in the musculoskeletal system and teaching. He has a first-degree black belt in Sho-Tae-Ryu martial arts and taught martial arts classes for his first job. He attended Cornell University in Ithaca, New York, where he was a Merrill Scholar, a Meinig Family Cornell National Scholar, president of the Preprofessional Association Toward Careers in Health (PATCH), and a counselor for the American Legion Boys Nation program. He completed his medical degree at The Johns Hopkins School of Medicine, where he also served as president of the Medical Student Senate. In his free time, he enjoys flying powered parachutes and SCUBA diving. Nathan credits much of his success to the support of his parents, Mark and Billie, and his siblings, Lissa, James, and Logan.

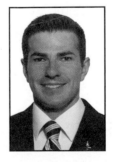

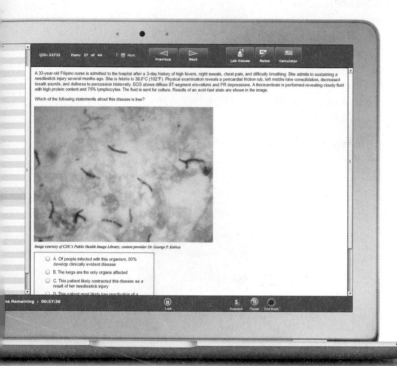
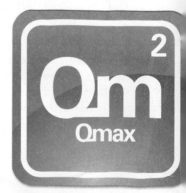